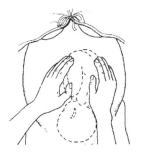

Maternal
and
Newborn Care

A complete guide for midwives and other health professionals

Editors:

Joanita de Kock
Dr Christa van der Walt

Consulting editor:

Sr Christa Mary Jones

JUTA
ACADEMIC

Project managed by Maylani Louw and Liesbet van Wyk
Editing by Maylani Louw
Proofreading and indexing by Ethné Clarke
Design, layout and typesetting in 9/12 pt Berkley Book by Mckore Graphics
Cover design by The Pumphaus Design Studio
Cover photograph courtesy of the Ngobeni family
Printed and bound in South Africa by Paarl Print

Preface

The midwife is the key provider of maternity services in South Africa. This textbook developed from the need for a concise source of information that would be accessible to midwives and midwifery students.

The authors, who bravely participated in the ambitious task to write this textbook, have a passion for the dedicated care of mother and child as an integral part of the childbearing family. We acknowledge the importance of the family and community in caring for women with healthy pregnancies, and therefore the needs of the childbearing family firmly remain the focus of the book. As caregivers we also value the importance of culturally appropriate care. It was our goal to refrain from the use of the terms 'normal' and 'abnormal' because we believe that a woman, and a child, should never be labelled, but cared for as a unique individual.

In South Africa, as in the rest of Africa, we strive to decrease maternal and neonatal mortalities and morbidities, and therefore need a scientifically sound knowledge base from which to direct our decisions. Due to the unique character of our country we aimed to involve as many people as possible from diverse backgrounds in order to incorporate the rich cultural diversity and contributions of our rainbow nation. Authors from all sectors (including universities, nursing colleges, government and the private sector) and most provinces contributed to this extensive source.

Our focus has been strongly evidence-based. To this end we included the national and international guidelines to make the textbook specific to the needs of women and newborn babies in South Africa, whilst at the same time accommodating global issues to facilitate the use of the book in other parts of Africa.

In **Section 1** the basic concepts of midwifery care are described in order to provide a background of the core of midwifery. The anatomy and physiology of reproduction are examined extensively in **Section 2** highlighting the relationship with midwifery care. The focus in **Section 3** falls on the principles of pregnancy care including preparation for pregnancy, childbirth and parenthood. In **Section 4** the birth process and midwifery care during this vulnerable period in life are reviewed, while also considering the care of the newborn baby at birth. Postnatal care is presented in **Section 5**.

In **Section 6** saving mothers has been used as a central theme. Our starting point was to address the major causes of maternal mortality and morbidity. A unique feature of this section is the chapter on perinatal loss, counselling and support.

Section 7 extensively covers the care of the healthy and the compromised newborn baby. Never before has comprehensive newborn care formed part of a local midwifery textbook and for that reason this part of the book is distinctive and significant.

As editors, we believe that this book will make a difference to the quality of midwifery education and patient care. We sincerely hope that all who engage with this book will greatly benefit from using it in their practice.

The editors

Acknowledgements

The editors and authors would like to thank the following colleagues for their valuable contributions:

Gustav Schellack – Checking all the pharmacology information
Tanya Heyns – Chapter 21 (General management of haemorrhage during pregnancy) and Chapter 22 (Proofreading of Trauma)
Carin Maree – Chapter 29 (Physical examination)
Adene van Zijl – Chapter 29 (The role of the family)
Anja Borain – General proofreading
Marlize Visser – General proofreading

Contents

Contributors

Joanita de Kock (editor)
M Cur (Midwifery and Neonatal Nursing
    Science) (RAU)
RN, RM, RCHN, RPN, RT, Adv Midwife
Lecturer, Department of Nursing Science
    University of Pretoria

Dr Christa van der Walt (editor)
BA et Sc, M Soc Sc (UFS), M Ed (UFS), D Cur
    (RAU)
RN, RM, RCHN, RT, RNA
Senior lecturer, Department of Nursing Science
    University of Pretoria

Christa Mary Jones (consulting editor)
RN, RM, RCHN, RNA, Adv Midwife
Lecturer/Facilitator Decentralised Ed
    Programme in Adv Midwifery and Neonatal
    Nursing Science
Director of the Catholic Medical Mission Board
    'Born to live' Prevention of Maternal to Child
    Transmission of HIV Programmes in SA and
    Consultant to Programme Development in
    Sub-Saharan Africa

Dr Gail Andrews
B Cur Hons (UWC), MPH (Univ of Wales), PhD
RN, RM, RCHN, RPN
Senior lecturer, School of Public Health,
    University of Pretoria

Joan Dippenaar
B Soc Sc Hons (UFS), M Cur (Midwifery and
    Neonatal Nursing Science) (RAU)
RN, RPN, RM, RCHN, RNA, RT, Adv Midwife
Senior lecturer, Medunsa

Antoinette du Preez
B Soc Sc Hons (UFS), BA Cur (Admin and
    Education) (Unisa), Dipl Advanced
    Midwifery and Neonatology (RAU), M Cur
    (Midwifery and Neonatal Nursing Science)
    (PU for CHE)
RN, RM, RCHN, RPN, RT, RNA, Adv Midwife
Senior lecturer, North-West University

Linda Greyling
B Cur, DNE, B Sc Hons (Anat), M Sc Anatomy
    (Pret)
Lecturer, Dept of Anatomy, University of
    Pretoria

Riana Hattingh
B Cur Hons (Advanced Midwifery and Neonatal
    Nursing Science) (Pret), BA Cur
    (Administration and Education) (Unisa),
    Dipl Perinatal Education (RAU)
RN, RM, RPN, RCHN, RT, RNA, Adv Midwife

Angie Hennessy
B Cur, Cert Neonatal Nursing Science, Dipl
    Advanced Neonatal Nursing Science, M Cur
    (Advanced Neonatal Nursing Science) (Pret)
RN, RM, RCHN, RPN, RT, Neo nurs
Part-time lecturer, Department of Nursing
    Science, University of Pretoria

Elizabeth Kaye-Petersen
BA Cur (Nursing Administration and
    Community Nursing Science) (UNISA), M
    Cur (Advanced Midwifery and Neonatal
    Nursing Science) (RAU)
RN, RM, RT, Adv Midwife
Senior Training and Development Specialist,
    Afrox Healthcare

Theresa Mabale

BA Cur (Unisa), DNA (Unisa), B Cur Hons
(Advanced Midwifery and Neonatal Nursing)
(Pret), Dipl Perinatal Education (RAU)

RN, RM, RNA, RCHN, RT, Adv Midwife

Unit manager, Labour ward, Kalafong Academic
Hospital

H Liesbeth Mangate

BA Cur Hons (Health Services Management and
Community Nursing) (UNISA), Diploma
(Advanced Midwifery) (McCord Hospital),

RN, RM, RNA, RCHN, RT, Adv Midwife

Assistent Director, Maternal Health, Department
of Health

Carin Maree

B Cur (Pret), BA Cur (UNISA), M Cur (RAU),
Dipl Child Health Nursing (Pret)

RN, RM, RPN, RCHN, CHN, RT, Neo nurs

Lecturer, University of Pretoria

Dr Patricia McInerney

BSc (Nursing) (Wits), MSc (Nursing) (Wits),
DNEd (Wits), Adv Dip Nursing (UNISA),
Dip Psychiatric Nursing (Wits), PhD (Wits)

RN, RM, RPN, RCHN, RT, RNA

Senior lecturer, University of KwaZulu-Natal

Karin (CS) Minnie

BArt et Scien (Nursing Science) (PU for CHE),
BA Hons, Dipl Adv Midwifery and Neonatal
Nursing Science (RAU), M Cur (Midwifery
and Neonatal Nursing Science) (PU for
CHE)

RN, RM, RCHN, RNA, RT, Adv Midwife

Senior Lecturer Midwifery, University of the
North-West

Kgabiso Rachel Mokhondo

BA Cur Hons (Unisa), Dipl Child Health, Dipl
Intensive Nursing Science, Cert Neonatology
(Pret)

RN, RM, RCHN, RNA, RT, Intensive Care, CHN

Nurse Researcher, MRC Unit for Maternal and
Infant Health Care Strategies, University of
Pretoria

Mpo Modjadji

BA Cur (Education and Community) (Unisa),
BA Cur Hons (Nursing Education) (Unisa),
Dipl Instructor Course, Dipl Advanced
Midwifery and Neonatal Nursing, Dipl
Occupational Health Nursing

RN, RM, RCHN, RT, Occup Health, Adv
Midwife

Lecturer, SG Lourens Nursing College, Pretoria

Edith Zodwa Moosa

BA Cur (Unisa), MA Cur (Maternal, Child and
Women's Health) (Natal)

Dipl Operating Theatre Nursing (Edendale),
Clinical Care Administration and Instruction
(Edendale), Adv Midwifery and Neonatal
Nursing Science (King Edward), Nursing
Education (Natal), Adv Nursing
Administration (Natal)

RN, RM, RCHN, RT, RNA, Adv Midwife, OTT,
CCAI

Formerly head of Midwifery department, Natal
College of Nursing (Addington Campus)

Dolly Nontuthuzelo Nyasulu

BA Cur (Comm Health Nursing and Nursing
Administration) (UNISA), M Soc Sc
(Maternal, Child & Women's Health Care)
(Natal)

RN, RM, RPN, Adv Midwife

Provincial Coordinator Maternal Health Care
KZN, Provincial Assessor Maternal Deaths
KZN, Co-facilitator of the Site Centred
Education Programme for Advanced
Midwives in KZN

Maternal, Child & Women's Health Sub-
Directorate, KwaZulu-Natal

Dr Bongi Noreen Nzama

BA Cur (Unisa), M Cur (UFH), M Cur
(Midwifery and Neonatal Nursing Science)
(RAU), Ed D (Boston)

RN, RM, RT, RCHN, Adv Midwife

Head of Department, Dept of Nursing Sciences,
University of Fort Hare

Dr Lou Pistorius

MBChB (Pret), FCOG (SA), M Med (O & G)
(Stell), Diploma in Fetal Medicine (Fetal
Medicine Foundation)
Private practice, Obstetrics & Fetal Medicine

Dr Solina M Richter

B Nurs (US), BA Cur (Unisa), M Cur (Adv
Community Nursing) (Pret), D Cur (RAU)
RN, RPN, RM, RCHN, RNA, RT
Assistant Professor, Faculty of Nursing,
University of Alberta, Canada

Seugnette Rossouw

B Cur Hons (Clinical nursing) (Pret)
Dipl Child Health Nursing, Dipl Patient
Assessment, Diagnosing, Treatment and Care
RN, RM, RCHN, RNA, RT, Child Health Nurs
Lecturer, Department of Nursing Science,
University of Pretoria

Section *1*

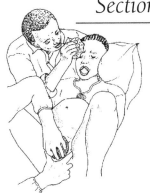

Midwifery concepts

Chapter *1*

Introduction to midwifery and neonatal nursing

Elizabeth Kaye-Petersen

Introduction

The aim of this chapter is to inform student midwives about matters that affect the practice of midwifery within the South African context, thus having a direct or indirect bearing on the woman, her family and the community in which she lives. Over and above national issues, student midwives must also be well informed about our country's links to international professional organisations such as the International Confederation of Midwives (ICM).

This chapter also places emphasis on ethical midwifery practice and the dominant values of the midwifery profession. Student midwives are also reminded of the caring ethos that is embraced by all midwives at national and international level.

Midwives of today trek into the frontier of the twenty-first century confronted with an era of continual restructuring of healthcare. Providing healthcare in this challenging age, midwives are discovering that computer technology, medical and scientific advances, increased consumer demand for quality healthcare and the new roles and responsibilities under managed healthcare systems have all escalated the need for continuing professional development and metamorphosis in their careers.

Definition

A midwife is a person who, having been regularly admitted to a midwifery educational programme, duly recognised in the country in which it is located, has successfully completed the prescribed course of studies in midwifery and has acquired the requisite qualifications to be registered and/or legally licensed to practise midwifery.

The midwife must be able to give the necessary supervision, care and advice to women during pregnancy, labour and the postpartum period, to conduct deliveries on her own responsibility and to care for the newborn and the infant. This care includes preventive measures, the detection of abnormal conditions in mother and child, the procurement of medical assistance and the execution of emergency measures in the absence of medical help. She has an important task in health counselling and education, not only for the women, but also within the family and the community. The work should involve antenatal education and preparation for parenthood and extends to certain areas of gynaecology, family planning and childcare. She may practise in hospitals, clinics, health units, and domiciliary conditions or in any other service.

Source: International Confederation of Midwives, 1992.

The midwife

In South Africa, the midwife is recognised as a practitioner in her own right and is accountable and responsible for her own acts and omissions. A midwife must, in terms of the Nursing Act (Act No 50 of 1978, as amended) be registered with the South African Nursing Council (SANC) to practise midwifery.

Legal aspects affecting the practice of midwifery

Midwifery is an autonomous, self-regulating profession that bases its practice on scientific principles. Midwifery is practised within a legal framework. In South Africa, the Nursing Act (Act No 50 of 1978) governs the practice of midwifery. In terms of this Act, the registered midwife/accoucheur is an independent practitioner, which means that she is accountable for all her acts and omissions. In terms of Chapter 2, Section 16 (1) of this Act it is a criminal offence to practise the profession of a midwife without being registered or enrolled with the SANC.

Over and above being registered or enrolled, practise of a profession requires knowledge of its scope of practice and the rules or conditions under which a person may practise. In midwifery, the scope of practice for midwives clearly defines the course of the daily professional activities of the midwife (Government Notice R2598 of 30 November 1984, as amended). Midwifery practice is based on a scientific process of assessment, planning, implementation, evaluation, education, counselling and fulfilling an advocacy role.

The rules setting out the acts and omissions are found in Government Notice R387 of 15 February 1985, as amended. Chapter 2, No 3 authorises midwives to carry out acts in respect of diagnosing, treatment, care, prescribing, collaborating, referral, co-ordinating and patient advocacy.

The SANC is duty bound to conduct inquiries into complaints received from various sources. Government Notice R373 of 13 March 1970, as amended authorises the SANC to investigate and when it deems necessary to conduct formal inquiries into the alleged misconduct of all nurses and midwives who are registered with the SANC to practise their professions. The SANC has conducted many such professional conduct hearings over the years. They have involved technical misdemeanours and criminal acts, as well as acts and omissions related to negligence and incompetence of an ethical and moral nature (SANC Professional Conduct Report, 1999:2).

Professional accountability and liability

Midwives are increasingly finding that their professional practice is open to scrutiny and may be legally challenged by consumers of healthcare. In some cases, consumers expect the perfect birth and when the unexpected happens they turn to the courts for redress. This practice results in defensive healthcare, in which procedures are done not because of the patient's needs but because of fear of potential litigation should something go wrong. The midwife must be aware of this aspect of contemporary healthcare and recognise that accountable and safe midwifery practice rests on a sound knowledge base, responsible communication, complete and accurate documentation of care and concerned action in the patient's best interest.

The International Confederation of Midwives (ICM)

The aim of the ICM is to improve the standard of care provided to women, babies and families throughout the world through the development, education and appropriate utilisation of the professional midwife.

The nursing process

The nursing process is the systematic application of the problem-solving process in clinical midwifery care. It enables the midwife to progress logically through actions and decisions aimed at resolving specific patient problems and to stay solution focused. The nursing process (in this book we prefer to refer to it as such) is usually described in five separate stages, namely, assessment, midwifery diagnosis, planning, implementation, evaluation and recording. The progression through the stages depends on the nature of the health problem or need, the setting, the available resources and the competencies (knowledge, skills, attitude and values) of the midwife and her patient.

Assessment

The midwife gathers both subjective and objective data from the woman and the family members as the need arises. Subjective data includes the information obtained from the woman and/or family members reflecting their perception of her health status or problem and its management. Objective data is measurable and includes physical assessment findings and laboratory test results.

Midwifery diagnosis

The data collected during assessment is processed through three phases to ensure that accurate and meaningful midwifery diagnoses are achieved:

▶ The data is first analysed to establish categories of concerns or needs.
▶ The data is then synthesised to look for patterns and relationships.
▶ Finally, the data is validated with the woman for relevance and completeness, with other midwives when appropriate and with a family member should the need arise.

The establishment of accurate midwifery diagnoses is crucial in guiding the selection and implementation of effective midwifery interventions. Unlike the medical diagnosis that remains the same throughout the woman's health problem, the midwifery diagnosis will reflect the changing response of the woman as her condition improves or worsens. The midwifery diagnosis has two elements: the identification of the woman and her family's needs or problems and their probable cause.

Planning

An essential aspect of planning care is the establishment of outcomes. Expected outcomes are derived from the problems identified during the diagnostic stage. The midwife relies on her knowledge and assessment skills to prioritise the midwifery care plan. In most instances the woman is not in a life-threatening situation, so the midwife must ensure that the woman and where possible, the family, are

The International Code of Ethics for Midwives

In keeping with its aim of woman's health and focus on the midwife, the ICM has formulated a code to guide the education, practice and research activities of the midwife.

Midwifery relationships:

a) Midwives respect a woman's informed right of choice and promote the woman's acceptance of responsibility for the outcomes of her choices.

b) Midwives work with women, supporting their right to participate actively in decisions about their care, and empowering women to speak for themselves on issues affecting the health of women and their families in their culture and society.

c) Midwives, together with women, work with policy and funding agencies to define women's needs for health services and to ensure that resources are fairly allocated considering priorities and availability.

d) Midwives support and sustain each other in their professional roles and actively nurture their own and others' sense of self-worth.

e) Midwives work with other health professionals, consulting and referring as necessary when the woman's need for care exceeds the competencies of the midwife.

f) Midwives recognise the human interdependence within their field of practice and actively seek to resolve inherent conflict.

g) The midwife has responsibilities to her or himself as a person of moral worth, including duties of moral self-respect and the preservation of integrity (Revised May, 1999).

Practice of midwifery:

a) Midwives provide care for women and childbearing families with respect for cultural diversity while also working to eliminate harmful practices within those same cultures.

b) Midwives encourage realistic expectations of childbirth by women within their own society, with the minimum expectation that conception or childbearing should harm no women.

c) Midwives use their professional knowledge to ensure safe birthing practices in all environments and cultures.

d) Midwives respond to the psychological, physical, emotional and spiritual needs of women seeking health care, whatever their circumstances.

e) Midwives act as effective role models in health promotion for women throughout their life cycle, for families and for other health professionals.

f) Midwives actively seek personal, intellectual and professional growth throughout their midwifery career, integrating this growth into their practice.

The professional responsibilities of midwives:

a) Midwives hold in confidence client information in order to protect the right to privacy and use judgement in sharing this information.

b) Midwives are responsible for their decisions and actions and are accountable for the related outcomes in their care of women.

c) Midwives may refuse to participate in activities for which they hold deep moral opposition, however, the emphasis on individual conscience should not deprive women of essential health services.

d) Midwives understand the adverse consequences that ethical and human rights violations have on the health of woman and infants, and will work to eliminate these violations (Revised May, 1999).

e) Midwives participate in the development and implementation of health policies that promote the health of all women and childbearing families.

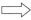

Advancement of midwifery knowledge and practice:

a) Midwives ensure that the advancement of midwifery knowledge is based on activities that protect the rights of women as persons.

b) Midwives develop and share midwifery knowledge through a variety of processes, such as peer review and research.

c) Midwives participate in the formal education of midwifery students and midwives.

Visit the ICM webpage: www.intlmidwives.org

Source: ICM Publication, May 1999.

involved in the planning and prioritising of her care. Cognisance is also taken of the midwife's scope of practice, other relevant regulations, protocols and guidelines that direct the midwifery care plan. The care plan is communicated to colleagues through verbal and written entries on the appropriate documentation.

Implementation

The midwife, together with the woman and her family, implements the plan to achieve the prioritised outcomes.

Evaluation

The midwife, woman and the family evaluate the woman's progress, or lack of progress, toward the identified outcomes. Evaluation is logical and continuous throughout every stage of the nursing process. The outcome of the evaluation determines the need for revising the expected outcomes, additional assessment data or modification of midwifery interventions.

Documentation and recording

The midwife must ensure that all records are accurate, complete and that they meet the policy requirements of the specific institution and the SANC. Accurate record keeping is one of the most important functions of the midwife as it serves as evidence of the midwifery care that was ministered. As midwives we make complex decisions about the woman's care, but our documentation does not always reflect these decision-making processes. Documen-tation must clearly communicate the midwife's judgement and evaluation. It is also used to inform other professionals involved in the woman's care.

From a legal perspective it is important that the midwife knows that any record documenting patient care may be used as evidence in a court of law or as part of an investigation or disciplinary procedure.

The context of midwifery practice

Family-centred midwifery

It is our philosophy that midwifery and neonatal nursing care should be family-centred care. It should focus on supporting the integrity of the family and individualising care, in order to promote individual and family health.

The effectiveness of family-centred midwifery care is attitudinal. Where the need arises, scientific method and medical technology should be combined with the knowledge and sensitivity needed to provide holistic and individualised care to women and their families. Table 1.1 outlines the principles of family-centred midwifery and Table 1.2 compares family-centred care with traditional care.

Much change is needed to accommodate family-centred care especially in the midst of intensive obstetric interventions. Women who are designated high-risk status also need the benefits of supportive individualised care to allay their fears and anxieties.

Community-based midwifery

Effective community-based midwifery care is of critical importance in developing countries and in South Africa in particular, where we are witnessing an increasing number of HIV

Table 1.1 Principles central to family-centred midwifery

Principle	The midwife's role
1. The family is capable of making decisions about care if given adequate information and support by the midwife and other members of the multi-professional team.	This principle requires the midwife to enter into a partnership with the family, rather than assuming an authorative role on which the family becomes dependent. Health education is important and the family is included in discussions about their care.
2. In the majority of cases childbirth is a normal, healthy event in the life of a family.	This principle focuses the midwife's attention on maintaining the health of the woman and her family. Pregnancy and birth are viewed as states of health that require preventive and supportive care, rather than a state of illness that must be treated. Health maintenance cannot occur without the active participation of the family members themselves.
3. Childbirth is the beginning of a new set of important family relationships.	This principle requires the midwife to organise care in a way that enhances positive interactions among parents, the infant and other family members. The midwife's concern extends beyond physical needs in recognition of the fact that holistic health care also has psychological and social dimensions.

infected women returning home with babies who are infected as well. The current economic climate, together with escalating healthcare costs, and hospital costs in particular, has resulted in shorter hospital stays and early discharge from hospitals. This requires that a well-developed community-based service be in place to ensure the continuity of care.

The essence of the notion of 'community' is a group of people who have relationships based on common interests and a shared identity. The commonalities that develop the sense of community can be geographic, ethnic, religious, political and ideological, or based on gender, ability, sexual identity or many of the other shared interests that bring people

Table 1.2 Features of family-centred care and traditional care

Family-centred care	Traditional care
▶ Provision made for antenatal and parenting classes.	▶ No provision made for antenatal and parenting classes.
▶ Attendance by the father or support person during labour and birth.	▶ Separation of the father or support person from the woman during labour and birth.
▶ Flexible policies with regard to routine procedures.	▶ Routine use of medication, episiotomies or other procedures.
▶ Presence of father or support person at complicated or caesarean birth, if circumstances permit.	▶ No presence of father or support person for complicated or caesarean birth, even if circumstances permit.
▶ Unrestricted family visitation.	▶ Restriction of family visitation in the post-birth period.
▶ Flexible rooming-in policy.	▶ A restrictive policy with regard to rooming-in.

together. Community-based midwifery practice occurs in the context of such shared commonalities. Community-based midwifery is also characterised by partnership and close, genuine collaboration between communities, midwives and other health professionals.

The most important aspect of building partnerships between midwives and community members would be the development of trust through relationships that mature over time. Partnership indicates joint participation in all aspects of project or programme planning, especially in decision-making. The next section makes some suggestions on how the midwife can facilitate such partnerships with communities.

Working with the community

The longer a midwife practices, the more she will find that there are many structural and cultural influences which prevent women from being healthy. Some of these include poverty, lack of access to healthcare and health services, lack of education, harmful beliefs or cultural practices and lack of support from their husbands, partners, or other family members. Since these problems are deeply embedded in the fabric of communities, solving them would require the involvement of the whole community.

> Ideas on methods that empower are outlined in an excellent book entitled *Helping health workers learn* (David Werner & Bill Bower, 1988).

To assist the community in working together, the midwife will need to find out:

▶ What other members in the community think about the problem (once the problem has been identified).
▶ Who is willing to work on the problem? Networking will help you with this or you can enlist the help of a community member to contact people.
▶ How do they see themselves or other community members dealing with their issues and concerns?

▶ What are the different members able to contribute? (People could contribute their ideas, time, skills, or a venue in which to meet, etc.)
▶ What are the conflicts of interest in the community? (Who are the people with power or money who might be helpful or problematic?)
▶ How will their involvement promote their self-esteem, strengthen their self-care skills, cultivate a sense of mastery and power, and enhance their capacity to act more effectively on their own behalf? (Fostering the empowerment of community members is central to getting them to work together or participate in health development, so this question should always be at the forefront.)

As far as possible, the midwife tries to link the woman with existing community resources and provides materials on these resources, which include postpartum support groups, baby clinics, infant feeding clinics and resource centres. The midwife also networks with individuals and groups (locally, nationally and internationally) who may be willing to assist in addressing some of the problems of the community in which she works.

Contemporary trends, issues and dilemmas in midwifery

It is sometimes difficult to meet the needs of women and their families and at the same time keep accurate and comprehensive notes. The recording of patient care should never be seen as an administrative task, it is an integral part of holistic midwifery care.

Midwifery is a dynamic healthcare profession. It is essential to stay in touch with the latest trends, dilemmas and issues that may influence our practice. The following contemporary issues influence the practice of midwifery in South Africa.

Education of women, families and informal caregivers

The spiralling healthcare costs have seen decreases in the length of hospital stay following childbirth. Much more preparation is therefore needed during pregnancy to prepare the woman and family for the birth, the hospital stay, and for the help they will need at home, following discharge from the hospital. It could be done through one-on-one instruction or formal antenatal classes, either by a midwife or an informal community caregiver (lay health worker) at various stages throughout the pregnancy (see Chapter 11).

Continuing professional development

Traditionally regulatory bodies, such as the SANC, meet their responsibility to protect the public by licensing qualified individuals, denying licences to the unqualified and ensuring professional discipline for those who are incompetent, negligent, or in violation of their principal Act and the regulations that emanate from the respective Acts. Regulatory bodies or professional councils are expected to establish mechanisms that ensure continued competence of their licencees. The most common measure adopted by health professional councils is Continuing Professional Development (CPD). CPD is the lifelong learning which takes place in a professional's career after the point of qualification and/or registration.

Society has a right to expect those who profess to a certain body of knowledge and skills to be able to deliver their 'goods', whether that be sound legal advice, knowledgeable and compassionate midwifery care, effective medicine, or efficient teaching.

Midwives are therefore compelled to continually improve their level of competence. If a professional does not keep abreast of developments in her field of practice, a backlog develops which will affect her professional effectiveness negatively. Each profession has certain competencies and specialty knowledge that must constantly be updated and enhanced. CPD must therefore provide for sufficient professional growth and self-actualisation.

Human rights

South Africa has in the past decades undergone a period of transformation from an autocratic to a democratic state. In the process, the country has developed a Constitution, which is hailed as the most liberal and a model of human freedom for the rest of the world to emulate. The 'Bill of Rights' is enshrined within the Constitutional Act (Act No 108 of 1996, Chapter 2). The Constitution as the law supreme governs every facet of South African life, including the practice of midwifery. The National Department of Health also developed the *Patients' Rights Charter* and the Batho Pele principles in an endeavour to promote the culture of a caring ethos.

Professional ethics is critical to the relationship between the professions and civil society. There is an honouring of an established social contract – a contract that is dependent on ethical practice and respect for human rights. Table 1.3 illustrates how human rights relate to safe motherhood. Midwives and other health professionals have been given a free hand to regulate themselves by society. In return for this right to self-regulation society expects them to protect the rights of patients, families and communities. It is also expected that the highest standard of care and professional conduct be maintained. However, this trust can be open to abuse.

Midwifery education and training programmes should ensure that student midwives acquire knowledge and an understanding of the following:

▶ The conceptual framework for human rights.
▶ The core principles of human rights.
▶ Her advocacy role for vulnerable women, families or groups in her care.
▶ How to facilitate the adoption of a human rights culture in her working environment.
▶ How to promote the ethical practice of midwifery that is firmly grounded in a human rights approach.
▶ The relevant codes related to human rights.

Table 1.3 Human rights related to safe motherhood

1. Rights relating to life, liberty and security of the person.	The right to life is being increasingly applied to require states to take positive measures to protect against preventable deaths – an application with clear implications for safe motherhood.
2. Rights relating to the foundation of families and of family life.	The promotion of women's rights to survive pregnancy and childbirth and to enjoy family life.
3. Rights relating to the highest attainable standard of health.	For women this includes the right to information and reproductive health services.
4. Rights to equality and non-discrimination on grounds of sex, marital status, race, age and class.	This human right can be used against laws or policies that require women seeking health services to obtain authorisation from their husbands, or that criminalise medical procedures that only women need, such as abortion. Laws must be in place to protect women and children against violence and sexual abuse.

Source: Adapted from Cook, 1997.

The midwife's role in reducing violence against adolescent girls and women

The first stage in the midwife's intervention is the acceptance that violence against adolescent girls and women is a human rights violation and has severe consequences on the achievement of safe motherhood. Midwives should not remain indifferent but should acquire knowledge and skills that will empower them to address this problem effectively.

Before midwives broach the subject of violence against adolescent girls and women, they should be encouraged to examine themselves and to confront any biases, misconceptions and fears that they may have about the issue.

An adolescent girl or woman who has been sexually assaulted can be victimised again through any forms of judgemental or indifferent behaviour. Mechanisms should be put in place to avoid these unacceptable behaviours. Aspects of sexual assault training should be incorporated into midwifery education and training programmes.

HIV/AIDS

HIV infection is not only one of the most significant health problems of the twentieth and twenty-first centuries, it is also one of the most significant social issues of our times. The social, political and economic issues raised by this disease are numerous and complex. There are three major areas of controversy surrounding the HIV/AIDS crisis that deserve careful consideration: testing, education and funding. The following thought-provoking questions arise in each of these areas:

▶ *Routine testing.* Should testing be voluntary or mandatory? Should test results be disclosed to others? If so, under what circumstances?

▶ *Education.* Is education an effective way to change high-risk behaviour? What should be included in such education programmes? At what age should these programmes be introduced?

▶ *Health service funding.* Who should bear the cost of HIV/AIDS treatment? Is healthcare a right of all individuals or accessible only to those who can afford to pay for it?

CRITICAL THINKING EXERCISES

1. Hold formal debates on current trends, issues and dilemmas in midwifery.
2. Conduct consultative interviews with midwives in practice, managers and policy makers.
3. Keep reflective journals on risk management, professional malpractice and the management thereof.
4. Read national and international literature and note the key trends discussed in publications.
5. Visit the web pages of the Department of Health, WHO and ICM.

Midwives, by virtue of their profession, deal with women and their families on a daily basis. Student midwives, through their formative period of professional growth, should be purposefully engaged in reflective and critical thinking and actively participate in community outreach programmes, so as to make a significant contribution towards addressing this scourge.

At the time of writing this book, the new Nursing Bill for nurses and midwives in South Africa was still being routed through legislative procedures. The scope of practice for nurses and midwives should integrate the primary healthcare approach and other national priorities, so that the provision and management of midwifery services optimises service delivery of these services.

Conclusion

This chapter has broadened the student midwife's outlook on what midwifery practice entails. Emphasis was placed on various aspects that influence safe midwifery practice. A midwife is trained and educated according to nationally prescribed norms. The Nursing Act (Act No 50 of 1978 as amended) forms the legal framework for midwifery practice and the SANC further frames regulations that govern the practice of the registered midwife. Midwives are professionally accountable and liable for their actions.

The ICM is an international body which aims to improve the standard of care for women, babies and families throughout the world. The International code of ethics for midwives guides education, practice and resesarch in midwifery.

Midwifery and neonatal nursing is family-centred in order to promote and support the integrity of the family. CPD refers to life-long learning and midwives are compelled to continuously improve their level of competence through CPD. Safe motherhood is a human rights issue and midwifes should become actively involved in reducing violence against adolescent girls and women. HIV/AIDS has definite implications for midwives as professionals and individuals.

References

Bobak, I. M. & Jensen M. D. 1993. *Maternity and gynaecologic care: The nurse and the family*. Fifth edition. St Louis: Mosby.

Fulbrook, S. 1998. Medical-legal insights – record keeping: Legally and professionally important. *British Journal of Theatre Nursing*, 7(12):10-11.

ICM (International Confederation of Midwives). 1993. International code of ethics for midwives (6 May 1993).

Klein, S. 1996. *A book for midwives*. California: MacMillan Education Ltd.

Krieger, J. & Ciske, S. 2000. The community as full partner in public health initiatives, *Washington Public Health,* Fall 2000:1-4.

Labonte, R. (Ed.) 1997. *Power, participation and partnerships for health promotion*. Melbourne: Victorian Health Promotion Foundation.

Ladewig, P. W., London, M. L. & Olds, S. B. 1994. *Maternal-newborn nursing*. Third edition. Redwood City: Addison-Wesley Nursing.

Lowdermilk, D. L., Perry, S. E. & Bobak, I. M. 1995. *Maternity and women's health care*. St Louis: Mosby.

Lyer, P. and Camp, N. 1995. *Nursing docu-*

mentation: A nursing process approach. Second edition. London: Mosby.

May, K. A. & Malmeister, L. R. 1994. *Maternal and neonatal nursing: Family-centred care*. Third edition. Philadelphia: J B Lippincott.

Morton-Cooper, J. D. 2000. *Action research in health care*. First edition. Oxford: Blackwell Science Ltd.

Pillitteri, A. 1999. *Maternal and child health nursing*. Third edition. Philadelphia: J B Lippincott.

Rodden, C. & Bell, M. 2002. Record keeping: Developing good practice. *Nursing Standard,* 19(1):40-42.

SANC (South African Nursing Council). 1985. Government Notice R387 Rules setting out the acts or omissions in respect of which the council may take disciplinary steps. 15 February 1985. Pretoria: SANC.

SANC (South African Nursing Council). 2000 Draft Document: A system for continuing professional development for nurses and midwives in South Africa. Pretoria: SANC.

SANC (South African Nursing Council). 1970. Government Notice R373 Regulations for the investigation of alleged misconduct and the conduct of inquiries. 13 March 1970. Pretoria: SANC.

South Africa. 1978: The Nursing Act 50 of 1978. Government Printer.

Wallerstein, N. (1992). Powerlessness, empowerment, and health: Implications for health promotion programs. *American Journal of Health Promotion*, 6(3):197-205.

Werner, D. & Bower, B. 1988. *Helping health workers learn*. California: Hesperian Foundation.

Publications

The official journal and newsletter, *International Midwifery* (published six times a year) contains updates on the ICM activities, reports from representatives and members, articles from midwives working in the international field and a section of news on topics of interest to midwives. A website, at www.intlmidwives.org provides information about ICM and related activities in the maternal and child area.

Chapter 2

Sociocultural aspects of maternity care

Dr Gail Andrews

Introduction

Whatever the cultural origins or religious beliefs and practices of the families we work with, they all have a need to feel respected, accepted and understood. This is especially important for people embarking on the adventure of parenthood. Pregnancy, birth and the transition to parenthood are very challenging life events that often leave individuals feeling very sensitive and vulnerable. The quality of care and the support that parents receive at this time significantly affect their response to these challenges. To provide the best possible care to pregnant women, their families and communities, it is imperative that the midwife has knowledge of the specific beliefs and cultural practices of the people in the community in which she works.

A critical life experience, childbearing often involves traditional beliefs and practices. The public health and anthropological literature indicate that understanding culture-specific factors is vital to the effectiveness of health interventions in general and that interventions fail when culture-specific factors are not considered.

This chapter explores the role of the midwife in addressing the sociocultural needs of families and communities. It examines the role of culture in defining and shaping who we are and how culture influences the healthcare practices in communities. Suggestions are offered on effective ways in which the midwife can approach cultural diversity in midwifery care. Because the family is regarded as the basic unit within a community with which the midwife would be concerned, it is necessary to start by defining what a family is, what purposes it serves and the various family forms that may be encountered in contemporary South Africa.

The family

Society defines families in many ways, and these definitions often involve family structure, function, composition and ties of affection. Some definitions emphasise the importance of emotional involvement and view the family as persons who are joined together by bonds of sharing and emotional closeness and who identify themselves as part of the family. Other definitions offer a broader interpretation. In these interpretations the family is 'who they say they are'. These definitions include a variety of family forms such as the extended family living in two or more households, cohabiting couples, blended families, childless families, gay and lesbian families, and single-parent families. Because many ethnic, religious, and cultural groups coexist in South Africa, the varying family forms are recognised and accepted in differing degrees. The midwife therefore has to be sensitive to this, as well as to the fact that not all mothers are part of an intact nuclear family. Others may not have an extended family to offer support during pregnancy, labour or the postnatal period. The next section briefly describes the various family forms in our society.

Nuclear family

The nuclear family consists of parents (husband and wife) and their dependent children. The family lives apart from the husband's or wife's family of origin and is usually economically independent. The 'idealised' two-parent, two-child nuclear family, in which the father is the sole provider and the mother primarily the homemaker, represents only a small number of contemporary South African families.

Extended family

The extended family includes the nuclear family and other people related by blood. Referred to as kin, these family members include great-grandparents, grandparents, aunts, uncles and cousins. Through its kinship network, the extended family is an important source of support to all its members.

Alternative family forms

Variations of the traditional nuclear and extended families have always existed, although they have not always been recognised. Indeed, most of these alternative family forms have been considered deviations from the norm in South Africa until quite recently. However, the emphasis on human rights following the advent of democracy in South Africa, and which is enshrined in the Constitution, has led to greater recognition and acceptance of these alternative family forms in our society.

Single-parent family

The single-parent family has been increasingly recognised and accepted by society. The emergence of single parenthood as a planned choice reflects the greater emphasis on women's reproductive rights as human rights. It also reflects a growing acceptance of the notion that a woman has the right to decide if and when to become pregnant and bear a child. On a broader level it also reflects the belief that each person has the right to choose to be a parent. For example, a gay man can now choose to be a parent.

The single-parent family may also result from the loss of a spouse by death, divorce, separation, or desertion; from an unplanned pregnancy or the birth of a child outside marriage; or from the adoption of a child. The single-parent family tends to be vulnerable economically and socially, especially in South Africa where up to 45% of households are headed by women.

The death of both parents as a result of HIV/AIDS has resulted in another type of single-parent family in South Africa – that headed by an aging grandmother. Yet another family form that is on the increase is the child-headed family, which is becoming increasingly common among the burgeoning orphan population where children have lost both parents as a result of death from HIV/AIDS. This poses a real challenge for the midwife. The high rate of teen pregnancies is exacerbated by high levels of sexual abuse of young girls, and in this regard orphans are especially vulnerable. The myth that an HIV-infected male can cure his disease by having sex with a virgin has resulted in an increase in forced sex between older men and young girls. The result is that many teens or very young girls find themselves with unplanned and unwanted pregnancies, and often without support from parents or the extended family. In these situations the midwife needs to play a key role in ensuring that these grandmothers and pregnant teens are linked up with the social security system (for social support grants). The effective co-ordination of care between the various levels (primary, secondary, tertiary) and by various health professionals (midwife, community nurse, social worker) is imperative.

Blended family

The blended family is also called a reconstituted, combined, or remarried family and it includes stepparents and stepchildren. Separation, divorce, and remarriage are common in South Africa, where approximately 60% of marriages end in divorce. Divorce and remarriage may occur at any time in the family life cycle and affect family function differently, depending on when they occur in the cycle. The midwife therefore needs to be sensitive and not make the assumption, for example, that she is dealing with a couple having their first child, since for one of the couple it may be the second or third.

Homosexual family

The rights of persons and equality are enshrined in the South African Constitution, and increasingly lesbian and gay families are receiving greater recognition. Children in such families are either the offspring of previous heterosexual unions, conceived by one member of a lesbian couple through artificial insemination or adopted. Although they still face resistance and discrimination, the constitutional court has increasingly ruled in the favour of gay and lesbian couples. The midwife should bear in mind that gay parents have the same biological and psychological needs as heterosexual parents.

Functions of the family

As the family progresses through its life cycle, it accomplishes certain functions for the well-being of its members. These functions have been described differently by various authors, but are essentially derived from five areas identified by the World Health Organisation (1978):

▶ *Biological* (reproduction and care of children)
▶ *Economic* (earning money to perform other functions)
▶ *Educational* (the teaching of skills, attitudes and knowledge)
▶ *Psychological* (common bonds of affection and coping with stress and crises)
▶ *Sociocultural* (which involves the socialisation of children).

The sociocultural area includes the transfer of values relating to behaviour, tradition, language, religion and moral attitudes, that is, the transmission of culture.

Culture

All communities, irrespective of their level of urbanisation and industrialisation, have evolved their own culture pattern. This can be defined as the common way of life shared by all members of the group that enables them to function cohesively. It includes their beliefs and values (morals), their customs (traditions), assumptions and perceptions, and their social and historical inheritance. Culture shapes how we think about the world and ourselves and it involves the way we develop and organise aspects of social life, including healthcare practices such as methods of childbirth. It includes the relationships between different members of a family, traditional ways of preparing food and approved methods of raising children.

Most of us grow up not being very conscious that we have a culture. This is because our culture, like the air we breathe, is around us from the day of our birth and we acquire almost all of it unconsciously in early childhood. Furthermore, we often find it hard to distinguish, even in ourselves, what is cultural from what is individual or personal. We may not realise that what we regard as normal, universal values and ways of behaving are in fact cultural and may therefore be normal only in our particular context.

Culture and gender

Gender is a social construct and refers to the identities, roles and relations of women and men that are formed by culture and society. Culture usually determines who has power and status in society. In Africa, as in many patriarchal societies, boys are more valued than girls. As indicated previously, the process of acculturisation begins at birth and is mediated by every contact the infant has with the world around him or her. This includes gender roles. Right from the cradle, girl babies are dressed in pink and boys in blue. The first question commonly asked after the birth of a child is 'is it a boy or a girl?' The sex of boys and girls then often determines how they are raised. Girls are socialised into caring, nurturing roles and to be mothers. Boys are seen as potential decision-makers, protectors of the family and socialised accordingly.

To a large extent, the patriarchy inherent in black societies has resulted in the low status of women, who are generally regarded as inferior. This ingrained gender structure has negatively affected the empowerment of women and undermined their options in various spheres of life, namely as in the workplace and in the home. At a personal level their lack of empowerment constrains women's ability to refuse sex or negotiate safer sex practices such as the use of condoms. This not only impacts negatively on the health of the woman but also affects her ability to care for her family.

Implications for the midwife

It is important for the midwife to realise that she has been moulded in her own habits and ideas by her own cultural pattern. As with every culture, our traditions and practices contain both 'rational' and 'irrational' elements. The midwife should develop the insight and sensitivity to recognise that the customs and practices of her own group are neither the only, nor necessarily the best but merely some of a range of possible alternatives. When we achieve this level of sensitivity, we are better able to respect differences, value diversity and appreciate the richness of the various ethnic traditions in our society.

Health workers (and midwives are no exception) have often been criticised for imposing their values and practices on patients, groups or communities. As midwives we will be more successful in the prevention and management of maternal and neonatal ill health if we pay greater attention to the sociocultural aspects. For example, the midwife should be aware of the root causes of disease that are often political, cultural, social or economic. She should recognise (or identify) the resources of the pregnant woman, her cultural pattern and the expectations of individuals, families and communities. The following aspects of cultural patterns are of particular and direct relevance to the midwife.

Patriarchy and patterns of household authority

As already previously mentioned, a woman's position in society has negative consequences for her health and that of her family. There is evidence that the slow decline in maternal mortality and morbidity in developing countries is rooted in the limited power of women and their unequal access to resources in families, societies and economic markets.

For most of its history, the public health field has evaded issues of sexuality and avoided recognising the role of power in sexual relationships between men and women. The 1994 Cairo Conference on Population and Development and the 1995 Beijing Women's Conference publicly ended this silence. The latter was achieved by focusing attention on how gender influences sexual relations and reproductive health decision-making. Where traditionally men have been excluded, there is now greater recognition of the need to involve men in reproductive health decision-making. This is significant since in most heterosexual unions, men wield more power and have greater authority, particularly in developing country contexts where patriarchy is still very entrenched.

While involving men, midwives should however continue to promote the rights of women, in particular the right of women to non-discrimination. The Convention on the Elimination of all forms of Discrimination Against Women (CEDAW) defines discrimination against women as:

> *Any distinction, exclusion or restriction made on the basis of sex which has the effect or purpose of impairing or nullifying the recognition, enjoyment or exercise by woman, of human rights and fundamental freedoms in the political, economic, social, cultural, civil or any other field.*

The midwife therefore looks well beyond the immediate precipitating medical causes of maternal morbidity and mortality, to the failures in health systems and the transcending failures in social justice that condemn women to a marginal, neglected and deprived status in their communities. The midwife understands that the most critical right underlying safe motherhood is women's right to equality with men. She recognises that many societies tolerate maternal morbidity and mortality with much more fatalism and composure than they tolerate avoidable deaths and disabilities that strike men and she participates in campaigns to help change these attitudes.

Furthermore, health promotion activities planned by the midwife should involve those who have authority or wield power in the household. For example, sexual health education about safer sex should involve men since women may have very little power in negotiating safe sex. In these sessions, the midwife uses the opportunity to sensitively and appropriately raise the consciousness of both men and women regarding gender issues and how these impact on the health and wellbeing of women and families.

Likewise, health education about childcare should not be directed at the mother only, since the grandmother might have an important role in child rearing. Nutrition education on the other hand, must be directed at the family members who purchase and cook the food. For example, in poor communities, where both parents may have died from AIDS, this is usually the grandmother, on whose pension the household survives.

Infant feeding and child-rearing practices

The duration of breastfeeding, time of weaning and types of foods considered suitable, depend largely on the cultural setting. Within the context of HIV/AIDS this poses an immense challenge for the midwife. For example, women in most African societies generally have a low status, are subservient and find it difficult to practise what is not the dominant cultural norm, for fear of being sanctioned. For example, HIV-positive mothers who are advised to exclusively breastfeed their babies find it difficult to do so because the norm is to give breastfeeding substitutes in between. Likewise, it is difficult for these mothers to practise exclusive bottle-feeding.

Marriage and childbirth

Sociocultural factors such as early marriages impact negatively on the health status of women and are as common in Africa as in most developing countries. In some instances marriage occurs as early as 10 to 12 years, as with the child brides in India. There are health complications that result from conception when the young girl's body is not fully grown. Early marriage also increases the risk of early and prolonged childbearing.

Coupled with the complications of child-birth, there is always a high likelihood of girls who marry at an early age facing nutritional problems and poverty. Especially because most of them are married at an age when they are not physically and mentally able to fend for themselves. Very often their lives depend heavily on their husbands who in many cases are polygamous. The young woman on whom the health of the family depends becomes trapped in this oppressive cycle at an early age, with negative consequences for her health and wellbeing.

Cultural attitudes to infertility

In most African societies fertility is highly valued, and giving birth is a key event that marks the transition of a young girl into woman-hood. Within the home, women's natural ability to bear children gives them a certain power and in some societies childbearing women are rewarded with places of honour. For most women, however, this has rarely translated into social and political power in the broader society. Indeed women's reproductive function has many negative consequences for their reproductive health and this has been well documented.

In some cultures proving one's fertility is traditionally more important than marriage. In cultures where childbearing is so highly valued, failure to father or bear a child can have serious social and emotional consequences for the couple. In cultures where motherhood is the primary and perhaps the only accepted role for women, infertility can be particularly painful and may lead to social isolation in the community, or worse, rejection – even by their husbands. Often women who are infertile are viewed as 'useless' by their husbands and dis-carded. It is not surprising therefore, that many customs are directed against infertility. For example, in the some ethnic groups (Shangaan and Pedi) in South Africa eating eggs in pregnancy is believed to result in abor-tion or sterility and is therefore taboo. The midwife needs an understanding of the beliefs of the people she cares for.

Beliefs and customs related to food and nutrition

Beliefs and customs related to food and nutri-tion in a community are of particular impor-tance and direct relevance to the midwife. Feeding practices that discriminate against girls in childhood may lead to iron deficiency anaemia, malnutrition, iodine deficiency, deformed pelvic bones and subsequent prob-lems in childbirth, such as obstructed labour, ruptured uterus and at times the death of a woman. In many communities a number of food taboos exist at various stages of the life of a woman. In particular, the midwife should explore beliefs about nutrition and food dur-ing pregnancy that could be harmful. In some cultures for example, deficient dietary intake is not considered a cause of protein energy malnutrition (PEM), but a mother's alleged infidelity may be. Beliefs such as these should be dealt with appropriately.

How to approach cultural diversity in midwifery practice

The midwife should strive to understand the local culture pattern of the community in which she works. This is imperative because firstly, it leads to an understanding of the cul-tural factors underlying disease patterns in the community.

Secondly, an understanding of culture pro-vides insight into people's values, knowledge of, and attitudes to health and disease, which in turn fosters an understanding of their health-care seeking behaviour. Often a women's deci-sion to seek care is guided by cultural percep-tions of what is considered normal or problem-atic. It is known that among the delays that lead to maternal mortality, the first delay, that is the decision to seek care, may in part be due to the failure to recognise the problem as poten-tially serious. In many instances this is related to the fact that cultural perceptions of what is normal and problematic differ from biomedical perceptions.

Thirdly, understanding the culture allows the midwife to approach cultural and religious aspects of maternity care with regard for women's choice. Respecting the human rights of women includes respecting their right to choice, especially in such a personal area as reproductive health. A woman's personal preferences about how her labour and birth should be managed should be assessed. This requires the midwife to validate the woman's cultural beliefs, especially since they may influence the following aspects of maternity care:

▶ It might determine who and how many people the woman wants with her for support during labour.

▶ It might determine the degree of involvement of the father and any needs he may have. In some cultures the father prefers not to be involved, with birthing being regarded as 'women's business'.

▶ In some instances provision may need to be made for religious observance including prayer and diet. For example, Muslims do not eat pork and practising Catholics usually do not eat meat on Fridays.

▶ Often the woman or family's attitudes to pain, pain relief and other interventions are influenced by religious or cultural traditions. Blood transfusions, for example, are not allowed among people of the Jehovah Witness faith.

▶ Culture might determine whether the mother has any preferences about disposing of the placenta. For example, among Muslims in the Cape it is customary to bury the placenta. The placenta is not disposed of by the midwife since the family usually want to bury it themselves. It is placed in a marked plastic bag to be taken away by the family.

▶ For some parents, the choice between burial and cremation is influenced by culture and religion. For example, Jewish law requires all bodies or remains, of whatever gestation, to be buried. Islam too, requires burial rather than cremation. Likewise, in African culture, when the mother dies there would be a preference that she be buried rather than cremated because of the belief in connecting with the ancestors.

Classification or categorisation of customs

At the risk of over-simplifying the complex, the approach proposed by Williams, Baumslag and Jelliffe (1994) has been found to be very helpful when dealing with an unfamiliar culture. It essentially consists of the three steps of exploration, analysis and categorisation, to which techniques and elaboration have been added as appropriate.

Exploration

Explore as far as possible the relevant customs and traditional practices of the women being cared for. To elicit the necessary cultural information or explanations about childbearing, the midwife may need to ask certain questions.

The following questions may be helpful:

▶ What do you and your family consider important for you to do to remain healthy during pregnancy?

▶ What are the things you can or cannot do to improve your health and the health of your infant?

▶ Who do you want to have with you during your labour?

▶ What beliefs or actions are important to you and your family after the infant's birth?

▶ What do you and your family expect from the midwife who will be caring for you?

▶ How will family members participate in your pregnancy, childbirth, and parenting?

Analysis

Once an understanding of the cultural preferences and patterns has been gained, the midwife analyses the effects of these customs and traditional practices on the health of both the mother and child.

Categorisation

Next the midwife categorises these customs and practices as beneficial, harmless, of uncertain value or as harmful. The midwife promotes and nurtures those beliefs, customs or practices that promote physical, emotional adaptation or social adaptation to childbearing. Those that might be harmful should be carefully and respectfully explored with the mother and family, using participatory approaches, or participatory action research methodology.

Beneficial

These are customs or traditions that appear to benefit the health of mothers and children, although they may differ from western practices, such as prolonged breastfeeding in rural African communities. Another cultural practice, which is once again gaining recognition by the Western healthcare system, is that of support by a layperson during labour (see Chapter 13 and 15).

Harmless

Included under the category of harmless would be customs that are neither beneficial nor harmful to the mother or child, such as 'rooming in' of mother and baby for a certain length of time in the postnatal period. Another example is a practice among Hindu women in the Indian community, of wearing a black dot on their forehead (the 'third eye') during pregnancy, because of the belief that it keeps off the 'evil spirit'. Hanging beads around a baby's neck or waist in the belief that it will keep the baby well, as practised in some African communities, is another. In some instances using a harmless method could result in a woman not using a more helpful or beneficial method, in which case it becomes harmful. For example, in some African communities women tie a string around their waist to prevent pregnancy. While this in itself does no harm, it does not prevent pregnancy. If a woman resorts to this practice instead of using a contraceptive method she will most likely get pregnant.

Uncertain value

Sometimes a midwife may encounter customs that are difficult to classify as either beneficial or harmful. In such instances, it is impossible to be certain of their value with a more focused analysis. For instance, the use of certain traditional medicines that are purported to boost the immune system of HIV-positive mothers. Without analysis it is not possible to know whether the practice is indeed a source of nutrients or a danger. With customs in this uncertain group, further observation and investigation is required before including it in nutrition education, for example.

Harmful customs

These are practices that impact negatively on the health and wellbeing of mothers and their children, such as putting certain herbal medicines into the vagina during labour. This can cause infection. As could the practice of placing a cow-dung dressing on the umbilical stump. Other examples of harmful practices are female circumcision and the practice of dry sex in some African communities. Using substances such as spirits or vinegar, or 'muti' prepared by traditional healers to dry out the vagina can disturb the bacterial balance of the vagina or cause tears that could make women more vulnerable to sexually transmitted infections and HIV infection.

By knowing the culture and classifying the cultural practices in this way, the midwife will help to improve maternal and neonatal services in the community. The aim of exploring and analysing the cultural practices in this way is to preserve the beneficial cultural practices and beliefs and integrate these into health promotion activities or sessions, while attempting to modify the harmful practices. The midwife should bear in mind that the observance of traditional beliefs and rituals, even if they appear to be unnecessary or irrational, helps people to identify with their family or community. For many people it engenders a sense of belonging. It also plays a central role in the maintenance of health and wellbeing and in building social capital and stability in communities.

Conclusion

This chapter explored the role of the midwife in addressing the sociocultural needs of families and communities in maternity care. It described the different family forms in contemporary South Africa and discussed the role of culture in defining and shaping who we are, and how culture influences the healthcare practices in communities. The family forms a social network that acts as an important support system for its members. Ideally, the family provides a safe, intimate environment for the development of its children and adult members.

Some important aspects of culture for the midwife were highlighted and suggestions were made on effective ways in which the midwife can approach cultural diversity in maternity care. A culture's economic, religious, kinship and political structures pervade its beliefs and practices regarding childbirth. The expression of parental roles and the way that children are viewed reflect cultural differences. Many ethnic, religious, and cultural groups coexist in South Africa, therefore varying family forms are recognised and accepted in differing degrees.

Knowledge of the specific beliefs, practices and choices of women is imperative for those who provide care to pregnant women and the midwife should, using participatory approaches, discourage harmful practices while encouraging those that are beneficial.

References

Kayne, M. A., Greulich. M. B. & Albers, L. L. 2001. Doulas: An alternative yet complementary addition to care during childbirth. *Cinical Obstetrics and Gynecology*, December 44(4):692–703.

Okolacha, C., Chiwuzie, J., Braimoh, S., Unuigbe, J. & Olumeko, P. 1998. Sociocultural factors in maternal morbidity and mortality: A study of a semi-urban community in Southern Nigeria. *Journal of Epidemiological Community Health*, 52:293–297.

The Prevention of Maternal Mortality Network. 1992. Barriers to treatment of obstetric emergencies in rural communities of West Africa. *Studies in Family Planning*, 23:279–291.

United Nations. 2000. Convention on the Elimination of All Forms of Discrimination Against Women.

Williams, C. D., Baumslag, N. & Jeliffe, D. B. 1994. *Mother and child health: Delivering the services*. New York: Oxford University Press.

WHO (World Health Organisation). 1978. *Health and the family: Studies in the demography of family life cycles and their health implication*. Geneva: WHO.

CRITICAL THINKING EXERCISES

1. Discuss in groups the various family forms found in contemporary South Africa.
2. Discuss some of the important aspects of culture for the midwife, and the ways in which a midwife can approach cultural diversity in midwifery practice.

Chapter 3

Quality in midwifery

Dr Christa van der Walt

Introduction

We encourage pregnant women to come to our clinics and hospitals [for antenatal care]. We offer this care because we believe we can give them the best opportunity of having a live, healthy baby. This is a very serious undertaking…

Many midwives and doctors are providing the best [antenatal] care possible. But there is evidence from the perinatal deaths reported to our Perinatal Review Meetings that some health workers are providing care that is of a very poor standard. As a result we are not fulfilling our responsibilities to our people (Philpott, 2001:68).

While we recognise the fact that safe motherhood interventions should be implemented in the context of broader health programmes (such as nutritional advice and micro-nutrient supplementation, child survival and development, immunisation, safe water and sanitation, family planning (fertility control), the avoidance of unwanted pregnancies, and the prevention of malaria and of HIV/AIDS and other sexually transmitted diseases), midwives have an important role to play in improving the outcomes. As midwives we have a moral and ethical, as well as professional responsibility towards the provision of quality midwifery care.

Maternal and perinatal deaths in South Africa continue to be unacceptably high, even with taking into account the effect of HIV/AIDS on this mortality rate (see Chapter 4). In South Africa the improvement in quality of healthcare has been identified as one of the key challenges facing the health sector in the next decade.

What is quality of care?

Quality of care is a function of the care rendered and the care received; the interface between provider and patient, between health services and the community. There are many definitions for 'quality of care', depending on whose perspective is taken. One commonly used definition is: 'Doing the right thing (i.e. providing effective care) right (i.e. efficiently), the right way (meeting patient expectations of prompt care).'

The definition of Avedis Donabedian, one of the earliest writers on this topic, divides quality of care into three elements:

▶ *Structures* include the physical characteristics of facilities (such as buildings and equipment, human resources (quantity and mix of staff), the availability of basic supplies (drugs) and management systems.

▶ *Processes* are the activities associated with providing and receiving care. They include aspects such as quality of diagnosis, interpersonal dimensions of care and rational drug use.

▶ *Outcomes* are the changes in health status such as perinatal index, patient satisfaction and improvement in maternal and neonatal mortality and morbidity.

Both the perspectives and the providers need to be taken into account when quality of maternity services is defined. Good quality care can therefore be defined as "care that meets acceptable technical standards as well as the needs and expectations of users and communities".

Quality of midwifery care is not a simple homogeneous variable but a complex construct incorporating values, beliefs and attitudes of individuals involved in the healthcare interaction. Hulton et al (2000:1) illustrate the complexity of quality of care as follows:

The existence of maternal health services does not guarantee their use by women. Neither does the use of maternal health services guarantee optimal outcomes for women.

The recognition that the quality of services has an impact on the use of services has given us a strong incentive to improve quality of midwifery care with the goal of greater acceptance and more substantial use thereof (Hulton et al, 2001).

Good quality maternal health services are those that meet the following criteria:

▶ They are accessible and available as close as possible to where women live, and at the lowest level facility that can provide the services safely and effectively.

▶ They are acceptable to potential users and responsive to cultural and social norms such as preferences for privacy, confidentiality and care by female health workers.

▶ They have on hand all essential supplies and equipment.

▶ They provide comprehensive care and/or links to other reproductive health services.

▶ They provide for continuity of care and follow-up care.

▶ They are staffed by technically competent healthcare providers who rely on clear guidelines and protocols for treatment.

▶ They are staffed by workers who provide caring, respectful and non-judgemental care that is responsive to women's needs.

▶ They provide information and counselling for clients on their health and health needs.

▶ The clients are involved in decision-making and seen as partners in healthcare who are also active participants in protecting their own health.

▶ They offer economic and social support to healthcare providers that enables them to do the best job they can.

Causes of poor quality of care

The World Health Organisation (WHO, 1998) identified the most common factors that contribute to poor quality care as substandard care, lack of drugs and supplies, delays in referrals, and poor interaction between clients and healthcare providers. This corresponds with the findings of the past three years' reports on Confidential Enquiries into Maternal Deaths in South Africa (DoH, 1998; 1999; 2000; 2001) as well as the Saving Babies Reports of 2000 and 2001 (MRC & DoH, 2001 & 2002).

Substandard care

Substandard care is often the result of staff being demotivated, poorly supervised, under-paid and overworked. Many have also not received adequate training or refresher cours-es to upgrade their skills.

Inconvenient operating hours, services organised around fixed or rigid timetables, and stipulations on who can accompany a woman to a health facility also detract from the quality of the service. If people have access to more than one facility, the quality of the services often becomes the key decision-making variable.

Supply shortages and infrastructure problems

Many facilities lack basic supplies and equip-ment. Frustration caused by a lack of basic supplies like gloves, antiseptics and pens, may affect our interactions with women seeking care.

Delays in referrals

Delays in referring women from community health facilities to hospitals is one of the most important and avoidable factors that prevent women from receiving the care that would save their lives. Staff at the community facili-ties may not recognise the seriousness of the problem. Even if they do, many rural health centres have no means of communication (telephone or radio) with health facilities offering more advanced care, or systems for transporting women to such services.

Avoidable factors

Avoidable factors within the health system contribute to a significant proportion of maternal deaths. Among the main causes identified by Fawcus et al (1996) were failures to identify women with severe conditions, including post-abortion complications and sepsis, and refer them for treatment at a high-er level of the healthcare system.

Client–provider interactions

Many studies have found that healthcare workers often treat women in an insensitive manner, not paying adequate attention to their concerns and treating them rudely, par-ticularly when they come late for treatment or do not comply with medical advice. Yet positive interactions between women and healthcare providers lead to client confi-dence and compliance. Clients and midwives may perceive quality of care differently. Midwives may be anxious to ensure technical correctness, whereas pregnant women may be more concerned with issues such as birthing position and social support. The two approaches must be reconciled in the search for quality of care.

General approaches to quality improvement

There are three different approaches to quali-ty improvement. Although indicators and the measurement thereof are central elements of all these approaches, the three approaches dif-fer fundamentally in how they assess and go about improving quality.

Quality Assurance (QA)

Detailed expectations and procedures are set out and periodically measured, usually by an external team. The aim is to get the units, meeting these standards, accredited by a national or organisational body such as the Council for Health Service Accreditation of South Africa (COHSASA). Facilities are awarded a certificate for a specific period of time. The fact that evaluation is done by an external party rather than by the staff them-selves, often leads to striving only to reach the 'standard' and not to improving the total qual-ity of care.

Continuous Quality Improvement (CQI)

This approach is continuous and participatory, involving staff at all levels in the collection and analysis of data and in the determination of pri-orities and standards. Strong features of this approach is team building, building of local cultures of quality, the implementation of activities on a continuous basis and the involvement of the perspectives of the service users. The processes of maternal and perinatal audits and measuring patient satisfaction by means of exit interview or focus group discussions are examples of this approach.

Total Quality Management (TQM)

The TQM approach is concerned with the fundamental reorientation of the healthcare system and its people towards 'total quality'. Quality is seen as a way of life, a way of viewing the health system as a whole. This means that quality is being made part of performance criteria for managers.

Strategies to improve the quality of care

The WHO emphasises that improving the quality of maternal health services does not require providing services only through sophisticated health facilities. *A few simple interventions can improve the quality of maternity care significantly and even more so, a caring attitude of midwives.*

Evidence-based healthcare and patient-centred healthcare are core elements of the quality improvement movement. The WHO estimates that 10 to 30% of healthcare interventions have no basis in evidence and are inappropriate. These interventions may compromise the safety of the mother and her unborn baby. Large variations in the quality of care delivered at different facilities and between private and public sectors, regions and provinces, suggest that maternity care is not always based on the best available knowledge.

The Guidelines for Maternity Care in South Africa is an evidence-based manual for healthcare providers, based on the best available evidence from published research, modified to suit local conditions. These guidelines are not cast in stone. They can be modified according to the experience of the practitioner and new evidence. Each woman is an individual and may not necessarily be served best by these

guidelines. Individual hospitals and community health centres should draw up their own protocols based on the contents and adjusted to their own particular circumstances.

Research has shown that many interventions performed routinely in the past may in fact not benefit the women and their babies. Examples of these include routine inductions, routine episiotomies, restricting the mother's position at birth, taking babies away from their mothers in the postnatal wards, and giving breastfed babies top-up feeds with formula milk (Proctor & Renfrew, 2001:1).

All of the guidelines and protocols directing maternity and neonatal care in South Africa are built on a strong evidence base. In South Africa a limited number of midwives have access to published evidence, other than in the form of guidelines and protocols.

Midwives should be actively involved in research, not only to recruit subjects but also to be real partners in research, and hereby build the research capacity of midwives. It is necessary to understand research before one can actually initiate new projects. Although a basic knowledge of research methods forms part of any Midwifery curriculum in South Africa (SANC, 1990), experience has shown that the best way to learn to do research is by participating actively in a good research project.

The value of audits and feedback on avoidable causes of maternal and perinatal mortality and morbidity has been discussed in Chapter 4. It is important to see this against the background of quality improvement. The Saving Mothers and Saving Babies Reports are examples of how South African healthcare professionals strive to improve the quality of care to mothers and babies through learning lessons from maternal and perinatal deaths 'despite the fact that each death represents an individual tragedy' (DoH, 2002).

Correct use of the partogram should be the norm in all institutions conducting births. Quality Assurance programmes should be implemented using an appropriate tool.

Practice check

The following six tests might be applied to any system of maternity care:

Availability: Does the system provide a service for all who need it?

Accessibility: Is it possible for all who need the service to make use of it easily?

Acceptability: Is the service provided in a way that is congenial to those who need it?

Effectiveness: Does the service meet its own stated aims and identified needs of those it seeks to serve?

Efficiency: Does the service make the best use of all available resources, including the resources of its consumers?

Economy: Are there sufficient resources available to provide a service that meets all the criteria above?

Quality Check

In order to assure high quality of care, maternal health services should be evaluated at regular intervals, from both service provider and client perspectives, and improved as needed (DoH, 2002).

The ability to make good decisions is an essential criterium for standards for 'best practice'. To ensure high standards of record keeping and decision-making we must check the quality of our work at regular intervals. The Quality Check instruments for antenatal care and intrapartum care have been developed and tested in clinics and hospitals in KwaZulu-Natal. It has been shown to help to improve the quality of information obtained and decisions made (DoH, 2001).

The Department of Health recommends that the following steps should be taken:

▶ Each month a 100 consecutive antenatal records of all clients who are 36 weeks or more pregnant, should be examined as they leave the clinic. The same should be done with partograms.

▶ For each antenatal care (ANC) record, give one point for each of the items listed on the Quality Check form that has been recorded or half when it is incomplete. This will give a maximum score of 25 points, which if multiplied by four will give a percentage score.

▶ Record the most common items missing on the records.

▶ Identify and record the major reasons for incomplete record keeping and/or incomplete decision-making.

▶ Decide what needs to be done to improve the quality of record keeping and decision-making.

Source: MRC & DoH, 2002.

CRITICAL THINKING EXERCISES

1. What is the ideal number of antenatal visits?
2. Why should women attend childbirth education classes?
3. What advice should be given to a woman regarding the use of traditional medicine for her and her baby?
4. Why are we using a 20 minutes CTG monitoring strip? Why 20 minutes?
5. Is it safe to use a Pinard stethoscope?
6. What is the best information to give a mother regarding cord care?
7. Is it true that colostrum applied to the nipples will prevent sore and cracked nipples?
8. What are the effects of aromatherapy during labour?

Conclusion

In this chapter we have provided an overview of quality in healthcare and more specifically, in midwifery care. The issues of conceptualising quality as well as measuring it were highlighted and the strategies used to improve the quality of our care were described. It is clear that midwives have to improve the quality of midwifery care through quality improvement strategies aiming at identifying avoidable causes of mortality and morbidity as well as patient satisfaction issues.

References

Adar, J. & Stevens, M. 2000. *Women's health.* Health Systems Trust 2000: SA Health Review.

DoH (Department of Health). 2002. *Saving mothers: Second report on confidential enquiries into maternal deaths in South Africa 1999–2001.* Pretoria: DoH.

DoH (Department of Health). 2000. *Guidelines for maternity care in South Africa: A manual for clinics, community health centres and district hospitals.* Pretoria: DoH.

Campbell, O., Koblinsky, M. & Taylor, P. 1995. Off to a rapid start: Appraising maternal mortality and services. *International Journal of Gynaecology and Obstetrics,* June supplement (48): S33–S52

Chalmers, B. 1997. *Overmedicalisation and appropriate technologies.* Presentation at Safe Motherhood Technical Consultation in Sri Lanka, October 1997.

Enkin, M., Keirse, M. J. N. C., Neilson, J., Crowther, C., Duley, L., Hodnett, E. & Hofmeyr, J. 2000. *A guide to effective care in pregnancy and childbirth.* Third edition. Oxford: Oxford University Press.

Fawcus, S. et al. 1996. A community-based investigation of avoidable factors for maternal mortality in Zimbabwe. *Studies in Family Planning,* 27(6):319–327.

Fonn, S. 1997. *Empower women, ensure choices: South African case study.* Presentation at Safe Motherhood Technical Consultation in Sri Lanka, October 1997.

Koblinsky, M., Campbell, O. & Heichelheim, J. 1997. *Quality of care: What does it mean for safe motherhood?* Presentation at Safe Motherhood Technical Consultation in Leslie, J. & Gupta, G. R. 1989: Utilisation of formal services for maternal nutrition and health care. Washington DC: International Center for Research on Women.

MRC & DoH. 2002. *Saving babies 2001: Second perinatal care survey of South Africa.* Pretoria: Department of Health.

Philpott, H. 2001. Quality assurance: Information for decision making in antenatal care. In: *Saving babies 2001: Second perinatal care survey of South Africa.* Pretoria: DoH.

Proctor, S. & Renfrew, M. (Eds.) 2001. *Linking research and practice in midwifery: A guide to evidence-based practice.* Edinburgh: Baillière Tindall.

Shorney, J. 1990. Preconception care: The embryo of health promotion. In: Alexander, J., Levy, V. & Roch, S. (Eds.) 1990. *Antenatal care: A research-based approach.* London: MacMillan.

Thaddeus, S. & Maine, D. 1994: Too far to walk: Maternal mortality in context. *Social Science and Medicine,* 38(8):1091–1110.

Thom, A. 2001. Quality of care. Paper delivered at the Health Summit 2001.

WHO (World Health Organisation). 1993. *Midwifery practice: Measuring, developing and mobilising quality care.* Report of a Collaborative WHO/ICM/UNICEF pre-congress workshop, Vancouver, Canada, May 1993. Geneva: WHO.

WHO (World Health Organisation). 1994. *Mother-baby package: Implementing safe motherhood in countries.* Geneva: WHO.

WHO (World Health Organisation). 1995. Quality of care: Doing things the right way. *Safe Motherhood Newsletter,* 17, March-June. Geneva: WHO.

Chapter *4*

Maternal and infant health profiles

H. Liesbeth Mangate

Introduction

Maternal and neonatal health profiles are important indicators in health services and the country at large. They are used to determine the health status of the country and the quality of care given to women and children as the most vulnerable groups worldwide. The low birth weight, neonatal and perinatal mortality rates in your services are important as these rates reflect the living conditions, standards of health and quality of perinatal healthcare services in that region. It is important that midwives have the necessary knowledge and skills to conduct effective maternal and neonatal morbidity and mortality audits.

Determining the status of maternal and perinatal health in South Africa

In terms of the National Policy Health Act, Act No 116 of 1990, deaths during pregnancy, childbirth and the puerperium were made notifiable events on 1 October 1997. The Minister of Health appointed a National Committee on Confidential Enquiries into Maternal Deaths (NCCEMD), which is responsible for the enquiry process. The notification and confidential enquiry process enables the country to identify major causes of maternal deaths and the avoidable factors contributing to maternal deaths. It is crucial

Table 4.1 Levels of care at public health services

Leve of care	Staff composition	Services provided
Level 1	▶ Clinics attended by registered midwives. ▶ Community health centres attended by midwives, midwives with an advanced diploma in midwifery and sometimes a physician. ▶ Sub-district hospitals staffed by midwives, doctors and a visiting specialist/obstetrician.	▶ Provide antenatal and postnatal care. ▶ Provide the services offered at the clinic, plus 24-hour delivery services. ▶ Provide the services offered at the community health centre, plus 24-hour caesarean sections.
Level 2	▶ District or secondary and regional hospitals with a staff complement consisting of midwives, physicians, and specialists.	▶ Provide the services offered at the sub-district hospital, plus services for complex deliveries and intensive care.
Level 3	▶ Tertiary, central or teaching hospitals with the staff complement of a level 2 hospital, plus specialists.	▶ Provide the services of a level 2 hospital, plus services for super-specialist care.

that all maternal deaths be notified for accurate statistics and analysis. Notification of maternal deaths in South Africa is constantly improving. There are, however, still some elements of under-reporting in some provinces.

Levels of care and the services provided at each level

Public healthcare services in South Africa are divided into levels of care. Table 4.1 illustrates the staff composition and the services to be provided in different levels.

The process of reporting on maternal mortality

The process followed for each maternal death in a facility is as follows:
▶ If a maternal death occurs, the maternal mortality meeting is held in the facility concerned and the maternal death notification form (MDNF) is completed.
▶ The form, together with a copy of the woman's bed letter or records, is then sent

to the provincial office within seven days of the maternal death.
▶ The provincial maternal, child and women's health co-ordinator then informs the secretariat of the NCCEMD at the Department of Health (DoH) that a death has occurred.
▶ The NCCEMD will issue a unique file number for the particular case.
▶ The provincial co-ordinator replaces the name of the woman with the unique number and sends all documentation to the provincial assessors.
▶ The provincial maternal, child and women's health (MCWH) co-ordinator informs the secretariat at the NCCEMD at the DoH.
▶ A team of provincial assessors, comprising the midwife and a physician, then critically analyse the case and complete the maternal death assessor's form (MDAF). The assessors will provide information on the primary, final and contributory causes of death and also establish whether there were avoidable

factors, missed opportunities or substandard care that may have contributed to the maternal death. The assessors then complete and return all the documentation to the province within 30 days.

▶ In cases where the woman received anaesthesia during the process, the documents are also sent to the provincial anaesthetic assessor who also assesses the anaesthetic management of the case and identifies the cause of death, avoidable factors, missed opportunities and substandard care relating to anaesthesia that may have contributed to the death.

▶ All documentation is then forwarded to the NCCEMD for collation and further analysis. Sending of data electronically direct to the NdoH from the assessors using the MaMMAS programme has now been introduced with the aim of reducing unnecessary delays. Issues of confidentiality have been looked into and thoroughly discussed. The programme does not include information from the anaesthetic assessor, however, and sending of data electronically and the use of hard copies run in parallel.

▶ The NCCEMD uses this data to compile the reports on maternal deaths in South Africa, entitled *Saving Mothers*. Once the comprehensive report is accepted, all data is destroyed and work begins on the next report. Comprehensive reports are produced every three years with yearly interim reports.

Measures of maternal mortality

The maternal mortality ratio (MMR) for developed countries is less than 15 per 100 000 live births. In 1998 the Demographic and Health Survey estimated the MMR for South Africa at 150 per 100 000 live births, which was in line with the findings of the *Saving Mothers Report* of 1998. However, recent findings suggest that the estimation might now be too low and that the most appropriate findings would be around 175 to 200 per 100 000 live births. It is important to note that for every maternal death, there are at least 27 perinatal deaths and more than 30 severe maternal morbidi-

ties. Measures of maternal mortality are critical as they reflect women's access to and use of essential healthcare services during pregnancy and childbirth, women's general health and nutritional status, access to financial resources and education, as well as access to reproductive care services, including family planning (fertility control).

The perinatal audit meeting

An effective audit process improves the quality of maternal healthcare services and lowers the maternal mortality and perinatal mortality rates (Philpott, 2001). A perinatal audit is a systematic review of current practice. It forms an integral part of modern midwifery and neonatal nursing science. Audit allows healthcare providers and administrators to identify problems in the health service. Problem identification is a crucial step in improving maternal and neonatal outcome. The audit process can be located at different levels within the healthcare sector.

The purpose of the perinatal audit meeting is to:

▶ Review the perinatal statistics for the month under review.
▶ Review the causes and preventable factors in the perinatal deaths.
▶ Determine corrective action.
▶ Advance the education and learning of healthcare professionals in the maternity service.
▶ Review all maternal (and neonatal) deaths.

All staff (physicians and midwives), managers, community health representatives and educators should attend these meetings. Good relationships, especially trust and respect between physicians and midwives, are essential elements of successful perinatal audit meetings.

Important definitions and concepts

There are a number of definitions provided by the DoH that should be known in order to understand the *Saving Mothers* and *Saving Babies* reports. Note, however, that it is not a full list and other definitions and concepts should be studied in conjunction when reading these reports.

Maternal mortality ratio (MMR)

Maternal death is defined as the death of a woman while pregnant or within 42 days of termination of pregnancy from any cause related to or aggravated by the pregnancy or its management, but not from accidental or incidental causes. The MMR is calculated as:

$$\frac{\text{Total number of maternal deaths x 100 000}}{\text{Total number of live births}}$$

Causes of maternal deaths

▶ *Direct causes of maternal death*: Deaths resulting from obstetric complications of the pregnancy (pregnancy, labour and puerperium), from interventions, omissions, incorrect management or from a chain of events resulting from any of the above.

▶ *Indirect causes of maternal deaths*: Deaths resulting from previous existing disease, or diseases that developed during pregnancy and which were not due to direct obstetric causes, but which were aggravated by the physiological effects of pregnancy.

▶ *Coincidental causes of maternal deaths*: Deaths from unrelated causes, which happen in the pregnancy or the puerperium.

▶ *Unknown*: Deaths during pregnancy, labour or puerperium where an underlying cause was not identified.

Neonatal death rate (NNDR)

Neonatal death is the death of a viable live born baby from birth to 28 days. These are divided into early (first seven days of life) and late (8 to 28 days). Early neonatal death (ENND) is an indicator of the quality of intrapartum care, whereas the late neonatal death of the quality of neonatal facilities in the health institutions concerned. The neonatal death rate is calculated as:

$$\frac{\text{Total number of neonatal deaths x 1 000}}{\text{Total number of live births}}$$

Stillbirth rate (SBR)

Stillbirth is used to define a viable baby born dead. They are divided into fresh and macerated stillbirths. The stillbirth rate is an indicator of the quality of midwifery and obstetric care in general. Fresh stillbirths usually reflect the quality of intrapartum care and macerated stillbirths reflect the quality of antenatal care. Stillbirth rate is calculated as:

$$\frac{\text{Total number of stillbirths x 1 000}}{\text{Total number of births}}$$

Perinatal mortality rate (PNMR)

The perinatal period begins at the age of fetal viability, that is from 28 weeks gestation or from the time the fetus weighs 1 000 g and above and ends on day seven after delivery. Death of the baby during this period is termed a perinatal death. It is calculated as the sum of stillbirths and early neonatal deaths. The PNMR is the most sensitive indicator of midwifery and obstetric care. For developed countries the PNMR for babies of 1 000 g or more is usually less than six per 1 000 births whereas for developing countries PNMR ranges from 30 to 200 per 1 000 births. Developed countries calculate the PNMR from 24 weeks gestation or 500 g. For South Africa, the PNMR for babies, 28 weeks gestation or more, or 1 000 g or more, is estimated to be 40 per 1 000 births, with major differences for different levels of facilities and provinces. The perinatal mortality ratio is calculated as:

$$\frac{\text{Total number of perinatal deaths x 1 000}}{\text{Total number of births}}$$

Low birth weight rate (LBWR)

A low birth weight baby is a baby weighing less than 2 500 g at birth. LBWR is an indicator of the socioeconomic and health status of the community and society in general. The LBWR for births in developed countries is around 7%, whereas in developing countries it is much higher, around 15%. The LBWR is calculated as:

$$\frac{\text{Total number of births} < 2\ 500\ \text{g} \times 100}{\text{Total number of births}}$$

Stillborn: neonatal death (SB:NND) ratio

The SB:NND ratio can also be calculated as another indicator of the perinatal environment. Developed countries have a SB:NND ratio of around one. In developing countries, the ratio is also around one with as many stillbirths as neonatal deaths. However, as care improves, that is, more births take place in institutions and labour, delivery and immediate care of the neonate is supervised, the NNDR declines and the SB:NND ratio increases. As antenatal care improves, the number of stillbirths declines and the ratio decreases again to one (MRC & DoH, 2002:4).

Perinatal care index (PCI)

The PCI takes into account the environmental factors. It is useful in comparing hospitals with similar circumstances or the same hospital over a period of time. It can also be used to compare the standard of care of various areas. A low PCI indicates good care because the PNMR is relatively low in relation to the LBWR, whereas a high PCI indicates poor care because the PNMR is relatively high in relation to the LBWR. The PCI is calculated as:

$$\frac{\text{Overall PNMR}}{\text{Percentage low birth weight babies}}$$

Booked status rate

A pregnant woman is regarded as booked if she has attended at least one visit to a general practitioner or the clinic prior to labour or developing a complication. In modern midwifery and obstetric practice, with the availability of on-site testing, a patient can be fully risk classified at the first visit and the antenatal care planned. The term 'booked' causes confusion. It would be more appropriate to use the term 'attended antenatal care'. The booking status rate reflects utilisation of health facilities. It is calculated as:

$$\frac{\text{Number of booked women}}{\text{(who have given birth)} \times 100}{\text{Total number of births}}$$

Other definitions often used is the caesarean section rate and the assisted delivery rate:

$$\text{Caesarean section (C/S) rate:}$$
$$\frac{\text{Number of C/Ss} \times 100}{\text{Total number of births}}$$

$$\text{Assisted delivery rate:}$$
$$\frac{\text{Number of assisted births} \times 100}{\text{Total number of births}}$$

Source: Adapted from the DoH (Department of Health), 2002:vii.

Causes of maternal deaths in South Africa

Demographic variables

Older women, especially women older than 35 years, are at a significantly higher risk than younger women. At the same time, primigravidae or women who have had five or more pregnancies are at greater risk of maternal death. Furthermore, it became clear that most of the emergency events leading to women's deaths occur in the puerperium and at level 1 and 2 hospitals. Poor attendance of antenatal care is associated with maternal deaths.

Primary obstetric causes of maternal deaths

According to the Department of Health (2002:7) for the period 1999 to 2001 the 'big five' causes of maternal deaths were:

◗ Non-pregnancy-related infections (31.4%).
◗ Complications of hypertension in pregnancy (20.7%)
◗ Obstetric haemorrhage (13.9%).
◗ Pregnancy-related sepsis (12.4%).
◗ Pre-existing medical conditions (7.0%).

Table 4.2 Primary obstetric causes of death (1999-2001)

Category	Number	Percentage %
Direct maternal deaths:	1462	59.8
Hypertension	507	20.7
Antepartum haemorrhage	100	4.1
Postpartum haemorrhage	240	9.8
Abortion	120	4.9
Ectopic pregnancy	27	1.1
Pregnancy-related sepsis	210	8.6
Anaesthetic related	76	3.1
Embolism	48	2.0
Acute collapse	134	5.5
Indirect causes of maternal deaths:	939	38.4
Non-pregnancy-related infections	768	31.4
Pre-existing medical diseases	171	7.0
Unknown:	44	1.8
Total	**2 445**	**100**
Coincidental:	45	

Source: Adapted from DoH, 2002:8.

Table 4.3 Common avoidable factors contributing to the high perinatal and maternal mortality in South Africa

Patient oriented factors	Administrative factors	Health care provider factors
▶ Not attending antenatal care. ▶ Infrequent antenatal care. ▶ Delay in seeking medical help. ▶ Self-induced termination of pregnancy. ▶ Failure to recognise dangerous complications.	▶ Transport problems from home to health care facilities. ▶ Transport problems between health care facilites. ▶ Barriers to entry. ▶ Lack of accessibility. ▶ Lack of health care facilities. ▶ Lack of personnel. ▶ Communication problems. ▶ Lack of appropriately trained staff.	▶ Problem with initial assessment and risk assessment or diagnosis. ▶ Delay in referring the patient. ▶ Incorrect management with incorrect diagnosis. ▶ Managing patients at an inappropriate level. ▶ Substandard management even with correct diagnosis. ▶ Not monitoring or infrequent monitoring of patients. ▶ Prolonged abnormal monitoring without action. ▶ Resuscitation problems.

Source: Adapted from DoH, 2002:8.

Non-pregnancy-related infections, especially AIDS, has increased by 8% from 23% in 1998 to 31.4% for the period 1999 to 2001. It is possible that, because of the under-reporting of AIDS, as much as 27.6% of maternal deaths could have been caused by HIV/AIDS. The five most common causes of maternal deaths accounted for 85.4% of the notified maternal deaths. Almost a third of the women (30.4%) who died received anaesthetic intervention at some point in time. There were 45 coincidental deaths, with motor vehicle accidents being the major cause of death and suicide the second most common cause of death. Table 4.2 summarises the primary obstetric causes of maternal deaths.

Avoidable factors, missed opportunities and substandard care

What remains important to us, as midwives, is the knowledge and understanding of the avoidable factors, missed opportunities and substandard care associated with maternal deaths in South Africa. Table 4.3 summarises the problems in care. In more than 50% of the cases there were healthcare provider related avoidable factors in the management of the event that lead to the woman's death. These figures are very important for us as midwives, as it directs us to major limitations in our quality of care.

Major problems relating to women are not attending antenatal care and delay in seeking help. Research is needed into the reasons for this. Transport problems may be a major contributory factor to most of the patient-related problems. Self-induced termination of pregnancy occurred in nearly 30% of women who died from complications of abortion. A lack of healthcare facilities including intensive care facilities, availability of blood for transfusion, drugs and laboratory facilities are common administrative factors associated with maternal deaths. It also seems that management of emergency events is associated with more that half of the cases of maternal deaths. These may include making the wrong diagnosis, not following the standard management protocol

(40.1%), lack of continued monitoring of women or response to abnormalities in the monitoring (22.2%). Other major problems are patients not being referred or managed at an inappropriate level of care. Resuscitation is also a major problem (22.7% of cases). The most common problem is inappropriate support of circulation by not giving sufficient fluids or giving too much and causing fluid overload.

Current status of neonatal health profile in South Africa

Neonatal health services have been a neglected area in maternal and childcare in South Africa. According to the Saving Babies 2001 report, the perinatal mortality rate for metropolitan, city and town and rural settings where 38.4, 43.4 and 25.5 per thousand births respectively.

The most common causes of perinatal deaths in South Africa were unexplained intra-uterine deaths, complications of hypertension in pregnancy, spontaneous preterm labour, antepartum haemorrhage, trauma

---

In a nutshell

▶ Maternal and neonatal health statistics are important evidence for public health interventions. Community-based information needs to be incorporated into a system for a comprehensive and practical approach.
▶ Midwifery training and education must empower the midwives with the necessary knowledge and skills to use maternal and neonatal indicators as a basis to improve maternal and neonatal health outcomes.
▶ However, major challenges still exist to help women with decision-making, to empower women and their families to adopt healthy behaviours, and to encourage men to support and promote women's health.

infections, fetal abnormalities and maternal diseases.

South Africa as a country has reasonable human resources which enable the provision of high quality care. Negative attitudes of midwives have been reported in various research reports. This is unacceptable and should be addressed by strict disciplinary actions. The following are measures to be put in place to improve maternal and neonatal outcome in different settings:

▶ Improve access to healthcare services.
▶ Improve curriculum of midwives and physicians to emphasise life-saving skills.
▶ Work with communities to address problems of transport.
▶ Improve general status of women.
▶ Target under-served groups.
▶ Focus on decentralisation of services.
▶ Work with communities to eliminate poverty and improve nutritional status of women.
▶ Focus on eliminating the unnecessary delays in providing quality maternal and neonatal services.

References

DoH (Department of Health). 2002. *Saving mothers: Second report on confidential enquiries into maternal deaths in South Africa 1999–2001*.Pretoria: DoH.

MRC & DoH (Department of Health). 2002. *Saving babies 2001: Second perinatal care survey of South Africa*. Pretoria: DoH.

Ransom, E. I. & Yinger, N.V. 2002. *Making motherhood safer, overcoming obstacles on the part way to care*. Population Reference Bureau.

JPHIEGO. 2001. Workshop report on implementing global maternal and neonatal health standards of care. (see: http://www.mnh.jhpiego.org)

WHO (World Health Organisation). 2002. Volume 1. *Beyond the numbers, Reviewing maternal deaths and complications to make pregnancy safer*. Geneva: WHO.

Philpott, H. 2001. Four components of a successful perinatal audit process. *Kwik-Skwiz no 29*. http://www.hst.org.sa/isds/-kwikskz/kwik29.htm, accessed on 2001/07/17.

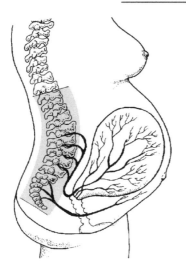

Anatomy and physiology of reproduction

Chapter 5

Female reproduction

Linda Greyling

Introduction

*Probably more important for the general
improvement of obstetrical practice was the
new knowledge of anatomy of the birth
canal … obstetric anatomy is the foundation for midwifery.*
(Roberts & Tomlinson, 1992)

The female reproductive organs may vary in
shape and size, even within their normal limits.
The midwife should be competent enough to
recognise 'normal' pelvic structures in the pregnant woman but, more importantly, she should
also be able to detect deviations from normal.

The bony pelvis

The pelvis forms a bony canal through which
the fetus passes during the normal process of
birth. If no abnormalities are present, the baby
of normal size will pass without difficulty.

The pelvic girdle

The pelvic girdle consists of four bones,
namely, two hipbones at the sides joining in
front, and the sacrum and coccyx behind.
Each hipbone consists of three parts, namely
the ilium, ischium and pubis.

The *ilium* is the large, prominent flared-out
part. The concave anterior surface is known as
the iliac fossa. The upper curved border is
called the iliac crest, with the anterior and posterior terminal points, known as the anterior
superior and posterior superior iliac spines.

The *ischium* is the lowest part of the hipbone. In the sitting position the body rests on
the rough ischial tuberosity. Posterior and
superior to the tuberosity is a projection called
the spine of the ischium, a useful landmark
when making a vaginal examination during
labour. The station (level) of the fetal head is
assessed in centimetres, measured above or
below the ischial spines.

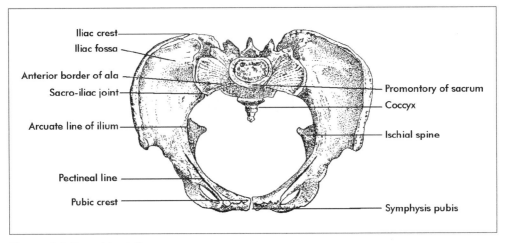

Figure 5.1 The pelvic girdle

The *pubis* consists of a body, and a superior and inferior ramus, with the two inferior rami forming the pubic arch. The two pubic bones meet at the symphysis pubis.

The sacrum is a triangular bone composed of five fused sacral vertebrae. The prominent rim of the upper surface of the first sacral vertebra is known as the promontory of the sacrum. Because it encroaches on the anterior-posterior diameter of the pelvic inlet and in some cases may prevent the fetal head from entering the brim, it is an important landmark. The anterior surface of the sacrum is smooth and concave, the posterior rough and convex.

The coccyx consists of four rudimentary coccygeal vertebrae.

Pelvic joints and ligaments

In the non-pregnant state there is very little movement in the pelvic joints. However, during the advance of pregnancy a certain amount of softening and stretching of the ligaments occurs, mainly under the influence of relaxin secreted by the corpus luteum, which results in slight separation of the joints and increased mobility, therefore increasing the diameter of the pelvic inlet.

The sacro-iliac joint

This is a plane joint. The joint is formed at the articulation of the sacrum with the ilium. It is partly cartilaginous and partly fibrous and is very strong.

The ligaments between the sacrum and ilium are the strongest in the entire body. Stability of this joint depends on the ligaments stabilising the joint, namely, the anterior and strong posterior ligaments, and the interosseous ligaments.

Additional ligaments stabilising the joint include the sacrotuberous and sacrospinous ligaments. The sacrotuberous ligament extends between the sacrum and the tuberosity of the ischium, with the sacrospinous ligament connecting the sacrum with the ischial spine. Both ligaments form the posterolateral wall of the pelvic outlet.

Limited backward and forward movement of the sacrum is allowed. However, late in pregnancy there is a great deal of strain on these joints as joint mobility increases with softening of the ligaments. Multiparous women frequently complain of backache at this time and in the weeks following childbirth.

Symphysis pubis

This is a cartilaginous joint. The joint is formed at the junction of the two pubic bones, united by fibrous cartilage.

The strong anterior ligament is further supported by the insertion of rectus abdominis

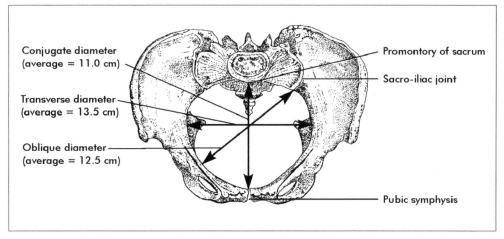

Figure 5.2 Diameters of the pelvic inlet (superior view)

and external oblique. The inferior ligament, or arcuate ligament, lies in the pubic arch.

This joint widens appreciably during the later months of pregnancy and the degree of movement permitted may give rise to pain on walking.

Sacrococcygeal joint

This cartilaginous joint is formed where the coccyx articulates with the apex of the sacrum.

This joint allows the coccyx to bend backwards when the fetus passes through the birth canal. Excessive stretching of the joint ligaments may result in pain, noticed by the woman on sitting.

Lumbosacral joint

This is the joint between the fifth lumbar vertebra and the sacrum. Considerable strain is placed on this joint late in pregnancy, because of the backward inclination of the sacrum.

The true and false pelvis

The bony pelvis is divided into two parts, namely the true and false pelvis. The false pelvis is the part above the pelvic brim (pelvic inlet) and consists mainly of the flared-out iliac bones. Although it has little obstetric importance, it contains some of the abdominal contents.

The true pelvis is the curved bony canal

through which the fetus must pass during birth. It consists of a pelvic inlet, cavity and outlet.

The inlet to the true pelvis is bordered posterior by the promontory and alae of the sacrum. The anterior border is formed by the symphysis pubis, the pubic crest and pubic tubercle. The linea terminalis, extending from the pubic tubercle to the sacro-iliac joint, forms a bony line between the sacrum and pubis.

Obstetrical measurements in the inlet include:
▸ The *anteroposterior diameter*, or obstetrical conjugate, measured between the back of the symphysis pubis and the sacral promontory is a distance of 12.5 cm. An accurate measurement can be made only by radiography. If 1.5 cm is deducted from the obstetrical conjugate, a fairly accurate assessment of this measurement, called the diagonal conjugate, can be made during a vaginal examination from the lower border of the symphysis pubis to the sacral promontory.
▸ The transverse diameter, measuring 13.5 cm, is taken at the widest part of the pelvic inlet, just behind the iliopectineal eminence.
▸ The left and right oblique diameters are measured from the left and right sacro-iliac joints to the opposite iliopectineal eminences respectively, and measures 12.5 cm.

The pelvic cavity

The pelvic cavity is the curved area between the pelvic inlet above and the outlet below. It is bordered by the pubic bones in front, with the posterior wall formed by the curve of the sacrum and coccyx. The upper part of the cavity is more spacious than the lower part, which is measured on the level of the ischial spines.

The importance of the ischial spines

The ischial spines are important landmarks, both as indicators of the type of pelvis, as well as reference points to indicate the station of the presenting part.

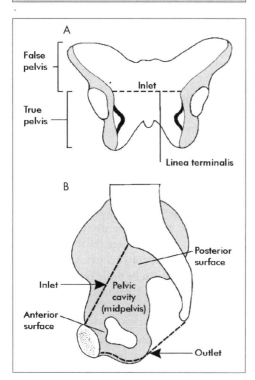

Figure 5.3 Female pelvis. A: True and false pelvis; B: Curved cavity of true pelvis

The pelvic outlet

The upper plane

The ischial spines lie approximately midway down the birth canal and represent the upper level of the pelvic outlet. It is assumed that the head is engaged when it has reached this point. The distance between the ischial spines, the interspinous diameter, measures between 10 to 10.5 cm, and is the narrowest part of the birth canal. The ischial spines can be palpated during a vaginal examination. This level also represents the point where the axis of the birth canal inclines to the front. It is more or less the plane of attachment of the pelvic floor (levator ani muscle).

The lower plane

The lower plane of the pelvic outlet, or perineum, is a diamond-shaped area, which becomes a slit-like area when the person is in the upright position. The borders of the perineum are as follows:

- *Anterior*: The subpubic arch.
- *Lateral*: The inferior pubic rami and ischial tuberosities.
- *Posterolateral*: The sacrotuberous ligament.
- *Posterior*: The sacrococcygeal joint.

The perineum is made up of two triangles, namely, an anterior or urogenital triangle and a posterior or anal triangle. The common line that divides the two triangles extends between the ischial tuberosities.

Obstetrical measurements in the outlet include:

- The anatomical anteroposterior diameter, measuring 9.5 cm, is the distance between the apex of the subpubic angle and the tip of the coccyx. The normal coccyx bends backward during delivery of the head. This action increases the diameter to 12.5 cm.
- The obstetrical diameter, measuring 11.5 cm, is measured from the subpubic angle to the lowest stable point, which is the sacrococcygeal joint.
- The transverse diameter, between the inner surfaces of the ischial tuberosities, measures approximately 11 cm.

Pelvic inclination

A lateral view of a woman in the standing position shows that her pelvis is not at a right angle, and forms an angle of 40 to 50° with

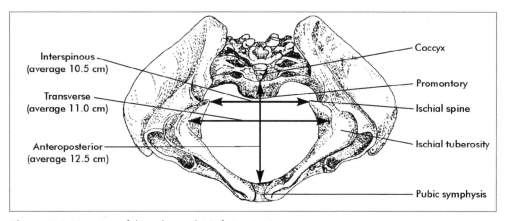

Figure 5.4 Diameters of the pelvic outlet (inferior view)

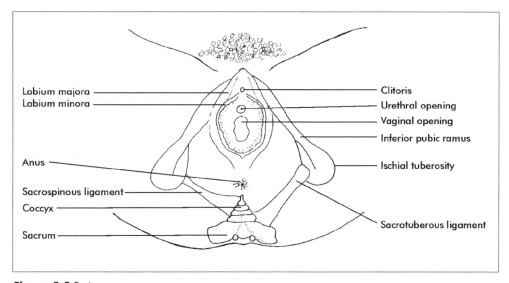

Figure 5.5 Perineum

the horizon. In this position, the inferior end of the sacrum is on the same level as the superior border of the symphysis pubis. The whole pelvis is thus tilted forwards and an axis extending through the pelvis will follow the natural curvature of the cavity (see Figure 5.6). At the outlet the inclination is 10°, or nearly horizontal.

In some ethnic groups, especially in southern Africa, the inclination of the plane of the brim may be closer to 90°, which could delay engagement of the head during labour.

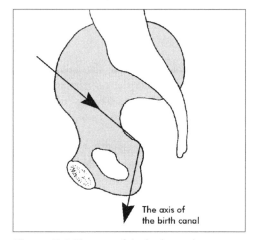

The axis of the birth canal

Figure 5.6 The axis of the birth canal

Axis of the birth canal

A line drawn at right angles to the planes of the inlet, cavity and outlet would represent the anatomical axis of the birth canal. During the actual birth the midwife facilitates the natural upward curving movement of the baby's head and body as they emerge from the birth canal.

The four basic types of pelvis

Variation in the shape of the female pelvis have been classified into four basic types:

Gynaecoid

The gynaecoid, or normal female pelvis, is found in a woman of average build whose hips are broader than her shoulders, has an average height and in whom no deformity is evident. The inlet of this type of pelvis is fairly round, with the transverse measurements larger than the anteroposterior measurements.

Android

The android pelvis is referred to as a male type of pelvis. It has a heart-shaped brim. The anteroposterior measurements are longer than the transverse measurements, resulting in a narrow anterior section, which further decreases the available space.

Anthropoid

The anthropoid pelvis has an oval brim with a small transverse diameter. The anterior segment is also small.

Platypelloid

The platypelloid, or simple flat pelvis has a transversely oval brim that is narrow in the anteroposterior diameter. This is usually a shallow pelvis with a capacious outlet.

It is not possible to clinically determine the type of pelvis that a woman has when she presents to the midwife during her pregnancy. However, the gynaecoid pelvis is the most favourable for normal labour; posterior fetal positions are more common with an anthropoid pelvis; perineal tears are more common

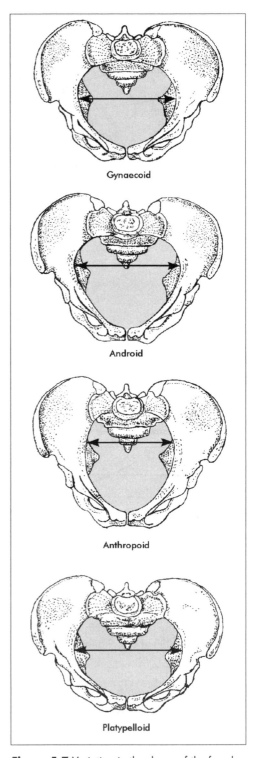

Gynaecoid

Android

Anthropoid

Platypelloid

Figure 5.7 Variation in the shape of the female pelvis

with an android pelvis and arrest of labour is more common in a platypelloid pelvis. In retrospect the pelvic shape can be suspected according to the course of labour.

The pelvic floor

The pelvic floor comprises a number of muscles, mostly sections of the levator ani muscle, which fills the pelvic outlet.

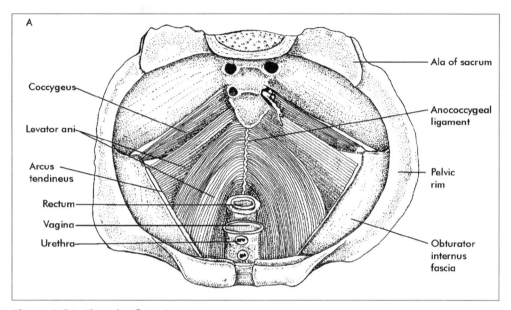

Figure 5.8A The pelvic floor: Superior view

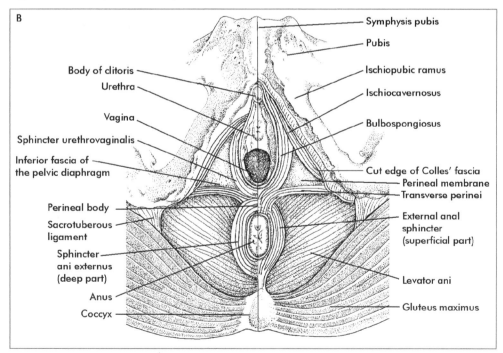

Figure 5.8B The pelvic floor: Inferior view

By their mode of attachment to the pelvis, the two levator ani muscles resemble a sling or hammock. In front they are attached to the lateral inside part of the pubis, to the fascia over the obturator internus muscle and at the back to the ischial spines and sides of the coccyx. The two levator ani muscles slope downward and medially to insert on the upper parts of the vagina, the perineal body, the anal canal, the anococcygeal ligament between the anus and coccyx, the coccyx and lower part of the sacrum. The gutter thus formed aids in anterior rotation of the fetal head during its descent in the birth canal. Three canals, namely the urethra, the vagina and rectum, perforate it.

Between the vagina and rectum, the superficial and deep muscles of the perineum, including the anal sphincter, decussate and join to form the strong perineal body.

A triangular shaped diaphragm (urogenital diaphragm) covers the anterior external aspect of the pelvic floor. It covers the area between the inferior borders of the ischiopubic rami in front and an imaginary line between the ischial tuberosities at the back. The urogenital diaphragm is made up of superficial and deep layers of fascia and a muscle layer in-between.

The urethra and vagina pass through the urogenital diaphragm. The external genital organs, the muscles associated with the external genitalia and skin of the perineum are superficial to the urogenital diaphragm.

The cervix, upper vagina, bladder and rectum are securely anchored to the superior (internal) surface of the pelvic floor. Connective tissue, muscle and strong fascial attachments support these organs. The connective tissue surrounding the uterus is known as the parametrium and merges with the fascia of the transverse cervical ligaments (Mackenrodt's ligament) and fibres of both levator ani muscles.

The external female genital organs

The external genital organs extend from the mons pubis to the perineum and are visible on inspection of the perineum.

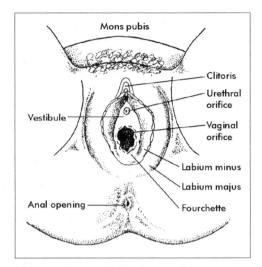

Figure 5.9 External female genital organs

The mons pubis is a fatty cushion situated superficial to the symphysis pubis. It is covered by hair.

The labia majora, or greater lips, are two elongated masses of fibrous tissue and fat, covered with skin and hair on their outer surfaces. The round ligaments of the uterus are inserted into the anterior portion of the labia majora.

The labia minora are two thin vascular skin folds enclosed by the labia majora. They fuse posterior to form a skin fold, the fourchette, or anterior edge of the perineum. In front, the labia minora enclose the clitoris to form the prepuce of the clitoris.

The clitoris is analogous to the penis in the male. It is situated above the external urethral orifice.

The vestibule is a triangular-shaped area, bounded anteriorly by the clitoris, laterally by the labia minora and posteriorly by the fourchette. The urethra and vagina open in it.

The clitoris serves as a useful landmark in locating the urethral orifice for catheterisation when, following childbirth, extensive bruising and laceration of the vulva are present. It is extremely sensitive and any contact with this area should be avoided when the midwife performs internal examinations.

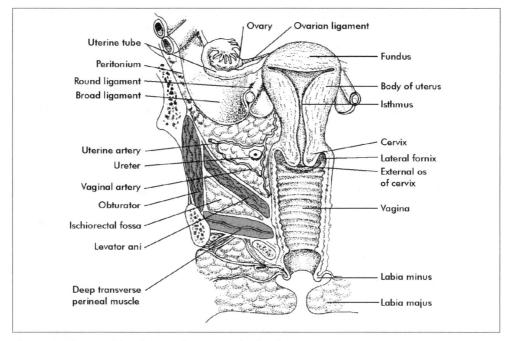

Figure 5.10 Internal female genital organs and pelvic floor

The internal female genital organs

The vagina

The vagina is a musculomembranous canal extending between the vestibule and cervix. It is 8 to12 cm in length, with a shorter anterior wall. The uterus lies almost at right angles to the vagina, in a position referred to as anteflexion. The upper end of the vagina is divided into four fornices by the cervix projecting into it. The largest fornix, or posterior fornix, is found behind the cervix, the one in front is the anterior fornix and on the right and left are the two lateral fornices.

Ridges or rugae, that tend to be obliterated with repeated childbearing, are seen on the

inner layer of the vagina. It is richly supplied with blood vessels, mainly from the vaginal arteries. The muscular layer is not well developed and the vagina is capable of great distension.

The lower half on the anterior wall of the vagina is in close contact with the urethra, while the upper half is in contact with the bladder.

The lower third of the posterior vaginal wall opposes the rectum. The upper part is in contact with the peritoneum at the base of the pouch of Douglas. On the lateral side, the vagina is in relation to the levator ani muscles.

The uterus

The uterus is a hollow, flattened, pear-shaped organ. It is situated in the true pelvis, behind the bladder and in front of the rectum. The uterus is covered externally by the peritoneum, except the lower anterior part where the peritoneum is reflected onto the superior surface of the bladder.

The non-pregnant uterus is about 7.5 cm

> **Note**
>
> If difficulty is encountered during labour to insert a catheter, a finger placed against the anterior wall of the vagina can be used as a guide to direct the catheter into the bladder and thus avoid injury to the urethra.

long. The rounded upper part of the corpus above the insertion of the uterine tubes is known as the fundus. The superolateral angle where the uterine tube is inserted is known as the cornu or horn.

The body, the greater part of the uterus, gradually tapers downwards and the constricted area immediately above the cervix is the isthmus.

> The isthmus distends to form the lower uterine segment during pregnancy. The incision for a caesarean section is made in the lower segment.

The downward continuation of the isthmus becomes the cervix, which is the lowest part of the uterus. The cervical canal is 2.5 cm long, and the constricted area where the cervix and isthmus meet forms the internal os, which leads into the uterine cavity. The cervix projects into the upper part of the vagina. The external os, which is a small round opening at the lowest point of the cervix, becomes a transverse slit and more gaping after childbirth.

In structure the cervix differs from the body of the uterus, containing fewer muscle cells and more collagen fibres. A mucous membrane, containing glands that secrete an alkaline mucus, lines the canal.

> The non-pregnant cervix has the firm consistency of the nose. The pregnant cervix has the soft consistency of the lips and appears bluish in colour.

The cavity of the uterus is triangular in a coronal section and communicates with the cervical canal by means of the internal os. This, in turn, opens into the vagina through the external os.

The endometrium lining the body of the uterus consists of columnar epithelium, glands that produce an alkaline secretion, and connective tissue cells capable of rapid regeneration following menstruation. The endometrium is richly supplied with blood.

The myometrium or muscle coat forms most of the thickness of the uterine wall and consists of three layers, an inner layer of circular fibres, a thick intermediate layer and outer longitudinal layer. The fibres of the intermediate layer form an encircling figure of eight arrangement around the blood vessels. By constricting them they control bleeding during the third stage of labour. The fibres of the outer muscle layer are four times more plentiful in the fundus of the uterus and the decreasing gradient aids in the expulsion of the fetus.

The perimetrium is a layer of peritoneum that covers the outside of the uterus except at the sides, beyond which it extends to form the broad ligaments. The perimetrium is firmly attached to the uterine wall except at the lower anterior part where, at the level of the isthmus, the peritoneum is reflected on the bladder.

Position of the uterus

The position of the uterus is almost horizontal when the woman stands upright. It leans forwards, forming an angle of approximately 90° to the vagina. This position is known as anteversion. It also bends forwards on itself with the fundus resting on the bladder, producing anteflexion. When this position of anteversion and anteflexion is maintained, prolapse of the uterus is less likely to occur. When the uterus is displaced backwards or retroverted, it lies in the same axis as the vagina and is more liable to prolapse. The uterus is maintained in position by four pairs of ligaments and indirectly by the pelvic floor.

Ligaments supporting the uterus

The broad ligament is a double fold of the peritoneum, extending outwards from the lateral surface of the uterus and attached to the lateral wall of the pelvis. The lower border of the broad ligament is thickened and strengthened with fascia, fibrous tissue and muscle to form the most important uterine support, called the transverse cervical ligament (cardinal ligaments). If this ligament is overstretched or damaged during labour, it cause the uterus to sag downwards. The lateral peritoneal end of the broad ligament continues

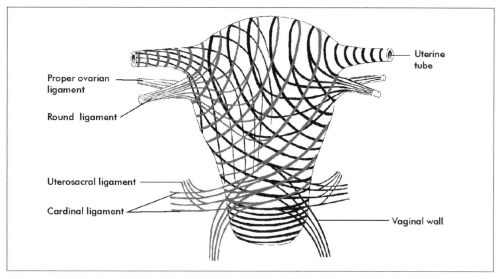

Figure 5.11 The myometrium: Schematic representation of the uterine musculature

onto the posterior abdominal wall as the suspensory ligament of the ovary, containing the ovarian artery and vein.

The round ligament arises in front and below the insertion of the uterine tube, runs between the folds of the broad ligament, passes through the inguinal canal and inserts deep to the labia majora. It has little value as a support, but tends to hold the uterus forwards in anteversion.

The uterosacral ligament consists of folds of peritoneum extending backward from the sides of the isthmus and attached to the sacrum. It forms the lateral border of the base of the recto-uterine pouch (pouch of Douglas). It helps to maintain uterine anteversion by pulling the cervix backwards.

The uterine blood supply
The vessels supplying blood to the uterus are the uterine and ovarian arteries. The uterine

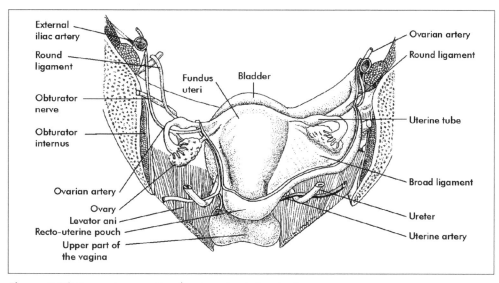

Figure 5.12 Ligaments supporting the uterus (posterior view)

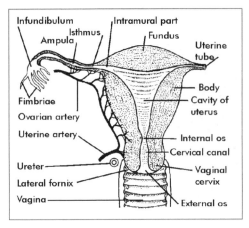

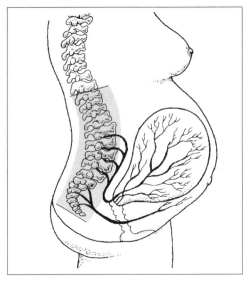

Figure 5.13 Uterine blood supply

Figure 5.14 Uterine nerve supply

artery, a branch of the internal iliac artery, is sheathed in the transverse cervical ligament and joins the uterus at the level of the isthmus. It sends a branch to the upper part of the vagina and cervix, but the larger branch runs up alongside the uterus between the folds of the broad ligament, giving off branches to the body of the uterus and eventually linking with the ovarian artery.

The ovarian artery is a branch of the abdominal aorta. It passes between the folds of the broad ligament, supplies the ovary and uterine tube and then the fundus of the uterus.

The uterine blood supply is increased during pregnancy. The fetus depends on a constant supply of oxygen, nutrients and metabolites via the maternal blood.

Nerve supply of the internal genital organs

The main nerve supply of the uterus comes from the pelvic autonomic system, both sympathetic and parasympathetic. Impulses transmitted by the sympathetic nerves can either stimulate or inhibit the uterus, depending on whether it is influenced by chemical agents or by hormonal factors in the fetoplacental unit.

Sympathetic nerve fibres pass to the pelvic plexus in the base of the uterosacral ligaments, from which the uterus, vagina, bladder

and rectum are supplied. Nerves from the pelvic plexus pass to the paracervical ganglia situated close to the cervix. The contact pressure on the cervix from a well-applied presenting part results in the transmission of a stimulus through the paracervical ganglia from the nerve endings in the cervix. These impulses result in stronger contractions of the muscle fibres in the upper uterine segment.

The uterine tubes (fallopian tubes)

The uterine tubes are two muscular canals, extending from the cornu of the uterus and opening into the peritoneal cavity near the ovaries. Each tube measures approximately 10 to 14 cm in length and is enclosed in the upper part of the broad ligament. The ciliated mucous membrane lining the tube and the rhythmic peristaltic movement of the muscle coat furthers the passage of the ovum from the ovary along the tube to the uterus.

The ovaries

The ovaries are paired almond-shaped organs, 2 to 4 cm in length, found on the posterior surface of the broad ligament to which they are attached by the mesovarium. The ovary is brought into contact with the uterine tube by one of the fimbrae extending from the fimbriated end of the uterine tube, the infundibulum.

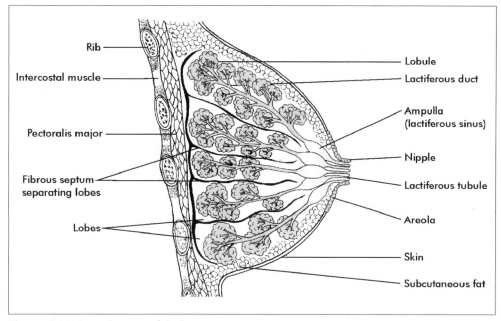

Figure 5.15 Sagittal section of the breast

The breast

The average adult female breast extends between the second and sixth ribs, and the lateral sternal border and anterior axillary fold. A triangular tongue-shaped tail of breast tissue, the axillary tail (Spence) extends toward the axilla.

The areola is a pigmented zone, varying from pale pink to deep brown in colour. The skin of the areola contains multiple sebaceous glands (Montgomery's tubercles) responsible for lubrication of the nipple. During the third trimester the sebaceous glands hypertrophy markedly.

The adult female breast contains glands and ducts, fibrous tissue that binds the individual lobes together and fatty tissue (about 80 to 85%) within and between the lobes. The breast tissue is joined to the overlying skin and subcutaneous tissue by fibrous strands, called Cooper's ligaments.

Each lobe in the breast consists of a group of lobules, and the many lactiferous ducts in each lobule unite to form a major duct that drains a lobe and converges toward the areola. Each of the major ducts widens to form an ampulla as it reaches the areola and then narrows for its individual opening on the nipple.

Physiological changes in the breasts during pregnancy

In the nonpregnant, nonlactating breast the alveoli are small and tightly packed. During pregnancy the alveoli enlarge, and during lactation the alveolar cells secrete milk. In response to progesterone secreted during pregnancy, the breast size and turgidity increase markedly. These changes are accompanied by deepening nipple and areolar pigmentation, nipple enlargement, areolar widening and increase in the number and size of the lubricating glands in the areola. The number of branches in the duct system increases and the ducts widen. After delivery the breasts start to secrete milk. With cessation of nursing the breast rapidly returns to its pre-pregnancy state.

References

Beischer, N. A. & Mackay, E. V. 1986. *Obstetrics and the newborn: An illustrated textbook*. Second edition. London: Baillière Tindall.

Ellis, H. 1992. *Clinical anatomy: A revision and applied anatomy for clinical students*. London: Blackwell Scientific Publications.

Lindner, H. H. 1989. *Clinical anatomy*. Norwalk: Appleton and Lange.

Llewellyn-Jones, D. 1999. *Fundamentals of obstetrics and gynaecology. Volume 1*. Third edition. London: Mosby.

Meyer, B. J. et al. 1988. *Die fisiologiese basis vir geneeskunde*. Pretoria: HAUM.

Roberts, K. B. & Tomlinson, J. D. W. 1992. *The fabric of the body: European traditions of anatomical illustration*. Oxford: Clarendon Press.

Williams, P. L. et al. 1995. *Gray's anatomy*. New York: Churchill Livingstone.

Chapter 6

Conception and fetal development

Linda Greyling

Introduction

The study of human embryology is important because it develops knowledge about the beginning of human life and the changes that occur during the developmental stages before birth. On the other hand, infants have always been born with defects and abnormalities. Records of human congenital malformations extend back into prehistoric times, but it was not until the seventeenth and eighteenth centuries that Harvey, the Hunters and their contemporaries even began to explain the causes of malformations (Williams, 1995:333).

Early development of the ovum

When ovulation takes place, the ovum is released into the peritoneal cavity and finds its way into the uterine tube. Under influence of

oestrogens at the time of ovulation, the uterine tube becomes arched and its fimbriated end is cupped underneath the ovary to receive the ovum from the ruptured Graafian follicle. The cilia and peristaltic muscular contractions of the uterine tube move the ovum along the uterine tube.

In preparation for fertilisation, both male and female cells undergo changes involving the chromosomes and cytoplasm. The purpose of this is:

▶ A reduction of the number of chromosomes to half the number found in somatic (body) cells, in other words, from 46 to 23. This is accomplished through meiotic division.
▶ Altering the shape of the germ cells in preparation for fertilisation. For example, the male cell loses much of its cytoplasm and develops a head, neck and tail during a process called spermatogenesis. The female

cell gradually becomes larger as a result of an increase in cytoplasm during a process called oogenesis.

Conception

Fusion of the ovum and spermatozoon is called conception or fertilisation and initiates the beginning of a new life. Normally, only one ovum is produced per month by the ovaries, but as many as 1x108 spermatozoa for each millilitre of seminal fluid are deposited in the vagina when coitus takes place. At this time the cervix secretes an alkaline mucus that attracts the spermatozoa. A limited number of sperm reach the uterine tube; a few may penetrate the zona pellucida, but only one fuses with the nucleus of the ovum.

The most likely period for conception to take place is immediately following ovulation, which is 14 days before the next menstrual period. The majority of women conceive between the 10th to 18th day of the menstrual cycle. Neither ovum nor spermatozoon is thought to be capable of fertilisation for longer than 48 hours.

The results of conception are as follows:
▶ Restoration of the diploid number (46) of chromosomes.
▶ Gender determination through the chromosomes (XX or XY).
▶ Variation of the human species.
▶ Initiation of the first cell division.

If conception occurs, the chorionic hormones secreted by the trophoblast prevent atrophy of the corpus luteum that, with further growth, becomes the corpus luteum of pregnancy.

Removal of the corpus luteum of pregnancy before the fourth month usually results in abortion.

Formation of the decidua

When conception takes place the endometrium becomes known as the decidua. The increased activity of the decidua is caused by the stimulus of oestrogenic hormones, and progesterone from the corpus luteum. The result is a soft, vascular, spongy bed in which the fertilised ovum can readily become implanted.

The three layers of the decidua

The outer layer, the compact layer, is made up of closely packed cells and the necks of the glands. It is the most superficial of the three layers and lies adjacent to the uterine cavity.

The middle or spongy layer is formed mainly of tortuous dilated glands and decidua cells.

The inner layer is called the basement layer and regenerates the new endometrium during the puerperium.

Embedding of the placenta in the decidua

Throughout pregnancy the placenta remains securely embedded in the decidua, but as soon as the baby is born the placenta must be shed. If the placental attachment is limited to the spongy layer, it will be possible for the placenta to become separated from the decidua. Should the placenta embed too deeply, it would be adhered to the muscular wall and so complicate the third stage of labour.

The decidua basalis is the area of decidua underneath the embedded ovum. Decidua found over the developing embryo is the decidua capsularis, and the remainder that lines the uterus is the decidua vera.

Development of the embryo
Developmental stages

The length of pregnancy or gestational period is divided into three periods of development:
▶ The pre-embryonic period that extends from fertilisation of the ovum to the formation of the three germinal layers. This period lasts from the first week to the end of the third week.
▶ The embryonic period, during which the germinal layers differentiate to form the

most important organ systems, is also called the period of organogenesis. This extends from the fourth to the eighth week.

▶ During the fetal period further growth of the tissues and organs occurs, as well as an increase in the size of the fetus. This stage extends from week nine to the end of pregnancy.

Development of the fertilised ovum

While being propelled along the uterine tube, cell division takes place and the fertilised cell, or zygote, divides through a process called mitosis. When it reaches the 16-cell stadium on the second day, the cluster of cells, called a morula, resembles a mulberry. Three to four days are required for the journey along the uterine tube to the uterus. A cavity or blastocele forms in the morula on the fourth day, which is now known as the blastocyst. Cells on the inner aspect of the blastocyst clump together, forming an inner cell mass or embryoblast that will give rise to the embryo. The remainder of the cells are pushed to the periphery, to be called the trophoblast cells. These cells will eventually form the placenta.

Implantation of the blastocyst

Six to ten days after fertilisation may elapse before the blastocyst is ready for implantation in the uterine wall. The blastocyst comes to rest on the decidua. The trophoblast cells associated with the embryoblast form two types of cells, namely an outer and inner layer of trophoblast cells. The outer layer is called the syncytiotrophoblast and has the power of breaking down tissue, thereby eroding the decidua and allowing the blastocyst to become embedded. The inner layer of trophoblast cells is then called the cytotrophoblast.

During implantation of the blastocyst slight vaginal bleeding may occur. Since implantation

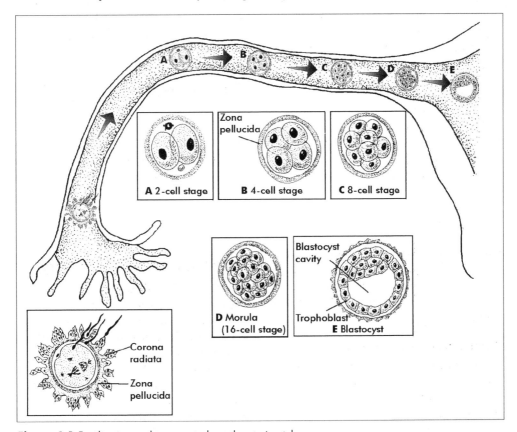

Figure 6.1 Fertilisation and transport along the uterine tube

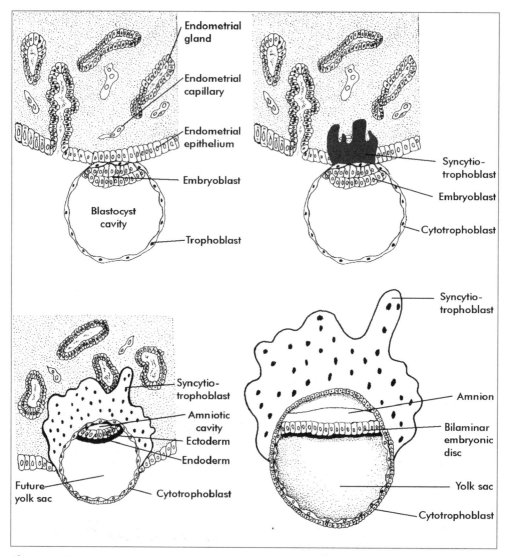

Figure 6.2 Stages in implantation of the blastocyst

Variation in implantation sites

Implantation normally occurs in the anterior or posterior walls of the uterus in the region of the fundus and body of the uterus. If implantation occurs in the region of the internal os of the cervix, the developed placenta could extend across the os (placenta praevia) and cause severe haemorrhaging during pregnancy and delivery. An implantation site outside the uterus is commonly referred to as an ectopic or extra-uterine pregnancy. This could be anywhere in the abdominal cavity, the uterine tubes or on the ovaries. An ectopic pregnancy usually results in the death of the embryo and/or severe haemorrhage.

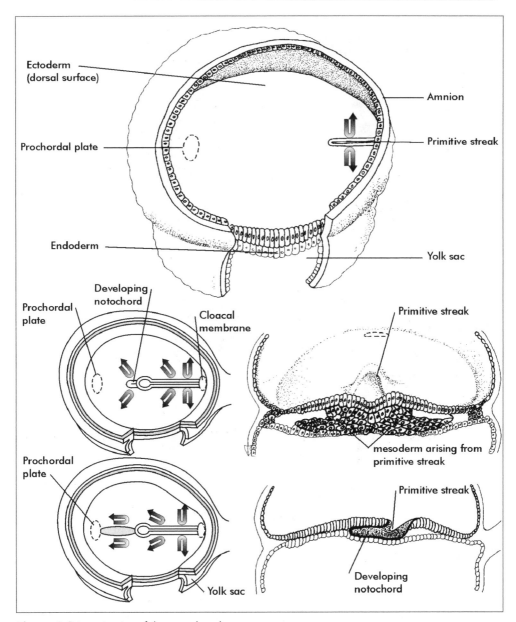

Figure 6.3 Invagination of the mesoderm layer

correlates with the date at which a normal menstrual cycle would have commenced (if fertilisation had not occurred), this slight bleeding might be mistaken for a menstrual period. By the eleventh or twelfth day after fertilisation decidual cells will have closed the opening, after which the blastocyst can only be seen as a slight protrusion into the lumen of the uterus.

Pre-embryological development

During the following stage the embryoblast develops into a two-layered structure, consisting of an ectodermal and endodermal layer, called the bilaminar embryo disc.

Two cavities develop, namely the amniotic sac opposite the ectodermal layer and below it, the yolk sac, associated with the endodermal

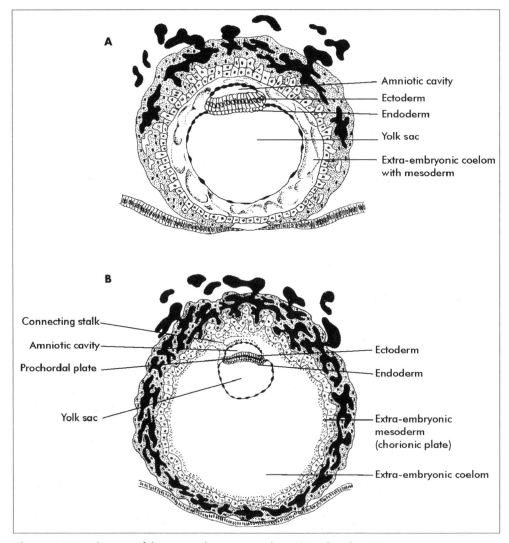

Figure 6.4 Development of the extra-embryonic mesoderm (A) and coelom (B)

layer. The amniotic sac is filled with amniotic fluid.

During the third week an additional layer, the mesoderm, invaginates between the ectodermal and endodermal layers. Mesodermal cells migrate from a caudal midline region called the primitive streak.

At this stage, a new group of cells that developed from the trophoblast, called the extra-embryonic mesoderm, completely fills the area between the inner surface of the cytotrophoblast and the outer surface of the yolk sac and amniotic cavity. Large cavities eventually form in the extra-embryonic mesoderm, except in the region of the developing body stalk, creating a new space called the extra-embryonic coelom. Later, the extra-embryonic coelom enlarges and becomes the chorionic cavity. Extra-embryonic mesodermal cells remaining on the inner surface of the cytotrophoblast are now known as the chorionic plate.

In a small midline area in the cephalic region of the embryo disc, called the prochordal plate, the ectodermal and endodermal layers remain firmly attached. This represents the future mouth area of the embryo. The

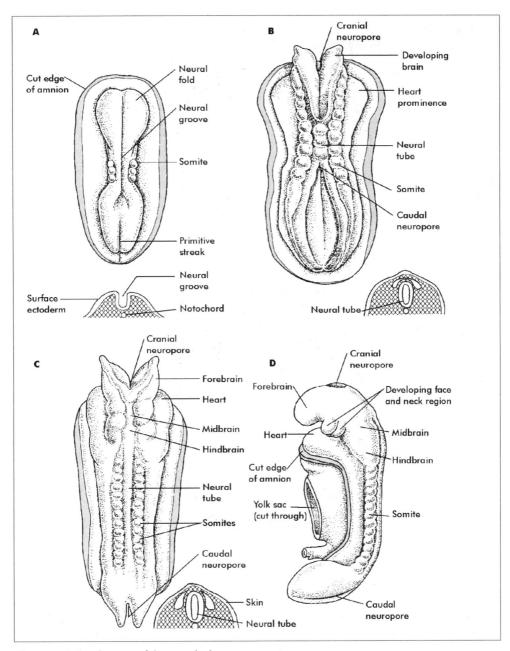

Figure 6.5 Development of the neural tube

cloacal membrane or future anus is established similarly in the caudal end of the embryo.

During further growth, the initially flat and almost round embryonic disc becomes elongated with a wider cephalic and narrow caudal end. A solid midline cell-axis called the notochord, develops cranial to the primitive streak and will eventually serve as the basis for the axial skeleton (see Figure 6.4).

The notochord persists in the vertebral column of the adult as the nucleus pulposis of the intervertebral discs.

In the midline region dorsal to the

Fetal development from the three layers of the embryoblast

From each particular layer parts of the embryo and fetus develop:

▶ The ectoderm forms the nervous system, skin and certain lining mucosa.

▶ The mesoderm forms bone, muscle, the circulatory system and certain internal organs.

▶ The endoderm forms the mucosa of the alimentary tract, the epithelium of the liver, pancreas, lungs and the bladder.

---

developing notochord, the ectodermal layer forms the basis of the central nervous system, during a process called neurilation. Initially, the cells arrange themselves to form a midline groove, called the neural groove. The walls of the neural groove then approach each other in the midline to form a neural tube. Closure of the neural tube begins near the middle of the embryo and progresses towards the cranial and caudal ends. This neural tube is the beginning of the brain and spinal cord.

Failure of the cranial end of the neural tube to close gives rise to a condition called anencephaly. At birth, there is an absence of the vault of the skull, and the brain can be seen as an exposed mass of tissue. The defect is often accompanied by an open spinal cord in the cervical region.

The mesodermal layers on both sides of the developing neural tube also undergo changes and paired cuboidal bodies, called somites, start to form (see Figure 6.5).

Cells from the somites give rise to most of the axial skeleton, namely the vertebral column, ribs, sternum and skull and the associated musculature, as well as the adjacent dermis of the skin.

The formation of blood vessels starts during the third week in the connecting stalk, the chorion and the embryo. The primitive heart, a tube-like structure, forms in the area cranial to the prochordal plate. By the end of the third week the heart tubes have joined blood vessels in the embryo, connecting stalk and chorion to form a primitive cardiovascular system. Circulation of blood already begins by the end of the third week.

Embryological development

From the fourth week onwards the beginnings of all major external and internal structures appear. By the end of the eighth week all the main organ systems have begun to develop, although function is still minimal.

This is the most critical period in the embryonic development because developmental disturbances during this period could give rise to congenital abnormalities.

By a process of lateral and longitudinal folding of the embryo the flat trilaminar disc is converted into a C-shaped cylindrical structure. During folding, the yolk sac is incorporated into the embryo as the primitive gut and both the lateral and ventral body walls are established.

Owing to folding of the head the future mouth area and primitive heart are moved ventrally to their anatomical positions, and the developing brain is now the most cranial structure in the embryo (see Figure 6.6). Tail-folding moves the cloacal membrane and body stalk to the ventral side of the embryo.

As a result of folding the amniotic sac eventually surrounds the embryo. As the amniotic cavity increases in size the amnion comes into contact with the chorionic plate to which it becomes adherent (see Figure 6.7).

The embryo is still attached to the developing placenta by a broad band of extra-embryonic mesoderm, the body stalk.

After development of blood vessels the connecting stalk becomes the umbilical cord, extending between the placenta and embryo.

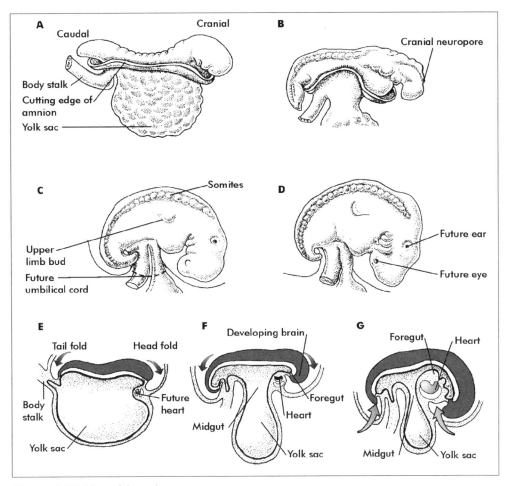

Figure 6.6 Folding of the embryo

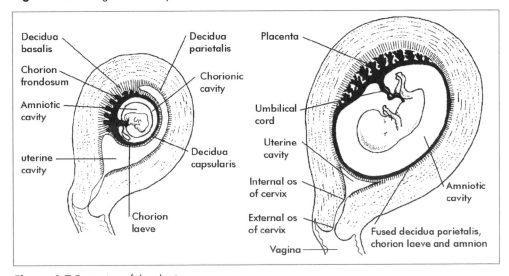

Figure 6.7 Formation of the chorion

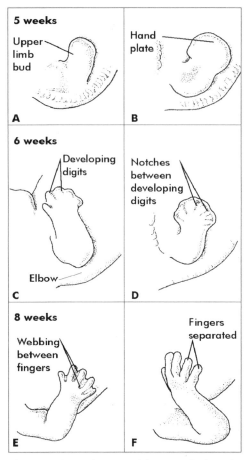

5 weeks

Upper limb bud

A

Hand plate

B

6 weeks

Developing digits

Elbow

C

Notches between developing digits

D

8 weeks

Webbing between fingers

E

Fingers separated

F

Figure 6.8 Development of the upper limb and digits

During this period the beginning of the future neck and face area becomes visible, as well as the beginnings of the future ear, the otic placode. The upper and lower limb buds can be seen as swellings on the lateral body wall.

Considerable growth occurs in the limbs during these weeks. The joint regions become identifiable, and by the end of the embryonic period the notches that have developed between the digits in the hand and footplate

Failure of the halves of one or more of the vertebral arches to fuse result in the development of varying degrees of a defect called spina bifida.

have separated the fingers and toes (see Figure 6.8).

Distinct growth of the head takes place as a result of the rapid development of the brain. By the fifth week most of the sections of the central nervous system have been established. The optic vesicles that will become the eyes develop as diverticulums from the brain during the fifth week.

The developing eyes, that have been open until now, develop eyelids. The eyelids approach each other and fuse. By the end of the eighth week the embryo has developed distinct human characteristics.

Although differentiation of the external genitalia has begun during the embryonal period, it is still not possible to determine the sex of the embryo from the appearance of the genitalia.

Fetal period (prominent stages)

Development during the fetal period is mainly concerned with growth of the body, but also with growth and differentiation of the tissues and organs.

Although the head still forms almost half of the fetus at the beginning of the fetal period (ninth week), by the end of the 12th week this distinction has been erased as a result of rapid growth in body and limb length. By the end of

Growth abnormalities

Abnormalities in the extremities vary enormously. It includes complete absence of a limb (amelia), limbs represented only by irregularly shaped bone (meromelia) and abnormally short limbs (micromelia). Abnormalities of the fingers and toes include extra fingers or toes (polydactyly), abnormal fusion of the fingers or toes (syndactyly) and a lobster claw, where the first and second and fourth and fifth digits are fused.

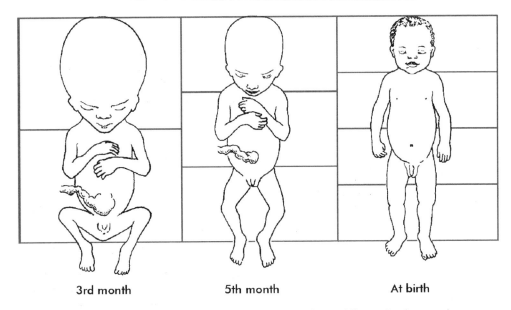

| 3rd month | 5th month | At birth |

Figure 6.9 Proportional growth of the head, limbs and body during different developmental ages

the 12th week the fetus begins to move, although at this stage the mother cannot feel the movements.

The external genitalia have developed into the adult shape during this phase. Urine formation also begins during the 9th to 12th weeks and is excreted into the amniotic fluid. The fetus absorbs some of the fluid after swallowing it, but the rest of the waste products pass into the maternal circulation through the placenta.

The 13th to 16th week period is characterised by more rapid growth of the body, with ossification centres, visible on radiographs of the fetus, appearing in the skeleton. By the end of this period the eyes and ears have moved to their definitive positions and the fetus appears even more human.

A prominent characteristic of the period extending between weeks 17 to 20 is the strong fetal movements felt by the woman (quickening). The skin of the fetus is now covered with *vernix caseosa,* which is a mixture of fatty secretions from the fetus and dead cells. This protects the fetus' skin, amongst others, from exposure to the amniotic fluid. By week 20 the body of the fetus is covered with very fine hair, called *lanugo,* and eyebrows and hair are also visible.

Substantial weight is gained during the period extending from 21 to 25 weeks. Blood in the capillaries is visible through the very thin skin, and the skin is usually wrinkled and pink to red in colour.

The lungs begin to secrete surfactant, the substance that facilitates expansion of the alveoli of the lungs, during the 24th week. A fetus born during this period can survive if given intensive care, although the chances of survival of the fetus increase minimally during the 26th to 29th week. This is primarily as a result of the ability of the lungs to function more independently.

The eyes re-open at the beginning of the period extending from 26 to 29 weeks. More fat is deposited below the skin and the fetus appears less wrinkled.

A fetus of 32 weeks and older usually survives if born preterm. Normal birth usually takes place 266 days or 38 weeks after fertilisation, or 280 days or 40 weeks after the beginning of the last menstrual period.

The mature fetus
The fetal skull

At this stage the skull is large in proportion to the rest of the skeleton. The bones of the fetal

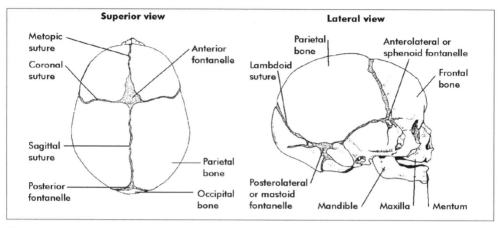

Figure 6.10 Fetal skull and fontanelles

skull are still very thin and ossification, with regard to the suture lines and sites of the fontanelles, is incomplete. Fontanelles form in the sutures at the junctions between the bones of the calvarium.

The main fontanelles present at this stage:
▶ The anterior fontanelle (or bregma) is a midline fontanelle formed at the junction between the frontal and parietal bones. This is the largest of the fontanelles and is a diamond-shaped area. Pulsation from the superior sagittal sinus directly below the fontanelle is transmitted through the over-lying skin. This fontanelle should be closed by 18 to 24 months of age.
▶ The posterior or occipital fontanelle is a

> ## Purpose of the fontanelles and sutures
>
> The fontanelles and sutures allow some compression (moulding) of the skull during birth and aid the midwife in determining the position of the head during labour.

triangular fontanelle at the junction of the occipital and parietal bones. This fontanelle closes during the second month.
▶ Lesser fontanelles include the paired sphenoid and mastoid fontanelles.
  ◆ The sphenoid or anterolateral fontanelles are at the junction between the frontal, parietal, temporal and sphenoid bones and should be closed by six months of age.
  ◆ The mastoid or posterolateral fontanelles

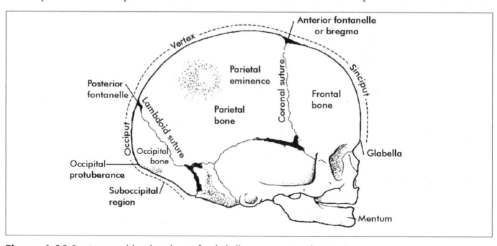

Figure 6.11 Regions and landmarks on fetal skull important to obstetrics

---

Fetal skull diameters

▶ The biparietal diameter of the fetal skull is of the greatest obstetric importance. This is the distance between the parietal eminences and represents the largest transverse diameter in the fetal skull, and measures 9.25 cm at term.

▶ The suboccipitobregmatic diameter (anterior-posterior diameter) extends from the occipital bone, an area close to the neck, to the bregma. When the fetal head is well flexed, this distance measures 9.5 cm.

▶ The occipitofrontal diameter extends from the back of the head (external occipital protuberance) to the glabella (on the frontal bone just above the orbits). When the fetal head is neither well flexed or well extended, but straight, the fetus is said to be in the 'military position'. This distance measures 11.7 cm.

▶ The mentovertical diameter extends from the tip of the mentum to the vertex. It is the longest diameter and measures 13.5 cm (seen in brow presentations).

▶ The submentobregmatic diameter is of importance during a facial presentation and measures 9.5 cm (see Figure 6.12).

---

are between the parietal, occipital and temporal bones. The latter should be closed by the second year.

A metopic suture (G. forehead), which represents the fusion line between the two frontal bones, is usually present at this age. This suture should be closed by age six to eight years. Other sutures include the sagittal suture between the parietal bones, the lambdoid suture between the parietal and occipital bones and the coronal suture between the frontal and parietal bones.

In anatomical terms, the highest point of the skull is the vertex, which lies near the middle of the sagittal suture. In obstetrics, the portion of the fetal skull between the bregma and posterior fontanelles represents the vertex. The bregma is the point where the coronal and sagittal sutures meet (anterior fontanelle), with the lambda at the junction between the sagittal and lambdoid sutures (posterior fontanelle). Occiput refers to the occipital region or back of the head and sinciput to the anterior part of the head just above and including the forehead.

Movements of the fetal skull accomplish descent of the fetus through the birth canal (pelvis). The particular diameter of the fetal skull will be determined by the degree of flexion or extension of the fetal head, in other

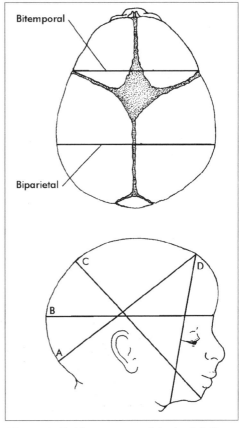

Figure 6.12 Measurements of the fetal skull
A: suboccipitobregmatic diameter
B: occipitofrontal diameter
C: mentovertical diameter, and
D: submentobregmatic diameter

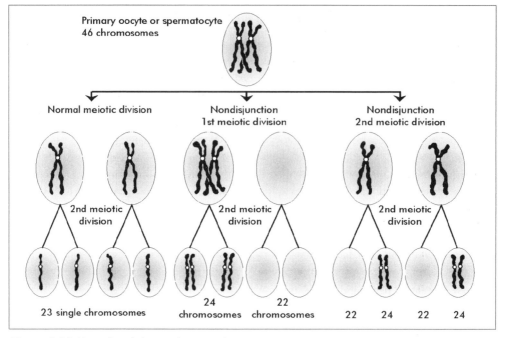

Figure 6.13 Normal and abnormal meiotic division

words, complete flexion or extension of the fetal head presents the smallest diameter of the fetal head and facilitates movement of the head through the pelvis.

Body size and length

The average length of the fetus during the last three months of pregnancy should be approximately 40, 45 and 50 cm with a weight of 2 kg, 2.5 kg and 3 to 3.5 kg respectively.

Skin

Progressive loss of *lanugo* occurs in the month or so preceding birth except for the hair on the eyelids, eyebrows and scalp. During this period the covering of *vernix caseosa* remains a prominent feature. At full term the *vernix caseosa* is reabsorbed and no longer so prominent. At birth the skin is still much thinner than that of, for example, a child.

Human genetics

All body (somatic) cells are descendants from one cell and therefore contain the same DNA.

DNA is duplicated before cell division, which means that a replica is made of each molecule and each of the DNA thus contains the chemical information about all cell activities. DNA is contained within a chromosome of which each somatic cell contains 46. The language the information is written in is the genetic code.

Duplication of the DNA and chromosomes in somatic cells occurs during a process called mitosis and in sex cells in a process called meiosis. During mitosis two identical daughter cells are created from the mother cell, in other words, they are duplicated with 46 chromosomes each. During meiosis, however, the daughter cells only contain half the number of chromosomes (23) in the mother cell and need to fuse with a cell with a similar number of chromosomes (23) to end up with the full complement of chromosomes (46).

Malformations (defects) present at birth are referred to as congenital (born with) malformations. The causes of congenital malformations include the following:

▶ Genetic factors that include both chromosomal and single gene defects.

▶ Environmental factors, including drugs, chemicals, infections and maternal disease.

▶ Multifactorial factors, such as the interaction of multiple genes with one or more environmental factors.

Genetic factors are some of the major causes of congenital malformations (approximately one third of all major congenital malformations).

These include:

▶ Numerical chromosomal malformations, such as nondisjunction, which means a failure of the chromosome pair to separate during mitosis or meiosis and both chromosomes pass to the same daughter cell. Examples of chromosomal abnormalities include trisomy 21 (extra chromosome no. 21) or Down's syndrome. Klinefelter's syndrome is an abnormality of the sex chromosomes and where the male is born with an extra X chromosome (47, XXY).

▶ Structural abnormalities result from chromosome breakage. The causes of the breakage could be radiation, a viral infection, drugs or chemicals. An example of such an abnormality is the *Cri du chat* syndrome in which there is a loss of an arm of the chromosome no. 5.

▶ Abnormalities caused by mutant genes could be a single gene error in the genetic make-up (genotype). The new gene is then called a mutant and gives rise to a defect called a mutation. Environmental agents, such as large doses of radiation, can accelerate the rate of mutation.

Environmental causes of congenital malformations also include those malformations caused by agents known as teratogens. Known human teratogens that produce or raise the incidence of congenital malformations, include drugs, chemicals, infectious agents and high levels of radiation. The organs or parts of an embryo most sensitive to these agents are those affected during a period of rapid development. During the first two weeks of development teratogens have either no known effect or the effects are so severe that the embryo is aborted.

During the fetal period teratogens may either produce only minor morphological defects, such as enlargement of, for example, the clitoris, or they could produce severe functional defects, as seen in alcohol abuse that is likely to cause mental retardation.

Multifactorial causes give rise to most congenital malformations, including neural tube defects and congenital heart malformations.

References

Meiring, J. H. et al. 1994. *Anatomie vir die medies-wetenskaplike student*. Pretoria: J. L. van Schaik Publishers.

May, K. A. & Mahlmeister, L. R. 1990. *Comprehensive maternity nursing: Nursing process and the childbearing family*. Philadelphia: Lippincott.

Meyer, B. J. et al. 1988. *Die fisiologiese basis vir geneeskunde*. Pretoria: HAUM.

Moore, K. L. 1988. *Essentials of human embryology*. Toronto: BC Decker.

Sadler, T. W. 2004. *Langman's medical embryology*. Baltimore: Williams & Wilkens.

Stedman's medical dictionary. 1990. Baltimore: Williams & Wilkens.

Thibodeau, G. A. & Patton, K. T. 1993. *Anatomy and physiology*. Baltimore: Mosby.

Williams, P. L. et al. 1995. *Gray's anatomy*. New York: Churchill Livingstone.

Chapter *7*

The placenta and amniotic fluid

Linda Greyling

Introduction

During early development the zygote and blastocyst obtain their nutriment at first from their own cytoplasm, and then from both tubal and uterine secretions until their implantation into the uterine wall. At this stage, nutrients are absorbed over the surface of the developing embryo. After implantation the nutritional needs of the embryo are met at first by the development of a primitive 'exchange system' between the maternal tissue and embryo and later by the highly sophisticated placenta.

The placenta

The developing placenta

As a rule, the placenta is attached to the posterior wall of the uterus near the fundus. The point where the blastocyst becomes embedded in the uterine wall determines the site of attachment.

At the end of the second week the develop-

ing syncytiotrophoblast cells surround the whole blastocyst and form rudimentary outgrowths, called chorionic villi (primary villi)

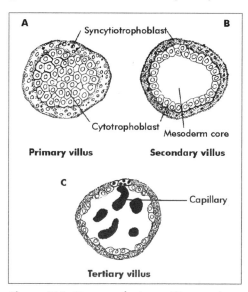

Figure 7.1 Structure of primary (A), secondary (B) and tertiary villi (C)

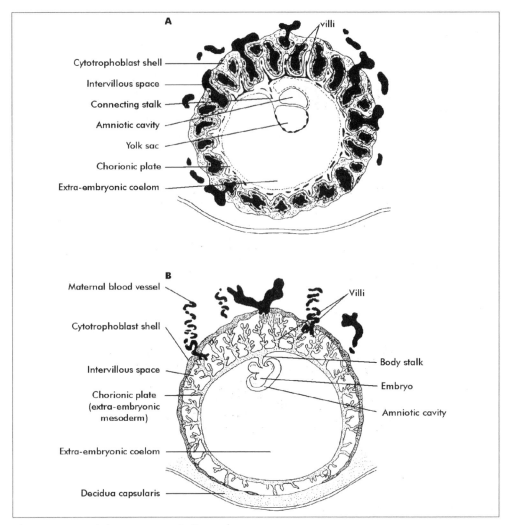

Figure 7.2 Radial appearance of villi

that contain no blood vessels. They absorb nutrients directly from the disintegrated cells in the implantation cavity.

During the third week radially arranged villi cover the entire outer surface of the chorionic plate. Those on the embryonic pole grow abundantly and are known as the chorion frondosum (bushy chorion), which ultimately forms the placenta. These chorionic villi penetrate the maternal blood vessels with which they come into contact, and become bathed in a lake of maternal blood. The opened maternal vessels become known as sinuses and the areas surrounding the villi as blood (intervil-

lous) spaces. These villi therefore 'float' in the slowly circulating maternal blood from which they absorb nutrients.

Some of the chorionic villi, called anchoring villi, are attached to the decidua. The villi on the remainder of the blastocyst, opposite the embryonic pole, degenerate, leaving the chorion laeve (bald chorion), which on its inner surface is adherent to the amnion and on its outer surface to the decidua capsularis, and after week 12 to the decidua vera (see Figure 6.7 in Chapter 6).

A villus is a branching structure that arises from the chorionic membrane as a single

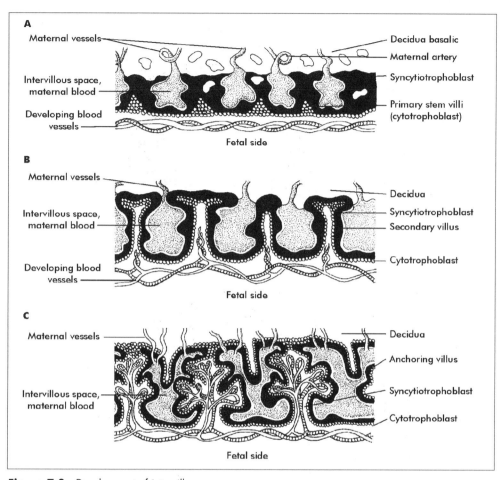

Figure 7.3 Development of intervillous spaces

stem, which divides and subdivides until it terminates in the fine filaments that are embedded in the decidua basalis. The first villi to appear have a cytotrophoblast core with an outer covering of syncytiotrophoblast. These are called the primary villi. When the core is gradually replaced by developing mesoderm, the villi become known as secondary villi. By their selective action, chorionic villi absorb the particular substances needed for the developing embryo from the maternal blood. During the subsequent stage, blood vessels, within which fetal blood circulates, develop in the mesodermal centre of the villus. This is then called a tertiary villus.

Eventually, the fetal heart will pump 500 ml of blood through the placenta per minute. The fetus develops its own blood and maternal blood never circulates in the fetus. In the placenta there are four layers of tissue between fetal and maternal blood, namely, syncytiotrophoblast, cytotrophoblast, mesoderm and the capillary wall. Unless some breakdown of the placenta occurs, fetal and maternal blood does not mix.

From weeks 12 to 20 the placenta weighs as much as and even more than the fetus, because at this stage it must deal with the metabolic processes of nutrition, with which the underdeveloped fetal organs are unable to cope. During the later weeks of pregnancy some of the fetal organs, such as the liver, begin to function, so the cytotrophoblast and the syncytio-trophoblast gradually degenerate and disappear.

The placenta at term

The placenta, or afterbirth, is a discoid structure, about 15 to 20 cm in diameter, 2.5 cm thick at the centre and weighs approximately one-sixth of the weight of the baby at term (more or less 500 g).

It is made up of chorionic plate facing the fetus (fetal surface) and a basal plate in contact with the decidua (maternal surface). The maternal surface is made up mainly of syncytiotrophoblast components with a thin layer of the decidua basalis attached to it. Tissue on the maternal surface is arranged in some 15 to 20 cotyledons or lobules that are separated by sulci or grooves. Maternal blood gives it a bluish-red colour, and a thin layer of trophoblastic cells covers the surface. Frequently some cotyledons have a whitish appearance that is caused by excessive fibrinoid formation resulting in infarction of a group of intervillous lakes.

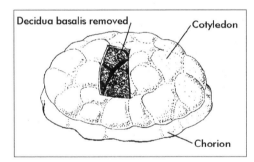

Figure 7.4 Maternal surface of the placenta

The fetal surface is smooth, white and shiny. On it the branches of the umbilical vein and arteries and the insertion of the umbilical cord can be seen. It is covered with two membranes, the chorion and amnion, which are continued beyond its outer edge to form the sac that contains the fetus and amniotic fluid.

The placenta separates from the uterine wall after delivery of the fetus and is expelled, together with the membranes. The process of separation requires the rupture of many uterine arteries. Their torn ends are closed by contraction of the uterine walls and, under normal circumstances, postpartum haemorrhage is limited.

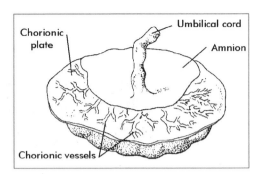

Figure 7.5 Fetal surface of the placenta

Placental circulation

The cotyledons receive their blood from the maternal arteries in the endometrium. These vessels pierce the decidua and then enter the intervillous spaces. In the intervillous spaces the villi are bathed in oxygenated blood. After the exchange of gases and other substances, blood returns to the endometrial veins and the maternal circulation.

Blood from the fetal heart circulates through the fetus and is carried by the arteries of the umbilical cord to the placenta. The umbilical arteries spread over the fetal surface of the placenta and subdivide until they terminate in the chorionic villi, which absorb the products of digestion, namely, amino acids, glucose, minerals, vitamins, and probably fatty acids from the mother's blood.

The fetal alimentary tract does not digest food, nor do the lungs inhale oxygen, therefore the placenta carries out the functions of the stomach, liver, intestines, lungs and kidneys.

Oxygen is taken from the mother's haemoglobin and carbon dioxide and other waste products are given off into the maternal blood, the interchange of substances taking place by osmosis and diffusion, as well as by the selective activation of the cytotrophoblast and the syncytiotrophoblast. The replenished oxygenated blood returns to the fetus via the umbilical vein.

Functions of the placenta

The placenta is a metabolic and incomplete endocrine organ, as well as the means through which the fetus obtains its needs. It not only

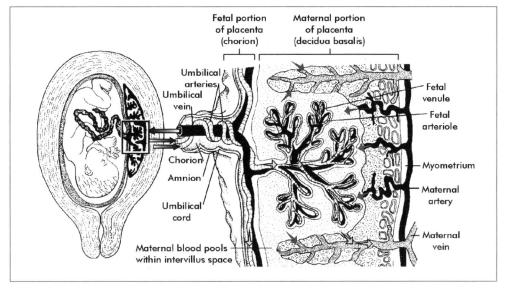

Figure 7.6 Placental circulation: The direction of blood flow is indicated by arrows. Maternal blood flows through the uterine arteries into the intervillus spaces. The blood returns through the uterine veins to the maternal circulation.

selects and transports the substances necessary for fetal life and growth from the mother's blood; it also changes some of these so that the fetus can utilise them. The efficiency of the placental functions depends on adequate uterine blood flow.

The placental barrier, which allows selective permeability by the placenta, is represented by the structures that separate the maternal and fetal blood. These include, amongst others, the endothelium of the fetal blood vessels, the tissue of the villi, and the trophoblast structures. The placental barrier allows water, oxygen and other nutritive substances and hormones from mother to fetus, and products of excretion from fetus to mother.

Placental functions can be classified as nutritional, respiratory, excretory, endocrine and protective.

Nutritional

The fetus requires amino-acids (proteins) for building tissue, glucose for growth and energy, calcium and phosphorus for the composition of bones and teeth, and water, vitamins, electrolytes, iron and other minerals for blood formation, growth and various body processes.

Until the fetal liver is sufficiently developed to function, the placenta metabolises glucose, stores it in the form of glycogen and converts it into glucose, as required. The products of digestion that are present in the mother's blood pass to the fetus via the placenta, mainly by enzymatic carriers. Fatty acids are believed to pass through the placenta. The fetus also converts glucose into fat. Minerals and vitamins are readily transported across the placenta to the fetus.

Fetal nutrition

It is the mother's food that provides fetal nutriment and only when her diet is inadequate are her tissues depleted. To meet fetal requirements and avoid maternal depletion a diet rich in the essential nutrients is imperative during pregnancy.

Respiratory

Actual pulmonary respiration does not occur in the fetus. The fetus obtains oxygen from the mother's haemoglobin by simple diffusion and gives off carbon dioxide into the maternal blood. Although fetal respiratory movements are believed to take place there is no pulmonary exchange of gases in utero.

Excretory

The fetus can only excrete metabolic waste products through the placenta. However, there is not a large amount of excretion from the fetus since its metabolism is mainly anabolic (building up).

Endocrine

Human chorionic gonadotrophin (HCG) is produced in the chorionic villi. This hormone forms the basis of the immunological and other pregnancy tests. Initially, HCG maintains the functions of the corpus luteum (secretion of oestrogen and progesterone), until the placenta is mature enough to take over the functions of the corpus luteum (more or less from days 50 to 70). Thus, large amounts of HCG are excreted during weeks 7 to 10, but after week 12 the peak period has passed and a low level is maintained until term.

The fetoplacental unit produces oestrogen from weeks 6 to 12 when the amount rises steadily until term. After expulsion of the placenta it falls and allows prolactin to initiate lactation. The fetus provides the placenta with the vital precursors for the production of oestrogen and as both placenta and fetus are concerned in the production of oestrogen excreted in urine during pregnancy, the amount is an index of fetoplacental function.

Human placental lactogen (HPL) affects carbohydrate metabolism and may be concerned with fetal growth. The level of HPL in the blood reflects placental function.

Most maternal hormones do not cross the placental barrier. Hormones that do cross are, for example, thyroxine (thyroid gland). Of some importance also are the synthetic progestins that could cause musculisation in female fetuses.

Protective

A very important function of the placenta is to inactivate a number of undesirable substances. The placenta can be compared to an ultrafilter that allows very small molecules to pass through the placenta but prevents large molecules from passing to the fetus. Most pathogenic and non-pathogenic organisms can only cross the placental barrier if the membranes have been damaged, for example, babies born with tuberculosis.

With the exception of certain viruses, few organisms can pass through the placenta to the fetus. *Treponema pallidum* (syphilis) passes readily through the placental barrier, the protozoa of malaria and toxoplasmosis also reach the fetal blood stream, as well as the *Rubella* virus.

Note

If the *Rubella* virus infects the woman during the eighth to 12th week of pregnancy the infant may suffer from cardiac defects, cataracts or deaf mutism.

Antibodies, but very few antigens, are transmitted across the placenta. This explains the passive immunity babies are born with that protects them against certain communicable diseases during the first six to 12 months. The condition, known as *erythroblastosis fetalis*, or haemolytic disease of the newborn, may result in intra-uterine death as a result of Rhesus allo-immunisation.

Sedative drugs and analgesic gases, for example, *morphine, chloroform* and *ether*, pass readily through the placenta to the fetus. If *morphine* is given to the mother within three hours of the birth of the baby, it could depress the fetal respiratory centre and make the establishment of respiration difficult. It is known that antibiotics pass through the placenta and antisyphylitic drugs given to the mother have the same beneficial action on the fetus. Teratogenic drugs pass through the placenta and cause fetal deformities. Examples are Roaccutane® (multiple birth defects) and *clomiphene* (female reproductive system).

Malformations and abnormal insertions of the placenta

There are several common malformations of the placenta and abnormal attachment or insertion of the umbilical cord to the placenta.

Battledore placenta

With a battledore placenta the umbilical cord is inserted at the edge of the placenta in the manner of a raquet. This condition is believed to be of no clinical significance.

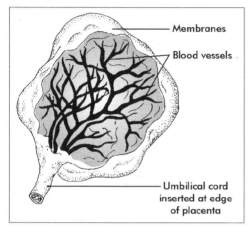

Figure 7.7 Battledore placenta

Placenta velamentosa

With placenta velamentosa the insertion of the umbilical cord is such that it ends in the membranes surrounding the placenta. The vessels traverse the membranes before reaching the placenta itself.

Succenturiate placenta

Succenturiate placenta (or accessory placenta) consists of an accessory lobe of placental tissue, situated in the fetal sac membrane with blood vessels running from the main placenta. It is formed by hypertrophy of some

> **Identifying a succenturiate lobe**
> If there is a hole in the membrane with blood vessels running to it, the midwife should know that a succenturiate lobe and not a piece of membrane has been retained.

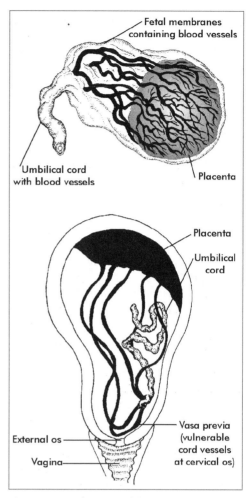

Figure 7.8 Placenta velamentosa

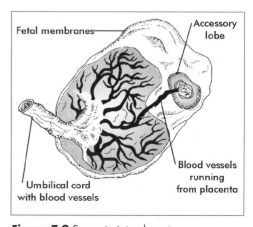

Figure 7.9 Succenturiate placenta

chorionic villi in the chorion laeve, that should have atrophied. Such a lobe is liable to be retained in utero and may give rise to profuse postpartum haemorrhage.

Bipartite and tripartite placenta

Bipartite and tripartite placenta is where there are two or three complete or almost complete lobes. Their blood vessels unite when joining the umbilical cord, whereas the succenturiate lobe does not directly join the cord vessels. In twin placentae there are two cords.

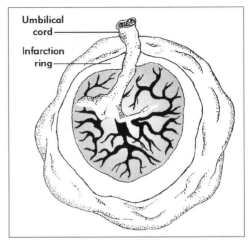

Figure 7.11   Placenta circumvallata

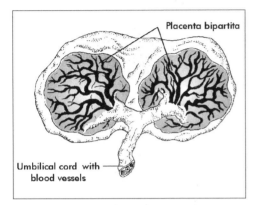

Figure 7.10   Bipartite placenta

Placenta circumvallata

Placenta circumvallata has a double layer of amnion and chorion that has undergone infarction. This is seen as an opaque ring on the fetal surface. It has little significance.

Diseases of the placenta

▶ *Hydantiform mole*: This is a cystic, degenerative proliferation of the chorionic villi.
▶ *Infarcts*: Infarcts are areas of necrosed chorionic villi, red in the early stage and white later with a solid cartilaginous consistency, produced by increased concentration of tissue thromboplastin. They are commonly seen on the maternal surface, but may be present on the fetal aspect. Calcareous degeneration, characterised by gritty particles that feel like sandpaper and sometimes form plaques on the maternal surface, is not infarction. It is associated with the normal degenerative processes of

the placenta at term. The small white areas often present around the periphery of the placenta are fibrin nodes and not true infarcts.
▶ *Oedema of the placenta*: Oedema of the placenta results in a large, pale placenta with water oozing from it. It is associated with *hydrops fetalis* and is due to haemolytic disease of the newborn, caused by Rhesus allo-immunisation.

The placenta in multiple births

The following types of placentae can occur (mostly in twins):
▶ Separation of the embryoblast and separate implantation sites, in other words separate amnion, chorion and placenta for each fetus (Figure 7.12A).
▶ Separate amniotic sacs but a single chorion and placenta are shared (Figure 7.12B).
▶ Two embryos sharing a single amnion, chorion and placenta (Figure 7.12C).
▶ Similar to the above-mentioned but incomplete or unequal separation of the embryoblast (Figure 7.12D).

The fetal sac

The sac enclosing the fetus consists of a double membrane, namely, the outer chorion and the inner amnion. Both the fetus and amniotic fluid are contained within this sac, which

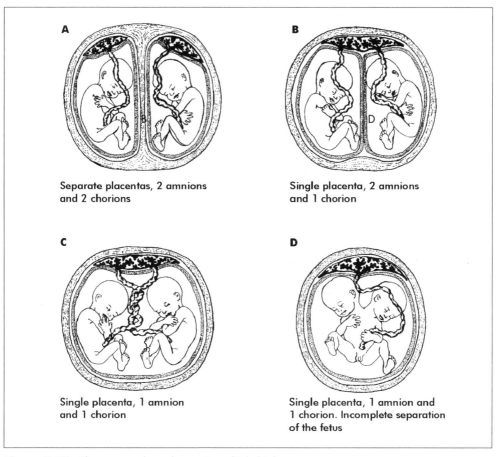

Figure 7.12 Placentae and membranes in multiple births

ruptures during labour to permit the expulsion of both.

The chorion is a thick, opaque, friable membrane and is adherent to the decidua vera on its outer aspect until the third stage of labour when it becomes detached during the expulsion of the placenta. As pieces of chorion may be retained in utero, it must always be carefully examined after being separated from the amnion. The chorion cannot be peeled off the fetal surface of the placenta because the placental chorionic villi are growing from it.

The amnion is a smooth, tough, translucent membrane, lining the chorion and is in direct contact with the amniotic fluid. The two membranes can be detached up to the insertion of the umbilical cord.

The umbilical cord

The thick connecting stalk becomes visible during the formation of the extra-embryonic coelom to form the link between the embryo and chorion. During lateral and head and tail folding, the amnion cavity that initially occupies the space dorsal to the embryo, expands to surround the embryo, obliterates the extra-embryonic coelom and comes to lie against the body stalk. Another result of folding is that the body stalk moves from a more caudal position to the ventral side of the embryo, close to the diminishing yolk sac. Umbilical vessels develop in this structure.

The umbilical cord extends from the fetal umbilicus to the fetal surface of the placenta. It is composed of an embryonic form of an

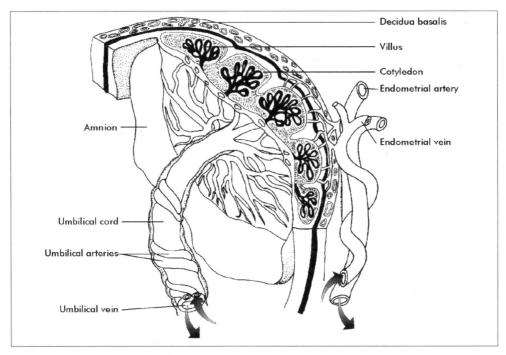

Figure 7.13 The umbilical cord

outer shell of amniotic cells with an inner mass of extra-embryonic mesoderm (body stalk) or Wharton's jelly. The cord carries two umbilical arteries and one vein. The two arteries contain impure blood going from the fetus to the placenta. The umbilical arteries are empty after birth and can be felt as fibrous cords. If one artery is shorter than the other artery the cord is twisted in a spiral fashion.

> **Note**
>
> A single artery is present in some cases and is often associated with other fetal abnormalities.

The umbilical vein in the cord contains blood returning to the fetus after having been oxygenated and replenished in the placenta. The vein can easily be seen and in cases where the baby needs urgent treatment after birth, drugs may be injected into the vein and milked into the circulation.

The average length of the cord is approximately 50 to 56 cm. If the length is less than 40 cm it is considered short. Cords as short as 15 cm have been seen, but fortunately are very rare. If the cord is looped around the fetus the descent of the fetus may be impeded and the placenta may separate prematurely, causing a haemorrhage, or the cord may break.

Cords of 1.5 m to 2 m have also been reported. A long cord may become coiled around the fetus and this happens during the middle months of the pregnancy when the ratio of amniotic fluid to fetus is so great that it can move about freely.

True knots in the cord occur when loops form through which the fetus can pass before or during labour. If drawn tight when the fetus descends during labour, it will lead to stillbirth due to hypoxia. *False knots* are merely Wharton's jelly heaping up and are not clinically significant.

The cord is commonly inserted in the centre of the fetal surface of the placenta. When the cord is inserted away from the centre yet not at the edge, it is termed a *lateral* insertion. A *battledore* insertion is one in which the cord is situated at the very edge of the placenta. A

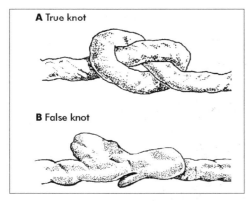

Figure 7.14 True knot (A) and false knot (B)

velamentous insertion exists when the cord is inserted into the membranes of the fetal sac, 5 to 10 cm from the edge of the placenta, but rarely as much as 15 to 20 cm, with the umbilical vessels running between placenta and cord. This form of insertion is more dangerous when the placenta is situated in the lower uterine segment because the vessels may lie over the internal os. The term *vasa praevia* is applied when fetal blood vessels pass through the membranes and lie over the internal os in front of the presenting part during labour. The vessels may be compressed or may rupture with slight bleeding, but if the bleeding is severe the fetus becomes exsanguinated. It is then usual to estimate the baby's haemoglobin immediately after birth.

Amniotic fluid (liquor amnii)

The clear pale straw-coloured fluid in which the fetus floats is present in the amniotic sac from the earliest weeks of pregnancy. The origin of amniotic fluid is thought to be both fetal and maternal. The most likely source is the amniotic epithelium covering the fetal surface of the placenta and umbilical cord, but also the fetal urine from the 10th week of gestation.

The amount increases until the quantity varies, at term, from 500 to 1 500 ml. It consists of 99% water, is alkaline in reaction, and various mineral salts are present, including urea, which is derived from urine passed by the fetus. A trace of protein (0.25%) is usually found in the amniotic fluid; therefore a voided specimen of urine from a woman whose membranes have ruptured may contain a trace of protein.

> ### Polyhydramnios and oligohydramnios
>
> If the amount of fluid is over 1 500 ml the condition is known as polyhydramnios, and if less than 300 ml, the term oligohydramnios is applied.

The fetus swallows the *liquor amnii*. The fluid is then absorbed through the intestinal tract of the fetus into the circulation and passed into the maternal blood via the placenta. Urine passed by the fetus into the amniotic fluid is mostly water since the placenta functions as an exchange for metabolic waste products.

The fluid distends the amniotic sac and allows for the growth and free movement of the fetus. It also acts as a shock absorber, protecting the fetus from jarring and injury. The fluid maintains the intra-uterine temperature. During labour it equalises uterine pressure and prevents marked interference with the placental circulation.

Amniotic fluid is regarded as an ultrafiltrate fetal serum that contains fetal cells. Up to the 12th week of pregnancy there is very little amniotic fluid, but it increases to 100 to 150 ml between the 12th and 14th week. Its maximum volume is reached during the 34th week, after which there is a decrease in its

> ### An excess of amniotic fluid
>
> In cases where the deglutition centre of the brain is not developed, as in some cases of anencephaly, an excess of amniotic fluid is present. This also occurs in cases where there is some malformation of the oesophagus, as in oesophageal atresia. Fetal malformations, monozygotic twins and diabetes are associated with an excess of fluid.

volume. Amniotic fluid is used for diagnostic purposes to determine lung maturity, certain fetal abnormalities and Rhesus allo-immunisation.

Discolouration of amniotic fluid

▶ *Normal discolouration*: Epidermal cells and *lanugo* from the skin of the full-term fetus are usually present and with *vernix caseosa* may give a turbid or milky appearance.
▶ *Meconium*: Amniotic fluid with a green colour indicates that meconium has been passed by the fetus and should be taken as a possible sign of fetal distress.
▶ *Brown discolouration*: Brown discolouration of the amniotic fluid is found during listeriosis, a rare and mostly fatal transplacental infection.
▶ *Yellow discolouration*: Yellow or golden discolouration of amniotic fluid and *vernix caseosa* is found during haemolytic disease (Rh allo-immunisation) in the fetus.

Protection against infection

Amniotic fluid contains lysozyme, a basic protein that functions as an antibacterial enzyme, as well as IgG antibodies.

Lung development

Alveoli in the lungs are filled with a fluid secreted by the lungs. The fluid may be involved in the alveolar development and expansion of the lungs at birth. It also contains surfactant, secreted by cells in the alveoli.

The fluid secreted by the alveoli differs from amniotic fluid regarding its pH, since it is more acid, and has a lower protein content. From time to time, small volumes of this fluid are dumped into the pharynx where it mixes with amniotic fluid. It is therefore possible to determine lung development, since small amounts of surfactant can be detected in the amniotic fluid at 28 weeks and after 36 weeks, a sufficient amount is secreted to maintain lung stability.

References

Ladewig, P. W., London, M. L. & Olds, S. B. 1998. *Maternal–newborn nursing care. The nurse, the family, and the community.* Fourth edition. Menlo Park, California: Addison Wesley Longman.

May, K. A. & Mahlmeister, L. R. 1990. *Comprehensive maternity nursing.* Second edition. Philadelphia: JB Lippincott.

Meyer, B. J. et al. 1988. *Die fisiologiese basis vir geneeskunde.* Pretoria: HAUM.

Moore, K. L. 1988. *Essentials of human embryology.* Toronto: BC Decker.

Sadler, T. W. 1985. *Langman's medical embryology.* Baltimore: Williams & Wilkens.

Williams, P. L. et al. 1995. *Gray's anatomy.* New York: Churchill Livingstone.

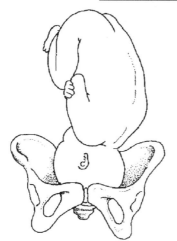

Pregnancy care

Chapter 8

Healthy adaptation to pregnancy

Elizabeth Kaye-Petersen

Introduction

The period from conception to the birth of the baby is about 40 weeks long. This chapter describes the changes in the structure and function of the various organs and systems of the body associated with pregnancy. These changes can usually be divided into those caused by hormonal changes and those caused by pressure, mainly because of the growth of the fetus and the uterus.

Physiological changes of pregnancy

Changes in the reproductive system

Ovaries and fallopian tubes

Following conception, follicular activity in the ovaries continues and the cells lining the ovaries become active in hormone produc-tion. The corpus luteum persists and produces progesterone until the 16th week of pregnan-cy when the placenta takes over the function of secreting oestrogen and progesterone. The corpus luteum, having no further function, regresses (see Chapters 5 and 6).

Uterus

Before pregnancy, the uterus is a small, pear-shaped organ measuring approximately 7.5 x 5 x 2.5 cm and weighs approximately 60 g. At the end of pregnancy the uterus measures approximately 28 x 24 x 21 cm and weighs up to 1 000 g. Its capacity increases from 10 ml to 5 litres or more. The cells increase 17 to 40 times their pre-pregnancy size as a result of oestrogen and the growing fetus.

The upper portion of the body of the

uterus (from the upper border of the isthmus to the fundus) enlarges and is known as the upper uterine segment. The isthmus softens and stretches and forms the lower uterine segment.

There is a marked increase in the fibrous cells between the muscle bands and this adds to the strength and elasticity of the uterine muscle layers. The blood circulation to the uterus increases as the fetus and the placenta develop. At the end of the third trimester one sixth of the maternal blood volume is contained within the vascular system of the uterus. Throughout pregnancy the uterus contracts painlessly and irregularly, thus stimulating the movement of blood through the intervillous spaces of the placenta (the so-called Braxton Hicks contractions).

Cervix

Oestrogen stimulates the growth and activity of the glandular tissue of the cervix. Thick, sticky mucus is secreted and accumulates to form a mucous plug, known as the operculum, which seals off the endocervical canal to prevent the ascent of bacteria into the uterus. This plug is expelled when the cervix dilates during labour.

The increase in blood vessels and blood flow through the cervix results in a purple discolouration known as the Chadwick sign.

Vagina and vulva

The vaginal epithelium increases in size, there is a thickening of the mucosa and an increase in the vaginal secretions. These changes are also oestrogen induced. The vaginal secretions are thick, white and acidic with a pH of 3.5 to 6.0. This low pH plays a significant role in preventing infections. It also favours the growth of yeast organisms, resulting in candidiase, a common infection in pregnancy.

The smooth muscle cells of the vagina also increase in size with an accompanying loosening of the connective tissue. By the end of pregnancy, the vaginal wall and the perineum have become sufficiently relaxed to accommodate the birthing process.

Breasts

Oestrogen and progesterone stimulate breast changes before or soon after the first menstrual period is missed. There is an increase in glandular tissue in preparation for lactation. By the end of the second month superficial veins are prominent on the skin and nipples are more erectile. Montgomery's tubercles are also enlarged and are visible on the areola. These sebaceous glands secrete sebum, which keeps the nipple and areola soft and supple. The pigmented area around the nipple darkens and is known as the primary areola. The mottled skin changes that often appear beyond the primary areola are known as the secondary areola. Colostrum is secreted from the breasts during the third trimester. This substance is rich in proteins, minerals and antibodies and continues to be secreted two to four days after the birth of the baby.

Respiratory system

Oestrogen-induced oedema and vascular congestion of the nasal mucosa result in a feeling of nasal stuffiness as the pregnancy progresses. At the same time the uterus enlarges and exerts pressure on the diaphragm, which is elevated and displaced by 4 cm. This causes the rib cage to widen and the chest circumference to increase by 6 cm. Despite the decrease in the vertical dimension of the thoracic cavity, the vital capacity (maximum volume of air exhaled following a maximum expiration) of the woman does not decrease because of the compensatory horizontal expansion of the chest wall. The upward displacement of the diaphragm and ultimately the lungs decreases the residual volume of the lungs up to 20%. The volume of air breathed in (tidal volume) is increased up to 40% from non-pregnant values at term, to ensure adequate oxygen exchange. Oxygen consumption increases to meet the needs of the mother and her growing fetus. Breathing changes from abdominal to thoracic as pregnancy advances. These respiratory changes are often experienced as a shortness of breath.

Haematological system

Composition of blood

Changes in the haematological system are one of the most prominent in the body of the pregnant woman. These changes may lead to iron and folate deficiency as the haemoglobin, serum iron and folate and red cell folate concentrations fall and the total iron-binding capacity rises. Enkin et al (2000:42) draw attention to the fact that in developed countries these changes do not need any interventions as they are physiological changes that the body can compensate for. On the contrary, in developing countries, the amount of iron and folate in the dietary sources may not meet the additional demands placed on the maternal iron and folate stores of the mother by the growing fetus, the placenta and the increased maternal red cell mass (see Chapter 22 for a discussion of anaemia).

Blood volume

The blood volume increases from early pregnancy to 40 to 45% above non-pregnancy values. The increase in blood volume is made up by an increase in plasma volume of 40 to 60% up to the 34th week.

Red blood cells

The total volume of red blood cells in the circulation increases in response to the increased oxygen requirements during pregnancy. The red blood cell volume increases to 20% above normal non-pregnancy values and in women taking iron supplementation there is an increase of 30%.

The normal haemoglobin values (12 to 16 g/dl) and haematocrit values (37 to 47%) decrease noticeably during the second semester, when a rapid expansion of blood volume occurs. As the plasma volume increase is much greater than the red cell mass, there is a haemodilution effect, which is most apparent from the 32nd to 34th week of pregnancy. This is referred to as the *physiological anaemia of pregnancy*. If the haemoglobin values drops to 10 to 11 g/dl or less and the haematocrit drops to 35 g/dl or less, anaemia is diagnosed.

White blood cells

The white cell count increases during the second and third trimesters of pregnancy from 3 000 to 15 000/mm³. During labour it can increase up to 30 000/mm³ and in the early postnatal period an increase of 25 000/mm³ may be reached. This physiological leucocytosis enhances the phagocytic and bacteriocidic properties of the blood.

Clotting factors

Although the bleeding and clotting times of pregnant women do not differ significantly from that of non-pregnant women, blood factors I and VII to X rise progressively. Factor XI and XIII levels, as well as platelets, drop to create a somewhat hypercoagulate state. The puerperium is regarded as the most dangerous period for the development of venous thrombosis.

Cardiovascular system

Cardiac position and size

The growing uterus exerts pressure on the diaphragm, pushing the heart upward and to the left. This lateral displacement makes the heart appear somewhat enlarged on X-ray examination. As a result of changes in the position and size of the heart, an increase in blood volume and cardiac output, auscultatory changes in the form of audible functional heart murmurs occur.

Cardiac output

The cardiac output increases by approximately 35% (from 5 to 7 litres per minute), mainly as a result of a response to increased demands for oxygen. Heart rate increases by 15 to 20 beats per minute. Although the average woman's heart can cope with these changes, strain is exerted on the heart of a pregnant woman with a co-existing cardiac condition.

The cardiac output can be influenced by maternal position. When lying on her back, the venous return is reduced due to pressure of the pregnant uterus on the inferior vena cava, resulting in reduced cardiac output and a consequent drop in blood pressure. This phenomenon, known as the *supine hypotension syndrome* or *vena cava syndrome*, is more prominent in the third trimester.

Blood pressure

The blood pressure decreases slightly with a diastolic decrease of 10 to 15 mm Hg, reaching its lowest point during the second trimester. This is because of a decrease in the peripheral vascular resistance due to the smooth muscle relaxing effect of progesterone. The venous pressure may be increased by as much as 25 cm H_2O in the lower limbs near term. This contributes to oedema of the legs and vulva, as well as aggravation of haemorrhoids.

> Many of these physiological changes may resemble the clinical picture of cardiac disease. The midwife needs to assess the pregnant woman vigilantly.

The femoral venous pressure slowly rises as the growing uterus exerts increasing pressure on the veins of the lower limbs. There is a tendency for blood to stagnate in the lower extremities with a resulting depending oedema and an increased susceptibility to developing varicosities in the legs, vulva and the rectum.

Gastrointestinal system

Nausea and vomiting, referred to as *morning sickness*, sets in during the first trimester of pregnancy. It may occur as a result of human chorionic gonadotrophin and increased oestrogen levels or because of decreased glucose levels due to increased glucose utilisation by the growing fetus.

As the uterus grows it displaces the stomach and intestines towards the back and the sides of the abdomen. This ultimately slows intestinal peristalsis and the emptying of the stomach, leading to heartburn, constipation and flatulence. Progesterone also affects the smooth muscle of the intestine thereby further slowing down intestinal motility. Heartburn may result from a reflux of stomach contents

into the oesophagus because of the upward displacement of the stomach by the uterus and a relaxed cardio-oesophageal sphincter due to the hormone relaxin.

Other changes include hypertrophy and softening of gum tissue due to a proliferation of local blood vessels. The gums bleed easily when mildly traumatised. Oestrogen may also cause increased saliva formation.

The slowing down of the gastrointestinal tract may also result in delayed emptying of bile from the gall bladder. This may lead to increased cholesterol levels and predispose the woman to gall stone formation.

Weight gain

The woman's pre-pregnancy weight should be determined. An average weight gain of 11.2 to 16 kg is acceptable for the entire duration of the pregnancy. Weight gain should average at 0.4 kg per month during the first trimester and 0.4 kg per week during the second and third trimesters.

Underweight women should gain slightly more, that is 0.5 kg per month during the first trimester and 0.5 kg per week during the second and third trimesters. An obese woman should not gain more than 0.3 kg per week.

> Women should be advised not to engage in weight loss programmes during pregnancy. A well-balanced diet that meets the fetal nutritional needs should be a priority.

Urinary system

Renal function

Renal function changes to a large extent during pregnancy as the kidneys handle an increased blood volume, metabolic products and also act as the primary excretory organ for the fetal waste products. The kidneys become heavier and larger as a result of the increased blood volume. Urinary output gradually increases. Glomerular filtration rate and renal plasma flow increase by 30 to 50% and remains at this level until term. The higher glomerular filtration rate leads to an increased filtration of glucose into the renal tubules. As tubular reabsorbtion of glucose occurs at a fixed rate there will be accidental spillage of glucose into the urine during pregnancy. However, the finding of more than a trace of glucose in a routine urine sample is considered abnormal until further testing proves otherwise and excludes gestational diabetes.

There is also increased excretion of other solutes due to the kidney's increased workload. These include vitamin B_{12}, folic acid, amino acids, uric acid and some other water-soluble vitamins. The rapid growth of bacteria in the urine is attributed to the excretion of these nutrients.

Fluid retention

The total body water increases to 7.5 litres. To maintain osmolarity, sodium reabsorbtion in the tubules is increased by progesterone and aldosterone. Fluid is retained to aid in the replacement of fluids should haemorrhage occur, and serves as a medium of transport for nutrients to the fetus. Physiological oedema is normal in pregnancy and usually occurs during the third trimester. Ankle oedema results from the dependent position of the legs, which favours the gravitation of fluid.

Ureters

The increased secretion of progesterone causes dilatation of the ureters and contributes to urinary stasis and the increased risk of infection. Retention of fluid and swelling (hydroureter) may occur and is more marked on the right side. The enlarged dextro-rotated uterus compresses the ureters as they pass over the pelvic brim especially on the right side (the sigmoid colon cushions the left ureter).

Bladder

Bladder irritability, nocturia, urinary frequency and urgency are reported in early pregnancy. Urinary frequency results from increased bladder sensitivity and later compression of the bladder. During the second trimester the bladder is pushed up into the abdomen. This displacement of the bladder results in the urethra being lengthened to 7.5 cm.

The increased vascularity in the pelvic region and decreased drainage of blood from the base of the bladder results in oedema of its tissue and renders the bladder more susceptible to trauma and infection during labour and the birthing process.

Skeletal adaptations

Relaxin and progesterone cause the gradual softening of the collagen in the body joints, thereby allowing for laxness in the lower spine, softening of the sacro-coccygeal joints and the symphysis pubis, and softening and widening of the pelvic joints. These changes facilitate the descent of the fetus and ultimately the birthing process.

As pregnancy advances and the uterus enlarges, the woman's upper spine is thrown backward to compensate for the heavy anterior weight of the uterus. This posture often causes backache because of the lumbar spine curving forwards (*lordosis*). The woman tends to stand straighter and taller, adopting what is referred to as the '*pride of pregnancy*' posture.

Calcium and phosphorus needs are increased to 1.2 g per day to meet the demands of the growing fetus.

The skin

General changes include hyperpigmentation, hair and nail growth, and increased activity of the sweat and sebaceous glands. Face and body pigmentation occurs from the 8th week of pregnancy as a result of melanocyte-stimulating hormone. *Chloasma gravidarum* (the face mask of pregnancy) is the brown pigmentation that appears on the forehead, nose and malar eminences.

The nipples, areola, vulva and thighs may darken. A dark, vertical line, known as the *linea nigra* may appear on the abdomen between the sternum and the symphysis pubis. *Striae gravidarum,* also referred to as stretch marks, appear in about 90% of women. They appear as reddish or purplish linear marks and may cause itching in some women. After delivery they recede to silverish marks but do not disappear completely.

Endocrinal system

Profound endocrinal changes occur that are essential for the maintenance of the pregnancy, normal fetal growth and postpartum recovery. Changes associated with the placental hormones are described in detail in Chapter 7.

Adrenal glands

The adrenals secrete increased levels of aldosterone and corticosteroids. The increased aldosterone aids in promoting sodium reabsorbtion to make up for the increased sodium excretion associated with progesterone. The corticosteroids regulate protein and carbohydrate metabolism.

Changes in the carbohydrate metabolism

Human placental lactogen (HPL) functions as a insulin antagonist and influences the following metabolic processes of pregnancy:

▶ Promotes the breakdown of fats (*lipolysis*) to raise the amounts of circulating free acids available for maternal metabolic use and fetal nutrition.

▶ It inhibits the use of maternal glucose and the production of glucose from non-carbohydrate sources such as proteins (*glucogenesis*). This 'sparing' effect is to ensure that adequate levels of glucose are available for fetal use especially for the periods between meals.

The risk of ketosis

If the pregnant woman does not eat adequate amounts of carbohydrates for a sustained period; ketosis develops from the metabolism of fat as an alternative source of energy. Fetal development may be impaired by constant exposure to ketosis.

In response to the increased level of corticosteroids, the pancreas produces higher levels of insulin. Oestrogen, progesterone and HPL counteract the effect of insulin during pregnancy,

therefore a diabetic woman who has been insulin dependent during her pre-pregnancy state will need more insulin during pregnancy (this must be monitored meticulously).

This insulin counteracting effect is a physiological adaptation to ensure a readily available source of glucose for activities of the fetus.

Immune system

Immunological responses seem to decrease during pregnancy. This occurs to prevent the woman's body from rejecting the fetus as if it were a transplanted organ. IgG production is decreased thus making the pregnant woman more prone to infection during pregnancy. The white blood cell increase may be compensatory to provide protection for the woman and the fetus.

Factors such as the overall health status, age, lifestyle, environment and nutrition affect the functioning of the immune system. The midwife carries out an ongoing assessment for factors that place the woman at risk and then implements appropriate interventions.

Psychological changes of pregnancy

Pregnancy and childbirth are events that touch almost every aspect of the human experience: biological, psychological, social and cultural. Individual adaptations to childbearing on each of these levels may be quite different, depending on the age, health, socio-economic status and cultural background of the woman and her family. Despite the natural variations, there are recurring themes and patterns that can guide the midwife in providing sensitive and effective care.

Acceptance of pregnancy

In the initial and during ongoing assessments of the antenatal period, the midwife should determine the woman's degree of readiness for the pregnancy and her acceptance thereof. A woman's response may range from excitement, biological fulfilment and high self-esteem to shock, disbelief and even despair. For the adolescent a crisis situation may develop as pregnancy can result from sexual experimentation and peer group pressure, or even rape.

The hormonal changes could also result in an emotional response such as increased irritability, outbursts of tears and anger that alternate with feelings of cheerfulness with little or no instigation. Even women who are pleased to be pregnant experience these conflicting feelings.

For many women pregnancy is regarded as one of the important goals of their lives and this affects their acceptance of pregnancy and eventual adaptation to motherhood. In contrast, other women have conflicting feelings, such as not wanting the pregnancy or deciding whether to maintain or relinquish a career or promotion opportunity.

Responses to change in body image

The woman's expanding abdomen may become a source of pride or conversely, an object of ridicule and shame. Her partner's response often affects the manner in which she will respond. Men respond in a variety of ways to their partner's changing shape. Some adopt a deep sense of admiration and pride that their manhood has been proven. Others may make derisive comments about the changes in her figure and show resentment.

The most important of the pregnant woman's significant others is the father of her child. There is increasing evidence that the woman who is nurtured by her partner during pregnancy has fewer emotional and physical symptoms, fewer labour and childbirth complications and a more successful postpartum adjustment. To most women the partner is a stabilising influence and a good listener to her doubts and fears.

Couples who do not understand the physiological and emotional changes of pregnancy can become distanced and upset by their partner's behaviour. A better understanding and appreciation of the partner's point of view can be fostered with increased communication. Couples are then able to identify problems, offer the necessary support and strengthen the bond between them as a result.

Adaptation of other family members

There are a variety of responses but reference will be made to only a few aspects.

The response of siblings to pregnancy varies with age and dependency needs. Younger children demonstrate more 'clinging' behaviour, for example, some revert to dependent behaviours in toilet training. School-age children are curious and ask numerous questions. Generally they are excited about the pregnancy and enjoy being included in preparations for the new baby.

Adolescents, on the other hand, are preoccupied with establishing their own sexual identity, so they seem to take on a more critical role. They have difficulty in accepting the evidence of their parents' sexual activity. Most grandparents are delighted with the prospect of a new addition to the family. Grandparents act as a potential resource for families. However, if parents are faced unexpectedly with grandparenthood they could respond with outbursts of anger and consequent estrangement.

During her assessment the midwife should identify these diverse situations and provide counselling, support and appropriate referral as the need arises.

> **CRITICAL THINKING EXERCISE**
> Interview a woman aproximately six weeks after the birth of her baby. Determine what sources of social support she is using, as well as any support systems that may need to be mobilised.

Conclusion

The South African society, often referred to as the 'rainbow nation' with a range of cultural diversities, provides a challenge for midwives who need to determine cultural beliefs and practices during the assessment of the pregnant woman.

There is widespread acculturation, in which some beliefs and practices are modified or dropped in favour of practices of the dominant culture. Over and above this, individuals also vary tremendously in their traditionalism or modernism, even within the same cultural group (see Chapter 2).

Midwives should be cautioned against imposing their own value systems on the women and their families. Assessment of psychosocial and cultural aspects is the foundation for a holistic approach to midwifery care.

References

Bobak, I. M. & Jensen, M. D. 1993. *Maternity and gynecologic care: The nurse and the family*. Fifth edition. St Louis: Mosby.

Fraser, D. M. & Cooper, M. A. (Eds.) 2003. *Myles textbook for midwives*. London: Churchill Livingstone.

Ladewig, P. W., London, M. L. & Olds, S. B. 1994. *Maternal–newborn nursing*. Third edition. Redwood City: Addison-Wesley Nursing.

May, K. A. & Mahlmeister, L. R. 1994. *Maternal and neonatal nursing: Family-centred care*. Third edition. Philadelphia: JB Lippincott.

Nolte, A. G. W. 1998. *A textbook for midwives*. First edition. Pretoria: J.L. van Schaik Publishers.

Pillitteri, A. 1999. *Maternal and child health nursing*. Third edition. Philadelphia: JB Lippincott.

Sellers, P. M. 1993. *Midwifery. Volume 1*. Cape Town: Juta.

Chapter 9

Antenatal assessment and care

Dr Christa van der Walt

Introduction

The approach to antenatal care presented in this book is based on the principles of the new World Health Organisation Antenatal Care Model (WHO, 2002), the Guidelines for Maternity Care in South Africa (DoH, 2002) and the principles of the Perinatal Self-education Programme (1998). These principles are developed for women with low-risk pregnancies. The care of women with pre-existing health problems, pregnancy-related problems and/or any risk factors are discussed in other chapters (see Section 6).

A sensitive approach by a skilled midwife will ensure appropriate care and will contribute towards a positive outcome, not only of the pregnancy and childbirth, but also with regard to the experience of the pregnancy.

Antenatal care should therefore focus on identification of risk factors, as well as on identifying and meeting the needs of families with regard to health promotion. The midwife is in a key position to guide women and their families through this period, pointing out sources of support and offering health information that can have a life-long effect on the families and communities.

The aim of antenatal care

Risk identification and health education remain the hallmark of antenatal care by the midwife. Women who receive antenatal care early in pregnancy and who have more antenatal visits tend to have lower maternal and perinatal mortality and better pregnancy outcomes.

The overall aims of antenatal care are therefore to:
▶ Support and encourage healthy adaptation, both physically and emotionally, to pregnancy, childbirth and parenting.
▶ Monitor the progress of pregnancy in order to ensure maternal health and normal fetal development and growth.
▶ Recognise deviations from normal to prevent the pregnancy from having a detrimental effect on maternal health.
▶ Ensure that the woman and her partner are prepared for childbirth and parenthood.
▶ Offer advice for future family planning (fertility control).
▶ Assist the woman in choosing a method to feed her baby.

These aims may be achieved by:
▶ Screening for pregnancy and other health problems and needs.
▶ Assessment of pregnancy risk status.
▶ Management of problems and needs that may arise during the antenatal period.
▶ Administration of medications that may improve the pregnancy outcome.
▶ Provision of health information to pregnant women, families and communities.

▶ Physical and psychological preparation for childbirth and parenthood.
▶ Empowering the woman (and the family and community) to take responsibility for her care by attending antenatal care and monitoring herself for the presence of danger signs that should be reported immediately.

The process of antenatal care

Antenatal care follows a problem-solving, solution-focused and action-oriented approach (See Table 9.1).

Who is responsible for antenatal care?

Midwives are responsible for the antenatal care of pregnant women with low risk for complication. Women with pre-existing conditions require specialist medical attention. Protocols and the scope of practice of the registered midwife should guide all referrals. Referral policies should be available at all facilities providing antenatal care. Feedback and support on the appropriateness of referrals should take place as part of total quality improvement.

Minimum staff requirements should be met in each clinic and hospital antenatal service. Advanced midwives play an important role as supervisors for the antenatal clinic.

In South Africa private midwives, general practitioners and obstetricians also provide antenatal care. Co-operation between these practitioners and practitioners from the public sector is essential to ensure continuity of care when a woman is referred or chooses to change caregivers. It is especially important to include the results of all special investigations so as to save valuable time and money by minimising the duplication of these tests.

Risk assessment

One of the principles of antenatal care is to screen pregnant women for risk factors to ensure that they get appropriate care and the correct

Table 9.1 The process of antenatal care

Assessment	Perform a holistic, systematic and thorough assessment:
Screening for health and socioeconomic conditions likely to increase the possibility of specific adverse outcomes.	▶ History ▶ Physical assessment ▶ Examination of all aspects of pregnancy that may pose a risk to the woman and/or her unborn baby. ▶ Socioeconomic, cultural, emotional and cognitive needs regarding pregnancy, childbirth and parenting. ▶ Identify risk factors and needs as a basis for planning individualised antenatal care.
Plan Providing preventive, promotive and therapeutic interventions known to be beneficial.	▶ Plan together with the woman and her support person or family. ▶ Record the needs and problems, as well as the plan to address these issues, on the antenatal card. ▶ Address future issues such as birth plan, emergencies, family planning, parenting and breastfeeding.
Evaluation	▶ Evaluate progress at follow-up visits. These visits must have clear objectives. ▶ Review the antenatal care plan and adapt where and when necessary.

level of health care, especially in a country like South Africa where transport in emergency is problematic.

Once a pregnancy has been diagnosed, the woman should be assessed for complications of pregnancy and for any risk factors that may threaten her and her unborn baby's wellbeing. This will also give an indication of when she must return for the follow-up visit and at which level her care will be the best. A woman with a risk factor must be followed up more frequently and evaluated with caution.

Women with risk factors for complications during childbirth only (such as a previous caesarean section), or those with a history or intrapartum complications but with otherwise normal pregnancies, should receive routine antenatal care. In such cases it is important that the place of birth should be selected carefully, arrangements should be made in advance to ensure that appropriate facilities for the birth of the baby and possible complications will be available and that the woman will be able to reach them in a timely manner.

The antenatal card

Good practitioners make good decisions based on good information (DoH, 2002). In busy antenatal clinics we may easily miss important information and fail to identify critical needs and problems of the women. Therefore, all ante-natal care should be recorded on the woman's antenatal card, which is issued at the first visit. The woman should be informed to bring this card with her, not only to the antenatal clinic, but also to any visit to a health care provider while she is pregnant. Complete records should be maintained at all times.

The antenatal card is completed at every visit and is retained by the woman until the birth of her baby, where after it is kept at the place of birth or final referral. Clinics do not need to keep a copy of this record, although information that is required to calculate quality of care should be kept in the clinic. These include a record of the number of first visits before 20 weeks, the number of first visits after 20 weeks, the total number of first visits, and the number of follow-up visits.

Essential information to be recorded on the antenatal card
- Name, age, parity and gravidity.
- Details of previous pregnancies, including causes of perinatal death, mode of delivery, indications for caesarean section and complications such as postpartum haemorrhage.
- Previous illnesses that might influence this pregnancy, including cardiac, renal and diabetic disease.
- History of the present pregnancy.
- The date of the first day of the last menstrual period (LMP) and the estimated date of delivery (EDD).
- The estimated period of gestation by dates (POGD) correctly recorded or plotted on the antenatal graph at each visit.
- Future methods of family planning (fertility control).

Examination
- Maternal height and weight.
- Blood pressure (recorded at each visit).
- Auscultation of the maternal heart for cardiac disease.
- Estimation of period of gestation by palpation (POGP) by utilising SFH (symphysis-fundal height) in centimetres, fetal size, hardness of the fetal head and the amount of liquor, recorded or plotted on the uterine growth graph.
- Estimation whether the gestational period by palpation correlates with the fetal size or whether there is evidence of intra-uterine growth restriction, recorded at each visit.
- Fetal presentation, recorded from 36 weeks onwards.
- Fetal heart heard or fetal movements felt.
- Urinalysis for proteinuria and glycosuria.
- Haemoglobin and Rh group.
- Syphilis test result recorded and treated if necessary.
- Counselling for HIV testing.
- Tetanus toxoid immunisation.

Furthermore, antenatal clinics should keep a record of mothers whose blood has been taken for a syphilis test, the results received, the percentage of positives and the percentage of women with syphilis who have completed the appropriate treatment (DoH, 2002).

The patient-carried antenatal card helps to overcome many of the obstacles in the way of achieving purposeful and effective antenatal care, especially with regard to continuity of care. These issues are particularly important in a migrant population. It also gives the pregnant woman more control during her pregnancy. When a woman comes to the clinic with a different version of the antenatal card, a new one should not be issued. Rather continue with the same card to keep a holistic picture of the woman's pregnancy.

Antenatal clinic record cards are not standardised throughout the country. However, they are very similar. Provision is made for important information to be recorded (see box). Every item is of great importance and must be recorded.

First antenatal visit

The first assessment of the pregnant woman should take place as early in the pregnancy as possible. All women should be encouraged to visit the antenatal clinic as soon as they miss a period, even as early as four to five weeks of gestation. Regardless of the duration of pregnancy at the first visit, all pregnant women coming to the clinic for antenatal care must be seen, registered (booked) and examined appropriately to the period of the pregnancy.

CRITICAL THINKING EXERCISES

1. Ask permission to sit in on an interview between a midwife and a pregnant woman during history taking.
2. Observe the non-verbal communication between the woman and the midwife during the interview, by noting eye contact, facial expression, posture, gestures or body movements, and other sounds, such as grunts and laughter.
3. On the basis of this information, what have you learned about the individuals being observed and the relationship that develops between them during the interview?
4. Did the midwife introduce herself to the woman? What information did she give to the woman about herself? Is she wearing a nametag?
5. How did the midwife address the woman? Was it appropriate?
6. Can you identify any attempt by the midwife to develop a rapport with the woman?
7. Did the midwife give an introduction or explanation about the purpose and function of the interview? Or did she go straight ahead and start requesting information from the woman?
8. How did the midwife obtain the information she required?
9. Would you say the midwife was controlling the interview or is there a more balanced exchange between the interviewer and the person being interviewed?
10. Did the midwife use language appropriate for the particular woman? Were any terms used which the woman may not have understood and which the midwife did not explain?
11. Were any techniques employed by the midwife to encourage the woman to talk more freely or in order to develop the conversation further?
12. Was the woman given an opportunity to ask questions?
13. In what way did the midwife draw the interview to a close?
14. Would you have handled the same situation any differently if you had been the interviewer, and if so, how and why?

In areas where late first visit bookings are a problem, it may be wise to start a pregnancy confirmation clinic, where women can drop in for urine tests. Late bookings often happen in South Africa because of various reasons, amongst others, fear of other women's jealousy. This phenomenon denies women the opportunity to receive advice early in pregnancy, as well as the support of the midwife at a stage when she is confused and uncomfortable because of morning sickness. A woman should never be required to make an appointment for a first antenatal visit at a later stage, as this often does not happen. Women who request termination of pregnancy should be counselled and referred appropriately.

The atmosphere in which the first antenatal visit takes place is very important in establishing a positive first impression of the health service in general. The midwife establishes a relationship of trust with the woman through a therapeutic interview during which a full history is taken. A welcoming, friendly attitude and respect are important factors to ensure that she will come back for further care. If a woman is likely to be a poor attender at subsequent follow-up visits, this visit may be crucial in affecting the future outcome of her pregnancy. Privacy for the interview should be fostered and interruptions should not be allowed.

The history

A comprehensive history should contain the following information:

▶ *Personal information.* Name, age, address,

Objectives of the first antenatal visit

▶ Assess the health of the woman by taking a full history, performing a physical examination and specific screening tests.
▶ Establish the duration of pregnancy and calculate the expected date of birth.
▶ The first assessment of risk factors must be done.
▶ Provide an opportunity for the woman and her family where they are present, to discuss their concerns and expectations.
▶ Offer advice on health and pregnancy-related matters.
▶ Establish a relationship of respect and trust with the woman and her family.
▶ Discuss the plan for antenatal care.
▶ The woman must be counselled regarding this pregnancy and issues of relevance to her at this stage.
▶ Explain the danger signs and signs of labour.

telephone contact number and medical aid information.

▶ *Socioeconomic status and lifestyle.* Request information on the woman's marital status, own and partner's occupations and educational levels, literacy levels, economic resources (currently employed), church denomination, housing (type, size, number of occupants), sanitary conditions (type of toilet, source of water), electricity and cooking facilities.

▶ *Health habits.* Ask the woman about tobacco smoking or chewing, use of alcohol or any other harmful substances, and her eating habits.

▶ *Current pregnancy.* The first day of the last normal menstruation must be determined as accurately as possible in order to calculate the expected date of birth of the baby. Remember not to coerce the woman into giving a date that she cannot remember. Also bear in mind that this date is only reliable if the woman had a regular menstrual cycle. The following factors should be taken into account in determining the reliability of the dates:

◆ The date of onset and the duration of the last menstrual period. If the last period was shorter in duration and earlier in onset than usual, it might have been an implantation bleed.

◆ Women using oral or injectable hormonal contraception must have menstruated normally after stopping the contraception.

▶ *Health or pregnancy-related problems since the start of the pregnancy.* The next step would be to determine if the woman experienced any illnesses accompanied with a high fever, with or without skin rashes, symptoms of a urinary tract infection or any vaginal bleeding. Give attention to any discomfort the woman may experience, such as nausea and vomiting, heartburn and constipation, and oedema of the ankles and hands (see Chapter 11 for advice on these conditions).

▶ *Planned or unplanned.* To support the woman in a holistic manner, it is important to determine whether this pregnancy is planned and wanted, and was there a period of infertility before she became pregnant.

▶ *Date of first antenatal visit.* Although examining the condition of the fetus is not routinely part of a first visit, many women come to the clinic for the first time very late in their pregnancies. Therefore the process should be adapted to include the condition of the fetus and any risks associated with that stage of pregnancy.

Previous obstetric history

An obstetric history consists of the following information:

▶ *Number of previous pregnancies:*

◆ Date (month, year) and outcomes of each pregnancy (live birth, stillbirth, abortion, ectopic pregnancy, hydatidiform mole).

◆ Find out whether the woman knows the cause of a previous perinatal death. If no

cause was found, the risk of recurrent
perinatal death is even higher.

✦ Specify preterm birth and type of abortion (elective, spontaneous, induced for other reasons). Remember that three or more successive first trimester abortions might suggest a possible genetic disorder. A previous mid-trimester abortion might suggest an incompetent cervical os.

✦ Grand multiparity (five or more previous pregnancies taken to viability).

✦ Multiple pregnancies: Non-identical twins tend to recur.

▶ *The birth weight, gestational age and method of birth of previous infants:*

✦ Previous low birth weight babies or spontaneous preterm labours tend to recur.

✦ Previous large babies (4 kg and more) may suggest maternal diabetes.

▶ *The type of birth:*

✦ A forceps delivery or vacuum extraction suggests that a degree of disproportion might have been present.

✦ If the woman had a previous caesarean section, determine if it was done for a recurrent cause, such as a 'contracted pelvis', or a non-recurrent cause, such as placenta praevia.

✦ The type of incision in the uterus is also important. The pregnant woman very seldom has the information but it may be found in the folder. Only a women with a transverse lower segment incision

for a non-recurrent cause should be allowed to attempt a vaginal birth.

▶ *Previous complications of pregnancy or labour.* This includes conditions such as pre-eclampsia, preterm labour, diabetes, antepartum haemorrhage, prolonged labour, shoulder dystocia, retained placenta, postpartum haemorrhage, uterine inversion and postpartum depression.

Medical history

Always remember that a medical condition may get worse during pregnancy. For example, a pregnant woman with a valvular lesion of the heart may go into cardiac failure. Some medical conditions may have an adverse effect in the pregnancy, for example a hypertensive pregnant woman is at high risk of developing pre-eclampsia (see Chapter 20). Ask the woman specifically about hypertension, diabetes mellitus, rheumatic or other heart disease, epilepsy, asthma, tuberculosis, psychiatric illness and any other illness such as porphyria or allergies. Ask about the regular use of any medication. This is often an indicator of an illness, which the woman has not mentioned. Certain drugs can be teratogenic during the first trimester, such as *retinoids* used for acne. Some drugs like *warfarin* are dangerous to the fetus late in pregnancy. The woman should be asked about allergies, especially about *penicillin* allergy. Ask about chronic renal disease, sexually transmitted infections, HIV status (if known and the woman is

Definitions

Gravida: A pregnant woman.
Primigravida: A woman who is pregnant for the first time
Multigravida: A woman who has been pregnant more than once.
Nullipara: A woman who has not given birth to a child yet, live or stilborn, excluding abortions.
Multipara: A woman who has given birth two or more times.

prepared to tell you) and other conditions depending on the prevalence in your region, such as malaria and hepatitis.

Surgical history

Question the woman regarding any surgery that might have implications for pregnancy, adverse reactions to anaesthesia, or abnormal bleeding and infection.

Family history

Find out whether the woman has any close family members with conditions that are known to be hereditary such as diabetes, multiple pregnancy, hypertension, bleeding tendencies and congenital abnormalities. These conditions increase the risk for both the mother and the baby.

The physical examination

A complete physical examination is done and the duration of the pregnancy is estimated by palpation. The latter should be clearly recorded on the antenatal card, indicating what method was used to do the final calculation. Careful and accurate estimation of the duration of the pregnancy at the first visit facilitates further management of the pregnancy. The first estimation of pregnancy duration with the expected date of birth will be used for the remainder of the pregnancy.

During the interview an overview of the general appearance and emotional status of the woman can be assessed to determine her general wellbeing. The woman's height and weight at the first visit is used to give an indication of her past and present nutritional status. These measurements are not routinely done, as there is insufficient evidence that it may influence the outcome of pregnancy (Enkin et al, 2000). Should it be the norm at your unit, make sure that you follow the protocol so as to increase the reliability of these measurements. Check for clinical signs of anaemia (pale complexion, fingernails, conjunctiva, oral mucosa, tip of the tongue) and shortness of breath.

During this general observation the woman can sit in a chair with her arm at the level of the heart for the blood pressure to be measured. Make sure that you follow the standard guidelines to measure a pregnant woman's blood pressure (see Chapter 20).

This is also the time to systematically inspect the oral cavity and teeth, to palpate the thyroid, auscultate the lungs, examine the vertebral column for tenderness, kyphosis, scoliosis and lordosis, and to test for tenderness at the renal angles. While the woman is lying on her back the heart and breasts can be examined (remember to tilt her pelvis slightly to prevent *vena cava syndrome*). Link the information gathered during the interview (history) to guide you during the physical examination. All systems need not be examined extensively. The following systems or organs should be examined.

Thyroid gland

A thyroid gland that is visibly enlarged and presents with a single palpable module or a modular goitre is possibly abnormal. This woman must be referred for further investigations. In pregnancy the thyroid is usually slightly, diffusely enlarged on palpation.

Breasts

A full examination of the breasts should be done. A palpable lump or a bloodstained discharge from the nipple is abnormal. It is always wise to use this moment during the antenatal visit to start the education process helping the women to make an informed choice about feeding her baby. Whenever possible women should be encouraged to breastfeed. They should also be encouraged to perform monthly breast self-examinations.

Auscultation of the chest and heart

Listen for abnormal murmurs. These women need to be referred to a tertiary institution urgently. Physiological murmurs are normal in pregnancy due to the increased cardiac output. A functional murmur is characterised by the fact that:

▶ It is mid-systolic.
▶ It is soft – not louder that 2/6.
▶ It is ejective in character.
▶ It does not radiate.
▶ It is usually heard over the mitral or aortic areas.

Abnormal breathing sounds in the upper lobes of the lungs may suggest tuberculosis. These women must be referred for further investigations. It is essential that a midwife is competent in examining the heart and lungs of a pregnant woman.

Abdomen

The woman should lie on her back with a pillow under her head. Always observe the woman's face during the procedure to determine the presence of a drop in the blood pressure, such as paleness, sweat on the upper lip and an anxious look on her face. Confirm that her bladder is empty.

Inspect the abdomen for scars, especially for previous caesarean sections and post-operative sepsis, and for fetal movements. Normal signs of pregnancy such as *striae gravidarum* and the *linea nigra* might be visible. Also observe the size and form of the abdomen. Palpate the abdomen for enlarged organs or masses.

An abdominal examination should be done specifically to determine:
▶ The size of the uterus
▶ Before 22 weeks: Anatomical landmarks are used in estimating the size of the uterus (see Figure 10.1).
▶ The height of the fundus from 22 weeks gestation.

Feel for the fundus of the uterus by gently palpating the abdomen until the fundus is clearly felt. The highest point of the fundus is regarded as the measuring point even if this is not in the midline of the abdomen. Retain an imaginary mark on the skin.

Measure the symphysis-fundal height (SFH) from the top of the symphysis pubis, over the curvature of the abdomen to the imaginary point on the fundus. The tape should not be stretched. Record this measurement on the antenatal card (Woods et al, 1998). Correlate the SFH with the dates and the size of the uterus. From 22 to 36 weeks the SFH is the most accurate reflection of fetal growth and it should be recorded on the symphysis-fundal growth curve to determine the profile of uterine growth. Correct use of this card is described in Chapter 10.

Abdominal palpation should be performed during the last trimester to determine the number of fetuses, fetal lie, position, presentation, estimated fetal weight, amniotic fluid volume, and fetal head above pelvis. Palpation of the fetal presentation and lie should be done from 34 weeks gestation to help the woman in planning the birth of her baby. Estimating the size of the fetus is often a guess but this skill can be improved with experience. The same applies for the volume of the amniotic fluid. Clinical estimation can serve only as a screening procedure for further investigations. Chapter 10 will describe the monitoring of fetal movements and fetal heart rate in detail.

External and internal genitalia

Look for signs of sexually transmitted infections such as shingles or multiple ulcers, a purulent discharge or enlarged inguinal lymph nodes. Pap smears are no longer routinely performed at antenatal clinics (national policy on cervical screening). Vaginal examinations are not done routinely. The same applies for pelvic assessments. For the midwife practising in a unit far from a referral hospital, it may be of value to do a pelvic assessment after 36 weeks in a primigravida to identify candidates for hospital births.

Bimanual examination to determine the size of the uterus can be done in early pregnancy if the duration cannot be determined in another way, for example, by sonar. Be on the look out for tenderness or masses in the adnexa.

Palpation of the fetus

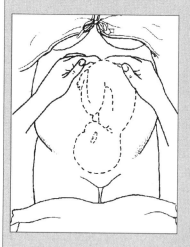

Fundal grip

Face the woman: Place both hands on the sides of the fundus to determine the fundal height. The highest point of the fundus will be used to measure the symphysis-fundal height.

The next objective is to determine the presentation of the fetus, such as cephalic (head), breech or transverse lie. A hard, firm a, ballotable head differs from a breech, being softer, irregular and less ballotable. Should no definite fundus be felt, consider the possibility of a transverse lie.

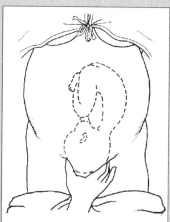

Pawlik grip

The next step is to determine the 'content' of the lower part of the uterus and to compare it with the finding of the fundal grip. This grip must be performed with care as it is often uncomfortable for the woman. As previously mentioned, try to distinguish between a fetal head and a breech. Taking both poles of the uterus in the hands helps to compare the two. The head is harder and can be ballotated, whereas the breech is softer and does not ballotate.

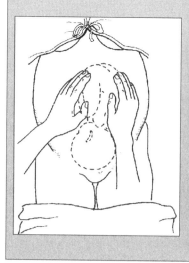

Lateral grip

The next objective is to determine the fetal position by determining to which side the back of the fetus is pointing. Move both hands downwards feeling the consistency of the sides of the uterus. The fetal back feels regular and offers greater resistance to pressure. On the opposite side of the fetal back it may be possible to feel fetal limbs.

You can use the palmar surfaces of the hands to systematically move from the fundus lower, or to move the hands over the umbilical region, 'walking over' the abdomen to feel the side that offers the greatest resistance.

Palpating the head above pelvis

The next step is to determine the degree of engagement of the fetal presenting part, usually the head, in terms of the number of fifths above the pelvic inlet (above symphysis pubis). This is only done when the woman is in labour and is discussed in Chapter 13.

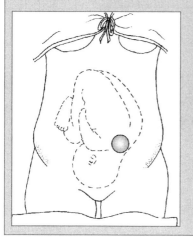

Auscultation of the fetus

The presence of the fetal heart is important in assessing life. It can be heard with a Pinard stethoscope from 22 to 24 weeks or by means of a Doptone from 12 to 14 weeks. Compare the fetal heart with the maternal pulse to ensure that you are hearing the fetal heart.

The fetal heart, can usually be heard best through the back of the fetus.

Other sounds that can be heard are the uterine soufflé (a murmur caused by maternal blood flow through the placenta) and the funic soufflé (the fetal blood flow through the placenta).

Determining the duration of the pregnancy

Use all the available information at this stage to make an as accurate as possible assessment of the duration of the pregnancy. The assessment of the period of gestation and fetal size by palpation require care, skill and experience:

▶ Last normal menstrual period: Last menstrual period (LMP) is only valid if the woman is sure about her dates, as well as where palpation of the uterus and measurement of SFH are compatible with the given dates. Use the 280-day rule (Naegele's rule) (first day of LMP – 3^m + 7 days). This will give you the expected date of delivery (EDD).

▶ The size of the uterus can be assessed by bimanual examination up to 12 weeks.

▶ The SFH measurement is currently seen as the most accurate method to determine the duration of the pregnancy. The SFH measurement is of less value at less than 20 cm and more than 36 cm (corresponding to less than 20 weeks and term respectively).

▶ The result of an early ultrasound examination, that is before 22 to 24 weeks.

▶ The estimated size of the fetus.

Ultrasound is extremely useful for measuring the duration of pregnancy and determining gestational age. An ultrasound of more than 24 weeks is less reliable and should be used together with other methods of gestational age estimation. It is probably still superior to palpation or measurement of SFH.

If there is no correlation between the gestational age according to the LMP and the clinical examination, the following can serve as a guideline:

▶ If the dates and the uterine size on bimanual or abdominal examination differ three weeks or more, then accept the uterine size as the more correct indicator of the duration of pregnancy.

▶ If the gestational age according to dates and the SFH measurement differ by four weeks or more, then the gestational age as determined by SFH measurement is a more correct indicator of the duration of pregnancy.

Conditions other than incorrect dates that cause a difference between dates and the size of the uterus are:

- Uterus bigger than dates may suggest multiple pregnancy, polyhydramnios, a large fetus for gestational age and/or maternal diabetes mellitus.
- Uterus smaller than dates may suggest intra-uterine growth restriction, oligohy-dram-nios, intra-uterine death and/or rupture of membranes.

Screening tests

As far as possible, any interventions or tests should be performed on the same day of the woman's visit. Only examinations and tests that serve an immediate purpose and that have been proven to be beneficial should be performed.

Essential screening tests

The following tests should be done routinely:
- *Syphilis serology*. Non-specific screening tests (RPR, VDRL) are performed using a rapid card test.
- *Rhesus (D) blood group*, using a rapid card test.
- *Haemoglobin (Hb)* screening using a portable Hb meter or copper sulphate screening test.
- *Human immunodeficiency virus (HIV) serology*. Testing must follow principles of counselling and voluntary testing. This is subject to national and provincial policy and available resources.
- *Urine dipstick* for protein and glucose.

Whenever possible, rapid and easy-to-perform tests should be used at the antenatal clinic or in a facility as close as possible to the clinic. Follow the guidelines provided with the kit. These procedures are discussed comprehensively in textbooks such as the Gynaecologic Self-Education Programme (the Department of Obstetrics and Gynaecology, University of Pretoria 2002). When test results are positive, treatment should be initiated at the clinic the same day. Should on-site testing not be available, women should come back to the clinic in two weeks' time for possible treatment should results be unfavourable.

Investigations that are not performed routinely

Screening tests that are available but not necessarily offered because of limited resources are tests for ABO blood group, Triple Test for Down's syndrome and neural tube defects, rubella serology, blood glucose screening, cervical smear, urine culture and mid-trimester ultrasound scan. The pregnant woman should be informed about this at the first visit.

Assessment of the family and social support system

During the antenatal visits, while the midwife is assessing the woman, she also needs to assess the psychological and cultural needs of not only the woman, but also that of her family, as it may influence a woman's acceptance of health care. Being culturally sensitive may help to midwife to render more holistic and therefore, more appropriate care.

Specific information to be obtained concerns cigarette smoking and the use of alcohol. Smoking may cause intra-uterine growth restriction while alcohol causes both growth restriction and congenital malformations. The single woman may need additional support to cope with the pregnancy and to plan for the care of her baby. Also try to identify other socioeconomic risk factors such as unemployment and poor housing. Overcrowding increases the risk of tuberculosis, malnutrition and intra-uterine growth restriction. Look out for any signs of violence and abuse.

During the antenatal period the midwife needs to familiarise herself with the family and overall support system for the woman, specifically with regard to health-related matters. The socioeconomic circumstances as reflected by housing, educational level, beliefs and values with regard to pregnancy and parenting, such as the father's involvement in this pregnancy, should be assessed. Their attitude and expectations towards this pregnancy, previous experiences, social support system and decision-making in the family are all factors that will guide the midwife in planning antenatal care with the woman. The task of the midwife is to help the woman to mobilise her social support system and to establish new ones where current ones are insufficient. Interpretation of the findings of the antenatal assessment means that one needs to sit back, look at all the findings and decide on the meaning or the significance of the findings. The correct action can be taken only if the information is interpreted correctly (MRC and DoH, 2001).

Information for pregnant women at the first visit

Certain information is seen as essential and should be offered to all pregnant women. Information leaflets with this information should be provided at hospitals and clinics. The information should be locally relevant and in the woman's own language. Illustrated cards and pamphlets can also be used, especially where the literacy level is low. This does not replace the need for effective spoken health messages.

Details on perinatal education and appropriate information are discussed in Chapter 11.

Ongoing antenatal care

Until further evidence becomes available, four antenatal visits appear to be the minimum that should be offered to pregnant women without identified risk factors (Enkin et al, 2000:19).

The principle is that the pregnant woman should be seen at regular intervals and with a specific aim.

▶ Should a woman visit the clinic for the first time and you cannot find any risk factors, schedule the next visit according to the clinic protocol and the woman's individual needs.

▶ Should any complications develop, change the woman's risk status clearly on her antenatal card and refer her to the high-risk clinic for follow-up. Her visits will then be scheduled more often according to an individual basis.

Essential information for all pregnant women

▶ Birth plan – estimated date of delivery and way of birth.
▶ Five danger signs and symptoms of pregnancy that should be reported immediately:
  ✦ severe headache
  ✦ abdominal pain (not discomfort)
  ✦ drainage of liquor from the vagina
  ✦ vaginal bleeding
  ✦ reduced fetal movements.
▶ Preparation for pregnancy, childbirth and parenthood.
▶ Special tests that cannot be offered at the facility.
▶ Emergency telephone numbers.
▶ Nearest clinic.
▶ Signs of labour.

▶ All pregnant women should be seen at 28, 34, and 40 weeks. Should they not have given birth yet, they should be seen at 41 weeks again.
▶ The wellbeing and growth of the fetus should be monitored continuously.

The 28th week visit

Assess the woman specifically with regard to the following:
▶ Antepartum haemorrhage.
▶ Signs of pre-eclampsia.
▶ Cervical changes in women with a risk for preterm labour, such as women with multiple pregnancies, a history of previous preterm labour and/or teenage pregnancy.
▶ Anaemia.
▶ Diabetes in women with excessive weight gain, weight of more than 85 kg, a family history of diabetes, previous baby of more than 4 kg and presence of polyhydramnios.
▶ Should the SFH fall below the 10th percentile, evaluate for causes of poor fundal growth.
▶ Should the SFH be higher than the 10th percentile, evaluate for causes of uterus larger than expected according to dates.

The 34th week visit

▶ Assess the woman for all the risks as mentioned for the 28th week visit.
▶ Determine the lie of the fetus. Refer women with breech and transverse lies for hospital delivery.
▶ Select women for hospital delivery such as women with previous caesarean sections and a small pelvis.

The 40th week visit

Should the woman not have delivered yet:
▶ These pregnancies should not be allowed to continue, especially if there are any signs of a compromised fetus.
▶ Low-risk women with no signs of fetal growth restriction may be allowed to wait for another week. This often happens in women with unsure dates. After a week, labour should be induced. It is better to refer these women to level 2 or 3 facilities.

Follow-up visits

The follow-up visits provide information of importance for subsequent care and for encouraging a healthy lifestyle. Perinatal education should be offered on individual or group basis.

Individualised antenatal care cannot be over-emphasised. The advice we offer has to be appropriate for the women and her choices. Religious and/or cultural preferences should be respected. In deciding to admit a woman to the hospital for special investigations, one needs to be sensitive to the effect this may have on her emotionally and on her social circumstances.

We know that there is a strong relationship between a woman's social situation and both her health and her utilisation of health services. Social and psychological support for women should be an integral part of high quality antenatal care (Enkin et al, 2000:22).

Medications and vaccines

In South Africa all women should be offered:
▶ Preconception until 12 weeks: Folic acid tablets 5 mg daily to prevent fetal neural tube defects.

> **The importance of antenatal care**
>
> *It is essential to understand the importance of antenatal care and realise that a poorly planned antenatal care programme is little better that no antenatal care.*
> (Theron, 1996:27)

▶ From 13 weeks: *Ferrous sulphate* tablets 200 mg daily or 30 mg elemental iron to prevent anaemia.
▶ *Tetanus toxoid* immunisation to prevent neonatal tetanus in areas where neonatal tetanus is still prevalent. The dosage is as follows: 0.5 ml intramuscularly followed by another dose four weeks later. A third dose should be given after another six months. A fourth dose should be given a year after the third dose and the fifth dose one to two years after the fourth dose.

Common ailments, such as sexually transmitted infections, common cold and heartburn, need to be treated according to the prescribed protocol and the available drugs. The midwife

> **CRITICAL THINKING EXERCISES**
>
> 1. What facilities are at present offered in the area in which you work to provide preconception care?
> 2. Does the DoH have leaflets, slides or videos on the importance of health prior to conception?
> 3. Are health professionals involved in the school curriculum on preparing for healthy parenthood?
> 4. Where are the local family planning (fertility control) facilities provided and are the physicians and health care workers aware of the importance of screening for health and giving preconception advice?
> 5. Where is your genetic counsellor located and what is the local system for referral?
> 6. Who is the best person to provide preconception care?

needs special training to prescribe or dispense these drugs (consult the latest legislation of the Council of Medicine Control).

In malaria endemic areas pregnant women should receive *sufadoxine/pyrimethadine*, three tablets once during the second trimester, which is repeated once in the third trimester.

Continuity of care

Remember that because of the structure and function of health care in South Africa, very often a woman will receive antenatal care from a variety of caregivers. We have to ensure in creative ways that the care she receives is not fragmented and impersonal. The value of the antenatal card that is kept by the woman has been highlighted already.

Access to care in case of need is an essential element of antenatal care with reduced visits. Written or oral information should be provided regarding where to go and whom to contact, on a 24-hour basis, in case they have concerns or emergencies (WHO, 2002).

In a nutshell

▶ The aim of antenatal care can never been reached if the service is not acceptable for the women and their families. As we are serving a diverse society, we need to develop sensitivity for their needs, expectations, beliefs and values regarding pregnancy, child-birth and parenthood.

▶ Communication skills are an essential prerequisite for overcoming the language and cultural barriers in our society.

▶ Involving women in their own care and giving them more control over the care they will receive is important. The patient-carried antenatal card is an excellent example of how this can happen. Antenatal care as should be individualised and planned, with the focus on problem identification and the search for solutions.

▶ Identify and record the risk factors and rate their severity and significance. If you are uncertain of your measurements and findings, and of their significance, call for help from a physician or an advanced midwife before going any further.

▶ Decide on appropriate action and record your action plan on the antenatal card. This will include interventions and referral if indicated. The appropriate intervention will be determined by the information gained thus far. The risk factors that require referral for further specialised management are discussed in Chapter 18. Again, if you are not absolutely sure that you are able to make the correct decision from the information available, you must consult someone more experienced.

▶ Discuss with the woman and her family, where appropriate, the best place for the birth of her baby (clinic or hospital) and record this on her card. Encourage the woman to organise transport in time.

▶ Discuss options available for future family planning (fertility control) and record her decision on the antenatal card.

▶ The findings at the first visit and the 36-week visit must be double-checked and counter-signed by an advanced midwife or physician or a senior, experienced midwife. The diagnosis has to be correct and the decisions about possible referral or treatment must be accurate. There are no second chances if something is missed. Decide when the woman needs to be seen again, and record the date on her card.

▶ Recording of all the findings should be made in legible, signed entries and clear instructions for ongoing care should be given.

⇒

▶ Good information is needed to make good clinical decisions. Therefore regular audits of records should be done and quality improvement programmes initiated which are driven by the midwives themselves.

▶ Health education that is appropriate and evidence-based, is the 'golden thread' woven through all contact with pregnant women and their families, throughout the perinatal period.

Source: The MRC Unit for Maternal and Infant Health Care Strategies, PPIP Users and the DoH, 2002. Saving Babies 2001: Second perinatal care survey of South Africa.

References

Alexander, J., Levy, V. & Roch, S. (Eds.) 1990. *Antenatal care: A research-based approach.* London: MacMillan.

Bennett, V. R. & Brown, L. K. (Eds.) 1999. *Myles textbook for midwives.* Thirteenth edition. Edinburgh: Churchill Livingstone.

DoH (Department of Health) 2002. *Guidelines for Maternity Care in South Africa.* Pretoria: DoH.

Enkin, M., Keirse, M. J. N., Neilson, J. et al 2000. *A guide to effective care in pregnancy and childbirth.* Third edition. London: Oxford University Press.

Gauteng Department of Health. 1998. *Antenatal care policy document.* Johannesburg: Gauteng DoH.

Nolte, A. G. W. (Ed.) 1998. *A textbook for midwives.* Pretoria: JL van Schaik.

Theron, G. B. 1996. Problem oriented antenatal care. In: Bassin, J. (Ed.) *Topics in obstetric and gynaecology.* Johannesburg: Julmar Communications.

Larsen, J. 1998. *Obstetrics in peripheral hospital.* DEPAM.

MRC Unit for Maternal and Infant Health Care Strategies, PPIP Users and the National Department of Health, 2002. *Saving Babies 2001 Second perinatal care survey of South Africa.* Pretoria: DoH.

Shorney, J. 1990. *Preconception care: The embryo of health promotion.* In: Alexander, J. & Levy, V. & Roch, S. (Eds.) 1990. *Antenatal care: A research-based approach.* London: MacMillan.

WHO (World Health Organisation). 2002. *The WHO antenatal care randomised trial: Manual for the implementation of the new model.* Geneva: WHO.

Woods, D. et al 1998. *Perinatal education programme. Manual 1, Maternal care.* Cape Town: Perinatal Education Trust.

Chapter 10

Fetal health, growth and wellbeing

Joan Dippenaar

Introduction

This chapter will focus on 'fetal surveillance' which encompasses common 'on site' monitoring of the wellbeing of the fetus. Some of the surveillance techniques are more invasive than others and it is therefore important to ensure that the benefit of the test does not outweigh the risk of the procedure. The assessment of the wellbeing of the fetus needs to be studied in conjunction with Chapters 6, 7, 13, 25 and other relevant chapters.

Assessment of perinatal risk factors

Risk scoring is an evaluation used to identify factors that put the health and life of the fetus in danger. Ideally this evaluation should take place prior to conception or at least before 22 weeks of pregnancy. Risk factors can be categorised as risks related to:

▶ *Maternal wellbeing* (maternal diseases and infections).
▶ *Fetal growth and development* (fetal and placental factors).
▶ *Fetal trauma* during *labour* (birth progress and trauma).
▶ *The postnatal period* (infections and respiratory distress).

Guided by these risk factors antenatal care plans should be guided by best practice protocols. The risks identified will determine the level of care, place of birth, level of healthcare worker, number of antenatal visits and special investigations required for a positive outcome of events.

All pregnant women should have routine assessment of fetal wellbeing assessment during the antenatal period. Special consideration should be given to two groups of women with a higher risk for compromised fetuses:

- Women with previously existing historical risk factors such as a previous stillbirth, neonatal death or medical disorders such as diabetes mellitus, hypertension or other illnesses.
- Lower risk women who develop obstetric complications such as antepartum haemorrhage, reduced fetal movements and fetal growth restriction.

The in-utero evaluation of the fetus depends on indirect information gathered since the fetus cannot be observed and felt or tested directly, with the exception of some invasive procedures (see Chapter 24). During pregnancy there are optimal times to gather information. For example, a pregnant woman who only registers for antenatal care after 22 weeks has missed the optimal time to evaluate for Down's syndrome at 16 weeks. The skills and knowledge of the midwife are a determining factor in the quality of the observation, analysis and decision-making process and the subsequent outcomes. Another important 'patient factor' which plays a vital role in the outcome of the pregnancy is the early registration for antenatal care. Baseline information gathered before 20 weeks of pregnancy is more accurate than gathered information later in pregnancy.

Assessment of the duration of pregnancy

The determination of the duration of pregnancy by dates and the expected date of birth has been explained in Chapter 9. As women in South Africa are often uncertain about the date of the last menstrual period, clinical assessment of the duration of the pregnancy is of utmost importance. The information gathered around the early period in pregnancy, as well as early determination of the size of the uterus is more accurate if the history and physical assessment is done before 20 weeks of pregnancy.

Clinical assessment of fetal growth and maturity

Clinically the best way to determine fetal growth is through the serial monitoring of uterine enlargement and symphysis fundal measurement.

Clinical assessment of the size of the uterus

Traditionally the size of the fetus was estimated against the clinical impression of the size of the uterus measured on abdominal palpation. This method is inaccurate after 24 weeks. The fundus of the uterus is palpable at the level of the symphysis pubis at 12 to 14 weeks, just below the umbilicus at 20 weeks, just above the umbilicus at 24 weeks, and just below the xiphisternum at 36 weeks (see Figure 10.1). The fetal heart can be heard with a Pinard stethoscope from 22 to 24 weeks. Fetal parts, the head and other parts are identifiable on palpation from 32 weeks. These findings may be used as a guideline but could be inaccurate in the presence of oligo/polihydramnios, multiple pregnancy, big head, unstable lie, fibroids and obesity. The assessment of the size of the uterus on abdominal palpation gives a crude guideline of the growth of the fetus after 24 weeks.

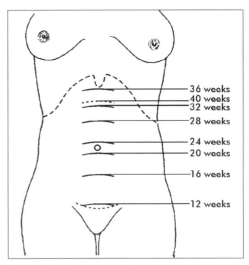

Figure 10.1 Duration of pregnancy as determined by the height of the fundus of the uterus according to landmarks on the abdomen

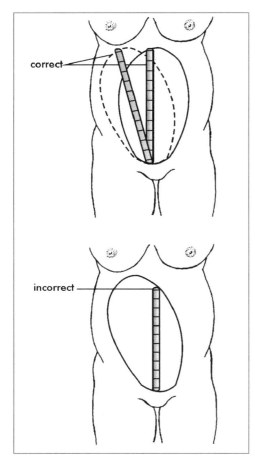

Figure 10.2 Measurement of the SFH

Symphysis fundus height (SFH) measurement

In non-obese women the distance in centimetres between the symphysis pubis and the fundus of the uterus is a more accurate reflection of the duration of pregnancy in the absence of the factors mentioned previously. The SFH is measured as described in Chapter 9 and plotted on the uterine growth card on the antenatal card. The SFH growth curve is compared with the duration of the pregnancy, usually according to the estimated dates. It is important that women receive care consistently from the same caregiver for accurate assessment, or that all caregivers use the same procedure.

Fetal growth cannot be established with a once-off measurement and needs a series of at least two to three measurements with at least two to three weeks between the measurements. According to the Guidelines for Maternity Care in South Africa (DoH, 2000:20) SFH is of little value before less than 20 weeks and after more than 35 weeks. The optimal time for measurement would be two or three measurements between 20 to 35 weeks of gestation. The expected fetal growth for a single pregnancy in a non-obese woman is a centimetre per week, thus a measurement of 28 cm will indicate a pregnancy of 28 weeks. Deviations from this standard if detected can indicate multiple pregnancy if the uterus is larger than expected, or fetal growth restriction if the uterus is smaller than expected. Two types of fetal growth restriction can be identified. *Asymmetrical growth restriction* is more common and is usually ascribed to inadequate supply of nutrition and insufficient blood flow to the fetus due to placental factors and maternal disease such as hypertension. These infants are usually small, with decreased soft tissue mass and disproportionately larger heads. This occurs because the fetus responds to the insufficient placental blood supply by redistributing the blood flow, more to the brain and heart and less to the liver and kidneys. Thus a progressive falling of abdominal diameter should be referred for sonography to determine the head diameter for conclusive diagnosis. *Symmetrical growth restriction,* which is diminished fetal body and head growth, is usually due to genetic or infectious causes, and is more serious in nature as the brain and heart of the fetus are also affected.

The solid line on the SFH growth card (see Figure 10.3) represents the 50th centile and the upper and lower dotted lines the 90th and 10th centiles. If the fetus is growing satisfactorily, the SFH measurements will fall between the 10th and 90th centiles. The woman should be referred for further investigations if:
▶ Two successive measurements are below the 10th centile.
▶ Three separate measurements are below the 10th centile.

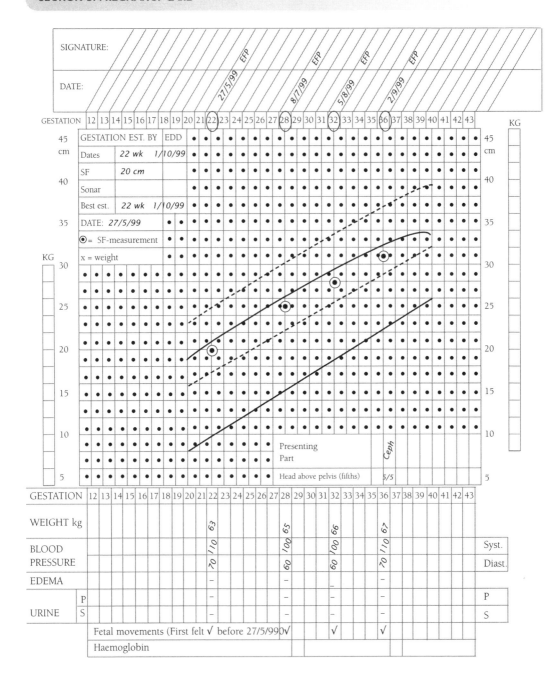

Figure 10.3 SFH graph of a woman with correct menstrual dates (DoH 2002)

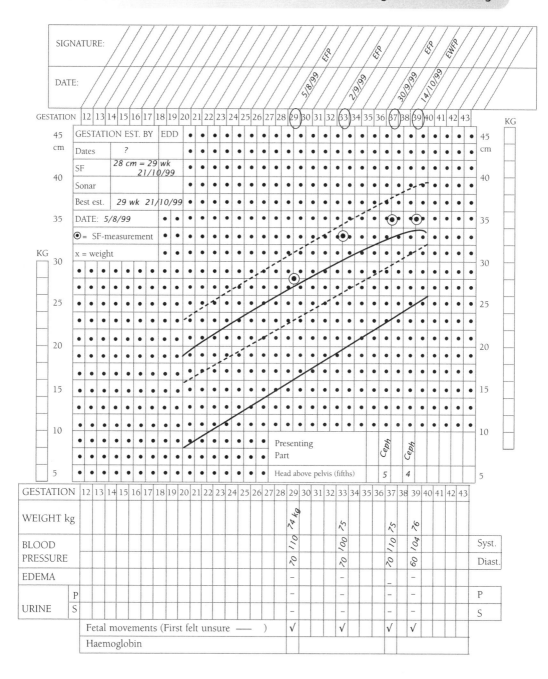

Figure 10.4 SFH graph of a woman whose menstrual dates are unknown (DoH 2002)

▶ Three successive measurements remain the same without necessarily crossing below the 10th centile.
▶ A measurement which is less than that of two previously recorded visits, without necessarily crossing below the 10th centile (see Figure 10.3).

Fetal movements

Fetal movements are first felt by primigravidae at about 20 weeks or by multigravidae by about 16 to 18 weeks. Because of variations between women, this information is not useful in the verification of the period of gestation. Women are aware of 80% of fetal movements, and because fetal movements are a reliable indicator of fetal wellbeing it can be monitored. All pregnant women should be made aware of fetal movements from 28 weeks onward. The DoH National Guidelines require that a woman who reports no fetal movement after 28 weeks must be transported by ambulance to the nearest hospital at once.

A fetal movement card can be used to record the frequency of fetal movements. These movements include kicking, rolling and turning movements (see Chapter 24). This card is not used as a routine but for situations where there is concern about the wellbeing of the fetus, in the presence of risk factors, or if there is a decrease in fetal movements. It is important to

---

Midwife's interventions with regard to decreased fetal movements

▶ Discuss the importance of fetal movement with the mother.
▶ Note the date of first movement.
▶ Educate about factors influencing movement such as nutrition, blood sugar, drugs and smoking.
▶ Discuss deviations (decreased movements from 28 weeks).
▶ Instruct the woman on the use of the fetal movement card.

---

inform the woman about fetal wake and sleep cycles, as well as other factors influencing the fetus, such as maternal blood sugar levels and drugs. The number of movements during an observation period is less important than a decrease in movements when compared to previous observation periods. If a fetus does not move much or the count falls to three or fewer per hour (excluding the rest periods), the fetus may be in danger and should be assessed with more sophisticated methods.

Monitoring of the fetal heart rate

Assessment of the fetal heart rate (FHR)

It is important to know that the fetus is alive in the first place. For this reason the fetal heart should be auscultated from 24 weeks and at each antenatal visit, although the presence of a fetal heart will not give an accurate indication of the neurological status of the fetus. If no fetal heart can be detected it may be a hydatidiform mole or an intra-uterine death, regardless whether the fetus is well or not. The Pinard stethoscope is still the norm in most clinics, but doptones are more available and they are more accurate. A normal increase of the uterus, together with an actively moving fetus, indicates fetal wellbeing independent of other risk factors. The detection of the FHR depends on the gestational age and position of the fetus.

Antenatal fetal heart rate monitoring

The electronic fetal monitoring (EFM) during the antenatal period, is utilised to perform the non-stress test (NST). It is a basic non-invasive screening for fetal wellbeing. The basis of the assessment is that a normal neurologically healthy fetus will have a characteristic heart rate pattern. Average baseline variability (more than 5 bpm) and accelerations in response to fetal movement are reassuring. It is costly to evaluate all pregnancies and a NST is usually only done if indicated.

Electronic fetal monitoring (EFM) is available in most maternity units, and level 2 and 3

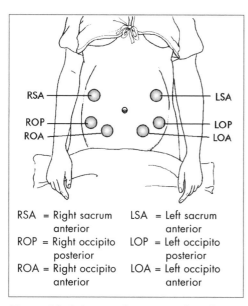

RSA = Right sacrum anterior LSA = Left sacrum anterior
ROP = Right occipito posterior LOP = Left occipito posterior
ROA = Right occipito anterior LOA = Left occipito anterior

Figure 10.5 Positions best to auscultate the fetal heart

facilities. If not, it may be necessary to refer the women to the nearest facility. Antenatal FHR monitoring is not done routinely and is only performed after 28 weeks of pregnancy in women not in labour (no stress or stimuli). It is indicated in the following situations:

▶ A woman with a viable fetus who reports a decrease in fetal movements or poor movements, which does not improve when the count is repeated.
▶ A woman with a high-risk condition that is being managed conservatively.
▶ If fetal growth restriction has been detected.

There are no contraindications for the test. The FHR monitoring is valuable in determining the integrity of the nervous system by measuring the reflex responses that control the fetal heart at that particular moment. An NST is one of the methods for differentiating between fetal distress and a healthy fetus. If the results of the test are equivocal more investigations are needed.

The procedure
First explain the procedure to the woman and then proceed with the test as follows:

▶ The woman is placed in a semi-lateral position (to avoid *supine hypotensive syndrome*), with her knees slightly bent.
▶ The blood pressure is checked in the left lateral position and recorded (and done periodically every ten minutes).
▶ Palpate the fetus to determine the position for the fetal heart monitoring (see Figure 10.5).
▶ Apply the external ultrasound transducer (using ultrasound gel) together with the toco transducer placed on the uterine fundus.
▶ Secure the transducers with abdominal belts.
▶ Set the recording at 1 cm per minute. Record over 10 to 20 minutes.
▶ Check the maternal pulse to make sure that the fetal heart is being observed and not that of the woman.
▶ Place the hand held event marker in the woman's hand. Every time she feels a movement she should press the button which will mark the event on the NST strip.
▶ The midwife should stay with the woman and make sure that the light flicks with each fetal heartbeat and that the recording is clear.
▶ The results are interpreted and recorded.

The midwife is responsible for the performing of the an NST according to established standards of care. Standard and appropriate intervention needs to follow depending on the results.

Interpretation of the NST strip
The fetus may be in a state of quiet sleep, characterised by reduced fetal heart rate variability. The active or rapid eye movement (REM) sleep state is characterised by increased body movements, heart rate variability and accelerations.

▶ *Variability* of the fetal heart rate of more than five beats per minute is an indication of a well-perfused central nervous system (see Figure 10.6).

▶ *Decelerations* of the fetal heart rate occur when placental perfusion is disturbed and the fetus becomes distressed. Vasoconstriction occurs in all major organs of the fetus, causing an increase in the peripheral resistance with a rise in arterial pressure and reflex vagal stimulation. This is then seen as a deceleration of the fetal heart rate. Intrapartum distress will be discussed in Chapter 13.

▶ *Reactive heart rate pattern.* A reactive heart rate pattern is defined as having a baseline of between 110 and 160 bpm with a normal variability (more than 5 bpm), absence of decelerations and at least two accelerations with an amplitude of 15 bpm and a duration of 15 seconds. Remember that a sleeping fetus may have a non-reactive pattern with poor variability, under which circumstances the electronic fetal heart rate monitoring can be repeated after 45 minutes (normal sleep period).

▶ *Non-reactive pattern.* A non-reactive pattern

Standard intervention

Refer for medical attention. Admit at once. Depending on the result, gestational period and risk factors follow the DoH guidelines for the management of fetal distress.
▶ Explain the problem to the woman.
▶ Position the woman in the left lateral position.
▶ Give oxygen by facemask (6 litres per minute).
▶ Start an intravenous infusion with Ringer's lactate at 240 ml per hour.
▶ Get medical assistance or accompany the woman by ambulance to the nearest facility.

Source: DoH, 2000:46

---

does not have the characteristics of either the reactive or the pathological patterns (absence of fetal movement with no acceleration of the FHR). It is best to

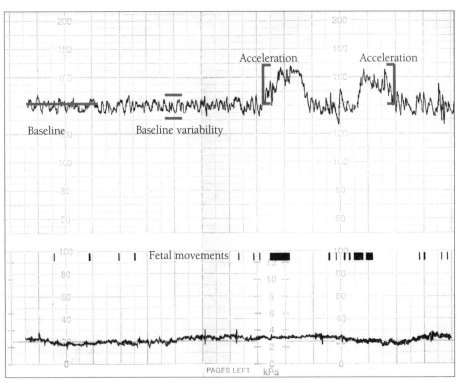

Figure 10.6 Terminology used to describe fetal heart rate patterns

repeat the test or to follow it up with more sophisticated methods (see Chapter 24).

▶ *Pathological pattern.* Decelerations of the FHR occur when placental perfusion is disturbed and the fetus becomes distressed. Vasoconstriction occurs in all major organs, causing an increase in the peripheral resistance with a rise in arterial pressure and reflex vagal stimulation. This is seen as a deceleration of the FHR. Warning signs that the fetus is in immediate danger are absent fetal movements, a baseline heart rate of less than 110 bpm or more than 160 bpm, greatly reduced heart rate variability (less than 5 bpm for more than 40 minutes), no accelerations, repeated late, prolonged (for more than 1 minute) and severe variable (more than 40 bpm) decelerations, which may be extremely shallow following Braxton Hicks contractions, and a sinusoidal pattern (see Chapter 13). Further evaluation is essential.

Conclusion

It is important to consider the costs of antenatal screening and special investigations in the national interest, versus the long-term costs for the caring of sick or abnormal infants. Routine screening of a fetal population can be very costly. The right intervention at the right time by skilled healthcare workers is the most cost-effective approach in antenatal care. All midwives should be skilled in the basic evaluation of fetal wellbeing. Guidelines for routine tests should be adapted for specific regions where specific risks are present. Since the perinatal mortality differs between provinces and rural and city areas, additional steps and protocols may be needed in different provinces to meet health needs in given situations.

CRITICAL THINKING EXERCISE

Identify the routine tests to be done on all women during pregnancy and determine the total cost for a low-risk pregnancy. Compare this with the cost of care of a premature infant 32 weeks of gestation.

References

Bassin, J. (Ed.) 1996. *Topics in obstetrics and gynaecology*. Johannesburg: Julmar Communications.

Boyles, M. 1996. Fetal assessment. *Midwives' practice guide*. No 4. Great Britain.

Cronje, H. S., Grobler, C. J. F. & Visser, A. A. 1996. *Verloskunde*. Pretoria: Academica.

DoH (Department of Health). 2002. *Human genetic policy guidelines for the management and prevention of genetic disorders, birth defects and disabilities*. Pretoria: DoH.

DoH (Department of Health), MRC Research Unit for Maternal and Infant Health Care Strategies and PIPP users 2001: *Saving Babies 2001. Second perinatal care survey of South Africa*. Pretoria: MRC Research Unit for Maternal and Infant Health Care Strategies.

Gibb, D. & Arulkumaran. 1998. *Fetal monitoring in practice*. Second edition. Oxford: Butterworth Heinemann.

Grant, A., Elbourne, D., Valentin, L. & Alexander, S. 1989. Routine formal foetal movement counting and risk of antepartum late death in normally formed singletons. *Lancet*, August 12, Vol 2.

Lindhard, A., Nielsen, P. V., Mouritsen, L. A., Zachariassen, A., Sorensen, H. U. & Roseno, H. 1990. The implications of introducing the symphyseal-fundal height-measurement. A prospective randomized controlled trial. *British Journal of Obstetrics and Gynaecology*. 97:675–680.

Liston, R. M., Bloom, K. & Zimmer, P. S. 1994. Controlled trial of fundal height measurement plotted on customised antenatal growth charts. *Birth*, 21(3)3:135–140.

Muri, J. H. 1998. The joint commission PRYX initiative: Implications of perinatal nursing and care. *Journal of Peri-Neonatal Nursing*. 2(1):1–10.

Simpson, K. R. & Knox, E. 1999. Strategies for developing an evidence based approach to perinatal care. *Maternal and Child Nursing*, May/June 24(3):122–131. http://www.Iprmvn.com

Theron, G. B. 1999. Effects of the maternal care manual from the perinatal education programme on the quality of antenatal and intrapartum care rendered by midwives. *South African Medical Journal*, 89(3):33–39.

Theron, G. B. 1996. Problem oriented antenatal care. In: Bassin, J. (Ed.) 1996. *Topics in Obstetrics and Gynaecology*. Johannesburg: Julmar Communications.

Woods, D. L. (Ed.) 1998. *Perinatal education programme. Manual 1. Maternal care*. Cape Town: Perinatal Education Trust.

Chapter 11

Preparation for pregnancy, childbirth and parenthood

Dr Solina Richter

Introduction

Childbirth education includes education concerning the pregnancy, birth, baby care and feeding, as well as parenthood and family planning (fertility control). It refers to the cognitive and affective needs of the pregnant woman and her family and aims at health promotion behaviour to ensure a healthy pregnancy, birth and postpartum period.

An historical perspective

Childbirth education is not new. It has always been available to women through the 'women's network'. Many women are still learning about childbirth and baby care from their own mothers, sisters and other female relatives. They learned through a tradition of women's wisdom, but also by attending births and helping rear babies and small children. Childbirth was seen as a central social event of which family and friends were part.

The nineteenth and early twentieth century were characterised by the Industrial Revolution, with its associated urbanisation, overcrowding and health problems. The nature of childbirth changed from being controlled by women to a male-dominated medical model. Women started giving birth in hospitals and birth changed from a once family-centred occasion to a lonely, sterile medical procedure. In the 1950s and 1960s the Lamaze method of preparation for childbirth was developed. Women pressed for more information about the birth process and insisted on greater involvement in decision-making. The emphasis was placed on active participation of the woman in the birth process and her choice to practise techniques to improve her 'performance'. The main aim of the midwife, according to this method, was to promote the belief that most women are able to give birth in a natural way.

During the 1980s many women experienced increased pressure because of the multidimensional role as wife, mother and professional person. Women increasingly started to delay pregnancy to further their careers. The family size decreased because of economic, social and cultural factors. Women had little experience of taking care of a baby and the need for childbirth education increased. Women did not question the medical model and passively accepted the childbirth practice of this era. The 1990s were characterised by a new trend in childbirth education which took on a more family-centred approach where active participation during the birth process was emphasised and the labour room again began to reflect a more homely atmosphere.

Now in the 21st century midwives can focus on preparing women for the high-quality technology birth or they can return to the model of less intervention. The medical profession should realise that childbirth education is an essential component of antenatal care.

A South African perspective

The multicultural composition of the South African population poses a unique challenge for childbirth education. A small section of the population has access to advanced technological medical services, while the majority live under poor socioeconomic situations with limited access to medical services. The maternal and perinatal mortality figures are high and there is also a high incidence of low birth weight babies. Furthermore, the South African healthcare system currently has a significantly reduced number of health personnel and services, which are not only insufficient but have also been found to be inaccessible, unavailable and unaffordable.

The section of the South African population with limited access to health services is also characterised by a high incidence of unmarried women, adolescent mothers and woman with a low socioeconomic status. It is unlikely that these women will have the opportunity to attend formal childbirth education classes. There are other obstacles to attending classes, such as lack of transport, low income and social isolation. Further, adolescent mothers are at risk of psychological and maternal behavioural problems that can be detrimental to both the mother's life and the baby's health. Adolescent mothers may experience a high degree of stress. They may be less responsive and less sensitive in their interaction with their babies and tend to provide less stimulation to their babies when compared to older mothers. The babies of these mothers are inclined to have poor health because it is unlikely that the mothers will exercise preventative behaviour, or will continue with breastfeeding and have their babies fully immunised. Different ways of advertising and presenting perinatal education will have to be followed to encourage a high attendance and interest from these women.

In South Africa there is a tendency to discharge women early after the delivery, which highlights the importance of childbirth education as an essential part of maternal and child healthcare. The private sector in South Africa follows a new management style. Managed healthcare aims to provide cost-effective administration, which includes the early discharge of the mother and baby. Due to a shortage of healthcare personnel and facilities early discharge also occurs in the public sector. Mothers and their babies are often discharged without being offered sufficient health education.

Childbirth education is thus extremely important, especially in the South African context, and can play an essential part in the reduction of maternal and perinatal morbidity and mortality. Factors such as delays in obtaining medical help, too many pregnancies, poor attendance of antenatal clinics and any poor health-seeking behaviour of pregnant women can be addressed through quality childbirth education.

A philosophy for childbirth education

A philosophy for childbirth education serves as a framework for action within the childbirth context. A philosophy should develop the midwife's ability to handle abstract ideas, answer pertinent questions, give direction to practice and provide a basis for ethical decision-making. To develop a philosophy of childbirth education, midwives have to examine their own beliefs and attitudes. The midwife should ask herself the following questions:

▶ What are my beliefs about childbirth and parenthood?
▶ What is the ultimate purpose of childbirth education?
▶ What is my role as midwife?
▶ What are my expectations of the women that attend classes?
▶ What are my beliefs about teaching and learning?
▶ Who controls the content of the childbirth education classes?

The purpose of childbirth education

Childbirth education should focus on ensuring a healthy baby and a healthy empowered mother, family and community.

Addressing women's needs for information will allow them to effectively participate in their own care. Childbirth education also gives rise to better parenting and the practice of preventive and promotive health behaviour. Childbirth education has a positive effect on the health of the baby. Mothers who have attended childbirth classes use less analgesics, which may have a negative effect on the baby during labour (Enkin et al, 2000).

The content of childbirth education

The content of the childbirth education programme should be adapted to the pregnant woman's circumstances. The pregnant woman and her family should be offered the information outlined in Table 11.1 during the antenatal, intrapartum and postpartum period.

The midwife should also adapt the educational materials to the specific needs of the pregnant woman, bearing in mind her existing knowledge, previous experience, age, attitude towards childbirth, learning style, socioeconomic status and religious beliefs. The themes should follow each other logically and the content and teaching strategies should focus on reaching the set objectives as best as possible.

An adult learner remembers content better if there is an opportunity for immediate feedback and discussion. Discussion with other class participants also fosters reassurance and the sense of community that comes from sharing experience and information.

Childbirth education should aim to ensure:

▶ A good experience of the antenatal, intrapartum and postpartum period for the mother.
▶ Optimum health for the mother.
▶ The necessary support system is in place for the mother and family.
▶ The mother is able to handle the baby with ease and confidence.
▶ The mother is educated to teach other women about care for a baby.
▶ The mother develops her own problem-solving and life skills.
▶ The mother is prepared to make informed decisions – decisions that are informed by evidence-based research results.
▶ The baby has the best opportunities for physical and psychological health.

Table 11.1 Content of childbirth education

Antenatal period:
▶ The physical changes that occur during pregnancy.
▶ The development of the fetus.
▶ General information and discussion about baby products and the myths surrounding pregnancy and childbirth.
▶ Prevention of a miscarriage and preterm labour.
▶ Diet during pregnancy.
▶ Permissible medication and the use of alcohol/drugs during pregnancy.
▶ Sex during the antenatal period.
▶ Antenatal visits and tests.
▶ The pregnancy-related complaints.
▶ The importance of certain warning signs and symptoms.
▶ Pregnancy-related ailments and problems:
  ◆ Hypertensive conditions during pregnancy
  ◆ Placenta praevia
  ◆ Preterm prelabour rupture of membranes
  ◆ Diabetes during pregnancy
  ◆ Management of pregnancy with previous mitral valve replacement
  ◆ Abruptio placentae.
▶ Exercise during pregnancy.
▶ Involvement of the spouse/partner during the antenatal period.

Intrapartum period:
▶ The first, second and third stages of labour.
▶ Progress of labour without interventions.
▶ Fetal monitoring.
▶ Signs of labour.
▶ Pain relief and comfort measures during the intrapartum period.
▶ The different types of delivery.
▶ Postoperative management of the woman after a caesarean section.
▶ Obstetric emergencies.
▶ Different procedures and instruments used during the intrapartum period.
▶ Support systems during the intrapartum period, such as a doula.

Period of hospital stay:
When the woman is hospitalised during the childbirth period:
▶ A tour of the hospital.
▶ Personal requirements for stay in hospital such as clothing.
▶ Hospital rules and regulations.
▶ Patients' Rights Charter.
▶ Identification of the baby.
▶ The complaints procedure.
▶ The safety and security measures of the hospital.

Postnatal period:
The care of the mother:
▶ Personal hygiene care.
▶ Suitable exercises.
▶ Emotional changes that occur during the postpartum period.
▶ Family planning (fertility control).
▶ Management of the family's needs.
▶ Sex during the postpartum period.
▶ Infant feeding choices.

⇨

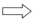

The care of the baby:
▶ Feeding needs of the baby.
▶ Care of the baby.
▶ The baby's appearance and behaviour.
▶ Minor problems that can be expected during the postpartum period.
▶ The immunisation of the baby.
▶ Prevention of cot death.
▶ Assessment of the development milestones.
▶ Developmental supportive care.
▶ Congenital abnormalities.
▶ Signs of illness.
▶ Registration of the baby's birth at the Department of Home Affairs.
▶ Physiological jaundice.
▶ Umbilical care.
▶ Different types of stools.
▶ 'Shaken baby syndrome'.

Educational needs that are specifically applicable to adolescent mothers:
▶ Discussing adoption.
▶ Emotional needs during the adoption process.
▶ Relationship with the adoptive parents.
▶ Single parenting.

Feedback from the class, self-evaluation and comments from various members of the health team provide the midwife with further opportunity to evaluate the effectiveness of the content and refinement of the teaching strategies.

The birth plan

A birth plan is a simple and clear way for the pregnant woman to communicate her wishes for labour and birth to the midwife. Writing a birth plan can be a wonderful guide to self-discovery and the process might help her, if shared with her support people, to understand her feelings and wishes about birth.

Being involved in all decisions about the birth processs is often the key for the pregnant woman to feel good about herself. Even a birth with many interventions can be a very positive experience if the woman is able to participate in the decisions around those interventions. A birth plan should not be seen

Table 11.2 Topics to be considered for the birth plan

The pregnant woman's wishes concerning:	The mother's wishes for the baby concerning:
▶ Place of birth.	▶ Vitamin K_1 injection/drops.
▶ Timing of departure for hospital or birth centre.	▶ Cleaning, weighing, warming, noise, light and examination.
▶ Invasive procedures such as the use of intravenous infusions and monitoring during labour.	▶ Antibiotic eye ointment.
▶ Details of who should be in attendance.	▶ Circumcision.
▶ Plans for pain relief.	▶ Separation from the mother/father.
▶ Birthing positions.	▶ Infant feeding method.
▶ Episiotomy.	

as a way for the pregnant woman to compel everyone around her to behave in a certain way. It is rather a way in which she can take responsibility for her own decisions, be fully informed and remain in control as far as possible. Table 11.2 outlines topics to be considered for a birth plan.

Preconception care

The appeal of pre-pregnancy advice is easy to understand. Whether a fetus is normal or malformed is usually determined by the time of the first antenatal visit. Antenatal care may permit detection of an abnormality, but pre-conceptional precautions may help to avoid it (Enkin et al, 2000:29).

Diet and nutrition

A preconception folic acid supplement can reduce the risk of neural tube defects by more than two-thirds, both for women who are at increased risk because of a previous occurrence of the condition during pregnancy and for women at normal risk. All women, but specifically women who are at increased risk, should be advised to follow a nutritious balanced diet and to start taking a folate supplement (5 mg per day) at least two months before the planned pregnancy. The supplementation should continue for the first three months of pregnancy.

Weight

It is advisable that women be at a normal weight for their build and height prior to conception. Women whose weight falls outside the optimal range may be subject to an increased risk of amenorrhoea and infertility. If a woman is underweight, there is evidence of an association with fetal abnormality, low birth weight and abortion. Overweight women have an increased risk of complications of pregnancy, such as hypertension.

Exercise and relaxation

A woman should be advised to establish a regular exercise programme, and if she is not accustomed to it, she should start at least three months before a planned pregnancy. It needs to provide cardiovascular exercise and general toning. Once an exercise programme is well established the woman is generally encouraged to continue during pregnancy. Exercise improves the circulation and general health and tones the muscles.

Smoking, alcohol and drugs

There is strong evidence that nicotine has harmful effects on the fetus and maternal smoking reduces birth weight. Smoking cessation programmes have a definite place in preconception care as long as they do not include the use of nicotine patches or gum to stop craving.

The damaging effects of excessive alcohol consumption in pregnancy include:

▶ Fetal growth restriction, mental retardation and *fetal alcohol syndrome* and altered neonatal behaviour. Developmental abnormalities have been associated with regular consumption of as little as 28.5 ml (two standard drinks) per day. Not only the regular drinker, but also the occasional drinker with the occasional binge are believed to be at risk. For this reason, women should be advised to reduce and preferably discontinue alcohol consumption before and during the pregnancy.

▶ Many drugs are known to have an adverse effect on pregnancy. They include self-medication such as cold remedies, painkillers, antacids, laxatives, as well as herbal and traditional medicine. However, their effect in the period before conception is not clearly known. The use of any medication during pregnancy should be carefully advised and expert knowledge should be consulted before use.

Family planning (fertility control)

A woman who takes a contraceptive pill is advised to have two to three normal menstrual cycles before falling pregnant. The exact date of conception can then also be determined which provides a more accurate expected date of birth. If an intra-uterine device is being used the woman should be advised to have it removed and wait a month before attempting to become pregnant. During the waiting period barrier methods of contraception can be used.

Infection

All women planning a pregnancy should have their immune status checked and be given a vaccine if necessary. Any pre-existing infection such as urinary tract infection, or a respiratory tract infection, or a sexually transmitted disease in either partner should be treated before conception is attempted.

Lead and chemicals

The association of lead poisoning with mental retardation and hyperactivity in children is well established and there is also evidence that it can result in congenital abnormalities and perinatal death. Any form of lead such as that found in petrol fumes, paint and solder should be avoided in the preconception period and thereafter.

Effects from radiation and chemicals such as gases, solvents, dusts and pesticides have been proven to affect the gonads of both men and women. Employers are obliged to tell their employees with which potential hazardous chemical they are working and ensure that they take the necessary precautions.

Basic medical screening

A basic physical examination should include a relaxed discussion with the woman about her dietary habits, lifestyle and risk of exposure to hazardous substances. It should include a general examination and height, weight, and blood pressure should be measured. A gynaecological examination should be done to screen for vaginal infections and a cervical smear should be performed. The following tests should also be administered:
- Urinalysis for a possible urinary tract infection.
- Blood tests for haemoglobin count, rubella immunity and syphilis.
- Stool sample tests for any possible

malabsorption or parasite infestations where these conditions are endemic.
- If subfertility or infertility is suspected a semen count can be requested. It should also be done if there is high alcohol consumption or the man has had a recent debilitating illness.

Pre-existing medical conditions

Drug therapy for existing medical conditions should be reduced to the minimum level for stabilisation of the condition before embarking on a pregnancy. A woman who has undergone major surgery or is receiving long-term medical treatment has to go for a thorough medical check-up and seek medical advice before falling pregnant.

Genetic counselling

Genetic counselling is advised if a close relative has had a child with an abnormality. If hereditary factors may play a part, the couple should be referred to a geneticist who will conduct further investigations and advise them about the likelihood of a recurrence. The couple can then make the decision whether to continue with the pregnancy or not.

Common discomforts associated with pregnancy

Pregnant women may experience a number of discomforts which the midwife should offer advice on for relief and intervention should it be needed.

Reproductive system

Breast tenderness and leakage of colostrum

The woman should wear a supportive bra, use absorbent pads and keep her nipples and areola dry. Soap should be avoided to prevent the skin around the nipple drying out (see Chapter 30).

Leucorrhoea

Leucorrhoea is the term used for the increased white, non-irritating vaginal discharge during pregnancy which is a normal physiological occurrence. Offer practical advice concerning personal hygiene, for example suggest that she wear loose cotton underwear and panty liners that should be changed regularly. However, any change in odour and colour, pruritus and dysuria should be reported to the midwife. Any infections such as *Trichomonas vaginalis* and *Candidiasis* need to be treated appropriately (see Chapter 19).

Frequency of micturition

In the early stages of pregnancy the woman may experience frequency of micturition due to the pressure of the growing uterus on the bladder. It also occurs in the later pregnancy when the fetal head enters the pelvis and reduces the available space. The midwife should advise the woman to drink water during the day but to limit fluid intake before bedtime.

Braxton Hicks contractions

Braxton Hicks contractions are infrequent and irregular contractions felt by the woman. These contractions facilitate the circulation of blood in the placental site and play a role in developing the lower segment of the uterus. Advise the woman to change position, walk for short periods and to practise relaxation techniques. It will also help if she keeps her bladder empty and increases her fluid intake. True labour should be excluded.

Oxygenation and circulation

Nasal congestion and epistaxis

The increased oestrogen levels may bring about hypertrophy and hyperaemia of the nasal mucosa which can result in epistaxis (nose-bleeds) or congestion. Using a humidifier or cool air vaporiser may offer some relief, as can the use of normal saline spray or drops.

Dyspnoea

Difficult breathing is a common symptom at 34 to 38 weeks and it is due to pressure on the diaphragm by the enlarging uterus. Primigravidae may experience lightening and relief in last weeks of pregnancy when the presenting part moves down in the pelvis.

The woman is advised to maintain a good posture, to use an extra pillow at night and to avoid large meals.

Faintness or dizziness

Faintness may be caused by postural hypotension due to pooling of blood in the dependent veins. A sudden change in position can also cause a sensation of dizziness. Advise the women to avoid sudden position change and to move slowly and carefully. It may also help to avoid warm, crowded areas and to exercise moderately to enhance venous return. Hypoglycaemia can be prevented by eating small, frequent meals.

Varicose veins

Varicose veins are caused by the vein walls relaxing due to the relaxin and progesterone hormones. Poor circulation in the lower extremities and prolonged standing or sitting may result in varicose veins in the legs and thighs. Pregnant women should avoid long periods of uninterrupted standing or sitting, constrictive clothing and crossing their legs. Performing moderate leg and foot exercises while sitting or standing, and resting with legs elevated may prevent varicose veins forming. While resting or sleeping the woman should assume a lateral position to enhance renal blood flow and urine formation. Any worsening of oedema, which persists after a night's sleep, and upper body or facial oedema should be reported immediately.

Nutrition, fluid and electrolytes

Nausea and vomiting

Nausea and vomiting occur between weeks 4 and 16 of gestation and it is believed to be caused by elevated human chorionic gonadotropin and changes in the carbohydrate metabolism. Severe and persistent vomiting (*hyperemesis gravidanum*) is discussed in Chapter 22. Support, explanation and reassurance rather than medication should be the initial approach for hyperemesis gravidarum. Helpful dietary advice is to avoid an empty stomach, as well as overeating. Frequent small meals (five or six meals per day) are recommended. Fatty, spicy, strongly seasoned or flavoured food and alcohol should be eliminated from the diet. It may help to eat a dry carbohydrate snack in the morning before getting out of bed.

Bleeding and tender gums

Increased oestrogen levels may bring about hypertrophy and hyperaemia of the mucous membranes. The woman should be advised to perform gentle and frequent oral care and to maintain good nutrition. Regular dental care should be obtained during pregnancy.

Heartburn (pyrosis)

Heartburn occurs mainly because of the displacement of the stomach by the enlarging uterus and the increase in progesterone and relaxin during the pregnancy which decrease the gastrointestinal motility and relax the oesophagus sphincter. The midwife should recommend limiting gas-forming, fatty and spicy foods. It may help if the woman retains an upright position for an hour after meals and maintains a good posture. An overdistended stomach can be avoided by eating smaller meals and sipping milk and herbal teas, while chewing gum and an antacid will help to relieve the symptoms.

Pica

Pica is the term used when a woman craves certain foods or unnatural substances of which the source is unknown. The midwife should be aware of the dangers if women crave a potentially harmful substance.

Ptyalism

Ptyalism is a rare discomfort of pregnancy characterised by an excessive saliva production which is often bitter tasting. This may occur from the eighth week of gestation and it is probably caused by the hormonal changes that occur during pregnancy. Advise the

woman to use mouthwashes regularly and maintain good oral hygiene.

Elimination

Constipation

Constipation may be caused by increased progesterone and relaxin levels and the increased displacement of the intestines due to the growth of the fetus. It can also be caused by the iron supplement that most women take during pregnancy. The midwife should advise on maintaining adequate fluid and daily roughage intake, moderate daily exercise and an established elimination pattern. Over-the-counter remedies should be avoided unless they have been approved by a physician, a midwife or a pharmacist.

Flatulence, bloating and belching

Decreased gastrointestinal motility and the pressure of the growing uterus on the large intestines can cause flatulence, bloating and belching. Air swallowing may also contribute to the problem. It may help to eat slowly and chew food thoroughly. Avoiding large meals, and gas forming, fatty and spicy foods will also reduce symptoms.

Haemorrhoids

During pregnancy, the enlarged uterus presses on the large abdominal veins and interferes with venous return, causing haemorrhoids. Symptoms of haemorrhoids include itching, swelling and bleeding which may be worsened by constipation and straining. Sitz-baths, medicated ointments and ice packs may provide relief and in the case of external haemorrhoids the patient should be shown how to gently reinsert the haemorrhoids while lying on her side.

Physical activity and rest

Fatigue and insomnia

Diminished energy levels usually occur during the first and last trimester of pregnancy. It may be due to a number of factors, such as the hormonal changes, the increased blood volume and workload of the heart, anaemia, incorrect posture or a lack of exercise. Advise the woman to take regular rest periods, to perform relaxation exercises and to follow a balanced diet.

Lower back pain

Many pregnant women experience lower back pain due to the exaggeration of the lumbosacral curve that occurs as the uterus enlarges. The midwife should educate the woman to understand her changing centre of gravity as the fetus grows. The use of good posture and proper body mechanics will prevent lower back pain.

Leg cramps

Painful muscular spasms of the gastrocnemius muscle may be due to ischaemia, a change in calcium and phosphorous ratio or the pressure of the enlarged uterus on the pelvic nerves. The midwife may recommend dorsiflexing the foot or standing or leaning forward on the affected foot. Warming and massaging of the affected area may also help. Including calcium-rich foods such as milk in the diet or supplementing with calcium carbonate or aluminium hydroxide gel can also be recommended. This stops the action of phosphorous on calcium and decreases the frequency and severity of cramps.

Round ligament pain

As the uterus enlarges and rises in the abdomen, the round ligaments stretch, hypertrophy and lengthen. The hormones may soften the ligaments to such an extent that some degree of support is needed. The first round ligament pain is often intense and causes a 'grabbing' pain in the lower abdomen and inguinal area. The midwife should warn the woman about the possible discomfort and reassure her. Wearing a maternity girdle will lift the abdomen and relieve the symptoms.

Skin and nervous system

Chloasma and pruritus gravidarum

Chloasma is a butterfly-shaped area of pigmentation that may occur over the face. The woman should be reassured that it will disappear after

the birth of the baby. It is also not uncommon for pregnant women to experience a generalised itching that often starts over the abdomen (*pruritus gravidarum*). This is thought to be due to the liver's response to the hormones and a slight rise in bilirubin levels. Advise the woman to use warm sodium bicarbonate or oatmeal baths and to avoid using soap and scratching the affected area. Water-based lotions may help to relieve the symptoms.

Carpal tunnel syndrome

Carpal tunnel syndrome causes a numbness, tingling or burning sensation on the hand near the thumb. It is due to compression of the median nerve in the carpal tunnel of the wrist and it usually occurs in the morning. Wearing a splint at night with the hand resting on two or more cushions may bring relief. Carpal tunnel syndrome usually clears up after birth. Any repetitive actions like knitting or crocheting should be avoided.

General lifestyle advice

Travelling

Travelling is unavoidable but the pregnant woman needs to stretch her legs at least every two hours, as well as take extra fluid and empty her bladder regularly. If travelling abroad she should check on any vaccinations needed, the safety of the drinking water and any possible endemic diseases in the area such as malaria. Sufficient preventive measures should be taken to avoid contracting the disease and the safety of this preventive measure should be discussed with the midwife. Travelling in a pressure-controlled plane is safe, however, long-distance travelling by air is not advisable in the third trimester, because of the danger of preterm labour. It also advisable for a woman to carry up-to-date details of her pregnancy so that should something unforeseen occur the information needed is readily available.

Clothing

Clothing should be loose and not constrictive in any way. Women who have large, pendulous abdomens may benefit by wearing a well-fitted maternity girdle. High-heeled shoes aggravate back pain, especially if a woman is already experiencing discomfort. Shoes should fit properly and feel comfortable. Any clothing that restricts the circulation of the lower extremities should be avoided.

Conclusion

The aim of childbirth education should be to share knowledge with all childbearing women and their partners so that they are able to make informed decisions and choices regarding their pregnancies while being guided by the honest experience of their midwifes. Women can thus become active participants rather than passive recipients of midwifery care.

References

Bennett, V. R. & Brown, L. K. 2000. *Myles textbook for midwives.* Edinburgh: Churchill Livingstone.

Creating your birth plan. *Things to think about before labor.* http://www.pregnantmothers-guide.com/library.philadelphia/EPHbirth-plan.html

Cronje, H. S., Grobler, C. J. F. & Visser, A. A. 1996. *Obstetrics in Southern Africa.* Pretoria: J.L. van Schaik Publishers.

Hale, M. F. *The birth plan: Helpful or troublesome?* http://pregnancytoday.com/reference/articles/birthplanarticle.html

Enkin, M., Keirse, J. N. C., Neilson, J. Growther, C. Duley, L., Hodnett, E., & Hofmeyr, J. 2000. *A guide to effective care in pregnancy and childbirth.* Oxford: Oxford University Press.

ICEA Position Paper: The Role of the Childbirth Educator and the Scope of Childbirth Education. 1999. *International Journal of Childbirth Education,* 14(4):33–39.

Ladewig, P. W., Landen, M. L. & Olds, S. B. 1998. *Maternal–newborn nursing care. The nurse, the family and the community.* Menlopark, California: Addison-Wesley Longman.

Lindell, S. G. 1988. Education for childbirth: A time for change. *Journal of Obstetric, Gynaecologic and Neonatal Nursing,* 17(2):108–112.

Lothian, J. 1997. Lamaze and Bradley childbirth classes. *Birth,* 24(2):133–134.

Nichols, F. H. & Humenick, S. S. 2000. *Childbirth education.* Philadelphia: W.B. Saunders Company.

Nolan, M. 1997. Antenatal education – where next? *Journal of Advanced Nursing,* 25(6):1198–1204.

Redman, S., Oak, S., Booth, P., Jensen, M. D. & Saxton, A. 1991. Evaluation of an antenatal education programme. Characteristics of attenders, changes in knowledge and satisfaction of participants. *Australian and New Zealand Journal of Obstetrics and Gynaecology,* 31(4):310–316.

Richter, M. S. 2000. Standaarde vir perinatale onderrig. Unpublished doctoral thesis. Johannesburg: Rand Afrikaans University.

Rollant, P. D., Hamlin, J. J. & Piotowski, K. A. 2001. *Mosby's rapid review series. Maternal–child nursing.* St Louis: Mosby.

Slade, P. 1996. In Niven, C. A. & Walker. A. *Conception, pregnancy and birth.* Oxford: Butterworth/Heinemann.

Tang, P. C. & Newcomb, C. 1998. Informing patients: A guide for providing patient health information. *Journal of the American Informatics Association,* 5(6):563–570.

Standing, T. S., El-Sabagh, N. & Brooter, D. 1998. Maternal education during the childbirth period. *Clinics in Perinatology,* 25(2):389–402.

Zwelling, E. 1996. Childbirth education in the 1990s and beyond. *Journal of Obstetric, Gynaecologic and Neonatal Nursing,* 25(5):425–431.

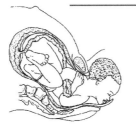

Labour and birth

The birth process

Mpho Modjadji

Introduction

Towards term there are physiological and anatomical changes in both the mother and the fetus in preparation for the process of labour and extra-uterine life. These changes will be discussed in this chapter.

The process of labour

Labour is the process in which the fetus, placenta and membranes are expelled from the uterus through the birth canal. It is a continuous process which includes involuntary co-ordination of uterine contractions leading to effacement and dilatation of the cervix, descent of the presenting part, and voluntary bearing-down effort of the woman, resulting in the birth of the infant.

Bennett and Brown define normal labour as follows: *Normal labour occurs at term and is spontaneous in onset with the fetus presenting by the vertex. The process is completed within 18 hours and no complications arise* (1998:392).

The duration and the outcome of the labour process are determined by five significant factors known as the 'P's:

▶ *Passage*. A birth passage which is adequate enough for the fetus to pass through.
▶ *Passenger*. The fetus must be in a favourable position and small enough to fit through the passage.
▶ *Powers*. Uterine contraction, which must be rhythmically coordinated, and efficient enough to efface and dilate the cervix.
▶ *Psyche*:.Maternal emotional wellbeing must be optimal to cope with the delivery of the fetus.
▶ *Maternal positioning*.

In the normal labour process these five factors act harmoniously and lead to a normal spontaneous vaginal delivery of the baby, placenta and membranes. If there is a deviation on one or more of these factors, poor progress of labour may take place. The rule of 'P's is discussed further in Chapter 26 (see Table 26.4).

Factors that influence the onset of labour

The exact cause of the onset of labour is unknown although we know it is influenced by a combination of various factors.

Progesterone

Progesterone is produced by the placenta and it has a relaxing effect on the uterine smooth muscle throughout pregnancy, thus inhibiting contractions. Towards term biochemical changes decrease the availability of progesterone to the uterine muscle cells. A subtle shift in the balance between progesterone and oestrogen takes place leading to oestrogen dominance.

Oestrogen

As progesterone levels drops towards term the oestrogen levels rise, causing contraction of the smooth muscle cells of the uterus. Oestrogen results in an increased sensitivity of the myometruim to oxytocin and also stimulates prostaglandin formation, causing uterine irritability and contractions. Oestrogen promotes the synthesis of prostaglandin in the decidua and amnion and chorion. This results in further stimulation of contractions due to the effect of prostaglandin on the smooth muscle cells.

Oxytocin

Oxytocin is produced by the posterior hypophysis and it stimulates contractions of the smooth muscle cells of the uterus. Towards term the uterus becomes increasingly sensitive to the effects of oxytocin. Oxytocin stimulates the release of prostaglandin. Oxytocin is not known for the initiation of labour but has an effect on the maintenance of labour.

Prostaglandin

Prostaglandin production increases just before labour, causing stimulation of contractions. It softens the cervix, stimulates oxytocin release and sensitises the myometrial cells to oxytocin, thus causing further contractions.

Fetal cortisol

The fetal production of cortisol near term decreases the relaxing effect that progesterone has on the uterus and at the same time increases the stimulating effect of prostaglandin.

Uterine distension

The uterine smooth muscles are gradually stretched as the pregnancy progresses. Usually smooth muscle contracts when stretched, but due to the relaxing effect of progesterone on the uterine smooth muscle cells, contracting does not take place. Due to the decreased availability of progesterone near term, the uterine smooth muscles react to the distension and contract.

True and false labour

False labour

Strong, frequent but irregular uterine contractions may be experienced. These are false labour pains which are also called Braxton Hicks contractions. Braxton Hicks contractions help to develop the neuromuscular pathway required for the coordinated contractions during true labour. They also assist in effacement of the cervix before labour begins.

True labour

Before labour begins, the woman will have a bloody cervical mucous discharge (show),

cervical ripening (effacement), and dilatation of the cervix may follow. Spontaneous rupture of membranes may take place before or after the onset of contractions, either by a leak or a gush of amniotic fluid. Uterine contractions usually start within 8 to 12 hours after the rupture of membranes. The differences between true labour and false labour are summarised in Table 12.1.

Stages of labour

Labour can be divided into four stages.

The first stage of labour

The first stage of labour starts from commencement of contractions and lasts until full dilatation of the cervix. This is a progressive process that can be divided into three different phases:
▶ The *latent phase* starts from the onset of labour until the cervix is dilated to 3 cm. During the latent phase there is more progress in effacement of the cervix and minimal descent of the presenting part.
▶ The *active phase* starts from 4 cm dilatation and lasts until full dilatation of the cervix (10 cm).
▶ The *transitional phase* forms part of the active phase and it is the period between 8 to 10 cm cervical dilatation. This is the most painful phase for the woman. During the active phase there is more rapid dilatation of the cervix and descent of the presenting

Table 12.1 Differences between true and false labour

True labour	False labour
▶ Regular contractions begin in the lumbar region and radiate around the abdomen.	▶ Lower abdominal pain is experienced as in dysmenorrhoea.
▶ The intervals between contractions shorten.	▶ The contractions are irregular.
▶ Walking may intensify the contractions.	▶ The contractions often lessen by walking.
▶ The duration of the contractions increase.	▶ There is no change in the duration of the contractions.
▶ Show is present and it increases as the cervix changes.	▶ No show is present.
▶ The cervix becomes effaced and dilates progressively.	▶ Effacement of the cervix takes place without any dilatation.

part. The contractions become stronger in intensity, duration increases to 40 to 60 seconds and frequency increases from two to three in ten minutes. There is often an increase in bloody show.

During the transitional phase the woman may experience an urge to bear down (push). Some women experience nausea, vomiting, irritability and even panic sensations as a result of the intense multiple stimuli. They may also experience a sense of helplessness and may often feel that they cannot continue any longer. Symptoms such as hyperventilation and restlessness may also be present.

The duration of the latent phase of labour differs so much between women that it is difficult to define the limits. False labour can also easily be mistaken for the latent phase. The progress during the active phase is monitored on the partogram on the principle of 1 cm per hour. Many women will give birth normally even at a dilatation rate of 0.5 cm per hour.

The second stage of labour

The second stage of labour lasts from full dilatation of the cervix to complete birth of the baby. For practical reasons the second stage of labour can also be divided into two phases:

▶ The first phase is when the cervix is fully dilated but the head is not yet on the perineum so there is not yet a desire to bear down.

▶ The second phase (also called the *expulsion phase*) is when the head has descended so as to press on the sacral nerves to the rectum, causing the urge to bear down. The combination of the intra-abdominal pressure and uterine contractions facilitate the descent of the presenting part. When the fetal head is crowning the woman may experience intense pain and either an increase or decrease in bearing-down effort.

The average duration of the second stage is 45 minutes for primiparous women and it can last up to two hours. The limitation of the length of the second stage depends entirely on the condition of the mother, the fetus and the progress of labour. In South Africa the parameters of 45 minutes for a primigravida and 30 minutes for a multigravida are used.

The third stage of labour

The third stage of labour lasts from the birth of the baby to the delivery of the placenta and membranes. After the birth of the baby the uterine muscles retract. The placental site starts to decrease in size, causing the non-elastic placenta to separate from the uterine wall. After separation, the uterus contracts and forces the placenta from the fundus into the lower uterine segment. The next contraction delivers the placenta and membranes.

Blood loss from the placental site is controlled by the contraction of the uterine muscles closing the maternal blood vessels.

The third stage usually lasts between 5 and 15 minutes. With passive (spontaneous) delivery of the placenta, it can last as long as 45 or even 60 minutes.

The fourth stage of labour

The fourth stage of labour lasts for about one hour after delivery of the placenta. During this period homeostasis is re-established.

Physiology of labour

Lightening

During the last few weeks before the onset of labour, lightening may occur when the lower segment of the uterus stretches allowing the fetus to move down into the pelvis. The uterine fundus does not press against the diaphragm any more, making maternal breathing easier and lessening her general discomfort.

Uterine contractions

Contraction is the response of the uterus to a stimulus to contract. Contractions are painful, involuntary and intermittent but have regular frequency. The uterus usually starts to contract in the fundal area and the contraction gradually spreads downwards, reaching the lower segment of the uterus approximately 15 seconds later, causing the longest period of contraction to be in the fundal area of the uterus. The contraction fades from all parts of the uterus simultaneously.

Uterine contractions have the following characteristics:

▶ *Wavelike appearance or sensation*. Each contraction has a wavelike appearance with a period of building the intensity (*increment*), peak or maximum intensity (*acme*) and a period of decreased intensity (*decrement*).
▶ *Basal tone*. The contraction is followed by the basal tone, a period of relaxation of the uterine muscles with a reduction in intra-amniotic pressure (5 to 12 mmHg).
▶ *Frequency*. The frequency of contractions gradually increases from about one contraction in 10 to 20 minutes at the onset of labour to three to four contractions per 10 minute period at the end of the first stage. If the contractions are too frequent, the uterus is not allowed enough resting time, which can lead to possible uterine rupture and/or fetal distress.

▶ *Duration*. The duration of a contraction is the time from the beginning of the contraction until it has completely ceased. At the onset of labour it can last 15 seconds and gradually increases to 40 to 60 seconds at the end of the first stage of labour.
▶ *Intensity*. Intensity is the strength of a contraction. During the active phase of labour the intra-amniotic pressure can rise from 25 to 60 mmHg above the basal tone. Contractions are described as mild, moderate or strong. The supine position affects contractions negatively, resulting in them being more frequent but of lower intensity. Contractions are stronger and more effective when the woman is in the upright position or lying on her side.

During contractions the intra-uterine pressure is increased, and when the pressure exceeds 30 mmHg, no new maternal blood enters the placenta, which leads to a reduction in

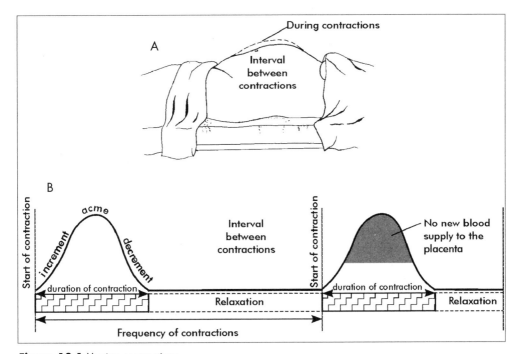

Figure 12.1 Uterine contractions
A: Changing of abdominal contour before and during the contraction
B: Wavelike pattern of contractions

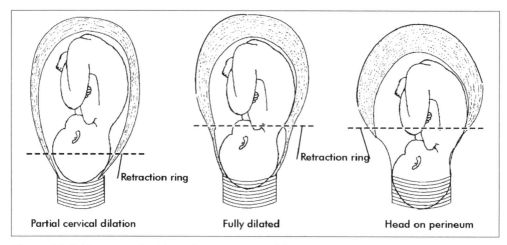

Partial cervical dilation   Fully dilated   Head on perineum

Figure 12.2 Normal or physiological retraction ring of the uterus.

placental perfusion. A healthy fetus can tolerate these periods of reduced perfusion (with subsequent decreased oxygenation) as long as there is enough resting time between contractions and the duration of the contraction is within normal limits.

Retraction

The uterine muscle has the unique property to retain some of the shortening that was obtained during the contraction without returning to its original length. This is called retraction. There is continuous shortening of the muscle fibres in the upper part of the uterus which causes thickening of the muscle tissue and a decrease in the size of the uterine cavity, which gradually forces the fetus downwards (descent).

Polarity

The upper segment of the uterus contracts and retracts pushing the fetus downwards, while the lower segment contracts slightly and dilates to allow expulsion to take place. This organised coordination of contraction and retraction of the upper and lower segments is termed polarity.

Formation of the retraction ring

The contraction of the upper uterine segment and retraction of the lower uterine segment lead to the formation of the boundaries between upper segment and lower segment known as the *physiological retraction ring*. During this process of retraction the lower segment becomes elongated and thinner (see Figure 12.2). In obstructed labour the ring becomes prominent and moves upwards in the uterus so that it can be palpated abdominally. This is known as a *pathological retraction ring* or *Bandl's ring*.

Cervical effacement

Effacement of the cervix is the softening, thinning and shortening of the cervical canal by taking up the internal os into the lower segment of the uterus. A woman presenting with an uneffaced cervix will have a cervical canal of up to 3 cm in length, whereas if the cervix is fully effaced, there will be no canal. Effacement and dilatation occur simultaneously in multigravida while in primigravida effacement occurs at the end of pregnancy and before cervical dilatation (see Figure 12.3).

Cervical dilatation

Dilatation of the cervix is the gradual widening of the external os from a tightly closed aperture until it is large enough (10 cm) to let the fetal head through. The uterine contractions result in the pressure of the presenting part and membranes on the cervix, causing it to dilate. The well-fitting presenting part will stimulate the uterus to contract better (Ferguson's reflex). A well-flexed fetal head, strong contractions, good application of the presenting part on the cervix and a relaxed woman favour cervical dilatation.

Bloody show

During pregnancy a mucous plug is formed due to cervical secretions that accumulate in the cervical canal. As a result of cervical effacement and dilatation the mucous plug is expelled. This is accompanied by minor bleeding from the exposed cervical capillaries. This bloodstained mucous discharge can be seen a few hours before or after the onset of labour. It is essential that the midwife is able to differentiate between heavy show and antepartum bleeding, or a blood-tinged discharge due to a vaginal examination.

Membranes and amniotic fluid

As the lower segment of the uterus stretches with cervical effacement and dilatation, the chorion becomes detached from the decidua vera causing the membrane to form a wedge filled with amniotic fluid. A well-flexed presenting head that fits well on the cervix will separate this amniotic fluid from the rest in the uterine cavity. The amniotic fluid between the intact membranes and the presenting part is called the *forewaters*, and it presses into the cervical canal, assisting in cervical dilatation during contractions.

The membranes can rupture before contractions start or during the first or second stage. After rupture of membranes (ROM) 70% of women will go into spontaneous labour within 24 hours. ROM leads to the pressure of each contraction being exerted directly on the placental area and it can lead to a reduced oxygen supply to the fetus. With intact membranes the uterine pressure will be evenly distributed, optimising oxygen supply to the fetus. Intact membranes also protect the fetus from infection.

Relationship of the fetus to the maternal uterus and pelvis

The position of the fetus in relation to the maternal uterus and pelvis is important because it enables the midwife to anticipate possible deviations in the labour process.

Fetal lie

The *fetal lie* refers to the long axis (spine) of the mother in relation to the long axis of the fetus:

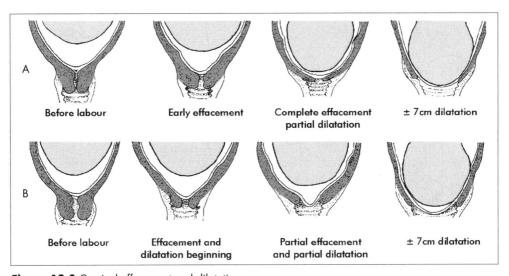

Figure 12.3 Cervical effacement and dilatation
A: Primigravida
B: Multigravida

▶ When the long axis of the fetus is parallel with the long axis of the mother, the lie is *longitudinal*.

▶ When the long axis of the fetus is at a right angle to the long axis of the mother, the lie is *transverse* or *oblique* (see Chapter 26, Figure 26.7).

Fetal presentation

Presentation refers to the part of the fetus that is situated over the pelvic inlet and will pass through the birth canal first (and will be felt during vaginal examination). The most common presentations are:

▶ Cephalic presentation (vertex or facial).

▶ Breech presentation.

▶ Shoulder presentation.

Cephalic presentations are further classified according to fetal attitude.

Fetal attitude

The *attitude* is the relationship of the fetal body parts to one another. The fetus is usually flexed in utero causing the chin to rest on the chest and the extremities to be folded against the body. In a cephalic presentation the attitude can be one of the following:

▶ *Flexion*. The normal and most preferred attitude with the smallest diameter. The chin rests on the chest with the occiput presenting.

▶ *Military attitude*. The vertex presents. Both fetal fontanelles can be felt on vaginal examination.

▶ *Extension*. The sinciput presents because the head is bent backwards. The largest diameter presents which will cause cephalopelvic disproportion in most cases. With hyperextension the face is presenting.

Fetal position

The *position* is the relation of the denominator to the maternal pelvis. There are different denominators used according to the specific presentation:

▶ In a cephalic presentation the denominator is the *occiput* (O).

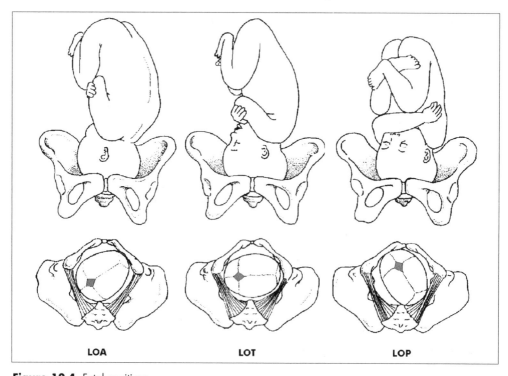

| LOA | LOT | LOP |

Figure 12.4 Fetal positions

- In a breech presentation the *sacrum* (S) is the denominator.
- In the facial presentation the *chin* or *mentum* (M) is used.

The fetal position is determined according the different areas of the maternal pelvis such as:
- left (L) or right (R)
- anterior (A) or posterior (P)
- lateral (L) or transverse (T)

For example, if the fetal position is LOA, it indicates that the occiput (O) is the denominator and the occiput is lying in the left (L) half of the maternal pelvis but also more anterior (A) than posterior.

Mechanism of labour

The mechanism of labour is a passive movement with changes in the posture of the fetus during labour. The fetus negotiates his pathway through the birth canal by means of uterine contractions and maternal bearing-down efforts. The postural changes the fetus undergoes are descent, flexion, internal rotation of the head, extension of the head, restitution, internal rotation of the shoulders while external rotation of the head takes place, and lastly, delivery of the shoulders and body in lateral flexion.

Except for descent and some flexion, all of the other changes take place during the second stage. There is a different mechanism of labour for each possible fetal position and presentation. It is important for the midwife to know and understand the normal mechanism of labour because abnormalities can then be detected easily.

The mechanism of labour will be described as it happens in the left occipitoanterior (LOA) position. Other features applicable to the LOA position are as follows:
- The lie is longitudinal (the long axis of the fetus is parallel to the long axis of the mother).
- The presentation is cephalic (occiput).
- The denominator is the occiput.
- The fetal back can easily be identified on

the left and anterior area of the abdomen; the limbs are on the right.
- The attitude is that of flexion.
- The sagittal suture is in the right oblique diameter with the anterior fontanelle right posterior and the posterior fontanelle left anterior.
- The fetal heart is heard clearly in the left lower quadrant of the woman's abdomen.

Descent

In a primigravida, descent often takes place from 36 weeks onwards, but due to the lax abdominal muscle tone in a multigravida it is delayed until the onset of labour. Descent is a continuous process during labour.

During the process of fetal descent the vagina stretches progressively. In addition the bladder is displaced upwards into the abdomen and the urethra stretched out. The presenting part descends with each contraction and retreats during relaxation. The pressure of the presenting part leads to stretching of the perineum and the vaginal introitus and vulva gradually open.

A normal anaesthesia is produced as a result of the decreased blood supply to the area. The anus averts, exposing the interior rectal wall (gaping) as the fetal head descends forward.

Engagement is a specific moment in the continuous process of descent. This is when the widest diameter of the fetal presenting part has passed through the pelvic brim.

Flexion

Flexion of the fetal head is the natural attitude of the fetus in utero as occurring before the onset of labour. Flexion increases as labour progresses due to the resistance from the pelvis, partially dilated cervix and the pelvic floor. The fetal spine is not centrally located on the fetal scull, but more posteriorly. As the head encounters resistance, more pressure is exerted on the longer anterior part, forcing the head to flex. A flexed head has a smaller diameter, which facilitates descent and negotiation through the pelvis. In a well-flexed head, the suboccipito-bregmatic diameter (9.5 cm) presents.

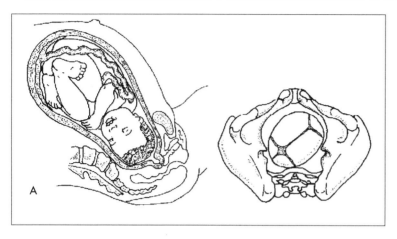

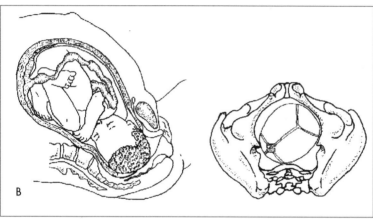

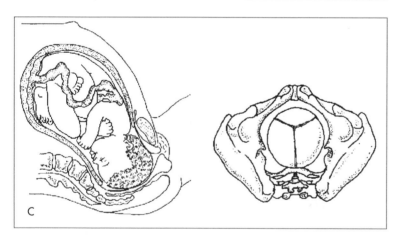

Figure 12.5 Mechanism of labour in a left occipitoanterior (LOA) position
A: Descent
B: Flexion
C: Internal rotation of the head

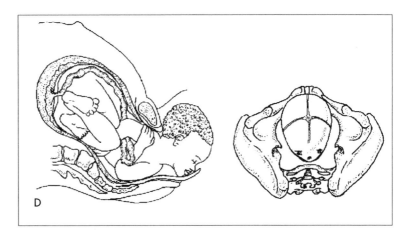

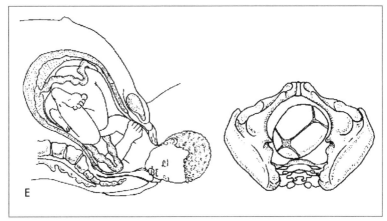

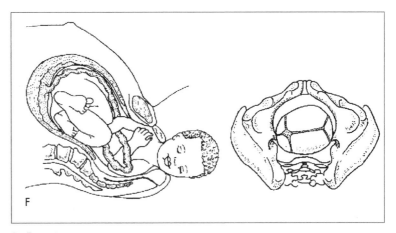

D: Extension
E: Restitution
F: External rotation of the head and internal rotation of the shoulders.

Internal rotation

The fetal head needs to rotate in order to pass through the pelvic outlet, which is widest in the anteroposterior diameter. In contrast to that, the pelvic inlet is widest in the transverse diameter. Internal rotation usually takes place during the second stage when the head reaches the pelvic floor. The occiput is the lowest part in a well-flexed fetal head and is the first to meet resistance from the pelvic floor. The levator ani muscles are gutter or boat shaped and slope down anteriorly. Whatever part meets the levator ani first (in this case it is the occiput), will rotate anteriorly (45°) until the sagittal suture lies in the anteroposterior pelvic diameter and the occiput lies directly behind the symphysis. Internal rotation of the head is not accompanied by internal rotation of the shoulders, which leaves the head and shoulders not in direct alignment any more. The head is now in the anteroposterior diameter, while the shoulders are usually still in the oblique diameter.

Internal rotation is often delayed following epidural anaesthesia due to the relaxing of the pelvic floor. Resistance caused by the pelvic floor is necessary for rotation to take place.

Extension

As the head continues to descend the perineum will bulge as the head passes through the vulval orifice (crowning). As the fetal head descends further and the crowning occurs, it pivots under the symphysis pubis and advances upwards. After the occiput, the vertex, sinciput, face and chin (momentum) sweep the perineum.

Extension is complete when the head is completely delivered. Extension takes place due to the uterine contractions, maternal bearing-down efforts and the resistance of the perineum.

Restitution

Once the head is completely delivered and is free of pelvic resistance, it returns to its original position (sagittal suture in the right oblique diameter). The head is again aligned with the shoulders as before internal rotation of the head took place.

Internal rotation of the shoulders and external rotation of the head

The fetal shoulders enter the pelvis in the oblique diameter. Similar to the head, the shoulders also rotate 45° to the anteroposterior diameter when reaching the pelvic floor, because the anteroposterior diameter is the widest diameter of the pelvic outlet. The anterior shoulder then lies under the symphysis pubis.

Together with the internal rotation of the shoulders, external rotation of the head takes place simultaneously in the same direction as restitution. This means that the fetal head rotates a further 45° after restitution so that the occiput lies laterally.

Delivery of the shoulders and body

The anterior shoulder is delivered first from behind the symphysis pubis, followed by the posterior shoulder that passes over the perineum. The rest of the baby's body is born without difficulty in *lateral flexion* as the vertebral column bends sideways through the curved birth canal.

It is important for the midwife to understand the mechanism of labour in order to work with it and to avoid complications through incorrect interventions.

> ### CRITICAL THINKING EXERCISE
> A primigravida asks how it is possible for her fetus (estimated at 3.5 kg) to pass through her pelvis. How would you respond?

Maternal adaptation during labour

Cardiovascular adaptation

With each contraction 300 to 500 ml blood is forced out of the uterus into the maternal vascular system. This results in an increased cardiac output of 10 to 15% during the first stage of labour and 30 to 50% during the second stage. Maternal anxiety and pain can increase the cardiac output even more.

Maternal blood pressure increases significantly during contractions in the first stage of labour. The contractions reduce the blood flow in the uterine artery, causing redirection to the peripheral vessels. The resistance leads to an increase in maternal blood pressure with an increase in pulse rate. Therefore the midwife should monitor the blood pressure between the contractions. During the second stage of labour the blood pressure rises even more, thereby increasing the risk for complications, such as cerebral haemorrhage in women at risk of hypertension.

Using the Valsalva manoeuvre for bearing down may increase the blood pressure at first, and then lead to a decrease in the pulse rate and later hypotension (see Chapter 14). Supine hypotension, analgesia and the vasodilating effect of epidural analgesia may contribute to hypotension.

Immune system

There is the likelihood of an increase in the white blood cell count (WBC) during labour and early puerperium. It is usually to between $14,000/mm^3$ and $16,000/mm^3$ but can increase up to $25,000/mm^3$. Although the mechanism leading to this increase in WBC is unknown, it may be due to an increase in neutrophils resulting from the physiological response to stress (physical or emotional) or tissue trauma. This increase makes it difficult to identify the presence of an infection.

Respiratory system

The increased physical activity leads to greater oxygen consumption with a subsequent increase in the respiratory rate. Anxiety further increases the oxygen consumption. During the second stage oxygen consumption nearly doubles.

Towards the end of the first stage of labour most women develop mild metabolic acidosis which is compensated for by respiratory alkalosis. During the second stage of labour the

woman's $PaCo_2$ level rises when breath holding accompanies bearing-down effort. These changes are potentially dangerous to the woman and fetus during labour.

In the fourth stage of labour the changes in the acid-base status that occurred during labour are quickly reversed because of the change in the woman's respiratory rate. By 24 hours after birth the acid-base levels should return to pregnancy levels and a few weeks after birth normal non-pregnant values can be expected.

Renal system

During the second trimester the urinary bladder becomes an abdominal organ, which can be palpated above the symphysis when full. During labour spontaneous voiding may be difficult because of sedation, embarrassment and tissue oedema caused by pressure from the presenting part. Proteinuria of 1+ may be present due to the response to the breakdown of muscle tissue from the physical work of labour.

Maternal renin, plasma renin activity and angiotensinogen are increased during labour.

Gastrointestinal system

During labour gastrointestinal motility and absorption of solid food are delayed which leads to a prolonged stomach emptying time. Although aspiration during general anaesthesia can take place, it plays a very small part in maternal mortality. Maternal morbidity does however occur. Fasting does not decrease the chance of aspiration, because it cannot ensure an empty stomach. No time interval since the last oral intake can guarantee a stomach volume of less than 100 ml. Nausea and vomiting is common and can announce full cervical dilatation.

The pH value of the gastric content will be less than 2.5 in more than half of women in labour.

Musculoskeletal system

The muscle activity during labour elevates body temperature and leads to an increase in diaphoreses (sweating), fatigue and evaporation to cool. With hyperventilation further evaporation takes place as the air must be humidified and warmed to the body temperature. Dehydration can therefore easily develop.

The increased joint laxity at term leads to backache and joint pain unrelated to fetal position. Leg cramps are also common.

Neurological adaptation

The behaviour of the woman will depend on her response to stress and the discomfort she encounters during labour. The response will differ from one stage of labour to the next. During the first stage of labour the woman may initially experience euphoria followed by seriousness. During the second stage of labour she may experience amnesia between contractions and fatigue after the birth. The woman is able to cope throughout labour due to endogenous endorphins (a naturally produced morphine-like chemical) and physiological anaesthesia of perineal tissues, caused by the pressure of the presenting part.

Endocrine system adaptation

Increased levels of oestrogen, prostaglandin and oxytocin, together with the reduction in progesterone levels, may trigger the onset of labour.

During contractions glucose is used as an energy source which results in a reduction in maternal blood glucose levels, with a subsequent reduction in insulin requirements.

Fetal adaptation during labour

Fetal heart rate

Fetal heart rate is a reliable indication of fetal wellbeing. The average fetal heart rate is 140 beats per minute. Throughout labour the baseline fetal heart rate should remain between 110 to 160 bpm with a variability of more than 5 bpm. Abnormalities of the fetal heart rate are discussed comprehensively in Chapter 13.

Fetal gas exchange

During uterine life the fetus uses the placenta for gas exchange. When the fetal body passes through the birth canal, fluid is expelled from the fetal lungs to enable the neonate to take his first breath after birth.

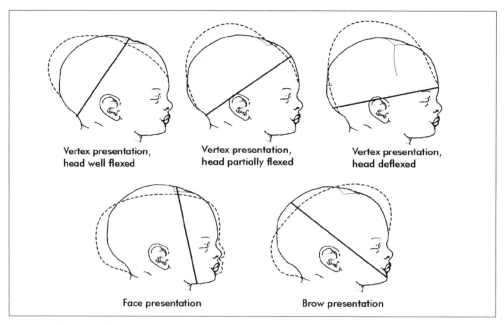

Figure 12.6 Moulding of the fetal skull. The moulding is indicated with a dotted line as it would appear in different presentations.

Fetal circulation

During labour several factors can affect fetal circulation, such as maternal position, uterine contractions, maternal blood pressure, placental perfusion and umbilical cord blood flow. The uterine contractions decrease circulation in the small uterine arteries and perfusion through the intervillous space. In a normal functioning placenta the fetal and placental reserves should be enough to prevent hypoxia during a contraction.

Integumentary adaptation

The fetus is exposed to the pressure in the birth canal during the process of labour. This may result in mild petechiae and oedema (caput succedaneum) of the presenting part (see Chapter 13).

Gastrointestinal system

During uterine life a fetus may pass meconium during hypoxic episodes, which may be swallowed and reabsorbed again. A fetus that passes meconium during labour is prone to low Apgar scores, lower pH values and higher perinatal morbidity and mortality.

Moulding

Moulding refers to the alteration of the shape and the diameters of the fetal head. It occurs as a result of the force of the uterine contractions and the pressure that is exerted by the passages on the fetal head as it is propelled through the pelvis. The suppleness of the fontanelles and the sutures within their membranous covering make it possible for the shape of the head to be modified to that of the bony canal without causing damage to the underlying structures. An observable characteristic of moulding is that the parietal bones slide under each other, while the occipital bone and the frontal bones move smoothly under the parietal bones.

References

Bennett, V. R. & Brown, L. K. (Eds.) 1999. *Myles textbook for midwives.* Thirteenth edition. Edinburgh: Churchill Livingstone.

In a nutshell

- The onset of labour is not due to one factor but due to the interaction between various factors.
- The fetus has to negotiate its pathway through the birth canal in a series of passive movements termed the mechanism of labour.
- During the process of labour both the mother and the fetus will undergo physiological changes to adapt. However, during the fourth stage homeostasis will be re-established.
- The midwife should be familiar with the normal process of labour in order to prevent complications, as well as to recognise deviations from the norm.

Burroughs, A. & Leifer, G. 2001. *Maternity nursing: An introductory text.* Eighth edition. Philadelphia: W.P. Sauders Company.

Coad, J. & Dunstall, M. 2001. *Anatomy and physiology for midwives.* London: Mosby.

Cronjé, H. S., Grobler, C. J. F. & Visser, A. A. 2000. *Obstetrics in South Africa.* Second edition. Pretoria: J. L. van Schaik.

Dickson, E., Silverman, B. & Shaults, M. 1994. *Maternity and gynaecological care.* Second edition. London: Mosby.

Enkin, M., Keirse, M. J. N. C., Neilson, J., Crowther, C., Duley, L. & Hofmeyr J. 2000. *A guide to effective care in pregnancy and childbirth.* Third edition. Oxford: Oxford University Press.

Gabbe, S.G., Niebyl, J. R. & Simpson, J. L. 1996. *Obstetrics: Normal and problem pregnancies.* Third edition. New York: Churchill Livingstone.

Gibb, D. & Arulkumaran, S. 1997. *Fetal monitoring in practice.* Second edition. Oxford: Butterworth-Heinemann.

Johnson, R. & Taylor, W., 2000. *Skills for midwifery practice.* London: Churchill.

Ladewig, P. W., London, M. L. & Olds, S. B. 1998. *Maternal-newborn nursing care. The nurse, the family, and the community.* Fourth edition. Menlo Park: Addison Wesley Longman Inc.

Lowdermilk, D. L., Perry, S. T. & Bobak, I. M. 1999. *Maternity nursing.* Fifth edition, St. Louis: Mosby.

May, K. A. & Mahlmeister, L. R. 1994. *Maternal and neonatal nursing family-centered care.* Third edition. Philadelphia: JB Lippincott.

Nolte, A. G. W. (Ed.) 1998. *A textbook for midwives.* Pretoria: JL van Schaik.

O'Gray, J. P., Gimovky, M. L. & Mcillhargie, C. J. 1995. *Operative obstetrics.* London: Williams & Wilkins.

Olds, S. B., London, M. L. & Ladewig, P. A. 2000. *Maternal newborn nursing: A family and community-based approach.* Sixth edition. New Jersey: Prentice Hall Health.

Pillitteri, A. 1995. *Maternal and child health nursing care of the childbearing and child rearing family.* Second edition. Philadelphia: JB Lippincott.

Sellers, P. M. 2001. *Midwifery.* Fourth edition. Cape Town: Juta.

Chapter *13*

First stage of labour

Dr Bongi Nzama, Joanita de Kock and Theresa Mabale

Introduction

The first stage of labour begins with the onset of regular painful uterine contractions accompanied by at least one of the following three indicators:

▶ Cervical effacement and dilatation.
▶ Rupture of the membranes.
▶ Show is present.

The first stage of labour culminates in full dilatation of the cervix.

13-1

The Better Births Initiative

Several hospitals and healthcare centres in South Africa and abroad incorporate the 'Better Births' principles when rendering care to women in labour. The overall goal of the Better Births Initiative is to improve the quality of care rendered to expectant women and their families by eliminating procedures that can be harmful, unpleasant or uncomfortable for the women. The Better Births Initiative supports the implementation of procedures and interventions that have been justified by scientific evidence, commonly referred to as evidence-based care. Only those interventions that are of benefit to women and their families are supported by this initiative. Reference will be made to these practices wherever applicable.

The principles of the Better Births Initiative

▶ *Humanity*. Women are to be treated with respect.
▶ *Benefit*. Care that is based on the best available evidence.
▶ *Commitment*. Health professionals are committed to improving care.
▶ *Action*. Effective strategies to change current practice.

Admission of the woman in labour

Several factors need to be considered when a woman is admitted to the labour ward.

Cultural and psychosocial considerations

Midwives should try to make women in labour feel at ease because many people experience a cultural shock in the hospital setting. Bauwens and Anderson (Stanhope & Lancaster, 1991) cite five factors that contribute to cultural shock:
▶ communication
▶ mechanical differences
▶ customs
▶ isolation
▶ attitudes and beliefs

Communication

Health professionals, as in any other professions, use specialised vocabulary among themselves. Women often feel left out of the conversation even though it concerns them. Every effort should be made to simplify the conversation, particularly when the woman is required to make important decisions. When interpreters are used, ensure that medical terms are translated accurately and that the woman understands their meaning. The Patients' Rights Charter (which also applies to labouring women) stresses the importance of providing a healthy and safe environment, access to healthcare, participation in decision-making and informed consent – all of which are dependent on good communication during labour.

Mechanical differences

Once admitted to the labour ward, the woman is often required to abide by the routines that may limit her mobility and decision-making. The labouring woman may interpret the institutional routines as restrictive, and they may have an intimidating effect on her, making her feel defenceless and at the 'mercy' of the health personnel.

On the other hand, home deliveries are less restrictive as they allow the woman to make her own decisions on matters such as assuming comfortable positions during labour, and in deciding what to eat or drink. The Better Births Initiative supports the use of a variety of birthing positions, and encourages medical practitioners and midwives to allow the women to assume those positions that they are most comfortable with (see Chapter 15 Figure 15.1).

Customs

South Africa is a country in which the various ethnic and racial groups have different customs relating to childbirth. Midwives need to show respect to all the women who are admitted to the labour ward irrespective of their cultural background. Providing adequate privacy is an essential aspect of labour ward practice that promotes a climate in which all women are treated with dignity and respect. The Patients' Rights Charter and the Batho Pele principles support the woman's right to confidentiality and privacy, an aspect that relates well to the respect of most people's customs. In instances where certain customary practices cannot be accommodated, an honest and truthful explanation of the reason therefore should be offered to the woman and her family. At all times, women should be treated with courtesy, dignity, patience, empathy and tolerance.

Isolation

Isolation of the woman is one of the limitations of institutionalised deliveries. The physical structure of most labour wards does not offer women the opportunity to be with their loved ones throughout labour and the prescriptive attitude of some medical practitioners and midwives can be as rigid as the structures. Women may feel very lonely and isolated from their spouses and other significant others at a time when they need them most (see also Companionship later in this chapter).

Another aspect of isolation has to do with the powerlessness women may feel in not being active participants in decision-making about their own care. Social inequalities may be another factor that contributes to the isolation of women. Language barriers can also cause isolation and midwives should assist the women to overcome their isolation by providing interpreters where possible.

Attitudes and beliefs

The attitudes and beliefs of midwives and medical practitioners have a major influence on how labouring women perceive their experience of birth. Due to different cultural and ethnic backgrounds, women differ in the manner in which they handle complications that arise during labour and in their expression of pain. Likewise, the midwives and medical practitioners may have their own expectations of how women in labour ought to behave. Midwives should be aware of their own prejudices and stereotypes regarding the women they admit to the labour ward.

Antenatal education may help to prepare women for delivery in a healthcare setting.

Screening for high-risk factors

Pregnancy and labour have potential risks for both the woman and the fetus. For this reason several screening phases should occur during pregnancy:

- The first screening phase occurs in the preconception period and it continues throughout the antenatal period.
- The second screening phase begins when the woman presents herself for admission at the labour ward. Examination of the woman in labour should be very thorough to identify possible risk factors so that she may be referred to an advanced midwife or medical practitioner, or be transferred to a level 2 or level 3 hospital if necessary. This will ensure that appropriate management and referral protocols are put in place timeously.
- The third screening phase takes place during the course of labour. It occurs mainly through accurate clinical observations and through the use of the partogram, both of which may lead to the early detection of unexpected fetal or maternal distress, or failure of labour to progress. Early interventions will reduce the risk of maternal or fetal/neonatal morbidity and mortality.

History taking

History taking marks the beginning of the second screening phase. A careful review of the antenatal card should be made to note any risk factors identified during the antenatal period, as they may have an influence on the progress of labour, and on the wellbeing of the fetus and the woman. There is a higher incidence of high-risk conditions in unbooked women, therefore they should be interviewed as during their first antenatal visit (see Chapter 9).

The woman should be asked about the following: What exactly brought her to the clinic or hospital? What is her presenting problem? The time of onset of the contractions, their frequency, intensity, approximate duration and where they are felt most. Information should also be sought regarding the presence of a show, the passage of liquor, fetal movement and any other relevant symptoms.

Essential information will include whether the woman has an infection of any kind or whether she is recovering from any illness, as this may impact on the progress of labour. According to the HIV/AIDS Policy Guidelines, genital infections, especially sexually transmitted infections (STIs) may result in chorio-amnionitis. Infection of the chorion or amnion may increase the chance of mother-to-child transmission (MTCT) of the virus.

Physical examination

A general examination must be conducted on admission of the woman in labour, which includes checking her general condition, vital signs, oedema, pallor, urine specimen and psychological state. Blood samples are taken in cases where these were not taken during the antenatal period, as in the case of unbooked women.

Observe for the presence of other untoward symptoms such as headaches, unusual pain and discomfort, general irritability, visual disturbances, dyspnoea, changes in the level of consciousness, convulsions and breathing difficulties or cyanosis. If abnormalities are detected, the midwife or medical practitioner in charge must be informed immediately and appropriate action should be taken.

Women may experience considerable levels of stress and fear at the onset of labour, particularly primigravidae who are usually apprehensive about the labouring experience. The levels of anxiety may be high in women who have been diagnosed as having a high-risk pregnancy, and in those who are admitted to health facilities that are far from their homes and loved ones. Midwives and other caregivers need to demonstrate sensitivity to the woman's psychological and emotional needs when conducting the physical examination. By doing so, they will help to reduce her anxiety considerably. A relaxed woman is likely to be more cooperative during labour.

Abdominal examination

The abdominal examination constitutes part of the physical assessment of the woman during labour. Abdominal palpation may aid in the diagnosis of the lie, presentation, position and attitude of the presenting part, all of which are then subsequently confirmed through a vaginal examination. The midwife should be guided by the following parameters when conducting an abdominal examination, which are discussed in detail in Chapter 9.

> **Aspects of the abdominal examination**
>
> ▶ Abdominal inspection.
> ▶ Symphysis-fundal height (SFH).
> ▶ Lie: The normal lie is longitudinal.
> ▶ Presentation: The normal presentation is cephalic.
> ▶ Attitude: The normal attitude is that of flexion of the head.
> ▶ Position.
> ▶ Amount of head above pelvis expressed in fifths.
> ▶ Estimation of fetal weight.
> ▶ Amount of amniotic fluid.
> ▶ Duration, strength and frequency of contractions.
> ▶ Auscultation of fetal heart rate before, during and after contractions.

The priorities of the abdominal examination during labour differ from those made during the antenatal period. Aspects that were earlier of less importance are now of utmost importance, such as determination of the presenting part, position and attitude of the presenting part and amount of head above pelvis. This information is important for planning the mode of delivery, for anticipating possible problems like slower progress due to posterior positions, and for identifying problems such as poor descent with subsequent poor progress of labour.

Vaginal examination

A vaginal examination is part of the screening for high-risk factors. It is conducted at the time of admission in order to set a baseline against which to measure progress of labour.

The vaginal examination is conducted in privacy, after obtaining consent to do so and after requesting the woman to empty her bladder. The woman is asked to lie in the dorsal or lithotomy position, with a slight left lateral tilt or in the Sim's position. The following factors should then be assessed:

The vulva and vagina. The condition of the vulva is inspected before the actual vaginal examination. The vulva is observed for the presence of any discharges, sores, oedema or varicose veins. As part of the precautionary measures to prevent MTCT, the vulva and vagina are cleansed using *chlorhexidine* 0.25%. However, any other appropriate disinfective agent, according to the unit policy may be used for this purpose.

The procedure for vaginal cleansing

With the middle and index fingers of one hand holding the labia apart, and effectively opening the vagina, the *chlorhexidine* is inserted into the vagina to disinfect and clean out any excess discharge. Following the cleansing, two fingers of the other hand are gently introduced into the vagina while taking care not to cause friction against the clitoral area, which is highly sensitive. This procedure is to be followed whenever a vaginal examination is to be conducted.

The cervix. The examining fingers then reach upwards and backward for the cervix. The *length* and *thickness* (effacement), *dilatation* and *consistency* of the cervix should be noted. The length and thickness (effacement) of the cervix are indicated in millimetres or centimetres. The dilatation of the cervix is indicated in centimetres and can be between 0 and 10 cm. The consistency can be firm, average or soft. The softer the cervix, the easier it dilates.

The *position* of the cervix should be noted and it may be posterior, central or anterior.

The examiner then determines the extent of *application* of the cervix to the presenting part and notes whether it is well applied, loosely applied or not applied at all. Good application favours dilatation of the cervix.

The Modified Bishop Score (see Table 13.1 on page 13-28) may be used as an accurate index of assessing the state of the cervix in a woman not yet in active labour.

The membranes. In order to assess the state of the membranes, one finger is passed through the external os and then through the internal os if the cervix permits. If the internal os is dilated, the state of the membranes is assessed whether intact or ruptured, and if ruptured, the colour of the liquor is assessed. The membranes should be felt for the existence of a presenting or prolapsed umbilical cord, which is characterised by the pulsation of the cord.

The presenting part. The vaginal examination allows for the positive *identification of the presenting part*, which may be a vertex (normal), face, brow, breech, shoulder or compound presentation. The *position* of the presenting part is determined by first locating the direction of the sagittal suture in relation to the pelvis, and then verifying the position of the anterior and/or posterior fontanelles (see Figure 12.4). In occipito-anterior positions, the posterior fontanelle is felt anteriorly, while in occipitoposterior positions, the anterior fontanelle is palpable anteriorly. The abnormal presentations are discussed in greater detail in Chapter 26.

In a normal vertex presentation the *attitude* of the fetal head is also determined (see Chapter 12).

The *station* of the presenting part is determined by drawing an imaginary line between the two ischial spines and estimating the lowest part of the presenting part against it (see Figure 13.1). If the lowest part of the presenting part is still above the imaginary line (expressed in centimetres), it will be indicated in negative symbols (for example –2). If the lowest level of the presenting part is on the

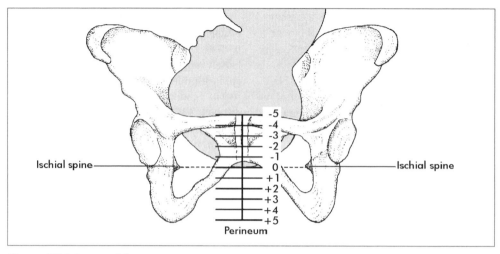

Ischial spine

-5
-4
-3
-2
-1
0
+1
+2
+3
+4
+5

Ischial spine

Perineum

Figure 13.1 Station of the presenting part

Note	Advantages of using the partogram during the labour process

Note

Vaginal examinations should not be conducted at random. They are conducted at four hourly intervals during the latent phase of labour, and at two hourly intervals during the active phase of labour.

Frequent vaginal examinations are uncomfortable for the woman and they may also expose her and the fetus to infection.

Risk factors such as placenta praevia should always be considered prior to conducting a vaginal examination. Therefore do not perform a vaginal examination if there is frank bleeding, as there may be the risk of dislodging a placenta praevia leading to a fatal haemorrhage.

Advantages of using the partogram during the labour process

▶ It is effective in the early detection of abnormal progress of labour and provides signals that prompt labour ward staff to make timely decisions on whether transfer or augmentation of labour is appropriate.

▶ It is an inexpensive, effective and pragmatic tool for detecting the various causes of prolonged labour and contributes to reducing operative intervention, thereby improving maternal and neonatal outcome.

▶ It is a useful referral tool as it sets norms of when midwives at a satellite clinic should transfer cases to the referral hospital to prevent the recordings from crossing the Action Line.

▶ It improves the handing over of cases transferred from the satellite clinic, and simplifies the takeover rounds at the end of each working shift. The smooth, efficient and effective handing over of cases diminishes the stress associated with working in the labour ward.

level of the imaginary line, it will be indicated as a station of 0. If the lowest part of the presenting part has passed the ischial spines, the station will be positive depending on the number of centimetres (for example +2).

The partogram

The partogram is a graphic recording of the progress of labour and the related condition of the woman and the fetus. It visually displays all the observations made during the first

Note

Use of the partogram does not substitute the need to screen all women as they arrive in labour to exclude pre-existing conditions that may require urgent attention or immediate transfer to hospital.

The goal in using the partogram is to manage labour effectively and to identify any risk factors that may arise during labour.

stage of labour in a manner that enables midwives and medical practitioners to recognise if the woman has moved into the high-risk category and to respond decisively to the identified problems.

If the partogram is used and interpreted correctly, it simplifies the management of labour and contributes to the reduction of maternal and fetal mortality and morbidity. Because of its profound benefits in the management of labour, the partogram should be used for all women who are admitted to the labour ward, whether in a community healthcare centre or in a hospital setting.

The partogram consists of three major features that are recorded graphically:
▶ The fetal condition.
▶ The progress of labour.
▶ The maternal condition.

The partogram also provides space for recording any drugs and intravenous infusions administered during labour. Failure to use a partogram during labour has been cautioned by the Department of Health to constitute substandard care (DoH, 2002:34).

Maternal condition and care

The assessment and management of the maternal condition are recorded on the partogram and relevant records.

Ambulation

Whenever possible, the woman in labour should be encouraged to walk around, take a warm bath or shower, sit, stand or assume any other position or activity that she feels comfortable with. The practice of giving birth in a warm bath of water is being used increasingly as it aids in relaxation, and helps to reduce the release of catecholamines. Contractions become more efficient, the periopd of labour shorter, labour augmentation less frequent, and fetal distress less common in cases where women remain active during labour. Lying in the supine position causes the uterus to compress the aorta and inferior vena cava, which reduces the blood flow in the uterus, and may lower the intensity of the uterine contractions. In addition, lying on the back may amplify the pain of labour, increase fetal distress, and lead to poor pelvic relaxation and to a higher incidence of operative deliveries. In low-risk cases women should not be confined to bed-rest during the first stage of labour, except in cases where the membranes have ruptured in the presence of a non-engaged fetal head. Other exceptions include women with a history of precipitate labour or women with vaginal bleeding.

Food and fluids during labour

Labour requires high-energy resources, which can be sustained by an adequate fluid and food intake. Therefore in all low-risk cases of normal labour there should be no restriction of oral intake. Many clinics and hospitals discourage the woman from taking oral fluids and food during labour out of fear that aspiration may occur if she has to undergo an emergency caesarean section. This practice should be discouraged as it can lead to dehydration and ketosis, which in turn reduces the intensity of the uterine contractions and slows the progress of labour. Restricting oral intake does not guarantee an empty stomach, and a complete reduction of the stomach contents is not possible. In most instances, labouring women show a preference for drinking fluids and instinctively avoid heavy meals. In instances where women appear to be dehydrated, they should be encouraged to take frequent sips of fluid. However, in cases where marked dehydration is evident, an intra-venous infusion should be set up.

Companionship

Labouring women benefit significantly from the presence of a spouse, partner, friend, rela-tive, caregiver or a voluntary 'doula' (woman trained to act as support companion to women during labour and delivery). Companionship provides unhurried care and attention, reassurance, motivation, comfort, encouragement and physical contact. Companions may help with relaxation and psycho-prophylactic techniques. The labour companion may help by rubbing the woman's back, timing the contractions, encouraging the woman to rest between contractions, and by attending to her breathing rhythm during labour. The companion could attend to other needs such as wiping the woman's face, or simply holding her hand.

Additional benefits of companionship include a shorter labour, fewer interventions, increased self-esteem and a positive outlook towards labour and the newborn baby.

Having private rooms that allow male com-panions may not always be possible in the labour wards of busy hospitals. In such situa-tions, it may be more desirable for the pregnant woman to arrange for a female com-panion. Midwives can adapt visiting hour restrictions or encourage women in early labour to meet with their relatives outside the labour unit.

Bowel action and the use of enemas

To date, there is no concrete evidence to sup-port the routine use of enemas during labour. There is no scientific evidence to support the beliefs that an empty bowel helps the fetal head to descent or that enemas diminish con-tamination during labour and therefore reduce the incidence of infection. Observations of the labouring process have shown that women who deliver without hav-ing had an enema pass faecal matter that is solid and easier to remove, while women who have had enemas pass more liquid and messier stools. The Better Births Initiative strongly discourages the use of enemas in labour, pointing out that enemas can be uncomfortable and embarrassing for the woman, and that they have the potential of damaging the bowel. In addition, an enema may be an added unnecessary cost for the woman or healthcare facility and it should only be administered if a woman requests it.

Emptying the bladder

A full bladder impedes the descent of the fetus; therefore the woman should be encour-aged to empty the bladder at frequent intervals throughout labour, preferably every two hours. A full bladder can be observed above the symphysis pubis, which on inspection looks elevated and can also be felt on palpation (see Figure 13.2). The distension causes immense pain and discomfort to the woman. A careful record should be kept regarding the time of voiding and the volume of urine passed. A decrease in the amount of urine and concentration of urine indicates inadequate fluid intake. Each specimen of urine should be tested for protein, ketones and glucose, and the findings entered on the par-togram. Sometimes, women in advanced labour may not recognise that the discomfort they are experiencing is associated with a full bladder, therefore midwives should be vigilant and monitor the urinary output frequently. Occasionally catheterisation may be necessary to relieve the woman's discomfort, but because of the associated risk of infection, it should only be carried out when absolutely necessary. Catheterisation may also be ordered prior to a forceps delivery or a caesarean section.

Pubic shaving

Shaving of the pubic hair is being discour-aged, as there is no evidence to support the claim that shaving reduces infection in women with perineal tears or episiotomies during labour. Skilled attendants are capable of perineal suturing with ease without shaving the pubic hair. Women experience pubic shaving as embarrassing and uncomfortable,

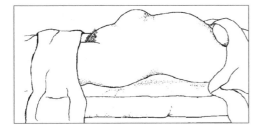

Figure 13.2 Illustration of a woman with a full bladder

with 'a prickly' sensation when the pubic hair begins to grow back. Other discomforts that follow shaving include a burning sensation and itching, redness and even superficial scratches of the vulva. Instead of shaving the pubic area, some institutions support the 'clipping' of thick perineal hair in cases where it is deemed necessary in preparation for performing an episiotomy.

Pain relief

Women in labour differ in their response and tolerance to pain. The management of pain and discomfort is discussed in detail in Chapter 15.

Vital signs

During the latent phase the woman's blood pressure and pulse should be monitored every two hours and her temperature measured every four hours. During the active phase of labour the blood pressure should be monitored at least hourly, pulse half-hourly and temperature every four hours.

Fetal condition

Assessment of the fetal heart rate during the first stage of labour can identify fetal complications, which if uncorrected may cause short- or long-term morbidity or even death. Evidence-based trials of monitoring fetal well-being have shown that constant observation of the woman in labour can avert these adverse outcomes.

The fetal heart rate (baseline rate) should be recorded every two hours during the latent phase and every 30 minutes during the active

phase on the partogram. The baseline variability and type of deceleration should also be indicated according to the institutional protocol. It is important to record these patterns on the partogram so that deviation can be picked up promptly and decisions are made in time to prevent fetal morbidity and mortality.

Methods of fetal monitoring during the first stage of labour

Intermittent fetal heart monitoring

Intermittent fetal heart monitoring is the predominant method of fetal assessment during labour, particularly in the low-risk pregnancies where less intervention is needed. Intermittent monitoring can be done using a fetoscope (Pinard's stethoscope) or a hand-held Doptone.

> **Note**
>
> Changes in fetal heart rate during or shortly after the contraction might give an early warning signal, therefore the emphasis is on monitoring the fetal heart rate 30 seconds before, during and until 30 seconds after the contraction. The possibility of monitoring the maternal pulse accidentally should be excluded by taking the maternal pulse at the same time as the fetal heart rate.

The following fetal heart rate patterns can be recognised using a fetoscope or hand-held Doptone and will be discussed later in the chapter:
◗ The normal fetal heart rate, which is between 110 to 160 beats per minute.
◗ Deceleration during a contraction.
◗ Late decelerations.
◗ Baseline tachycardia.
◗ Baseline bradycardia.

Continuous cardiotocograph monitoring

The use of continuous cardiotocograph (CTG) fetal monitoring is not necessary in low-risk pregnancies and should always have a proper indication.

Indications for continuous CTG monitoring in labour

▶ Antepartum haemorrhage
▶ Pre-eclampsia
▶ Multiple pregnancy
▶ Previous stillbirth of 38 weeks gestation
▶ Suspected fetal distress
▶ Intra-uterine growth restriction
▶ Meconium stained liquor amnii
▶ Prolonged rupture of membranes (more than 24 hours)
▶ Chorio-amnionitis/amniotic fluid infection syndrome
▶ Induced labour
▶ Previous caesarean section
▶ Prolonged labour (crosses Action Line)

Women's views of electronic fetal monitoring

Besides being the most expensive method, CTG monitoring also restricts the woman's movement by strapping her to the bed all the time, the woman may feel disempowered and helpless, and may even be afraid to ask to move around because she is concerned that she will disturb the monitor. Some women fear that if the monitor is used it means that there is something wrong with their baby.

According to Enkin et al in the studies conducted to assess women's views of fetal monitoring there were no clear differences between the group with fetal assessment with auscultation and the group with electronic fetal monitoring, except that the auscultation group showed more positive experience of labour.

Women on electronic fetal monitoring tend to be left alone more often. In some institutions the monitors are attached to a central station were midwives can view the CTG of different rooms simultaneously and pick up problems accordingly.

Source: Enkin et al, 2000:272.

Although electronic monitoring is supposed to be more reliable and accurate, false results can still arise, especially when the midwives and obstetricians are not skilled in the interpretation of the traces. The transducers may be wrongly applied and the maternal pulse monitored, which may lead to an inappropriate diagnosis of fetal distress and unnecessary caesarean section or a false reassuring pattern. To exclude this possibility the maternal pulse should always be assessed when applying the ultrasound transducer.

More caesarean sections are done when continuous CTG monitoring is used especially without the supportive use of scalp pH. The only advantage of continuous CTG monitoring for the neonate is a 50% reduction in the risk of neonatal seizures.

The admission test

Intrapartum fetal distress commonly reflects a problem preceding the onset of labour. For this reason some institutions which have access to electronic fetal monitors have embarked on a careful risk assessment of all the women who are admitted to the labour ward.

A short ten minute period of electronic fetal heart monitoring upon admission in labour is done on all women as a screening test for both low- and high-risk women. The rationale for this practice is that it helps to identify a fetus that needs more intensive monitoring in labour or a fetus that is already compromised.

The most crucial point in this policy is whether the test is interpreted accurately and whether it is acted upon appropriately. When there is some uncertainty the most senior obstetrician or midwife should be consulted. In Midwife Obstetric Units (MOU) where there is no obstetrician, the midwives have set protocols of patient referral to hospital.

The assessment of the amniotic fluid

It is important to assess the colour of the liquor amnii after the membranes have ruptured. A straw colour is normal but yellow may indicate haemolytic disease, such as Rhesus alloimmunisation, and a port-wine colour may be due to abruptio placentae. Fetal hypoxia causes relaxation of the fetal anal sphincter and a reflex passage of meconium intra-uterine. The fetus can aspirate the meconium either intra-uterine during 'gasping' movements or during the delivery. Meconium-stained liquor (greenish colour) is therefore associated with an increased risk of intrapartum and neonatal death, lower Apgar scores and lower acid-base status.

If meconium is present at the onset of labour, it indicates a hypoxic incident prior to the onset of labour. Thick, undiluted meconium carries the worst prognosis and it is associated with five to seven times increased risk of perinatal death. Thick meconium is also an indicator of reduced amniotic fluid, which is associated with impaired placental function. Although the risk seems smaller with light meconium-stained amniotic fluid, the fetus is still possibly at risk of meconium aspiration. Meconium-stained amniotic fluid combined with fetal heart rate abnormalities has an increased risk of perinatal mortality and morbidity. An amnioinfusion can be performed to dilute the amniotic fluid and reduce the chance of meconium aspiration.

If the breech is presenting and is compacted in the pelvis, meconium may be passed due to compression on the fetus. A breech fetus is also subjected to fetal distress and may pass meconium due to hypoxia.

The normal amount of amniotic fluid is about 1000 ml but in cases of polyhydramnios the woman may drain liquor in excess of 2000 ml. When this occurs, it should be recorded on the partogram.

If the membranes are intact, they must not be ruptured artificially as this can expose the woman and the fetus to infection. If, however, the membranes are ruptured at the time of admission, the duration of the rupture must be accurately recorded on the partogram. The presence of any foul odour or elevated temperature must be noted.

After rupture of membranes the colour of the drained liquor should be recorded every two hours. Three alphabetical letters are used to indicate the condition of the liquor on the partogram (see Figure 13.10):

▶ **I**: to denote intactness of the membranes.
▶ **C**: if the liquor is clear.
▶ **M**: if the liquor is meconium stained.

Fetal scalp blood sampling
Fetal scalp blood sampling is the assessment of the pH value of the fetal scalp blood. A scalpel blade is passed through the cervical os to make an incision on the fetal scalp. A blood sample is drawn in a capillary tube and the specimen is sent for laboratory analysis to determine the fetal acid base status. The values should be interpreted as follows: At or above 7.25 is normal, 7.20 to 7.24 is acidotic and below 7.20 indicates serious acidosis.

If the values are below 7.20, strict fetal heart rate observation is required. When used in combination with fetal heart rate monitoring it reduces the ceasarean section rate for fetal distress, without compromising the neonatal outcome. However, the procedure is no longer practised in some institutions due to the increased risk of HIV infections. It is a very difficult procedure, which requires a highly skilled obstetrician, and it is uncomfortable for the woman.

Fetal heart rate in relation to uterine contractions
The fetal heart rate (FHR) should be evaluated in relation to the uterine contractions during the intrapartum period. Uterine contractions increase myometrial pressure, which reduces the placental blood flow with a subsequent reduction in fetal oxygenation. A compromised fetus can be identified by fetal heart rate abnormalities but the fetal heart rate abnormalities cannot be properly classified without simultaneous monitoring of the contractions.

When the midwife uses the fetoscope or hand-held Doptone to count the fetal heart rate, one hand should be placed on the fundus of the uterus to feel the contractions in order to compare the fetal heart rate with the contractions.

When the woman is on CTG monitoring, the monitor automatically picks up the

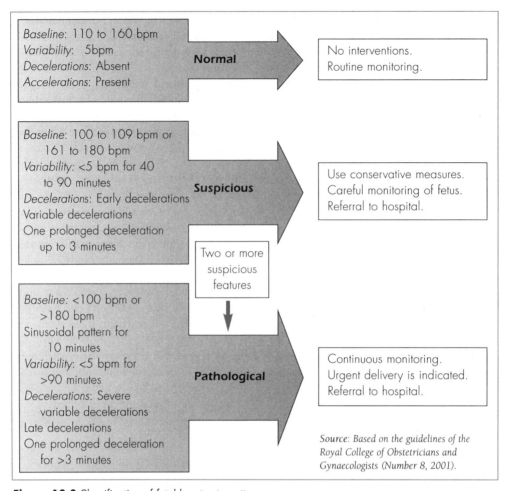

Figure 13.3 Classification of fetal heart rate patterns

contractions via the tocograph transducer and displays them as a graphic representation. The exact duration, intensity and resting tone cannot be evaluated according to the paper recording when using an external tocograph transducer. This will only be accurate when using an internal tocograph transducer. The external tocograph transducer may be negatively influenced by maternal obesity and a restless woman. Only the frequency of the contractions can be determined from the paper recording when a clear recording with minimal interference is maintained. Electronic monitoring can also pick up Braxton Hicks contractions.

Technique of electronic fetal monitoring

External CTG monitoring is measured through ultrasound. An external transducer is placed on the maternal abdomen and the moment-by-moment FHR is displayed graphically on paper. External monitoring is the only method to be used antenatally, as well as when the membranes are still intact or with minimal cervical dilatation. In countries where the risk of mother-to-child transmission of HIV is high, external CTG monitoring is preferred over internal CTG.

Internal CTG monitoring is performed by the application of an internal electrode on the fetal scalp. It is much more reliable but can be used only when the membranes have ruptured and the cervix has dilated at least 2 to 3 cm. In areas where the possibility of MTCT of HIV is minimal, internal CTG monitoring is still used.

Both fetal and uterine transducers should be applied simultaneously as the uterine activity can influence the fetal heart rate. The *tocograph transducer* is placed without the application of jelly on the fundal area of the uterus, as this is where the contractions originate and are at their strongest.

An *intra-uterine pressure monitor* can be used where a catheter is placed inside the uterus. This method is very accurate for measuring the number, length and strength of the contractions, but the membranes should be

ruptured and the cervix 2 to 3 cm dilated. It is seldom used in South Africa, possibly because of the high cost and the need for ruptured membranes.

The speed of the graph paper can be set to 1, 2 or 3 cm per minute, which should be taken into consideration when the graph is interpreted. In South Africa the 1 cm per minute setting is mainly used.

Interpretation of fetal heart rate patterns

The *baseline heart rate* is the mean rate excluding accelerations and decelerations and is determined over a time period of five to ten minutes.

Variability is the alteration in the baseline

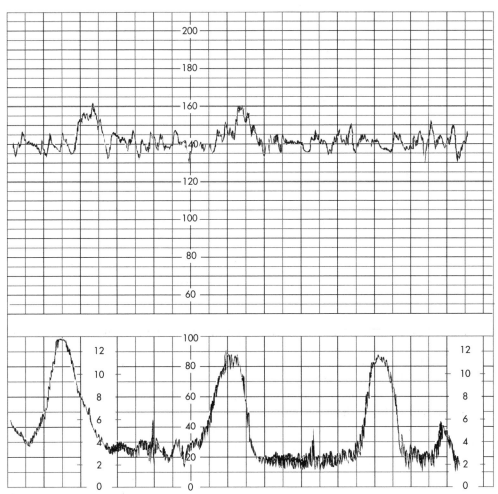

Figure 13.4 The normal fetal heart rate pattern

heart rate, measured over a period of one minute. The difference in heart rate between the highest peak and lowest trough (amplitude of oscillations) is determined and expressed in beats per minute (bpm).

The baseline variability normally exceeds 5 bpm giving the baseline a spiky appearance. A loss or reduction in baseline variability to below 5 bpm gives a flat baseline and this may indicate fetal distress. It may also be due to the fetus sleeping, or the administration of analgesia or a sedative such as *pethidine*.

It is important for midwives to understand the fetal heart rate pattern and to acquire the skills to interpret, describe and classify the pattern correctly so that the appropriate intervention can be taken as needed for the individual woman. Midwives should therefore be able to identify when a pattern is normal, suspicious or pathological.

Abnormalities of fetal heart rate baseline

Baseline tachycardia

A baseline tachycardia is a baseline fetal heart rate of more than 160 bpm.

- A *moderate tachycardia* is 161 to 180 bpm.
- *Severe tachycardia* is above 180 bpm.

A moderate tachycardia is usually not serious but should be evaluated further for absence of accelerations, poor baseline variability and

---

> **Possible causes of baseline bradycardia**
>
> - Late fetal hypoxia.
> - Intense maternal hypotension.
> - Prolonged umbilical cord compression.
> - Fetal heart block.

decelerations. It is usually not the baseline tachycardia itself that poses a problem, but its combination with other abnormalities. The management of the situation will depend on the aetiological factors and other pathological features.

Baseline bradycardia

A baseline bradycardia is a baseline fetal heart rate of less than 110 bpm.

- A *moderate bradycardia*, with between 100 to 109 bpm with good baseline variability, accelerations and no decelerations is no cause for alarm.
- *Severe baseline bradycardia* (less than 100 bpm) with reduced baseline variability and/or late decelerations is a sign of advanced fetal distress.

The possibility of monitoring the maternal pulse instead of fetal heart rate should be excluded. Severe baseline bradycardia should be managed as fetal distress.

> **Possible causes of baseline tachycardia**
>
> - Maternal pyrexia that increases the fetal metabolism.
> - Maternal dehydration.
> - *Hexoprenaline* (Ipradol®) administration which has a cardiac stimulant effect.
> - Infection of the placenta and membranes (chorio-amnionitis/amniotic fluid infection syndrome).
> - Fetal haemorrhage or anaemia. The fetus attempts to compensate to increase tissue perfusion.
> - Maternal heroin addiction.
> - Moderate compression of the cord.
> - Early fetal hypoxia. The sympathetic system is stimulated as the fetus attempts to compensate for the reduced blood flow.
> - Maternal hyperthyroidism where the thyroid-stimulating hormone crosses the placenta and stimulates the fetal heart rate.
> - Idiopathic.

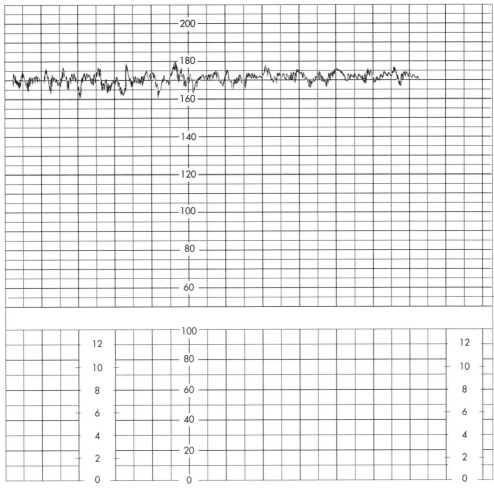

Figure 13.5 Fetal tachycardia

Sinusoidal pattern

The baseline can be within normal limits with a sinusoidal waveform appearance. The frequency is 2 to 5 waves or cycles per minute and the amplitude 5 to 15 bpm. This pattern should persist for at least 10 to 20 minutes (see Figure 24.2). The sinusoidal pattern is associated with hypoxia and anaemia (for example hydrops fetalis and abruptio placentae).

Decelerations of fetal heart rate

A deceleration is a transient decrease of the fetal heart rate below the baseline level of at least 15 bpm and lasting at least 15 seconds. The exception to the rule is the grossly abnormal trace of a baseline rate (usually within

normal limits) with decreased variability (<5 bpm) accompanied by repeated shallow late decelerations of less than 15 bpm.

Decelerations can be divided into four types, namely early, late, variable and prolonged decelerations. Identifying the type of deceleration may give an indication of the possible cause thereof, however, in some cases it is very difficult to determine the type of deceleration. One should be careful not to spend unnecessary time on this when the other features may indicate a grossly abnormal trace.

Early decelerations

Early decelerations are characterised by the slowing of the fetal heart rate, starting at the

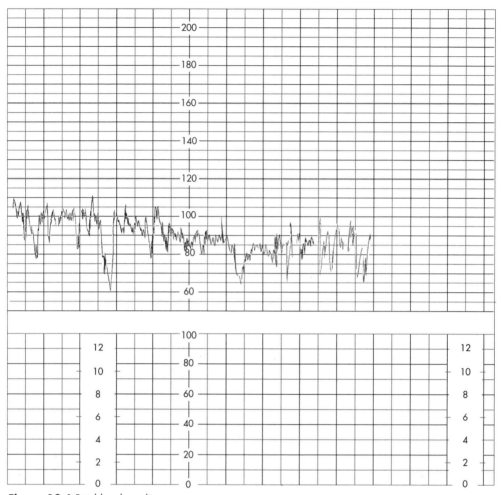

Figure 13.6 Fetal bradycardia

onset of the contractions and returning to normal by the end of the contractions. They are
symmetrical, repetitive and bell-shaped. The
lowest point of the deceleration occurs at the
peak of the contraction therefore they are said
to be a 'mirror image' of the contractions.
Early decelerations usually appear in the later
stage of the first stage of labour and are associated with the descent of the presenting part.
They are usually due to compression of the
fetal head, resulting in increased vagal stimulation which causes the fetal heart to decrease
during a contraction. As soon as the strength
of the contraction decreases, the compression
on the fetal head decreases with less vagal
stimulation.

Evidence of good baseline variability with
early decelerations is reassuring because it
indicates that the fetus is not hypoxic. Early
decelerations are not a sign of fetal distress but
the fetus is at high risk of becoming distressed, which means the situation should be
monitored more carefully. Early decelerations
will be of great concern with a breech presentation or a fetal head that is not well engaged
in the pelvis as vagal stimulation cannot be
responsible for the decelerations.

Due to the cause of early decelerations no
interventions are necessary, but the fetal heart
should be closely monitored. Where the
decelerations cannot be connected to the
cause of early decelerations (such as an
unengaged head), fetal distress should be
considered with appropriate management.

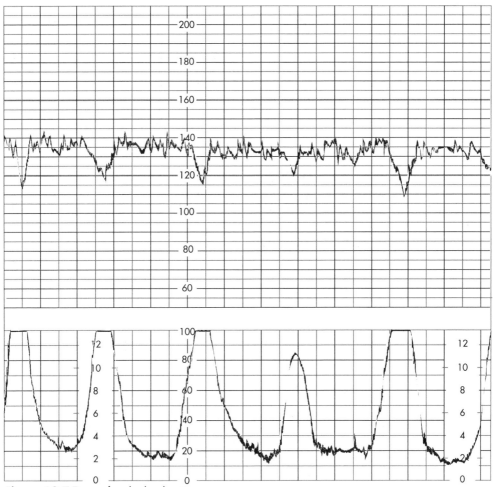

Figure 13.7 Trace of early decelerations

Late decelerations

Late deceleration is characterised by the consistent slowing of the fetal heart rate, starting after the onset of each contraction, and not returning to the baseline by the time the contraction has ended. The lowest point of the deceleration is more than 20 seconds after the peak of the contraction. The decelerations are uniform in shape and tend to reflect associated uterine contractions.

The retroplacental space has a reservoir of oxygenated blood which supplies the fetus with oxygen during a contraction. This retroplacental space is smaller in intra-uterine growth restriction and the blood supply may be poorer. After the onset of a contraction, the fetus first uses all the available oxygen in the

retroplacental space and when no oxygen is available any more, a hypoxic deceleration will start. This is why the deceleration starts later in the contraction. This deceleration will continue throughout until some time after the contraction and will only recover after oxygenation has been restored. Increased hypoxia will cause reduced variability.

Late deceleration is a sign of fetal distress due to the fetal hypoxia. The degree to which the heart rate slows is not important. One of the most worrying patterns is late decelerations (less than 15 bpm) with baseline variability of less than 5 bpm.

With late decelerations an obstetrician should be notified or the woman should be transferred to a higher-level hospital. In the

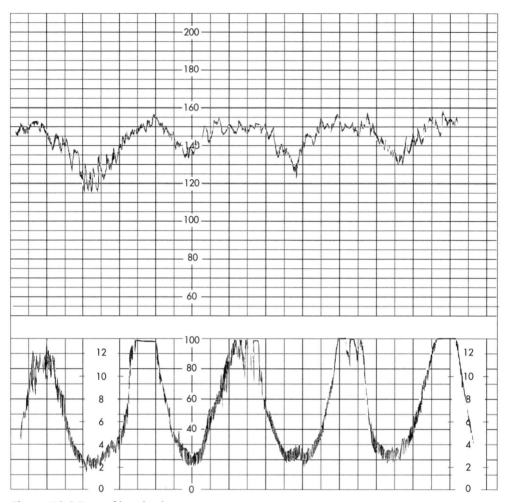

Figure 13.8 Trace of late decelerations

meantime intra-uterine resuscitation should be implemented (see Management of fetal distress later in the chapter.)

Variable decelerations

Variable decelerations are the most common decelerations and they can easily be mistaken for early decelerations. The decelerations vary in appearance (shape and size) and are not always related to the commencement or duration of the contractions. There is a sudden drop of fetal heart rate with a quick return. Variable decelerations are caused by compression of the umbilical cord. The cord may be around the fetal neck, limbs or body, or there may be a true knot in the cord or

cord prolapse. The cord may not necessarily be compressed in exactly the same way during each contraction which may result in a variable pattern of compressions.

The fetal heart usually responds well to the correct interventions such as amnioinfusion and maternal positional changes. Due to an increased risk of fetal distress the fetus should be monitored with care. One of the most important evaluations that should be made is the change of the trace over a time period. Certain pre-pathological or pathological features can develop over time and should be recognised.

The management will depend on the classification of the variable deceleration. (See Classification of variable decelerations on

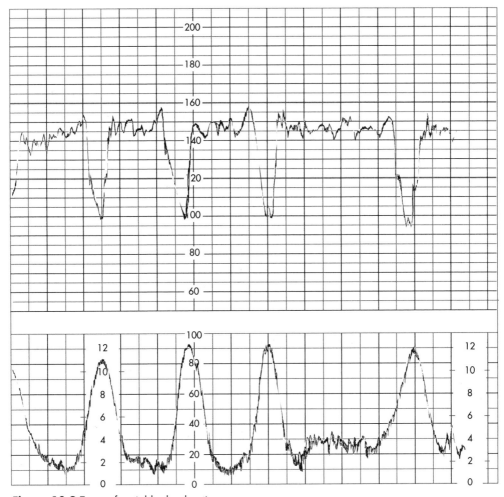

Figure 13.9 Trace of variable decelerations

page 13-20.) Normal variable decelerations should be carefully monitored. For the management of pre-pathological variable decelerations the clinical picture should be taken into consideration (such as the degree of cervical dilatation), and an amnioinfusion may then be considered. Pathological variable decelerations should be managed as fetal distress.

Prolonged decelerations

A prolonged deceleration (FHR less than 100 bpm for three minutes or less than 80 bpm for two minutes) that is not related to a contraction indicates bradycardia rather than a deceleration. Possible causes of prolonged decelerations include:

▶ abruptio placentae
▶ uterine hyperstimulation
▶ cord compression or prolapse
▶ scar dehiscence
▶ epidural analgesia
▶ vaginal examination

The clinical picture will indicate the most probable cause that can be corrected like stopping *oxytocin* infusion. In most cases the FHR will show signs of recovery to the baseline rate within six minutes. A scalp blood sample can be of value. Good baseline variability at the time of the bradycardia and during recovery is a reassuring sign. When bradycardia persists for longer than three to six minutes, hypoxia

---

Classification of variable decelerations

Normal variable deceleration pattern: Shouldering is small accelerations immediately before and after a deceleration and indicates that the fetus can still compensate for the effect of cord compression.

Pre-pathological variable deceleration patterns: Amplifying of shouldering (also called overshooting when the acceleration after the contraction is bigger than the one before the contraction).

Pathological variable deceleration patterns: .
▶ The loss of shouldering.
▶ Reduced variability during the deceleration (smooth pattern), which is also associated with baseline variability.
▶ Slow recovery to the baseline.
▶ Biphasic deceleration when the deceleration takes on the shape of a 'W' (halfway returning to the baseline and starting decelerating again before finally returning to the baseline).
▶ The duration of deceleration is longer than 60 seconds and the depth is greater than 60 bpm.

Source: Adapted from Gibb & Arulkumaran, 1997:38.

---

should be considered with an immediate delivery of the fetus.

Management of fetal distress (pathological patterns)

The specific management will depend on the severity and cause of the abnormal trace. The following guidelines should be followed:
▶ Inform the woman about the problem.
▶ Perform intra-uterine resuscitation:
 ✦ Turn the woman to the left lateral position (to exclude supine hypotension and increase placental perfusion).
 ✦ Administer oxygen with a facemask at 6 litres per minute for a maximum of ten minutes.
 ✦ Ensure adequate maternal hydration to increase placental perfusion with Ringer's lactate infusion at a rate of 240 ml per hour.

Research highlight

The current available evidence suggests that prolonged oxygen administration during labour is ineffective or even harmful.

Source: Hofmeyer, 2003; RCOG Clinical Effectiveness Support Unit, 2001.

 ✦ Where applicable, discontinue *oxytocin* infusion to decrease the uterine contractions.
 ✦ Perform amnioinfusion when severe variable decelerations are present to decrease the cord compression.
▶ Exclude vaginal bleeding.
▶ Perform a vaginal examination to exclude full dilatation, cord prolapse or presentation. Deliver immediately if cervix is fully dilated.
▶ If immediate delivery is not possible, administer *hexoprenaline* 10 micrograms IV.
▶ Prepare for caesarean section and notify the available obstetrician or arrange an urgent transfer to a hospital with theatre facilities.

Amnioinfusion

Amnioinfusion is a technique where luke-warm, sterile normal saline is infused into the uterus. A rubber or plastic catheter is inserted into the uterus via a partly dilated cervix (membranes need to be ruptured). An initial 800 ml normal saline is infused over one hour through a 15-dropper IV set, followed by 180 ml per hour.

An amnioinfusion is performed to correct oligohydramnios, which increases the risk of umbilical cord compression (identified by variable decelerations). It can also be used to dilute thick meconium in the amniotic fluid to minimise the risk of fetal meconium aspiration.

Progress of labour

The progress of labour is best monitored by using the partogram.

Drawing the Alert and Action Line

Zero time

Zero time must be noted as the time of admission of the woman to the labour ward. It does not denote the time at which the high-risk factors may have been initially identified.

Alert Line

As soon as the active phase of labour is diagnosed, an Alert Line is drawn on the partogram at a slope of 1 cm per hour from the first cervical dilatation that is greater than 3 cm. In cases where the partogram has a pre-drawn Alert Line, the cervical dilatation should be moved up to coincide with the Alert Line. It is important to record both the actual time that the woman has been in labour, and the number of hours following admission to the labour ward, so as to alert the midwife and the medical practitioner to the passage of time. When the cervical dilatation crosses the Alert Line, it is an indication that labour may be prolonged. The midwife

should react immediately and not wait for it to cross the Action Line. A decision should be taken whether to transfer the woman to the referral hospital if adequate facilities and expertise are not available to deal with obstetric emergencies.

Action Line

The Action Line is drawn two hours to the right and parallel to the Alert Line. Previously labour wards in Level 2 and 3 hospitals used an Action Line that is four hours to the right of the Alert Line. The National Department of Health (2002:34) cautions that while this practice may be acceptable in hospitals because they can respond promptly to an obstetrical emergency, it may be unsafe for community healthcare centres. Therefore the community centres should refer immediately when cervical dilatation reaches the Alert Line. The maternal case record should accompany the woman to the hospital.

If the plotting of the recordings crosses the Action Line it denotes excessively poor progress of labour and immediate interventions need to be put in place in order to prevent maternal and fetal morbidity. There are two indicators which are used to judge the progress of labour: the rate of cervical dilatation and the descent of the fetal head. When there is arrest of fetal descent or the cervical dilatation crosses the Action Line, immediate action should follow. Progress of labour should be evaluated according to the 'Rule of Ps' (see Chapter 26) and appropriate action should be taken, such as augmentation of labour or caesarean section.

According to the Report on Confidential Enquiries into Maternal Deaths in South Africa (2002) strong emphasis should be placed on the use of the partogram and on the implementation of appropriate management and referral protocols.

Cervical dilatation and effacement

Cervical effacement and dilatation are important parameters for measuring the progress of

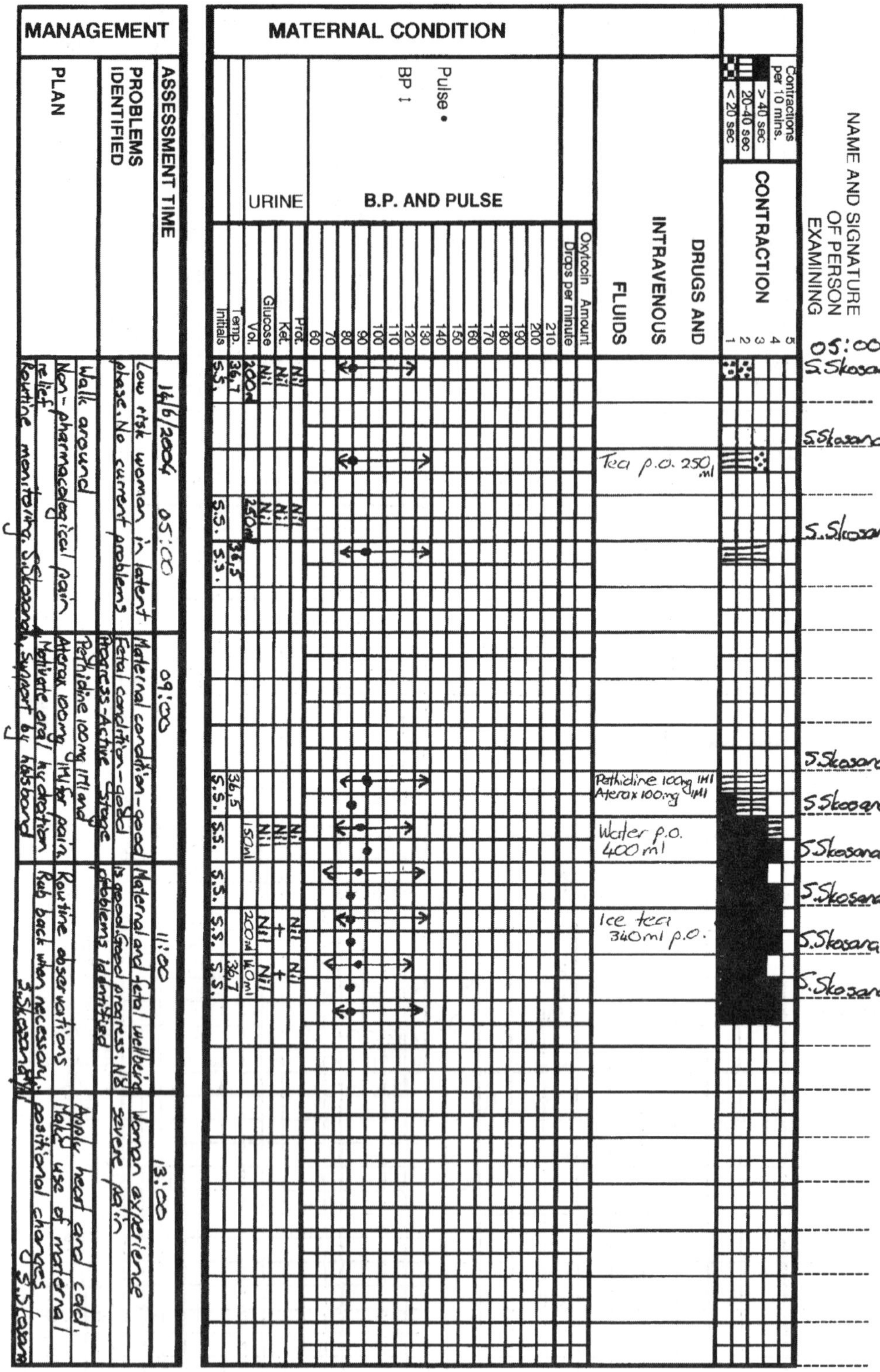

MANAGEMENT

PLAN | PROBLEMS IDENTIFIED | ASSESSMENT TIME

MATERNAL CONDITION

Pulse • BP ↑

URINE | B.P. AND PULSE

Temp. / Initials / Vol. / Glucose / Ket. / Prot.

60 70 80 90 100 110 120 130 140 150 160 170 180 190 200 210

Drops per minute | Oxytocin Amount

DRUGS AND INTRAVENOUS FLUIDS

CONTRACTION — Contractions per 10 mins.
- > 40 sec
- 20–40 sec
- < 20 sec

NAME AND SIGNATURE OF PERSON EXAMINING

05:00 S. Skosana R/N
S. Skosana R/N
S. Skosana R/N
S. Skosana R/N
S. Skosana R/N
S. Skosana R/N
S. Skosana R/N
S. Skosana R/N

14/6/2004 05:00 — Low risk woman in latent phase. No current problems — Non-pharmacological pain relief — Routine monitoring. S.Skosana. Support by husband. — Walk around

09:00 — Maternal condition-good. Fetal condition-good. Progress: Active stage — Pethidine 100mg IMI for pain. Aterax oral hydration. — Ratidine 100mg little oral — Motivate oral hydration. Rub back when necessary. S.Skosana R/N

11:00 — Maternal and fetal wellbeing is good. Good progress. N.B. No problems identified — Routine observations — Tea p.o. 250 ml / Pethidine 100mg IMI / Aterax 100mg IMI / Water p.o. 400 ml / Ice tea 340 ml p.o.

13:00 — Woman experience severe pain — Apply heat and cold. Make use of maternal positional changes. S.Skosana R/N

Figure 13.10 Example of completed partogram

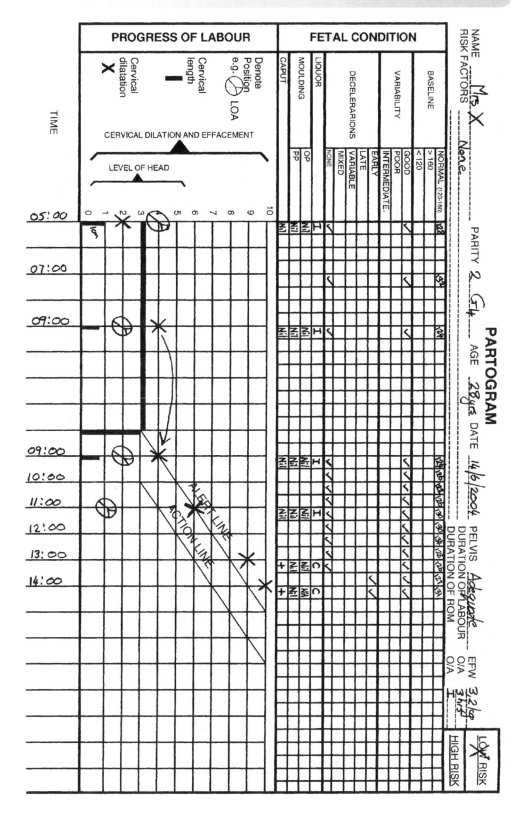

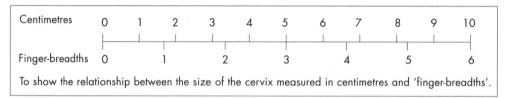

Centimetres	0	1	2	3	4	5	6	7	8	9	10
Finger-breadths	0		1		2		3		4	5	6

To show the relationship between the size of the cervix measured in centimetres and 'finger-breadths'.

Figure 13.11 Cervical dilatation in centimetres

labour (see Chapter 12 for the physiology of dilatation and effacement of the cervix).

With the first vaginal examination, the cervical dilatation is plotted as a 'x' at zero time on the partogram. The results of subsequent cervical examinations are recorded progressively at stipulated intervals along the 24-hour time scale. During the latent phase (3 cm cervical dilatation) vaginal examination should be conducted every four hours. In active labour (more than 3 cm cervical dilatation) it should be conducted every two hours. In cases where the plotting of the cervical dilatation has crossed the Alert Line, close monitoring should continue. Note the recording of the cervical dilatation on the partogram in Figure 13.10.

Descent of the fetal head

Two interrelated motions occur when the head enters the pelvic brim: descent and engagement of the head. The descent of the fetal head is described in relation to the pelvic brim and expressed in fifths. Ordinarily, the fetal head accommodates the full width of five (5) fingers.

In order to measure the descent, the midwife places her hand on the woman's abdomen and feels for the occiput and the sinciput.

▶ A head that is five-fifths (5/5) above the brim has not yet entered the pelvic brim, and is completely mobile on palpation.
▶ A head that is four-fifths above the pelvis is just beginning to enter the pelvic brim.
▶ At three-fifths above the brim, the head has partially entered the pelvic brim and

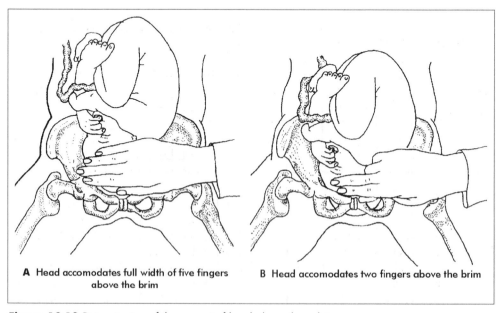

A Head accomodates full width of five fingers above the brim

B Head accomodates two fingers above the brim

Figure 13.12 Determination of the amount of head above the pelvis

on abdominal palpation, the hand can still partially encircle the fetal head.

▶ When the head is two-fifths above the pelvic brim, almost the entire occiput and more than half of the head will have entered the pelvic brim.

▶ Once the head has descended to the extent that only one-fifth remains above the pelvic brim, only the sinciput can be palpated abdominally.

▶ When the whole head has entered the pelvic brim, neither the sinciput nor the occiput can be palpated abdominally. This finding is recorded as nought-fifths (0/5) above the brim.

The better the descent, the better the progress of labour. Arrest in descent indicates a possible problem and further investigation should be made. Descent of the presenting part (felt on abdominal palpation) is a better parameter to use than station of the presenting part on vaginal examination. The descent of the fetal head is plotted as a circle on the partogram (see Figure 13.10).

If no excessive moulding takes place, the amount of head palpatable above the pelvis will correlate with the station of the presenting part.

Moulding of the fetal head

Moulding is the ability of the bones of the scull to overlap in order to pass through the birth canal (see Chapter 12). Excessive moulding is a key indicator of cephalopelvic disproportion. Moulding can be assessed during a vaginal examination where both interparietal and parieto-occipital moulding can be detected. The degree of moulding should be assessed and the information recorded on the partogram using the following taxonomy:

−   The bones are separated normally.
+   The bones are touching each other.
++ The bones are overlapping but can be easily separated with digital pressure.
+++ The bones are overlapping and cannot be separated with digital pressure. It is a sign of cephalopelvic disproportion.

It must be noted that moulding does not occur in post-term pregnancies. In such cases the fontanelles are less palpable.

Caput

On vaginal examination caput succedaneum may be felt. This is a swelling of the tissues over the presenting part of the fetal head which is caused by pressure during labour. With each contraction the presenting part is forced down onto the dilating cervix and during this time circulation to the scalp is reduced and swelling develops. Caput can be felt during vaginal examination and should be indicated on the partogram, if present.

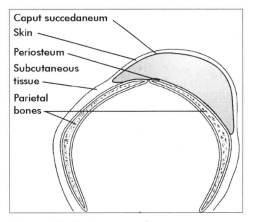

Figure 13.13 Caput succedaneum

Uterine contractions

Observing the uterine contractions is an important aspect of monitoring the progress of labour. The intensity, frequency and duration of the uterine contractions are monitored every two hours during the latent phase and every 30 minutes during the active phase, and plotted on the partogram directly below the cervicograph. The contractions are monitored during the last ten minutes of each half hour period. The characteristics of contractions are discussed in Chapter 12.

The duration of the contractions are graded into three categories and a different type of symbol is used to represent each category:

CRITICAL THINKING EXERCISES

1. Record the following contractions on a blank partogram:
   a) Pattern of contractions that would indicate uterine hypotonia.
   b) Pattern of contractions that would indicate uterine hypertonia.
2. What would the midwife's responsibility be in each of the above cases?
3. Plot the information of each of the following cases on a blank partogram. Analyse each case and indicate the type of labour outcome you expect.

Case A – *Linda, admitted at 14.00:*
▶ Level of head, 4/5
▶ Cervical dilatation, 4 cm
▶ Contractions 3 in 10 minutes, each lasting 30 seconds

At 18.00:
▶ Level of head, 3/5
▶ Cervical dilatation, 6 cm
▶ Contractions 4 in 10 minutes, each lasting 40 seconds

Case B – *Lindiwe, admitted at 08.00:*
▶ Level of head, 4/5
▶ Cervical dilatation, 4 cm
▶ Contractions 3 in 10 minutes, each lasting 40 seconds

At 12.00 noon:
▶ Level of head, 4/5
▶ Cervical dilatation, 4 cm
▶ Contractions 2 in 10 minutes, each lasting 20 seconds

Case C – *Varshika, admitted at 15.00:*
▶ Level of head, 3/5
▶ Cervical dilatation, 4 cm
▶ Contractions 3 in 10 minutes, each lasting 40 seconds

At 19.00:
▶ Level of head, 1/5
▶ Cervical dilatation, 8 cm
▶ Contractions 5 in 10 minutes, each lasting 50 seconds

Contractions lasting less than 20 seconds:

Contractions lasting 20 to 40 seconds:

Contractions lasting more than 40 seconds:

Refer to Figure 13.10 for details on how the duration and frequency of uterine contractions should be recorded on the partogram.

Artificial rupture of the membranes

For decades the artificial rupturing of membranes (AROM) was conducted as a routine procedure aimed at enhancing the progress of labour. This practice is now being discouraged as it has the potential risk of increasing mother-to-child transmission (MTCT) of HIV. The rupture of membranes for longer than four hours prior to delivery is associated with increased MTCT. According to the HIV/AIDS Policy Guidelines, routine AROM should be avoided in both HIV-positive and -negative women. The guidelines further stipulate that AROM should be done only if there are specific obstetric indications and then as late as possible.

Prophylactic antibiotics should be administered in women with CD4 counts of less than 200 cells/μL. However, most delivery units do not have the facilities to check the CD4 counts. It would be wise to provide prophylactic antibiotics in women who exhibit signs of severe immune deficiency, or if the rupture of membranes has exceeded four hours prior to delivery.

Intrapartum referral criteria

Women with pre-existing conditions identified through antenatal screening should be referred by midwives at satellite clinics when they are admitted to the labour ward. Screening for high-risk conditions is discussed in Chapters 9 and 18.

Some conditions may not be present

during pregnancy, but may manifest themselves only during labour. Midwives working at satellite clinics in particular should be vigilant and immediately refer women presenting with any of the problems listed in the box below. The unit's referral protocols should be followed closely and any pre-referral and in-transit management protocols implemented. Proper recording should be maintained throughout the transfer.

Induction of labour

Induction of labour is the initiation of labour by artificial method. Labour is induced when the benefits of delivering the fetus outweigh those of continuing with the pregnancy. An induction should be performed at a hospital.

Prerequisites and conditions for induction of labour

The duration of the pregnancy is a very important aspect when considering an induction of labour. The closer the gestation to term the more effective the procedure will be with the least amount of neonatal complications for the baby.

A favourable cervix responds to uterine contractions and cervical dilatation will follow. *Oxytocin* administration when the cervix

---

Indications for referral during the intrapartum period

- Eclampsia.
- Hypertension of 150/100 mmHg or more.
- Haemorrhage.
- Fetal distress: Decelerations or meconium stained liquor.
- Preterm labour or preterm prelabour rupture of membranes.
- Prelabour rupture of membranes for more than 12 hours.
- Pyrexia over 37.5 °C in labour.
- Malpresentations.
- Slow progress:
  - Prolonged latent phase – labour lasting longer than eight hours.
  - Cervical dilatation on partogram reaches the Action Line in the active phase.
  - Cervical dilatation on partogram crosses the Alert Line in the following cases: a grande multipara, teenage primigravida, or a woman who has a small or borderline pelvis.
  - Prolonged second stage. An experienced midwife should accompany such cases (see Chapter 14).
  - Placenta retained over one hour.

Indications for induction of labour

Maternal indications:
- Post-term pregnancy (42 weeks of gestation or more).
- Hypertensive disorders, including pre-eclampsia and eclampsia.
- Prelabour rupture of membranes at or after 34 weeks gestation, when onset of labour does not occur within 12 to 24 hours after the rupture of membranes.
- Abruptio placentae, depending on the severity of the condition.
- Maternal medical problems such as renal, respiratory or cardiac conditions.
- Elective induction on the request of the woman due to psychological reasons.
- Diabetes in pregnancy prior to the expected date of delivery to prevent perinatal mortality and macrosomia.
- Intra-uterine death to relieve the woman of the psychological stress of carrying a dead fetus, and also to prevent diffuse intravascular coagulopathy (DIC) four to five weeks later.
- A previous poor obstetric history such as stillbirth.

Fetal indications:
- Intra-uterine growth restriction.
- Diminished fetal movement.

Table 13.1 Modified Bishop Scoring system for assessing cervical ripening

Score	0	1	2	3
Dilatation of cervix in cm	<1	1–2	2–4	>4
Effacement of cervix in cm	>4	2–4	1–2	<1
Consistency of cervix	Firm	Average	Soft	–
Position of cervix	Posterior	Mid-anterior	–	–
Station of fetal head	–3	–2	–1 to 0	+1 to +2

is unripe (unfavourable) has been known to lead to a higher incidence of failure of induction, caesarean sections, infections and other complications. The cervix should first be assessed according to the Bishop score. A Bishop score of >7 indicates a favourable cervix which needs no ripening and labour can be induced by *oxytocin* alone. An unfavourable cervix (with a Bishop score of 6) first needs ripening by methods such as the use of prostaglandin. *Oxytocin* can then be introduced afterwards if needed to ensure regular contractions.

Methods of induction of labour

Sweeping/stripping of the membranes
Sweeping/stripping of the membranes involves separation of the membranes from the lower uterine segment through the cervical os. This

---

Contraindications for induction of labour

▶ Cephalopelvic disproportion.
▶ A severe fetal compromise such as fetal distress.
▶ Placenta praevia.
▶ Cord presentation or cord prolapse with a live fetus.
▶ Previous caesarean section due to fear of uterine rupture (relative contraindication).
▶ Congenital abnormalities of the uterus.
▶ Abnormal fetal presentation, lie and attitude.
▶ Grande multiparity (relative contraindication).

---

procedure is said to stimulate prostaglandin synthesis, which brings about cervical changes. Although this method is uncomfortable for the woman, it does reduce the need for other more formal methods of induction.

Amniotomy
An amniotomy is the artificial rupture of membranes with an amnion hook. The possibility of cord prolapse should always be excluded after the rupture of membranes. The amniotomy causes prostaglandin synthesis, which should bring about effacement and dilatation of the cervix. However, an amniotomy should never be performed when the presenting part is high, an unfavourable cervix is present or HIV/AIDS has been diagnosed.

Complications of an amniotomy may include the following:
▶ Cord prolapse, particularly when the presenting part is still high.
▶ Early decelerations of the fetal heart.
▶ Ascending infection (including MTCT of HIV).
▶ Vaginal bleeding due to trauma to the cervix.

Prostaglandins
There are other methods of cervical ripening for induction, but the group of prostaglandin compounds are found to be most effective and therefore more widely recommended. Prostaglandin use has resulted in higher incidence of uterine over-stimulation but negative infant outcome has not been reported.

- *Oral prostaglandins.* Synthetic *prostaglandin E₁*, analog *misoprostol*, can be administered orally and it has been found to be more effective in cervical ripening and the inducing of labour than *prostaglandin E₂* (PGE₂). Although this is a very promising and cost-effective method the optimal dosage still needs to be determined and the safety of the drug has not yet been confirmed.
- *Vaginal prostaglandins.* A maximum of four tablets PGE₂ (0.5 mg per tablet) may be administered vaginally by placing them in the posterior fornix. However, the tablets are no longer widely used and the modern method is to insert 1 mg or 2 mg of PGE₂ in a gel form (Prandin Gel®) in the posterior fornix, which has been found to be far more potent than the tablets.
- *Endocervical prostaglandins.* The use of 0.5 mg PGE₂ gel (Prepedil Gel®) endocervically is very effective for the ripening of the cervix even though the dosage of prostaglandin is lower than found in the vaginal preparates.
- *Extra-/intra-amniotic prostaglandins. Prostin F2 Alpha* 5 mg was previously used, but due to a high incidence of side-effects it is no longer being used. However, it is still used sometimes in the control of postpartum haemorrhage.
- Oral tablets are used in women with ruptured membranes and vaginal administration is preferred in women with intact membranes. The course of *prostaglandin E₂* tablets may be repeated twice if the first dose does not have any effect.

Oxytocin

Oxytocin is a hormone extract from the posterior pituitary gland. It acts at cell level on the smooth muscles of the myometrium and initiates uterine contraction. *Oxytocin* is found in 2 IU/ml, 5 IU/ml and 10 IU/ml. Intramuscular administration is not recommended during labour, but it can be used in the postpartum period to stimulate the contraction of the uterus to control postpartum haemorrhage.

Oxytocin regime for induction or augmentation of labour

1. Add 2 IU of *oxytocin* to 1000 ml Ringer's lactate.
2. Using a 15 drop/ml set, start the infusion at a rate of 15 drops per minute (60 ml per hour).
3. Increase the amount every 30 minutes by 15 drops per minute until three strong contractions of at least 40 seconds are obtained in a 10 minute period.
4. The maximum infusion rate is 60 drops per minute.
5. If the maximum infusion rate of 60 drops per minute is reached without achieving adequate contractions, the dosage should be increased. Start an infusion with 4 IU of *oxytocin* in 1000 ml at a rate of 45 drops per minute (120 ml per hour), increasing if needed after 30 minutes to 60 drops per minute.

Source: *DoH, Guidelines for maternity care in South Africa, 2002:42.*

Induction with *oxytocin* in the multiparous woman should be done with caution due to the higher risk of uterine rupture.

The rate of administration should be controlled and titrated against the uterine contractions. The administration rate should maintain effective well-spaced contractions. The contractions should not exceed three to five contractions per 10 minutes and they should not last longer than 45 to 50 seconds each. It is of utmost importance that the administration of the drug is recorded on the partogram and the woman should be monitored closely.

Possible side-effects of *oxytocin* administration include hyper-stimulation of the uterus, decreased placental perfusion that may lead to fetal distress, as well as uterine rupture. Rapid labour and birth can also cause cervical and vaginal lacerations and postpartum haemorrhage. Water intoxication and hyponatremia may develop due to the slight antidiuretic

Midwifery considerations during oxytocin administration

▶ The woman needs constant observation.
▶ The obstetrician should prescribe the drug or the institution should have a protocol of administration which includes clear and easy to follow guidelines for administering the drug.
▶ The correct dose should be given to the right woman, for example, multiparae should not receive the same dose as primigravidae.
▶ The oxytocin is added to a 1000 ml Ringer's lactate and it should be mixed well to ensure that the correct amount is administered consistently. The vacolitre should be labelled with the amount of oxytocin added, the time, date and signature of the person who performed the administration.
▶ The administration should be controlled by an infusion pump in order to give the accurate amount of oxytocin per minute.
▶ Each time the rate is increased it should be recorded properly on the partogram.
▶ The uterine activity and fetal heart rate should be monitored with continuous CTG.
▶ The contractions should be monitored every half hour by the midwife. They should not exceed three to five in 10 minutes and should not last longer than 45 to 50 seconds each. If the woman develops over-stimulation of the uterus, the infusion rate should be decreased or stopped.
▶ Any abnormal fetal heart rate pattern after oxytocin administration should be reported and the oxytocin administration should be stopped.

effect of the drug but this is more common where large quantities of oxytocin are administered over a long period of time. Water intoxication may cause confusion, vomiting, convulsions, coma or even maternal death.

Amniotomy combined with oxytocin drug

The intravenous administration of oxytocin after an amniotomy was the most widely used method, however, with the prevalence of HIV infection the practice has declined. After amniotomy, the intravenous oxytocin will shorten the time between rupture of membranes and delivery. Women who receive oxytocin from the time the membranes are ruptured are more likely to deliver within 12 to 24 hours of the administration of oxytocin. They are also less likely to undergo an assisted delivery or caesarean section.

Other methods of induction of labour

If all the above methods of induction have failed, the insertion of an indwelling catheter may be the last resort, particularly in cases where the induction has been indicated due to intra-uterine death. The indwelling catheter with a 30 ml water bulb is inserted into the cervix and traction is applied to stimulate dilatation.

The Lamicel® tent, a hygroscopic seaweed preparation, is inserted into the cervix to absorb moisture and swell up, thus dilating the cervix. However, most institutions no longer use Lamicel®.

Augmentation of labour

Augmentation of labour is an intervention performed to correct the poor progress of labour.

Induction versus augmentation

It is important to understand the difference between induction and augmentation of labour: With induction of labour, the woman is not yet in labour and labour is initiated by using methods to ripen the cervix and/or oxytocin is administered to introduce regular contractions. In augmentation the labour has started spontaneously but the uterine contractions need strengthening.

In a nutshell

▸ By using the principles of the Better Births initiative the quality of care rendered to women is improved.

▸ Every woman in labour should be thoroughly screened for high risk factors.

▸ Failure to use the partogram during labour constitutes substandard care.

▸ The three major aspects that should be monitored during labour are the maternal condition, the fetal condition and the progress of labour.

▸ During labour the fetal heart rate should be monitored from 30 seconds before, during and until 30 seconds after a contraction.

▸ The possibility of accidentally monitoring the maternal pulse should be excluded by taking the maternal pulse at the same time as the fetal heart rate.

Uterine hypotonia may be present with subsequent poor progress of labour. Augmentation is sometimes needed with epidural anaesthesia because it tends to inhibit uterine contractions. The two methods that are mainly used for augmentation is amniotomy (in the absence of HIV/AIDS) and *oxytocin*. Augmentation through the administration of *oxytocin* may be required in order to strengthen, regulate, and maintain the contractions. The regime for *oxytocin* administration and monitoring of the woman and fetus is the same as during induction of labour (see page 13-29).

References

Adams, T. J. & Douglas, M. J. 1995. Maternal oxygen administration and fetal wellbeing. *American Journal of Obstetrics and Gynecology,* September 173(3):974.

Alfirevic, Z. 2001. Oral misoprostol for induction of labour (Cochrane Review). *The Cochrane Library,* Issue 2. Oxford: Update Software.

Bennett, V. R. & Brown, L. K.(Eds.) 1999. *Myles textbook for midwives.* Thirteenth edition. Edinburgh: Churchill Livingstone.

Boulvain, M., Stan, C. & Irion, O. 2001. Elective delivery in diabetic pregnant women (Cochrane Review). *The Cochrane Library,* Issue 2. Oxford: Update Software.

Boulvain, M., Stan, C. & Irion, O. 2001. Membrane sweeping for induction of labour (Cochrane Review). *The Cochrane Library,* Issue 2. Oxford: Update Software.

Butnarescu, G. F. & Tillotson, D. M. 1983. *Maternity nursing. Theory to practice.* New York: John Wiley & Sons.

Cefalo, R. C. 2002. Effects of high-inspired oxygen fraction during elective caesarean section under spinal anaesthesia on maternal and fetal oxygenation and lipid peroxidation. *Obstetrical Gynecological Survey,* July 57(7):424–425.

DoH (Department of Health). 1998. *First interim report of confidential enquiries into maternal deaths in South Africa.* Pretoria: Department of Health.

DoH (Department of Health). 1999. *Second interim report of confidential enquiries into maternal deaths in South Africa.* Pretoria: Department of Health.

DoH (Department of Health). 2000. *Third interim report on confidential enquiries into maternal deaths in South Africa.* Pretoria: Department of Health.

DoH (Department of Health). 2002. *HIV/AIDS policy guideline. Prevention of mother-to-child HIV transmission and management of HIV positive pregnant women.* Pretoria: Department of Health.

DoH (Department of Health). 2002. *HIV/AIDS policy guideline. Prevention and treatment of opportunistic and HIV related diseases in adults.* Pretoria: Department of Health.

DoH (Department of Health). 2002. *Guidelines for maternity care in South Africa.* Second edition. Pretoria: Department of Health.

DoH (Department of Health). 2002. *Second report of confidential enquiries into maternal deaths in South Africa* 1999–2001. Pretoria: Department of Health.

Enkin, M., Keirse, M. J. N. C., Neilson, J., Crowther, C., Duley, L., Hodnett, E. & Hofmeyr, J. 2000. *A guide to effective care in pregnancy and childbirth*. Third edition. Oxford: Oxford University Press.

Gibb, D. & Arulkumaran, S. 1997. *Fetal monitoring in practice*. Second edition. Oxford: Butterworth-Heinemann.

Hamilton, P. M. 1989. *Basic maternity nursing*. Sixth edition. St. Louis: Mosby.

Hofmeyr, G. J. 2003. Amnioinfusion for meconium-stained liquor in labour (Cochrane Review). *The Cochrane Library*, Issue 1. Oxford: Update Software.

Hofmeyr G. J. 2003. Maternal oxygen administration for fetal distress (Cochrane Review). *The Cochrane Library*, Issue 2. Oxford: Update Software.

Hofmeyr, G. J. & Gülmezoglu, A. M. 2003. Vaginal misoprostol for cervical ripening and induction of labour (Cochrane Review). *The Cochrane Library*, Issue 1. Oxford: Update Software.

Howarth, G. R. & Botha, D.J. 2001. Amniotomy plus intravenous oxytocin for induction of labour (Cochrane Review). *The Cochrane Library*, Issue 3. Oxford: Update Software.

International Federation of Gynaecology & Obstetrics. 1987. FIGO News: Guidelines for the use of fetal monitoring. *International Journal of Gynaecology and Obstetrics*, 25:159–167.

Ladewig, P. W., London, M. L. & Olds, S. B. 1998. *Maternal–newborn nursing care: The nurse, the family, and the community*. Fourth edition. Menlo Park California: Addison Wesley Longman.

Larsen, J. 1999. *Obstetrics in peripheral hospitals: A South African manual for doctors and midwives*. Durban: Department of Paediatrics, University of Natal.

Luckas, M. & Bricher, L. 2000. Intravenous prostaglandin for induction of labour (Cochrane Review). *The Cochrane Library*, Issue 4. Oxford: Update Software.

Llewellyn-Jones D. 1982. *Fundamentals of obstetrics and gynaecology*. Volume 1. Third edition. London: Faber & Faber.

Nel, J. T. 1998. *Core obstetrics and gynaecology*. Durban: Butterworth Publishers.

Nolte, A. G. W. (Ed.) 1998. *A textbook for midwives*. Pretoria: J. L. van Schaik Publishers.

Oxorn H. 1986. *Human labor and birth*. Fifth edition. London: Appleton-Century-Crofts.

Peirce, B. T., Napolitano, P. F., Pierce, L. M. et al. 2001. The effects of hypoxia on fetal-placental vascular tone and inflammatory cytokine production. *American Journal of Obstetrics and Gynecology*, 185(5): 1068–1072.

Phillips, C. R. 1991. *Family-centered maternity/newborn care*. Third edition. St. Louis: Mosby.

RCOG Clinical Effectiveness Support Unit. 2001. *The use of electronic fetal monitoring, Evidence-based clinical guideline Number 8*. London: Royal College of Obstetricians and Gynaecologists.

Reeder, S. J., Mastroianni, L. & Martin, L. L. 1983. *Maternity nursing*. Fifteenth edition, London: J.B. Lippincot.

Sellers, P. M. 1993. *Midwifery*. Volume 2. Kenwyn: Juta.

Stanhope, M. & Lancaster, J. 1991. *Community health nursing: Process and practice for promoting health*. St. Louis: Mosby.

Williams, J. & Blanchard, J. 1996. *Electronic monitoring of the fetal heart*. Cheshire: Books for Midwives Press.

Woods, D. (Ed.) 1995. *Perinatal Education Programme: Maternal manual*. Cape Town: Perinatal Education Trust.

WHO (World Health Organisation). 1993. WHO/FHE/MSM/93.8. *Maternal health and safe motherhood programme. Preventing prolonged labour: A practical guide. The partograph part I: Principles and strategy*. Geneva: WHO Division of Family Health.

WHO (World Health Organisation). 1993. WHO/FHE/MSM/93.9. *Maternal health and safe motherhood programme. Preventing prolonged labour: A practical guide. The partograph part II: User's manual.* Geneva: WHO Division of Family Health.

WHO (World Health Organisation). 1993. WHO/FHE/MSM/93.10. *Maternal health and safe motherhood programme. Preventing prolonged labour: A practical guide. The partograph part III: Facilitator's guide.* Geneva: WHO Division of Family Health.

WHO (World Health Organisation). 1993. WHO/FHE/MSM/93.11. *Maternal health and safe motherhood programme. Preventing prolonged labour: A practical guide. The partograph part IV: Guidelines for operations research.* Geneva: WHO Division of Family Health.

WHO (World Health Organisation). 1993. WHO/FHE/MSM/93.12. *Maternal health and safe motherhood programme. Midwifery practice: Measuring, developing and mobilizing quality care.* Report of a collaborative WHO/ICM/UNICEF pre-congress workshop. Vancouver, Canada. Geneva: WHO Division of Family Health.

Chapter 14

Second and third stages of labour

Joanita de Kock

Introduction

During the second stage of labour the focus moves from a passive woman, experiencing a lot of pain, to a more physically involved woman. The tempo is fast with several events happening at the same time. Many emotions are involved as this is the moment that the parents have been waiting for. The woman will actively bear down and deliver her baby. During the third stage of labour the mother's focus shifts to bonding with her newborn, while the placenta is delivered and perineal repair is performed, where necessary.

The midwife's role during the second and third stage of labour is to conduct the birth of the baby and placenta, which includes the prevention and early detection of any complications. The parents should be supported emotionally and parent–infant bonding should be promoted at this time.

Onset and duration of the second stage of labour

The second stage of labour begins when the cervix is fully dilated (10 cm) and ends with the birth of the baby. For practical reasons, the second stage of labour can also be divided into two phases:

▶ The *first phase* is when the cervix is fully dilated, but the presenting part is not yet on the perineum and there is not yet a desire to bear down.

▶ The *second phase* (expulsion phase) is when the presenting part has descended and it exerts pressure on the sacral nerves to the rectum, causing the urge to bear down.

According to the WHO, the mean duration of the second stage of labour in primiparous women (who have delivered one viable child) is 45 minutes. The policy to limit the duration of the second stage of labour for a better maternal and fetal outcome has been evaluated in several studies and it has been found that except for higher pH values in the umbilical artery, there is really no other evidence that the practice benefits the baby (WHO, 1996). Rigid limitation of the second stage to an hour increases the possibility of interventions with a subsequent increased chance of complications. If the mother's condition is satisfactory, there is no sign of fetal distress and there is evidence of progress in the descent of the presenting head, then there is no need for any interventions. There is, however, a much slimmer chance of spontaneous delivery after a second stage of more than two hours in nulliparous women and more than one hour in multiparous women. In these cases assistance in the safe delivery of the child should be considered.

The only definite sign of the onset of the second stage is full dilatation of the cervix. In many cases the exact time is difficult to determine unless a vaginal examination is performed at that specific moment. Possible signs that the cervix might be fully dilated do not always appear immediately after full dilatation but only after descent of the head

(expulsion phase). These signs include involuntary bearing down, dilatation and gaping of the anus, restlessness and vomiting.

Midwifery care during the second stage of labour

The midwife plays a major part in the assistance and support of the woman and her family during the second stage of labour. She needs to guide the parents who may be feeling uncertain and anxious. Through showing unconditional acceptance and a caring attitude the midwife can enhance the positive experience of the birth for the woman and her family.

Preparation for the delivery

Preparations for the delivery include ensuring a comfortable environment, adequate lighting, sterile delivery equipment, protective clothing, and oxytocic agent. Enough extra stock and equipment should be available in the event of any possible emergencies.

Maternal assessment and care

The maternal pulse and blood pressure should be assessed every 30 minutes, provided that these are within the normal limits. The pattern of the contractions will change in the second stage of labour. They tend to be stronger and longer, lasting for one minute with a longer resting time between them. The contractions should be monitored continuously for strength, length and frequency.

The woman should also be observed continuously for signs of vaginal bleeding and this should be reported to a medical officer if bleeding is present, but a heavy show (blood mixed with mucus) is normal.

The bladder and urethra become traumatised during descent of the head, especially when the bladder is full or during prolonged labour. For these reasons the woman must be encouraged to empty her bladder spontaneously during the first stage or at the beginning of the second stage of labour. Routine emptying of the bladder by catheterisation is indicated only when the woman cannot void spontaneously. Catheterisation may cause infections of the urinary tract and it is technically difficult to perform at this stage, so great care must be taken to avoid injury. This is particularly important in the immunocompromised woman.

The progress of labour is evaluated by noting the descent of the presenting part. This is done by comparing the amount of head palpable above the pelvis to progression of the station determined during a vaginal examination. Descent of the presenting part could be very rapid in multigravidae. If descent is taking place, a further vaginal examination is unnecessary. If poor progress is suspected, a repeat vaginal examination is needed to evaluate the cause of the poor progress.

CRITICAL THINKING EXERCISE

A woman is bearing down and the fetal head is on the perineum. The fetal heart rate is 140 bpm before contractions and 110 bpm for the first 30 seconds after contractions. Should you be concerned about the fetal condition?

Fetal assessment during the second stage of labour

The midwife should examine the *liquor amnii* for meconium staining, which may indicate possible fetal hypoxia. The fetal heart rate should be assessed at five-minute intervals immediately after the contraction to rule out any possible fetal distress.

Signs of fetal hypoxia during the second stage of labour

▶ Gradual tachycardia.
▶ Reduced baseline variability between and during decelerations.
▶ Additional late decelerations.
▶ A fetal heart rate that fails to return to the baseline rate after decelerations.

Early decelerations detected by fetoscope or cardiotocograph (CTG), which can gradually become deeper and develop variable features, are common in the second stage of labour. They are usually benign and are seen when the head is on the perineum. Increased intracranial pressure results in changes in the cerebral blood flow. This will stimulate the vagal centres, resulting in a deceleration of the heart rate. However, a rapid return of the fetal heart rate to the baseline after each deceleration, with a normal baseline rate and normal variability, should reassure the midwife. Due to its difficulty in the second stage, continuous CTG monitoring would be necessary only in exceptionally high-risk cases.

Psychological support

It is essential to build a relationship of trust with the woman during the earlier stages of labour. If the woman trusts the midwife, she will feel safe and secure. In situations where the woman has no companion, the supporting role of the midwife will be of even greater importance.

The woman needs a lot of encouragement and support. Her ability to cope emotionally should be appraised throughout the labour.

The possibility of the father (or any other suitable person) supporting the mother should be discussed prior to the delivery itself. This will give the person enough time for psychological preparation for the delivery. If the father decides not to be present his wish should be respected and the woman should be allowed to select another companion of her choice. Both the woman and her partner will need a lot of information, guidance and support from the midwife. Their ability to cope emotionally should be evaluated and praised, where applicable.

Positions

The birthing position will depend mainly on the woman's preference. If any maternal or fetal risk factors are present continuous fetal monitoring will be needed, which will limit the choice of positions. The midwife's confidence and experience when she is using a less common position will be important. The woman might change her position between the first phase of the second stage and the expulsion phase when she is actively bearing down. When using upright positions the benefits are that labour is shorter, the episodes of severe pain are experienced less frequently and abnormal fetal heart rate patterns are observed less frequently. However, an increase in blood loss (more than 500 ml) is more common in upright positions.

Semi-sitting position
The semi-sitting position is commonly encouraged in western cultures. The woman's thighs are abducted and her back is supported by a wedged pillow or by her partner. In this position the midwife can clearly see and access the perineum. The disadvantage of this position is that as a result of the woman's weight on her sacrum, the coccyx is directed forwards which reduces the pelvic outlet.

Supine position
The supine position (also known as recumbent or dorsal position) is not recommended because pressure on the inferior vena cava is increased when the woman is lying on her back. This results in fetal heart rate abnormalities due to decreased uterine perfusion. Most women do not choose this position, because it is very uncomfortable. Progress is also slower.

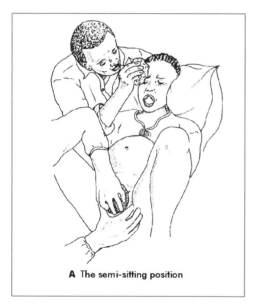

A The semi-sitting position

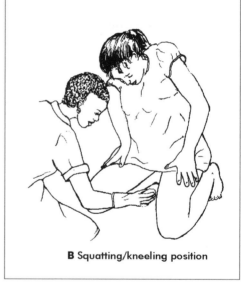

B Squatting/kneeling position

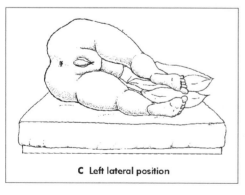

C Left lateral position

Figure 14.1 Maternal positions during the second stage of labour

Lithotomy position

The lithotomy position is used for better exposure of the perineum in situations such as breech presentations, twins or assisted deliveries and suturing the perineum. The woman's legs are placed in stirrups. Care must be taken to ensure that the woman's legs are not opened too wide or that one leg is not positioned higher than the other, as the abnormal traction forces on the perineum will result in severe perineal trauma. The stirrups can also cause excessive pressure on the legs. The woman may also feel uncomfortable and embarrassed in this position. Furthermore, the blood pressure can drop which will lead to a diminished supply of oxygen to the fetus. The frequency and intensity of the contractions may also be influenced and the woman has to push against gravity. Elevation of the woman's back by 30 to 40 degrees will lessen these disadvantages slightly.

Afterwards the woman's legs should be released gently and simultaneously from the stirrups.

Squatting/kneeling position

This is a very effective position which makes positive use of gravity. It facilitates the descent of the presenting part and enhances the woman's bearing-down efforts. A benefit of the squatting position is that the size of the pelvic outlet increases, which improves the speed and ease of delivery. In this position the transverse diameter of the pelvis can be increased by 1 cm and the anteroposterior diameter by 2 cm. The woman will need the support of a squatting bar or a companion though. Midwives often object to this position because the perineum is inaccessible, which makes the support of the perineum, the administration of analgesia or control of the delivery more difficult. However, most of these disadvantages can be overcome by encouraging the woman to use the squatting/kneeling position for swift descent of the presenting part and then, when the head is crowning, to change her position to semi-sitting so the midwife has easier access to the perineum and can control the delivery.

Left lateral position

The woman lies on her left side with her right knee pulled upwards for the left lateral position. An assistant might be needed to support her right thigh. Women find this position more comfortable and the perineum can be viewed clearly. Fewer episiotomies are required because the perineum is more relaxed. But it is more difficult to cut and repair an episiotomy in this position.

Hands and knees position

Advantages of the hands and knees position are that it can help the fetus to rotate from a posterior to an anterior position, it increases placental perfusion and may facilitate the birth of the shoulders. Perineal trauma is reduced and the midwife can easily observe the perineum in this position. The disadvantages include decreased contact between the midwife and the woman, the risk of faecal contamination and difficulty with interventions, such as perineal repair.

> **CRITICAL THINKING EXERCISE**
> A woman has asked you if she will be allowed to deliver in a kneeling position. How do you respond?

Pushing or bearing down

When to start pushing

The desire to bear down usually starts in the second phase of the second stage (expulsion phase) when the presenting part is pressing on the rectum. In multigravidae, descent is usually more rapid than in primigravidae. In many institutions women are advised to start bearing down as soon as the cervix is fully dilated. However, this may result in a prolonged period of bearing down with subsequent increase in maternal and fetal complications. The incidence of instrument-assisted deliveries increases significantly when bearing down commences early.

It is therefore better to delay pushing until the woman experiences the involuntary, spontaneous urge to bear down. The woman can remain in a comfortable position (such as left lateral) and wait for descent of the presenting part. She will only start pushing once the presenting part is pressing on the rectum and causing the urge to bear down. It has been found that delayed pushing has no dangerous effect on fetal or neonatal outcome.

In a posterior position the woman may experience the urge to bear down before full dilatation. Strategies such as 'panting' should only be implemented when the cervix is tight (not soft and retracting) and cervical dilatation is less than 8 cm. Self-administered Entonox® (a mixture of 48% oxygen and 52% nitrous oxide) is extremely helpful at this stage.

How to push

The Valsalva manoeuvre is commonly used in many labour wards. The woman is directed to push from the start of the contraction for as long as possible (10 to 30 seconds) while holding her breath (closed glottis). The procedure is then repeated throughout the contraction. The increased intrathoracic pressure results in haemodynamic changes. Blood is forced from the pulmonary circulation into the left heart chambers, causing a rise in blood pressure. If the woman continues to hold her breath, it will cause decreased maternal oxygenation and the blood pressure will start to fall steadily. Especially if the woman is lying on her back, it will add to the drop in blood pressure with a subsequent decrease in placental perfusion and fetal oxygenation. This may result in prolonged fetal heart rate decelerations, bradycardia, decreased fetal blood pH and lower Apgar scores.

Although sustained bearing down accompanied by the woman holding her breath decreases the duration of the second stage, it does not appear to be of any benefit but rather seems to compromise maternal-fetal gas exchange.

Alternatively the woman's own spontaneous pattern of bearing-down efforts can be supported. As the contractions increase in intensity, the woman will follow the natural urge to bear down. She will start pushing when the contractions are strong enough to evoke an involuntary urge to bear down. Several relatively short (4 to 6 seconds) pushing efforts will follow during each contraction. During bearing down the woman exhales slightly (exhalatory bearing-down efforts), which results in fewer haemodynamic changes and less intrathoracic pressure with a minimal drop in blood pressure.

This method is also beneficial for perineal relaxation and a slow delivery of the fetal head. Several trials that compared this method to the Valsalva method found that using shorter spontaneous efforts are better.

Supporting the woman's bearing-down efforts, rather than directing them, has been associated with spontaneous births and positive birth outcomes. Some women, however, will need guidance during their bearing-down efforts.

The woman will feel hot and sweaty, due to the warm environment and her bearing-down efforts, so she may find it soothing if wiped with a damp cloth. Small sips of water or ice should be offered to ease her thirst.

When the perineum is bulging severely and the fetal head is crowning, the method of bearing down should change slightly. A controlled and unhurried delivery can be

> **Fundal pressure should not be used**
>
> Fundal pressure is the application of an external force to the fundus in the direction of the birth canal in an attempt to shorten the duration of the second stage of labour. Midwives or obstetricians should not use fundal pressure because this method causes an increase in maternal discomfort. Up to date there is no standard technique and evidence reports harm to the uterus, perineum and fetus. In the case of shoulder dystocia, other methods such as suprapubic pressure and maternal position changes should be used (see Chapter 27).
> *Source: Simpson, 2001:64–70.*

achieved by guiding the woman on moderate short pushing efforts with periods of panting in between. This will give the perineal tissue time to stretch gradually.

Conducting the vertex delivery

The role of the midwife during the delivery is to minimise maternal trauma and to ensure safe delivery of the baby, which can be achieved through constant support and assessment. Having a good knowledge of what is normal during labour will enable the midwife to identify problems and intervene when abnormalities arise.

Asepsis

The midwives coming into direct contact with the woman during the delivery should wear protective clothing at all times, including an apron, gown, cap, protective glasses, face mask and gloves.

The midwife should reduce the risk of infection to the mother and baby as much as possible by aseptic hand washing immediately before putting on sterile gloves for the delivery. An aseptic technique should also be used when preparing the sterile equipment for the delivery. After the woman is placed in the desired position the vulvae and perineal area are cleaned with a cleansing agent to wipe away any bloodstained discharge. The technique of swabbing by starting at the outer areas and moving gradually inwards is shown in Figure 14.2. Contamination can be prevented by not using the same swab twice and not wiping from the anal area upward towards the vagina. The delivery area should be draped with sterile cloths. Cover the anus with a swab to prevent faecal contamination of the midwife's gloves, but leave the perineal area exposed so that it can be freely observed.

Delivery of the head

With each contraction there is increased bulging of the perineum and the vulvovaginal opening becomes more dilated by the presenting head. The head recedes between contractions, leaving the opening smaller. This allows

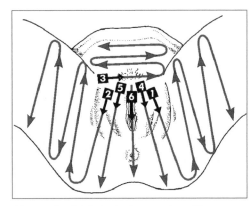

Figure 14.2 Method of perineal swabbing

the perineum to gradually flatten out. More and more of the head can be seen with each contraction until crowning of the head, which is when the vulva encircles the widest diameter of the head (biparietal diameter).

The midwife places the fingers of her one hand (hand nearest to the mother) on the fetal head. The speed of crowning should be controlled in order to prevent sudden expulsion of the head, which may cause intracranial injury or severe maternal lacerations. These lacerations can extend through the anal sphincter and into the rectum. A controlled birth will be accomplished with the correct bearing-down efforts (as previously discussed) together with light pressure on the head. At the same time, the perineum should be supported with the midwife's other hand.

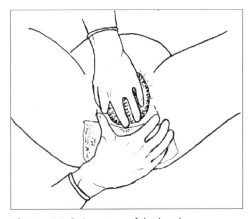

Figure 14.3 Crowning of the head

Research highlight

A large randomised clinical trial compared the support of the perineum with implementing the hands-off policy. The results showed that both methods have the same outcome in terms of perineal tears, but there was significantly less perineal pain on the tenth postpartum day with support of the perineum.

Source: *McCandlish et al, 1998:1267–1272*

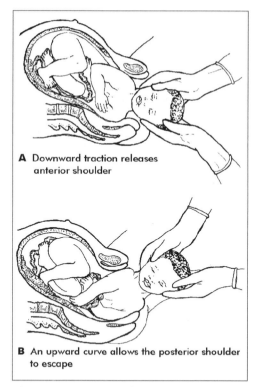

A Downward traction releases anterior shoulder

B An upward curve allows the posterior shoulder to escape

Figure 14.4 Delivery of the shoulders

The midwife should evaluate the stretching of the perineum throughout the descent of the head and infiltrate the perineum in advance when an episiotomy is needed or perineal trauma is anticipated. If an episiotomy is required, it should be made when 3 to 4 cm of the head is visible (see page 14-12).

Once the head is delivered the midwife should check whether the cord is around the neck. If it is loosely around the neck it can be slipped over the baby's head. If the cord is too tight, however, it should be clamped with two artery forceps 2 to 3 cm apart and then cut between the two. Preferably, the cord should be shielded when cut to prevent the blood from spraying. When the cord is looped around the baby's neck more than once, all the loops should be caught with the artery forceps and cut simultaneously. The forceps are then moved out of the way and the delivery continued normally. The baby's face can be wiped with a swab but the mouth and nose should be suctioned only when meconium is present in the amniotic fluid.

Delivery of the shoulder

The midwife should wait for spontaneous rotation of the shoulders into the anteroposterior axis before delivering the shoulders, which will ensure safe delivery of the shoulders and avoid perineal trauma. When the woman is in the squatting or kneeling position, the posterior shoulder may be released first. In the semi-sitting position the anterior shoulder will be released first. In the semi-sitting postion the head is held gently

between the hands and the anterior shoulder is then delivered with slight posterior traction, combined with the woman's bearing-down efforts. When the axillary crease in visible, the head is lifted towards the symphysis pubis to deliver the posterior shoulder over the perineum. The baby is then grasped around the shoulders and delivered towards the mother's abdomen. The baby can be placed near the vaginal introitus but if it is healthy the baby should be placed on the mother's abdomen, which enables the mother to see her baby and allows skin-to-skin contact. The time of birth when the entire baby is delivered should be recorded.

An oxytocic agent should be administered immediately after delivery of the anterior shoulder or after delivery of the baby. If there is the slightest uncertainty about whether it is a single pregnancy, it is safer to exclude the possibility of an undiagnosed twin abdominally after the delivery of the first baby and before administering the oxytocic agent.

Midwifery care during the third stage of labour

The third stage of labour commences when the baby is born and lasts until delivery of the placenta and membranes, which is usually after five minutes and seldom exceeds 30 minutes. The mother's focus shifts from her bearing-down efforts towards her newborn baby. The midwife should try to minimise the interference of physiological processes at this moment and encourage bonding between mother and baby. The third (and fourth) stage, however, is a period of great risk for postpartum haemorrhage. It is essential that the midwife detects this complication early and manages the situation carefully.

Clamping the umbilical cord

If the cord has not been clamped yet because it was not looped around the baby's neck, a plastic cord clamp should be applied 2 to 3 cm from the baby's umbilicus. An artery forceps should also be applied a bit further away and the cord must be cut between the two, at about 1 cm from the plastic cord clamp. The baby is then dried, warmly wrapped and given to the mother (see Chapter 16).

Delivery of the placenta

▶ *Expectant (passive) management* of the third stage of labour involves waiting for a spontaneous delivery of the placenta, without administering an oxytocic agent or applying controlled cord traction. Gravity or breast-feeding may be used to aid the delivery.
▶ *Active management* of the third stage of labour involves the routine administration of an oxytocic agent before the placental delivery, early cord clamping and delivery of the placenta with the use of controlled cord traction (with counter-pressure).

The preferred method is active management because there is a lower mean blood loss, less mild or severe postpartum haemorrhage, a shorter third stage of labour, and less use of therapeutic oxytocics. This method should be used in hospital settings, as well as home deliveries.

The oxytocic agent used during active management can either be Syntometrine® or *oxytocin* (Syntocinon®) 10 IU. Syntometrine® is a combination of 0.5 mg *ergometrine* and *oxytocin* 5 IU. In South Africa the drug of choice to be administered is *oxytocin* 10 IU. Although there is a slightly higher blood loss when compared to Syntometrine®, it is safer since it is not associated with hypertension (caused by the *ergometrine*), which is dangerous for women with pre-eclampsia, eclampsia and any cardiac conditions. Syntometrine® also has an increased incidence of vomiting. The use of *oxytocin* 5 IU alone is not recommended, however, because there is a higher risk of postpartum haemorrhage.

As previously mentioned, early clamping of the cord is performed. The *oxytocin* should be given time to act and the midwife checks for the following signs of placental separation:
▶ The fundus becomes rounder, smaller and lifts as the placenta moves into the lower uterine segment.
▶ There may be a sudden gushing of blood from the introitus.
▶ The cord lengthens as the placenta moves closer to the introitus.

No manipulation of the uterus should be done before it is fully contracted. Once the uterus is contracted, the umbilical cord is clamped closer to the introitus. Controlled cord traction is then applied as follows:
▶ The midwife grasps the cord firmly with one hand and applies light, controlled, steady traction in a downward and backward direction following the curve of the birth canal.
▶ The other hand is placed on the uterus above the symphysis pubis exerting a counter-pressure in an upward direction.
▶ When the manoeuvre is unsuccessful the midwife discontinues the traction. It is important to first release the traction on the cord before uterine counter-action is released.
▶ Before attempting the manoeuvre again,

uterine contraction should first be confirmed. Traction without a contracted uterus or a counter-action applied on the uterus may result in uterine inversion, which is a serious, life-threatening obstetrical emergency (see Chapter 21).

When the placenta is visible, the cord should be lifted anteriorly in order to follow the curve of the birth canal. As the placenta emerges, care should be taken not to tear the membranes as pieces will be left in the uterus. An artery forceps clamped to the membranes can also be used, and the membranes then gradually milked out, or the woman can be asked to cough. Immediately after delivery of the placenta and membranes, the midwife should check that the uterus is well contracted without any active bleeding. The perineum and vagina are carefully and gently inspected for possible lacerations (see page 14-13 for perineal repair instructions). The vulvae, perineum and surrounding areas are cleaned with warm water and/or a disinfectant solution, and a sterile sanitary pad is placed in position.

The blood loss should be measured as accurately as possible. Blood loss is often underestimated. The number of swabs and sanitary pads soaked with blood should also be taken into consideration. Blood loss should be less than 500 ml within the first 24 hours after delivery. Most women will cope with a blood loss of 500 ml, but it may be life threatening for women with severe anaemia.

Midwifery care during the fourth stage of labour

The fourth stage of labour is defined as the first hour after birth. This is a potentially dangerous period because of the possibility of a haemorrhage. Continuous assessment of the uterus should be made to ensure that the uterus stays firmly contracted. If the uterus is boggy (atonic) the fundus should be massaged until it is firmly contracted. The most significant source of bleeding is from the area where the placenta was implanted. A well-contracted uterus will clamp off the uterine vessels and prevent a haemorrhage. Bleeding should not exceed one soaked pad per hour. The fundus should be firm in the midline and below the level of the umbilicus. A uterus displaced upwards or laterally is an indication of a full bladder. The woman should be encouraged to void and if she is unable to, catheterisation will be necessary.

The midwife should assess the fundus and vaginal bleeding during the first hour. Furthermore, an assessment should be performed of the woman's general wellbeing and vital signs, and any abnormalities should be reported or referred.

The woman may experience tremors and uncontrollable shivering immediately after the delivery. A heated blanket and a warm drink tend to alleviate the problem.

The parents should be allowed enough private time to explore and bond with their baby. In the absence of any contraindications, the woman should be encouraged to breastfeed. Breastfeeding will cause uterine contraction and reduce the blood loss.

Following the delivery of the placenta the episiotomy or lacerations should be sutured, if necessary. The placenta should be examined to confirm that it is normal and complete. At the end of the fourth stage the woman can be given something to eat. After completion of the birth records the woman and her baby are then transferred to a postnatal ward.

Examination of the placenta

The placenta should be examined for completeness and any possible abnormalities. Also refer to the possible abnormalities described in Chapter 7. In order to recognise abnormalities of the placenta the following guidelines should be used.

Umbilical cord

▶ The length of the cord (including the segment left on the newborn) should be between 40 to 100 cm.

▶ The presence of two arteries and one vein.

▶ Check that there are no true knots in the cord.
▶ Central, lateral or Battledore insertion of the cord (Velamentous insertion is abnormal).

Membranes

Both the amnion and chorion should be present and complete. This can be determined by placing the placenta, with the maternal surface facing upward, on a flat surface. Insert one hand into the hole in the membranes through which the baby has been delivered. While the hand is inside the membrane, stretch it out to visualise the completeness thereof. Holding the placenta up by its cord while inserting your hand into the membranes is not recommended, because it increases the chance of blood spatter. Every effort should be made to determine whether the membranes are complete. Products left behind may predispose the woman to postpartum haemorrhage. Lastly, peel the amnion from the chorion to confirm the presence of both.

Pale and grey membranes, commonly accompanied by an offensive smell, suggest chorio-amnionitis/amniotic fluid infection syndrome.

Fetal surface of the placenta

▶ The colour of the fetal surface should not be green or opaque.
▶ All blood vessels should stop before reaching the end of the placenta. A blood vessel that radiates beyond the edge could indicate a placenta succenturiata and the extra lobe could easily have remained behind in the uterus.

Maternal surface of the placenta

▶ Check that all cotyledons are present. Placental remains in the uterus may cause postpartum haemorrhage, delayed involution or infection.
▶ Assess the maternal surface for any infarctions (firm areas of dead tissue). Recent infarctions are bright red and old infarctions form grey patches. Infarctions are only abnormal if they are extensive (50% of placenta).

▶ Calcification which appears as sandy white patches indicates degeneration of a full-term placenta.
▶ Any dark red areas or blood clots attached to the maternal surface are abnormal and indicate abruptio placentae. The severity of the abruptio is determined by the percentage of surface area affected.

Size and mass

▶ The normal size is approximately 15 to 20 cm diameter by 2.5 cm thickness, however, this can vary.
▶ The placental weight can vary according to the time of clamping of the umbilical cord. Early clamping will result in a placenta that is one-fifth of the birth weight and late clamping will result in a placenta that is one-sixth of the birth weight of the baby.
▶ An irregular shape may be due to a scarred or abnormal uterus.

If any abnormalities are noted, the obstetrician should be informed and the placenta kept for further examining. If there are indications that the placenta is incomplete, the uterine cavity should be explored by the obstetrician. It is usually not necessary to explore the uterine cavity if there are any parts missing from the membranes. All findings (normal and abnormal) should be recorded in the woman's records. Certain cultures, such as Muslims, have specific customs regarding the handling of the placenta and their wishes should be accommodated. In other cases the placenta can be disposed of by incineration or mechanical disposal.

Blood sampling

Fetal blood sampling can be obtained for various tests such as blood grouping and Rh, HIV, thyroid stimulating hormone and syphilis. Blood sampling should be performed by unclamping the artery forceps (before delivery of the placenta) and collecting a fetal blood sample in a bowl. After delivery of the placenta a syringe with a needle can be inserted into the blood vessels on the fetal side of the placenta to collect blood.

Episiotomy

An episiotomy is a surgical incision made into the perineal tissue to enlarge the vaginal outlet. The use of routine episiotomies has decreased dramatically over the past 20 years and now depends more on the individual circumstances.

Midline versus mediolateral episiotomy

There are two main episiotomy incisions, namely, a midline episiotomy and a mediolateral episiotomy.

The *midline episiotomy* is an incision from the midpoint of the fourchette downward but not through the anus. Less tissue is involved and it is therefore associated with less blood loss, easier repair, better healing and less postoperative pain and dyspareunia. There is, however, a higher incidence of third and fourth degree tears.

A *mediolateral episiotomy* is an incision from the midpoint of the fourchette towards the left or right ischial tuberosity. The incision should be more than 2 cm from the anus. Compared

---

Research highlight

Carroli and Belizan did a Cochrane review where they compared the effects of the restrictive use of an episiotomy with routine use of an episiotomy during vaginal birth. They found that there are more advantages in the restrictive use of an episiotomy such as a lower risk of posterior perineal trauma, less need for suturing perineal trauma and fewer healing problems at seven days postpartum. There are no differences in the risk of severe vaginal or perineal trauma (for example, third or fourth degree tears) or in the outcomes of pain, dyspareunia or urinary incontinence. There is, however, an increase in the risk for anterior perineal trauma in the restrictive use of an episiotomy. However, it is clear from the evidence that the restrictive use of an episiotomy is recommended.

Source: Carroli & Belizan, 2002.

---

to the midline incision, there is a reduced incidence of damage to the anal sphincter. This incision is the one most commonly used in South Africa.

Technique

The timing of the episiotomy is very important. It should be performed when the perineum is bulging and 3 cm to 4 cm of the head is visible. If performed too early, unnecessary blood loss will occur. If it is performed too late, perineal trauma may not have been prevented.

Indications for an episiotomy

▶ Fetal distress in the second stage of labour.
▶ Shoulder dystocia.
▶ Breech delivery.
▶ Assisted delivery.
▶ Persistent occipitoposterior position.
▶ Prevention of severe perineal trauma or a previous third-degree tear.
▶ Severe maternal exhaustion or poor maternal effort.
▶ Maternal conditions such as cardiac valve lesion.

Infiltration of the perineum

It is difficult to determine when to infiltrate the perineum. It is, however, preferable to infiltrate without performing an episiotomy rather than to infiltrate too late. *Lignocaine 1%* solution is used in a maximum dose of 20 ml. Before infiltration the midwife should insert the index and middle finger of her one hand into the vagina in the direction of her planned incision. The presenting part should be protected from accidental injection of the anaesthetic because it can cause fetal bradycardia. The midwife should also take care to avoid a needle-stick injury. The needle is inserted 4 to 5 cm into the perineum, just beneath the skin and in the direction of the planned incision. Before injecting the local anaesthetic, the back part of the syringe (plunger) is pulled back to determine whether the needle has been inserted into a blood vessel. If blood can be withdrawn, the needle should be repositioned and checked again until it is certain that it is not in a blood vessel. Approximately 5 to 7 ml of the local anaesthetic is injected into the perineum while the needle is slowly withdrawn. Shortly before the needle reaches the point of entry, the direction is changed and the perineum is injected for a second and third time, once on each side of the initial injection.

Incision of the perineum

While the midwife's two fingers are still in the vagina to protect the presenting part, a pair of blunt-ended, sharp scissors is inserted. During the height of a contraction a single incision of 4 to 5 cm is made on the infiltrated line. The presenting part will deliver immediately thereafter. Care should be taken to control the delivery of the presenting part and to support the perineum to prevent extension of the episiotomy into the anal sphincter. When there is a delay in the delivery of the presenting part, pressure should be exerted on the incision between contractions to reduce the blood loss.

Perineal repair

After the delivery the perineum should be inspected for lacerations, which usually occur during the delivery of the fetal head. Lacerations can occur even if an episiotomy was performed. The midwife should assess whether the sphincter muscle or rectal mucosa is intact. The midwife may suture an episiotomy and first- and second-degree tears, but a woman with third- and fourth-degree tears should be referred to an obstetrician for suturing. Minor lacerations need not be repaired as long as they are not bleeding. Repair of a laceration or episiotomy should be performed directly after delivery of the placenta.

Types of laceration

Posterior perineal lacerations

▶ A *first-degree* tear involves the perineal skin and/or the vaginal epithelium and/or fourchette without involving the muscles.

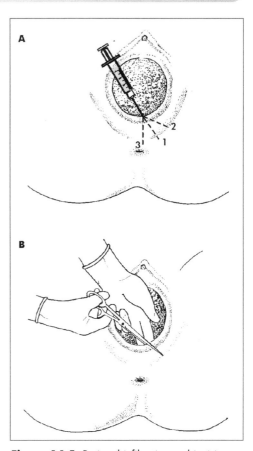

Figure 14.5 Perineal infiltration and incision

▶ A *second-degree* tear extends through the muscles of the perineal body.
▶ A *third-degree* tear involves all of the above, as well as the anal sphincter.
▶ A *fourth-degree* tear also involves the anterior rectal wall.

Anterior laceration

Anterior laceration may involve the labia minora below the pubic rami and to the side of the urethra and clitoris.

Cervical tear

This can include small tears in the cervix, which are very common but can also be larger and involve the entire cervix up to the lower uterine segment. It may be considered a possibility when continued bleeding with a well-contracted uterus is present (see Chapter 21).

Possible complications of an episiotomy

▶ Increased blood loss (especially when performed too early).
▶ Extension of an incision to a third- or fourth-degree tear (more common after midline incisions).
▶ Haematoma formation.
▶ Infection.
▶ Potential poor repair.
▶ Dyspareunia. The extent of the problem will depend on the type of suturing material as well as the method used.
▶ Rectovaginal fistula.
▶ Anal incontinence.

Technique of repair

The woman is placed in the lithotomy position or recumbent position (see page 14-4 to 14-5). Before suturing the laceration or episiotomy, ensure adequate anaesthesia. A vaginal tampon with a tail can be inserted to prevent blood coming from the uterus obscuring the midwife's vision. The vagina should not be packed with loose swabs as they may be left behind and increase the risk of infection.

Research shows that using absorbable sutures (Dexon®) causes less pain, reduced use of analgesia in the post-delivery period and requires less resuturing than non-absorbable skin sutures (silk, nylon or Supramid®). When the different absorbable sutures were compared, evidence was found that synthetic sutures (Dexon®, Vicryl®) are associated with less short-term pain and reduced use of analgesia when compared with chromic catgut. Although the absorbable synthetic sutures may cause irritation in some women that will lead to removal of the sutures, it is still the recommended material for all layers of repair (Kettle & Johanson, 2003).

Vaginal epithelium

The apex of the incision is identified and the first stitch is placed at or above this point. The vaginal epithelium is then repaired from the apex downwards up to the fourchette. Care should be taken that the vaginal opening is properly aligned. An atraumatic round-bodied needle is used because a cutting needle may lacerate the blood vessels. A continuous stitch affords better haemostasis. Care must be taken not to pull the suture too tight because oedema will still develop over the next 24 to 48 hours.

Perineal muscles

The second layer (perineal muscles) should be sutured with interrupted single or figure-of-eight stitches. Good approximation of tissue, leaving no dead spaces, is important to prevent the formation of haematomas, which will lead to infection and pain. The rectal mucosa should be excluded from the suturing.

Perineal skin

The perineal skin can be sutured with interrupted single stitches or a single subcuticular suture. The latter is more difficult to perform, but leads to fewer short-term problems than interrupted transcutaneous stitches. When using interrupted single stitches, they should be approximately 1 cm apart and not deeper than the layers of the skin.

After completion of the repair the genital area should be inspected to confirm complete haemostasis. The vaginal tampon can then carefully be removed and uterine contraction ensured. After warning the woman, a routine rectal examination should be performed gently to ensure that no stitches have penetrated the rectal mucosa. These stitches can cause fistula formation and, when present, the wound should be reopened and the stitches removed. The laceration or episiotomy should then be sutured again. After successful completion of the repair, the area is cleaned and a sterile sanitary pad applied. If the lithotomy position was used, the woman's legs should be released gently and simultaneously from the stirrups. She should be made comfortable and given information about the nature of the trauma, repair and aftercare.

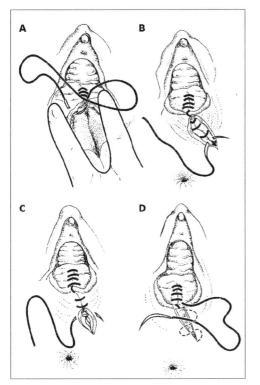

Figure 14.6 Episiotomy suturing

Record-keeping

It is the responsibility of the midwife conducting the delivery to ensure that all the records are completed before transferring the woman or leaving the mother after a home delivery. Complete records provide future caregivers information about the progress of labour and birth, as well as any complications and the management thereof. Information to be included in the woman's records will include:

▶ All the observations on the partogram.
▶ The duration and progress through all the stages of labour and birth.
▶ The drugs administered throughout labour and birth.
▶ The reason for performing an episiotomy, if required, as well as information regarding the perineal repair.
▶ The Apgar score of the baby and possible resuscitation or interventions should also be recorded.
▶ Many institutions include the brief physical examination of the newborn.
▶ The accurate recording of the volume of maternal blood loss is very important.
▶ The normal as well as the abnormal findings on the examination of the placenta, membranes and cord should be recorded.

The records are legal documents that should reflect all the events that have taken place. The reports should be concise, legible and signed.

In a nutshell

▶ In the absence of any abnormalities, the woman should only start bearing down when she is experiencing the involuntary spontaneous urge to do so.
▶ When the woman is bearing down, the fetal heart rate should be monitored every five minutes immediately after contractions.
▶ Using the supine position during birth has the most disadvantages for both the woman and her fetus.
▶ Exhalatory bearing-down effort is superior to the Valsalva manoeuvre.
▶ If the woman's condition is satisfactory, there is no fetal distress and continuous descent of the presenting part takes place, limitation of the duration of the second stage of labour is unnecessary.
▶ The recommended method of placental delivery is administration of oxytocin 10 IU together with controlled cord traction.
▶ The biggest complication of the fourth stage of labour is haemorrhage.

References

Bennett, V. R. & Brown, L. K. (Eds.) 1999. *Myles textbook for midwives*. Thirteenth edition. Edinburgh: Churchill Livingstone.

Bowes, W. A. (Jr) 2002. The effect of fundal pressure manoeuvre on intrauterine pressure in the second stage of labour. *Obstetrical & Gynecological Survey*, November 57(11):727–728.

Carroli, G. & Belizan, J. 2002. Episiotomy for vaginal birth (Cohrane Review). *The Cochrane Library*, Issue 3. Oxford: Update Software.

Cunningham, F. G., Gant, N. F., Leveno, K. J., Gilstrap III, L. C., Hauth, J. C. & Wenstrom, K. D. 2001. *Williams obstetrics*. Twenty first edition. New York: McGraw-Hill.

Dickason, E. J., Silverman, B. L. & Schult, M. O. 1994. *Maternal–infant nursing care*. Second edition. St Louis: Mosby.

Elbourne, D. R., Prendiville, W. J., Carroli, G., Wood, J. & McDonald, S. 2003. Prophylactic use of oxytocin in the third stage of labour (Cochrane review). *The Cochrane Library*, Issue 1. Oxford: Update Software.

Enkin, M., Keirse, M. J. N. C., Neilson, J., Crowther, C., Duley, L. & Hofmeyr J. 2000. *A guide to effective care in pregnancy and childbirth*. Third edition. Oxford: Oxford University Press.

Gibb, D. & Arulkumaran, S. 1997. *Fetal monitoring in practice*. Second edition. Oxford: Butterworth-Heinemann.

Gupta, J. K. & Nikodem, V. C. 2002. Position for women during second stage of labour (Cochrane review). *The Cochrane Library*, Issue 4. Oxford: Update Software.

Hofmeyr, G. J. & Kulier, R. 2003. Hands/knees posture in late pregnancy or labour for fetal malposition (lateral or posterior) (Cochrane review). *The Cochrane Library*, Issue 1. Oxford: Update Software.

Hofmeyr, G. J. & Kulier, R. 2002. Tocolysis for preventing fetal distress in second stage of labour (Cochrane review). *The Cochrane Library*, Issue 3. Oxford: Update Software.

Kaplan, C. G. 1996. Postpartum examination of the placenta, *Clinical Obstetrics & Gynecology*, September 39(3):535–548.

Kettle, C. & Johanson, R. B. 2003. Absorbable synthetic versus catgut suture material for perineal repair. (Cohrane Review). *The Cochrane Library*, Issue 1. Oxford: Update Software.

Kettle, C. & Johanson, R. B. 2003. Continuous versus interrupted sutures for perineal repair (Cohrane Review). *The Cochrane Library*, Issue 1. Oxford: Update Software.

Khan, G. Q., John, I. S., Wani, S., Doherty, T. & Sibai, M. 1997. Controlled cord traction versus minimal intervention techniques in delivery of the placenta: A randomised controlled trial, *American Journal of Obstetrics and Gynecology*, October 177(4):770–774.

Ladewig, P. W., London, M. L. & Olds, S. B. 1998. *Maternal–newborn nursing care. The nurse, the family, and the community*. Fourth edition. Menlo Park California: Addison Wesley Longman.

Lowdermilk, D. L., Perry, S. E. & Bobak, I. M. 1999. *Maternity nursing*. Fifth edition. St. Louis: Mosby.

Lundquist, M., Olsson, A., Nissen, E. & Norman, M. 2002. Is it necessary to suture all lacerations after a vaginal delivery? *Birth*, June 27(2):78–85.

McCandlish, R., Bowler, U., Van Asten, H. et al. 1998. A randomised controlled trial of care of the perineum during second stage of normal labour. *British Journal of Obstetrics & Gynaecology*, 105:1262–1272.

McDonald, S., Prendiville W. J. & Elbourne, D. 2003. Prophylactic syntometrine versus oxytocin for delivery of the placenta (Cohrane Review). *The Cochrane Library*, Issue 1. Oxford: Update Software.

Menticoglou, S. M., Manning, F., Harman, C. & Morrison, I. 1995. Obstetrics. Perinatal oucome in relation to second-stage duration. *American Journal of Obstetrics & Gynecology,* September 173(3):906–912.

Nolte, A. G. W. (Ed.) 1998. *A textbook for midwives.* Pretoria: J.L. van Schaik.

Prendiville, W. J., Elbourne, D. & McKonald, S. 2002. Active versus expectant management in the third stage of labour (Cochrane review). *The Cochrane Library,* Issue 3. Oxford: Update Software.

Righard, L. 2001. Making childbirth a normal process, *Birth,* March 28(1):1–4.

Roberts, J. E. 2002. The 'push' for evidence: Management of the second stage. *Journal of Midwifery & Women's Health,* January/ February 47(1):2–15.

Simpson, K. R. 2001. Fundal pressure during the second stage of labour. *American Journal of Maternal Child Nursing,* 26(2):64–70.

WHO (World Health Organisation). 1996. *Care in normal birth: Report of a technical working group.* Chapters 1, 4 & 5. WHO/FRH/MSM/96.24. www.who.int/reproductive-health/.

Williams, E., Van Dalen, S. C., Botha, D. E. & Louw G. 1997. *Prosedurehandleiding by Verloskunde,* geredigeer deur E. Williams. Derde uitgawe. Pretoria: Kagiso Tersiêr.

Woolley, R. J. 1995. Benefits and risks of episiotomy: A review of the English-language literature since 1980. Part I (CME review article). *Obstetrical & Gynecological Survey,* November 50(11):806–820.

Woods, D. L. (Ed.) 1993. *Perinatale self-onderrig program: Verloskunde.* Kaapstad: PEP.

Chapter 15

Pain and discomfort

Riana Hattingh

Introduction

The pain of childbirth is perhaps the most crucial challenge women and midwives have to cope with. This is due to the considerable variation in the way pain is reported and the different factors that influence the woman's experience of pain and labour. A woman's perception of this experience may have a long-term effect on her behaviour as a mother and on the relationship with her partner.

The standard approaches to labour pain management may not meet the complexity and individuality of this experience. Therefore it is desirable that the woman be allowed to make an informed choice about the variety of methods available to enable her to individualise her pain-related care.

Understanding the pain of childbirth

The experience of labour pain is a phenomenon integral to the most basic and fundamental of life's experiences – the bringing forth of new life. Unlike other pain experiences, the pain of normal labour is not associated with pathology.

The nature of labour pain has been described as cramping, tearing, nauseating, stabbing, burning, sharp, excruciating, throbbing and similar to dysmenorrhea but much worse. The pain may be experienced as local, with a tearing or bursting sensation because of distention and laceration of the cervix, vagina or perineal tissues, or it may be referred, with the discomfort felt in the back, sides or thighs. Although almost all labouring women experience lower abdominal pain during contractions, many women experience lower back pain during contractions that for some is continuous, even between contractions.

Midwives and medical practitioners can cause or increase the pain during labour by performing certain obstetric interventions and procedures.

Women who undergo induction of labour, report a more abrupt initiation of active labour

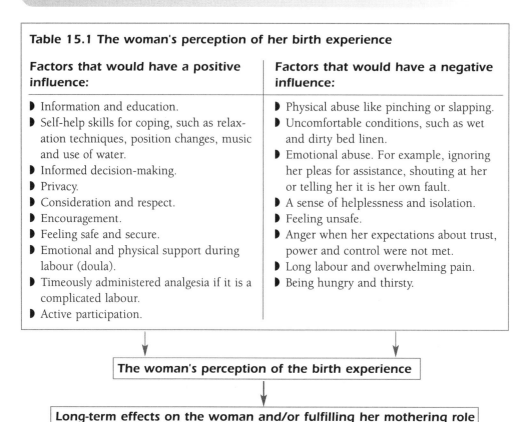

Table 15.1 The woman's perception of her birth experience

Factors that would have a positive influence:	Factors that would have a negative influence:
▶ Information and education. ▶ Self-help skills for coping, such as relaxation techniques, position changes, music and use of water. ▶ Informed decision-making. ▶ Privacy. ▶ Consideration and respect. ▶ Encouragement. ▶ Feeling safe and secure. ▶ Emotional and physical support during labour (doula). ▶ Timeously administered analgesia if it is a complicated labour. ▶ Active participation.	▶ Physical abuse like pinching or slapping. ▶ Uncomfortable conditions, such as wet and dirty bed linen. ▶ Emotional abuse. For example, ignoring her pleas for assistance, shouting at her or telling her it is her own fault. ▶ A sense of helplessness and isolation. ▶ Feeling unsafe. ▶ Anger when her expectations about trust, power and control were not met. ▶ Long labour and overwhelming pain. ▶ Being hungry and thirsty.

The woman's perception of the birth experience

Long-term effects on the woman and/or fulfilling her mothering role

Source: Adapted from Nichols and Humenick, 2000:69.

with stronger contractions that tend to peak more rapidly than spontaneous labour. They also report more pain during their vaginal examinations. They may also experience an increase in the strength and discomfort of contractions after amniotomy. Many complain of discomfort from tight abdominal fetal monitors, and that their pain increased when hospital staff told them to remain still during labour so as not to disturb the monitors. Other obvious sources of short-lived pain include the needles used to administer pain-relieving medications and intravenous solutions. Forceps, vacuum extractions and episiotomies can all be painful too.

Pain management theories

These theories were developed by studying pain transmission and its modulation. They have been applied in a variety of non-pharma-

cological and pharmacological approaches to relieve the pain of childbirth.

The endorphin system theory

The discovery of the endorphin system in 1975 helped us to understand why and how certain techniques to control pain during childbirth work, as well as why these same techniques under different circumstances appear to be ineffective.

Kimball found opiate receptor sites in the brain that led to the identification of endogenous chemicals (encephalins and endorphins) that are released from the brainstem and pituitary gland (1979:127–131). Endorphins have become more generally associated with these natural pain inhibitors. They act by travelling to the opiate receptors, where they fit like a key in a lock and block transmission of the pain impulse. The endorphin levels of a woman in labour have been found to be much higher than those of a non-labouring woman. The woman often feels relaxed and drowsy, which enhances her sense of wellbeing.

When a woman in labour feels that her or her baby's safety is being threatened, she becomes anxious and reacts by producing catecholamines (adrenalin and nor-adrenalin). This triggers the 'fight or flight' syndrome, which in turn causes the endorphin levels to fall. They will only rise again when the source of the disturbance is removed. Iatrogenic sources of pain and discomfort often trigger this type of reaction.

The gate control theory

The gate control theory was described by Melzak and Wall and states that the pain stimulus can be modified as it travels through the spinal cord (1965:971–979). The neural fibres that transmit pain are thin in comparison with those that transmit other sensations such as massage, heat and cold. These larger fibres will allow impulses to travel faster than the pain impulses in the thin fibres and will interfere with the transmission of the pain impulse, thus closing a hypothetical 'gate'.

During labour the pain can be reduced by using harmless stimulation to interfere with the transmission of the pain impulse. Techniques such as the application of superficial heat and cold, immersion in water, as well as touch and massage have been used successfully. In addition, activities such as regular position changes, standing, walking, hugging, rolling the hips, pelvic rocks and counter-pressure will activate receptors in the joints that will reduce painful stimuli.

Cognitive control theory

It is possible to enhance the descending inhibitory pathways and Handfield suggests the following three strategies:
▶ The woman replaces feelings of anxiety and fear of pain with knowledge, which includes childbirth education, reading books on the subject, birth rehearsals (acting out different scenarios of births that are normal as well as variations thereof),

modelling (an informative video that models coping with a realistic labour) and a trusting relationship with her care provider.
▶ Controlling mind and body activity with systematic relaxation, visualisation, paced breathing, music and self-hypnosis.
▶ Modifying the woman's reaction to pain through techniques such as conscious release, attention focusing, guided imagery, distraction or physical activity (1996:25).

Non-pharmacological methods of pain relief

These methods of pain relief are relevant to virtually all childbearing women but especially for the following:
▶ The woman who chooses to use the most effective medications possible but needs help before they can take effect.
▶ The woman who is almost fully dilated when the effect of the drug wears off.
▶ The woman who welcomes drug-free measures for pain relief as a complement to less effective medications.
▶ The woman who prefers to avoid pharmacological methods of pain relief during childbirth, as long as the pain does not overwhelm her. A number of women express a need to participate fully in the birth experience and they are concerned about the negative effects of medication on them, as well as their babies. For these women, as well as those who have little or no access to pharmacological methods of analgesia in childbirth, non-pharmacological pain relief methods that reduce pain seem to be helpful.

Techniques that reduce painful stimuli

Maternal movement and position changes
Women in labour experience less pain in some positions than in others. The effects of maternal position on pain are influenced by the fetal size and position, the relationship between the fetal

Figure 15.1 Effective maternal positions during the first stage of labour

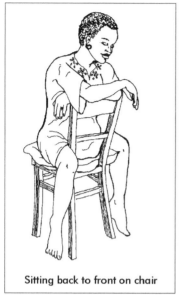

Sitting back to front on chair

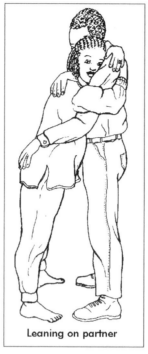

Leaning on partner

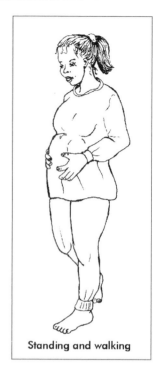

Standing and walking

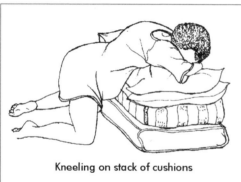

Kneeling on stack of cushions

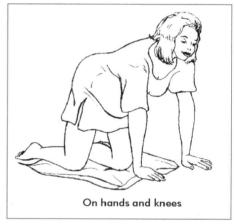

On hands and knees

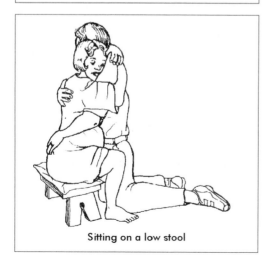

Sitting on a low stool

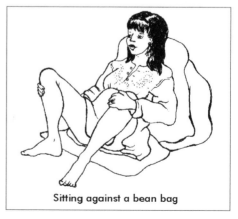

Sitting against a bean bag

head and the maternal pelvis, and the strength of the uterine contractions. Midwives should try not to restrict women, but support and help them to seek comfortable positions. Figure 15.1 shows possible positions that can be used during the first stage of labour. Some can even be useful during the second stage of labour. Trust the woman's judgement in deciding on a position. She should change positions frequently, every 20 to 30 minutes or when she feels like it. Women seem to adopt upright positions, such as walking, standing and sitting during the earlier stages of labour, then often return to a more recumbent position in advanced labour.

Pressure
Counter-pressure works well for those with back pain. The support person or midwife uses the heel of the hand, fist or firm object to apply constant firm steady pressure to the sacral area of the lower back. Counter-pressure can also be applied concurrently with the application of heat or cold.

Techniques that activate peripheral sensory receptors
Superficial heat and cold
Heat is generated from hot or warm objects, such as hot water bottles, electric heating pads, heated silica gel packs, warm blankets, baths, showers and warm moist towels.

How to use warm moist towels
- Immerse towels or towel nappies in very hot water and wring them out so they do not drip.
- Apply the hot towel over whatever area it is needed – all over her back and down her buttocks by overlapping them or rolled up and positioned over the vulva or lower abdomen.
- Wringing out towels for extended periods is exhausting for the support person, therefore it is helpful to save this form of pain relief until the transitional phase when it will be most appreciated.

Blocks of ice, frozen silica gel pack and towels soaked in cool or ice water can be used to bring cooling relief. These comfort measures have not been evaluated in randomised controlled trials but studies done through observation suggest that both the application of heat and cold may be effective (Enkin et al, 2000:316).

Using water during labour for pain relief
According to an experimental controlled trial done at Coronation Hospital in Johannesburg, the group of women who were immersed in the water experienced statistically less pain than the control group (Taha, Nolte, Hofmeyr & Dörfling, 2001). These researchers recommended that water should be an option available to all women during labour.

Touch and massage
According to Enkin et al, touch, in various forms, can convey pain-reducing messages, depending on the nature and circumstances of the touch (2000:318). The following ways of touch convey to the recipient a message of caring, of wanting to be with her and to help her.

Massage can be done by using light or firm stroking, vibration, kneading, deep circular pressure, continual steady pressure and joint manipulation. Because adaptation occurs after a while it makes good sense to make use of intermittent massage, or variation in the type of stroke and location of the touch.

Some women, at certain times, do not want to be touched, especially during transition, when the contractions are very close together. Always ask her permission before touching her.

Intracutaneous injection of sterile water
The injection of small amounts (0.1 ml) of sterile water at four spots in the lower-back area, have shown in well-designed controlled trials to achieve rapid (within two minutes), dramatic and often complete relief of back pain. The analgesic effect lasts 60 to 90 minutes. It works either by the gate control theory or through the release of endorphins.

Research highlight

The method of intracutaneous injection of sterile water is described in detail in Reynolds J. L. 1994. Intracutaneous sterile water for back pain in labour.

Source: Canadian Family Physician, October 40:1785–1791).

Support for women during childbirth

Continuous support during labour from care-givers (midwives or lay support people) appears to have a number of benefits for the mother and her baby and does not appear to be harmful in any way.

Pharmacological methods of pain relief

When labour becomes complicated, for example, the baby is in a posterior position, labour takes longer than expected, an induction is needed, the woman is extremely tired and anxious, or when the woman requests it, the situation may arise where it is necessary to administer medication.

Research highlight

A systematic review, done by Hodnett (1999), involving more than 5 000 women in 14 trials, assessed the effects of continuous support during labour. The continuous support included comforting touch and words of praise and encouragement. The results revealed that the continuous presence of a support person reduced the likelihood of needing medication for pain relief, operative vaginal delivery, caesarean birth and a five-minute Apgar score of less than seven. Continuous support was also associated with a slight reduction in the length of labour. When evaluating the effects of support on the mothers' view of their childbirth experiences the results were positive in the group who had received continuous support.

These medications are commonly given during labour and have side effects and complications that range from unpleasant to serious. It is therefore necessary to consider the advantages and disadvantages of each medication and utilise what is available to the woman's best advantage. The timing for the administration of any medication to relieve pain is important as it may influence the progress of labour as well as the condition of the woman and/or the fetus.

The medical practitioner prescribes the medication (or the authorised policies of the labour and delivery unit determine them). However, it is usually the midwife who administers it as she is the healthcare provider who is in constant attendance and is best able to assess each woman individually. The use of medication should be discussed with the woman and her informed consent must be obtained. By doing this, the midwife takes the woman's preferences into consideration, thereby enhancing her feeling of being in control of the birth process.

Sedatives and tranquilisers

These systemic agents are sometimes given to a woman in false labour or during the latent phase of labour if she is experiencing painful contractions but with little or no cervical effacement and/or dilatation. *Hydroxyzine* (Aterax®) is commonly used in the labour ward.

Hydroxyzine is an antihistamine that acts as a tranquiliser, sedative and, to a lesser extent, an anti-emetic while producing minimal circulatory and respiratory depression. Administration of *hydroxyzine* usually occurs in latent and active labour, often together with *pethidine*. This combination can provide some pain relief and alleviate anxiety. In some instances it may normalise uterine contractions in women with incoordinated uterine action. A medical practitioner's prescription is necessary.

Dosage

In labour *hydroxyzine* is given as an intramuscular injection of 50 to 100 mg (1 mg per kg) every four hours as needed. The woman should be informed about the discomfort it causes at the injection site.

Side effects
Hydroxyzine causes drowsiness in the woman and it improves the effect of the opioid (such as *pethidine*).

Opioids
Opioids (*pethidine*) can provide some pain relief. *Pethidine* does not take the pain away but it alters the woman's perception of the pain. If it is given during the latent phase, uterine activity and hence rate of cervical dilation may decrease. If given once labour is well established, the relief of pain and anxiety may make the uterine contractions more efficient. Its peak effect is 40 to 50 minutes after an intramascular injection and five to 10 minutes after an intravenous injection. Opioids may only be administered with a medical practitioner's prescription.

Dosage
Usually 100 mg of *pethidine* is administered intramuscularly (with *hydroxyzine* as previously mentioned) every four to six hours. An intravenous dosage of *pethidine* 25 mg may be administered *slowly*. This may be repeated after four hours if so indicated. It has been found that self-administered intravenous *pethidine*, using a specialised controller (patient-controlled analgesia), results in better pain relief and a lower total dosage of opioids than when it is administered intramuscularly by a care provider.

Side effects
The side effects of *pethidine* are dose related. Maternal side-effects include orthostatic hypotension, nausea, vomiting, dizziness and delayed gastric emptying.

Opioids cross the placenta virtually unhindered and they frequently cause respiratory suppression in the neonate. It is often accompanied by feeding problems and suppression of certain neuro-behavioural responses. The

half-life of the drug in adults is three hours, but in the neonate it is 22.7 hours. The greatest effect on the fetus is observed within 1.5 hours after an intramuscular injection. Lower Apgar scores, as well as more neonatal behavioural abnormalities, can be expected in the babies of women who received opioids during labour.

After birth the administration of narcotic antagonists such as *naloxone* (0.04 mg per kg) in particular to the neonate will improve breathing, feeding and neuro-behavioural response for 48 hours. It can also be administered intravenously or via the umbilical vein.

Inhalation analgesia
The most commonly used inhalation analgesic agent is Entonox®. Entonox® is a combination of premixed nitrous oxide, in a 52% concentration with 48% oxygen in a single pressurised cylinder (Entonox® apparatus). Inhalation needs to begin when the uterus has begun to tighten (even before the woman is aware of the contraction). The timing of the inhalation needs to be determined by the midwife, but the Entonox® is self-administered with a mask that has a non-return demand valve. This ensures that the woman is never able to render herself totally unconscious. When she becomes drowsy the mask will fall from her face and she will return to a wakeful state.

The use of Entonox® is reserved mainly for the last part of the first stage of labour (transitional phase). However, it is very helpful when women are very tense and require internal examination during the difficult delivery of a placenta or as an adjunct to local analgesia when suturing the perineum or episiotomy. Some women experience faintness and/or nausea while breathing. Entonox® has no clinically important side effects on the fetus.

Epidural analgesia and anaesthesia
Epidural analgesia and anaesthesia have emerged as the major approach to pain relief for women in labour, operative vaginal deliveries and caesarean births. During this procedure

a drug is injected through a catheter inserted into the second or third lumbar interspace by an anaethetist or gynaecologist who is sufficiently experienced in the technique. The drug can be administered by continuous administration with an infusion device or it can be topped up as required. It is very effective in relieving pain and the woman remains conscious.

Regional anaesthetic agents (*bupivacaine, lignocaine* and *ropivacaine*) and opioid analgesics (*fentanyl* and *sufentanil*) may be administered alone or in combination via the epidural route.

Side effects

There appears to be an increased length of first and second stage labour, an increased use of *oxytocin* to augment labour and a greater likelihood of fetal malposition and instrumental vaginal delivery, because the woman loses the desire and ability to bear down during the second stage.

During the second stage of labour, pushing should be delayed until the fetal head is visible at the introitus. This may reduce the risk of a difficult or instrumental delivery. Using upright positions, under controlled circumstances, seems to aid fetal decent, increase uterine contractibility, decrease length of labour and increase women's satisfaction with the birth process.

There is also a strong trend toward increased caesarean delivery with epidural analgesia. If administered during labour, it should be administered during the active phase of the first stage of labour (when the cervix is about 4 to 6 cm dilated) to lower the possibility of an operative delivery.

Localised short-term backache is another side effect. Although many women feel pleased with the pain-relieving effect of an epidural, some might feel disappointed emotionally, as though they have missed out on something.

Complications

An inadvertent dural puncture might result from epidural analgesia which causes a severe headache due to leaking of cerebrospinal fluid. These headaches require the woman to lie down as horizontal as possible. A blood patch may seal the defect in the dura.

Postlumbar dural punctures and unrecognised intravenous injection of anaesthetics that cause acute systemic toxicity and result in seizures and cardiac arrest are rare but they do occur. Then there is the complication of hypotension with associated shivering, pruritis, voiding inability, nausea and vomiting.

Effects on the fetus

The fetus may suffer complications as a result of maternal effects like hypotension or an allergy to the drug. Hypotension in the mother will lower blood flow and thus oxygen to the placenta. As a result the baby may develop fetal heart rate abnormalities. After the administration of an epidural the woman should never be lying on her back (dorsal position) but rather on her sides and preferably on her left side.

Midwifery care

There are several implications for midwifery care:

▶ The woman should be given the necessary information by the anaethetist or gynaecologist doing the procedure and give her informed consent. It is important that the midwife ensures that the woman really understands what is being said as there is often a language barrier between anaethetist or gynaecologist and the woman.
▶ No contraindications should be present.
▶ Before the epidural block, a loading dose of 500 ml to one litre of a balanced physiological solution (Ringer's lactate) must be given intravenously in order to prevent hypotension. An epidural block results in a sympathetic block and vasodilatation of the veins in the lower extremities, which results in profound hypotension.
▶ Assist the woman into the correct position for insertion of the catheter and explain the need to avoid movement during insertion.
▶ Baseline observations of the mother and

her fetus must be completed before the procedure is done. During and after the procedure the blood pressure must be measured every two minutes for the first six minutes; every five minutes for the next 20 minutes; every quarter of an hour for the next hour, and half-hourly thereafter. This must be repeated every time a top-up of the epidural is administered by a anaethetist or gynaecologist.

▶ To ensure that the level of the epidural anaesthesia does not go higher and paralyse the diaphragm and muscles used for breathing, the level of the block must be evaluated every half-hour using an ice cube or alcohol swab on the woman's back.

▶ Monitor fetal heart rate, uterine activity and cervical dilation during the procedure. Alert the anaethetist or gynaecologist administering the epidural, to the onset of a contraction so that the block can be administered between contractions. If the woman is receiving an *oxytocin* infusion, the infusion should be discontinued during the procedure.

▶ Bladder distention, due to sensory loss and the administration of large amounts of intravenous fluid over a short time period, will necessitate the insertion of a urinary drainage catheter.

▶ Since sensory and motor function is diminished or lost, care should be taken to avoid injury to the lower extremities. The woman must be turned every hour to ensure even distribution of the block. She will also need assistance to bear down during the second stage of labour.

▶ Provide emotional and physical support throughout the procedure and thereafter.

Contraindications

▶ Sepsis in the area where the needle will be inserted.
▶ Previous injury, operations or congenital malformations of the spinal column in the area where the needle will be inserted.
▶ Bleeding tendencies and previous administration of an anticlotting agent.
▶ Pathology of the central nervous system.
▶ Hypovolaemia.
▶ Gross obesity.

In a nutshell

▶ A woman's perception of the pain she experiences during labour is a balance between the emotional and physical elements and it also involves her past experiences of pain, her feeling of being in control and the meaning of the experience to herself (see Table 15.1).
▶ Her perception of her birth experience will in turn influence her mothering behaviour, her relationship with significant others and her self-esteem.
▶ Women need to receive adequate and balanced information about pharmacological and non-pharmacological pain management strategies to enable them to make an informed choice.
▶ In prepared, normal childbirth, non-pharmacological (supportive) pain management strategies are emphasised as the first line of action. Pharmacological intervention should therefore augment supportive strategies rather than become a substitute for them.
▶ Given the clear benefits and the absence of known risks associated with continuous intrapartum support (with hands-on comfort and verbal encouragement), every effort should be made to ensure that all labouring women receive support from those close to them, but also from experienced midwives.

References

Browning, A. J. 1983. Maternal and cord plasma concentrations of beta-lipotrophin, beta-endorphin, and gamma-lipotrophin at delivery. *British Journal of Obstetrics and Gynaecology*, 90:1152–1158.

Caton D., Corry M. P., Frigoletto F. D. et al. 2002. The nature and management of labor pain: Executive summary. *American Journal of Obstetrics and Gynecology*, May supplement 186(5):S1–S15.

Enkin E., Keirse M. J. N. C., Neilson J. et al. 2000. *A guide to effective care in pregnancy and childbirth*. Third edition. New York: Oxford University Press.

Handfield, B. 1996. *Thrown in at the deep end*. St. Kilda: Handfield and Bell.

Hodnett, E. D. 1999. Caregiver support for women during childbirth. Cochrane Review. *The Cochrane Library*, Issue 3. Oxford: Update Software.

Ketterhagen, D., VandeVusse, L. & Berner, M. A. 2002. Self-hypnosis. *Maternal Child Nursing*, November/December 27(6):335–338.

Kimball, C. 1979. Do endorphin residues of beta-lipotrophin in hormone reinforce reproductive functions? *American Journal of Obstetrics and Gynecology*, 134:127–131.

Labrecque, M., Nouwen, A., Bergeron, M. & Rancourt, J. F. 1999. A randomized controlled trial of nonpharmacologic approaches for relief of low back pain during labor. *Journal Family Practitioner*, 48:259–263.

Lowe, N. K. 2002. The nature of labor pain. *American Journal of Obstetrics and Gynecology*, supplement 186(5):S16-S25.

Mayberry, L. J., Clemmens, D. & De, A. 2002. Epidural Analgesia side-effects, co-interventions, and care of women during childbirth: A systematic review. *American Journal of Obstetrics and Gynecology*, supplement 186(5):S81-S93.

Melzak, R. & Wall, P. 1965. Pain mechnisms: A new theory. *Science*, 150:971–979.

McCaffery, M. 1972. *Nursing management of the patient with pain*. Philadelphia: JB Lippincott.

Nichols, F. H. & Humenick, S. S. 2000. *Childbirth education: Practice research and theory*. Philadelphia: WB Saunders.

Nolte, A.(Ed.) 1998. *A textbook for midwives*. Pretoria: J. L. van Schaik.

Perez, P. 1997. *The nurturing touch at birth*. Bauxhall: Cutting Edge Press.

Robertson, A. 1997. *Empowering women*. Camperdown: ACE Graphics.

Reynolds, J. L. 1994. Intracutaneous sterile water for back pain in labour. *Canadian Family Physician*, October 40:1785–1791.

Simpkin, P. & O'Hara, M. A. 2002. Non-pharmacological relief of pain during labor: Systematic reviews of five methods. *American Journal of Obstetrics and Gynecology*, supplement 186(5):S131–SS59.

Taha, M., Nolte, A. G. W., Hofmeyr, G. J. & Dörfling, C. S. 2001. Water as a method of pain relief. Proceedings of the twentieth conference on Priorities in Perinatal Care in South Africa. Presented at Drakensberg Gardens: Underberg.

Chapter 16

Care of the newborn baby at birth

Joanita de Kock and Rachel Mokhondo

Introduction

In most cases the condition of the baby after birth is satisfactory and does not need any interventions, which allows for early mother–infant bonding. The baby can be placed on the mother immediately after birth so the mother and her companion can see and hold the baby, as well as initiate early feeding. There are some babies, however, who will need additional interventions in order to adapt successfully to extra-uterine life.

The midwife plays an essential role in the initial care of the newborn and in facilitating parent–infant bonding and early feeding. The midwife should assess the condition of the baby and act promptly and effectively if resuscitation is needed.

Preparation for reception of the baby

The parents

The parents can easily be shocked by the appearance of a newborn baby due to the presence of blood, vernix, caput succedaneum and extensive moulding. They should be prepared for this so that it does not interfere with the bonding experience with their baby.

Healthcare personnel

In some instances the need for resuscitation of a newborn can be anticipated (for example, fetal distress, a difficult second stage or preterm labour). There are, however, many times that a baby might need resuscitation without any prior warning. Every midwife should therefore

---

Essential basic resuscitation equipment

▶ A neonatal ventilation bag (ambubag).
▶ Two infant face masks (size 1 for a normal newborn and size 0 for a small newborn).
▶ A mucus extractor and a portable or wall-mounted suctioning apparatus with suctioning tubes for small and bigger babies. A thicker tube (FG 10) is used in cases where there is meconium-stained amniotic fluid.
▶ Humidified oxygen (if available) or medical air with flow meters and tubing.
▶ Laryngoscope and endotracheal tubes in case advanced resuscitation is necessary.
▶ A second set of equipment should be available for possible multiple births or if the first set fails.

---

be skilled and equipped to intervene in situations where the newborn fails to initiate spontaneous breathing. Regular in-service training and up-to-date knowledge of the institution's policy on resuscitation are essential.

In addition to the midwife attending to the birth, a second midwife should be available to attend to the newborn.

Where resuscitation of the newborn is anticipated, two midwives are needed for resuscitation of whom at least one should be skilled and experienced in neonatal resuscitation. Midwives should protect themselves from possible infections, such as HIV, by wearing gloves at all times when handling the newborn until after his first bath.

The environment

The room temperature should be comfortable for the labouring woman and at the same time, be warm enough for the newborn baby. It is suggested that the environmental temperature be about 24 °C and free of draughts from windows or air-conditioning vents. Additional heat can be generated with safely mounted heaters, light bulbs or an overhead heater.

Two clean blankets or towels should be available to be used to receive the newborn, one for initial wrapping and drying, and the second one for covering the newborn to prevent heat loss. In a cold environment more blankets will be needed. The blankets or towels should be kept warm by placing them on any safe, non-flammable heat source available.

Other equipment available should be two newborn identification bands and documentation records, including the Road to Health card. A clock is also necessary to note the exact time of birth and Apgar scoring.

Equipment

It is essential to have the neonatal resuscitation equipment checked and functioning properly at all times in the labour unit. Although there may be variations because of policies, the essential components of any neonatal resuscitation area are listed in the box.

Care of the baby during and immediately after birth

After the birth of the head excess mucus may be wiped from the baby's mouth. When meconium is present in the amniotic fluid, the midwife responsible for the neonate should suction the baby before the birth of the shoulders to prevent meconium aspiration. This is done by first suctioning the mouth and then the nose.

Routine suctioning of all neonates is discouraged because the delicate mucous membranes of the neonate can be traumatised, which may increase the risk of mother-to-child transmission (MTCT) of HIV. There is also the risk of vagus stimulation with subsequent apnoea bradycardia with routine suctioning.

As the baby is born a rapid inspection should be made to ensure that there are no gross congenital abnormalities and then, ideally, the baby should be shown to the mother to confirm its gender and placed in a warm towel on the mother's abdomen. The midwife attending to the baby immediately dries the baby, which will also stimulate breathing and prevent any heat loss. The wet towel should be replaced with a warm dry one while the midwife attending to the birth ensures the cord is adequately clamped. It is particularly important to dry and cover the head of the baby for heat is lost when he is wet or uncovered. A hat can also be used. The one-minute Apgar can be assessed while these procedures are being performed.

Early identification of the neonate is essential. The institutional policy will determine the information needed on the identification bands and the midwife and the mother (where possible) should verify it before tying them to the baby. Care should be taken not to injure the baby while fastening the bands. Two identification bands should be secured, one on the infant's wrist and one on the ankle.

Assessment of the need for resuscitation (Apgar scoring)

Immediate assessment of the baby is done after birth to ensure that he is safely making the transition to extra-uterine life. This is done by Apgar scoring followed by an initial swift and gentle physical and neurological examination by the midwife while she is drying and wrapping the newborn baby.

Apgar scoring is performed one minute after the birth of the baby, followed by checks at five minutes and every five minutes thereafter until the score is 7. It is an objective measure of the condition of the baby in the first minutes after birth. It also serves as a guide for the method and vigour of resuscitation the baby may require. The five factors assessed are the heart rate, breathing efforts, muscle tone, response to stimulation and colour. Each factor receives a score of 0, 1 or 2 (see Table 16.1). Although the weight of scoring is the same, the heart rate and breathing efforts are the most important factors, and the colour is the least important.

A baby will be in good condition when he is actively crying or has an Apgar score of 7 or above. It is very rare for an infant to get an Apgar score of more than 9 at one minute after birth because most infants' hands and feet will still be blue.

Assistance with transition to breathing

There is no need for assistance with breathing when the neonate is crying. If no crying is

Table 16.1 Apgar score

Factors	Score allocated		
	0	1	2
Heart rate	Absent	Less than 100 bpm.	More than 100 bpm.
Breathing efforts	Absent	Slow and irregular.	Breathing actively or crying loudly.
Muscle tone	Absent	Some flexion of the extremities.	Arms and legs in flexion. Active movement at times.
Response to stimulation	Absent	Grimace.	Cough, sneeze or cry.
Colour	Pallor or central cyanosis.	Body pink and the extremities are cyanosed.	Body and the extremities are pink.

present, assess the breathing. If the chest is rising symmetrically with frequency of more than 30 per minute, no interventions are necessary. If no breathing is present or the infant is gasping, resuscitation should be started immediately.

Preventing heat loss

As previously mentioned, a *warm environment* and *drying the baby* are essential elements to preventing heat loss. Gentle rubbing will also stimulate breathing. During resuscitation the baby should be kept covered with only the chest exposed. Hypothermia exacerbates hypoxia as essential oxygen and glucose are then used for heat production and cold haemoglobin cannot release oxygen to the cells.

Airway

▶ *Position* the baby on his back on a flat surface with his head slightly extended ('sniffing' position). A folded cloth under the shoulders can help with the correct positioning.
▶ *Clear the airway* by suctioning first the mouth and then the nose. Avoid damaging the naso-oro pharynx. Special care should be taken when blood or meconium is present in the mouth and/or nose. The suctioning provides additional stimulation and the newborn might start breathing spontaneously. If no breathing is present, resuscitation should be continued.

Breathing

▶ *Confirm the correct position* ('sniffing' position).
▶ *Select an appropriate mask* according to the size of the baby (size 1 for a normal weight baby and size 0 for a small baby).
▶ *Correct placement of the mask* is when it covers the baby's chin, mouth and nose and there is a proper seal between the mask and the baby's face.
▶ *Ventilate the neonate* by pressing the ambubag two or three times while observing for the chest rising (adequate pressure

will cause the chest to rise). Failure of the chest to rise might be due to an incorrect head position, poor seal between face and mask, insufficient volume of air ventilated or an airway blocked with blood, mucus or meconium. Warm and humidified 100% oxygen should be used where available; otherwise positive pressure with air is also effective.
▶ *Ventilation speed* should be about 30 to 40 breaths per minute.
▶ *Re-evaluate spontaneous breathing* by stopping ventilation after one minute without removing the mask. If the breathing is absent, weak, slow or severe indrawing is present, resuscitation should be continued. Confirm chest rising with ventilations. Stop resuscitation when infant is crying or breathing at a rate of 30 to 60 breaths per minute with no chest or costal indrawing and no grunting for a period of one minute. Continue observing this baby.

If the baby's condition and breathing is still insufficient, continue with *advanced resuscitation* as discussed in detail in Chapter 31. Arrange for the transfer of the baby to a centre which specialises in high-risk neonatal care. Continue with mechanical ventilation while keeping the baby warm.

A skilled person can consider performing intubation and circulatory assistance by cardiac compression when the heart rate is less than 80 beats per minute (see Chapter 31).

CRITICAL THINKING EXERCISE

One minute after birth a baby's condition is as follows: His heart rate is more than 100 beats per minute and his breathing is irregular and slow. His hands, feet and body are blue. He grimaces if touched and shows signs of some flexion of his extremities.
1. Determine the first Apgar score.
2. Manage the baby according to his Apgar score.

Facilitation of parent–infant bonding

The moment of mother and child meeting for the first time is precious and will be remembered by the mother for the rest of her life. It is the midwife's privilege to hand the baby to the mother (and father) and then to withdraw, allowing this time to be private and personal. Should the midwife sense any hesitancy she can gently assist the woman to hold and touch her new baby. By so doing, she does not shame the woman into thinking she is incapable of caring for her child, but supports her as she explores her new role as mother. These first minutes can determine the quality of mother–child bonding in the future.

Any routine examinations or treatment should be delayed until the parents have had adequate time to meet their baby and the mother has had a chance to feed her baby for the first time.

Establishment of early infant feeding

Early infant feeding helps with mother–infant bonding. It also prevents neonatal hypoglycaemia and reduces the risk of physiological jaundice.

With the increase in HIV infection, many women will have to make a difficult decision about how they will feed their babies to prevent postpartum transmission of HIV. Some may opt to formula feed, while others may choose heat treatment of expressed breast milk or breastfeeding exclusively. Due to the delicacy of the situation the midwife needs to be sensitive to the mother's wishes without being dogmatic or judgemental.

If the mother has chosen to breastfeed she needs to be encouraged as she and the baby learn the art of breastfeeding. During the first hour the baby is usually awake and alert. The baby should be placed skin-to-skin on the mother's chest as soon after birth as possible and put to the breast as soon as possible. This early skin stimulation and suckling on the nipple helps to release the prolactin hormone which promotes the production of immunologically rich and nourishing colostrum as well as oxytocin. Oxytocin stimulates the breast to release the milk and at the same time stimulates the uterus to contract. An exclusively breastfed baby should not be given water, gripe water, glucose solutions or formula feeding. Breastfeeding is discussed in Chapter 30.

Mothers who have chosen to formula feed should know which formula they will use and bring it with them when they are in labour. If the mother came unprepared, she has to be assisted in her choice. A bottle should be prepared and available to the mother to feed her child within the first hour after birth so that she too, can begin to gain confidence in feeding her child.

Initial assessment of the newborn

Except for the screening for gross abnormalities that takes place during the first few minutes while determining the Apgar score and wrapping the baby, the assessment of the baby can be delayed until after meeting and bonding with the parents. Some institutions adapt the policy of a brief initial assessment of the newborn in the labour ward, which is then followed by a comprehensive assessment in the postnatal ward. This will exclude any possibility of overlooking important aspects in the labour ward. The comprehensive assessment can also be done in the labour ward if enough personnel and time is available.

Where possible, the baby should be examined in the presence of the mother. This provides the midwife with the opportunity to talk to the parents and explain her findings. It can also promote bonding. Although the baby should be uncovered during the examination, hypothermia should still be prevented with a warm, draught-free environment and by limiting the time of exposure.

The full examination will be discussed in

Chapter 29 but the following aspects are particularly important in the labour ward:
▶ The presence of vernix (which may be wiped off during handling).
▶ Normal respiration and colour.
▶ Birth injuries.
▶ Foul-smelling neonate due to chorio-amnionitis/amniotic fluid infection syndrome.
▶ Physical abnormalities.

Early identification of problems or abnormalities will make it possible to prevent further complications, as well as arrange an early transfer. When abnormalities are present that are not life-threatening (such as polydactylia) early identification will give the midwife time to inform the parents in a sensitive manner and take the extra care to promote parent–infant bonding.

The length, head circumference and weight of the neonate can be determined in the labour ward (if facilities allow it) or later in the postnatal ward. A detailed recording of the examination findings should be made on the maternal and neonatal charts.

References

Barkin, R. M. & Rosen, P. 1999. *Emergency pediatrics: A guide to ambulatory care*. Fifth edition. St. Louis: Mosby.

Bennett, V. R. & Brown, L. K. 1999. *Myles textbook for midwives*. Thirteenth edition. Edinburgh: Churchill Livingstone.

Coovadia, H. M. & Wittenberg, D. F. 1999. *Paediatrics and child health care. A manual for health professionals in the third world*. Fourth edition. Cape Town: Oxford University Press.

Cronje, H. S., Grobler, C. J. F. & Visser, A. A. 1996. *Obstetrics in Southern Africa*. Pretoria: J. L. van Schaik Publishers.

> ### In a nutshell
> ▶ All midwives should be skilled and equipped to manage the unexpected neonate who fails to start breathing spontaneously.
> ▶ Early mother–infant bonding is important.
> ▶ Infant feeding should be initiated within the first hour after birth.
> ▶ A baby is in a good condition when he is actively crying or has an Apgar score of 7 or above.
> ▶ Measures to prevent heat loss after birth should be in place as it compromises the newborn baby's health in various ways, including causing or worsening respiratory problems.

Deacon, J. & O'Neill, P. 1999. *Core curriculum for neonatal intensive care nusing*. Second edition. Philadelphia: WB Saunders Company.

DoH (Department of Health). 2002. *Guidelines for maternity care in South Africa*. Second edition. Pretoria: Department of Health.

Henning, P. A. 2002. *The examination of the newborn baby*. Pretoria: J. L. van Schaik.

Merenstein, G. B. & Gardner, S. L. 1998. *Handbook of neonatal intensive care*. Fourth edition. St. Louis: Mosby.

Nolte, A. (Ed.) 1998. *A textbook for midwives*. First edition. Pretoria: J. L. van Schaik.

World Health Organisation (WHO). 1998. *Basic newborn resuscitation: A practical guide*. Chapter 1. WHO/RHT/MSM/98.1. www.who.int/reproductive-health. Geneva: WHO.

Wood, D. L. (Ed.) 1996. *Perinatal education programme. Manual 2. Newborn care*. Cape Town: PEP.

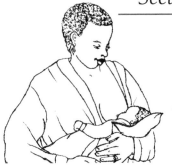

Section **5**

Postnatal care

Chapter *17*

Postnatal assessment and care

Elizabeth Kaye-Petersen and Dr Bongi Nzama

Introduction

The puerperium or postnatal period refers to the six weeks following the birth of the infant and the expulsion of the placenta and membranes. During this time, the woman's body undergoes significant changes. Physiological changes include the repair of injuries to the birth canal, involution of the uterus, and the gradual return of all the systems to their pregravid state. The woman cannot control her emotions. She undergoes psychological adaptations such as establishing a relationship with her infant, adapting to a changed relationship with her partner, as well as assuming and sharing the parenting role. Psychological problems that may occur include postpartum blues, depression and psychosis, all of which are discussed in Chapter 23.

There is evidence that maternal and neonatal acute morbidities and mortalities occur primarily during the postnatal period. The midwife should therefore be on the alert for warning signs.

The purpose of postpartum care

The overall purpose of postpartum care is to fulfil the holistic needs of the woman and her family. It provides for the early detection and treatment of complications, and advice and support with regard to breastfeeding, birth spacing, immunisation and maternal nutrition (WHO, 1998).

Physiological changes
The cardiovascular system

The 30 to 45% increase in circulating blood volume as a result of pregnancy allows the woman to withstand the normal blood loss at birth without ill effect. The diuresis that occurs between the second and fifth days postnatal, plus the loss of blood at birth, reduce the increased blood volume. This results in the blood volume returning to its pre-pregnancy state by the end of the first or second postpartum week. With each 250 ml of blood loss the haematocrit drops by four points and the haemoglobin value drops by 1 g/dl. If a woman enters labour with a haematocrit of 37%, it may decrease to approximately 33% on the first postnatal day and haemoglobin of 12 g/dl will drop to about 11 g/dl. The midwife should be cautioned that if an anaemic woman goes into labour her condition could become compromised with an average blood loss.

Maternal blood pressure should remain stable after birth. It must however be noted that a change from a supine to a sitting position could result in a drop of 20 mm Hg in systolic pressure. This is referred to as *orthostatic hypotension* and is due to the decreased vascular resistance in the pelvic area. A drop in blood pressure unassociated with a change in position may reflect continuing blood loss and demands immediate assessment. On the other hand, an increase in systolic pressure of 30 mm Hg and a diastolic of 15 mm Hg, especially when accompanied by a headache and visual changes, may suggest *pre-eclampsia*. Once again the midwife should be cautioned to assess the blood pressure always first when a woman complains of a headache and not simply resort to administering analgesia.

The body's blood clotting mechanisms are activated in the early postnatal period. A high level of plasma fibrinogen persists during the first few postnatal weeks to serve as a protective measure should postpartum haemorrhage occur, but this also has an adverse effect in that it increases the risk of thrombophlebitis. The midwife should routinely observe for signs of thrombosis as discussed further on in this chapter.

The white blood cell count may increase to 30 000, particularly the granulocytes, to

Our approach to postpartum care is based on a 'wellness' model, which views the woman as an active participant in her overall care, as opposed to an illness model in which the woman is viewed as a 'patient' who is dependent on others for care. In South Africa, the length of stay in public sector facilities, including primary health clinics and midwife obstetric units, has been significantly reduced to a minimum of six hours. At most, women who have had normal birthing processes, and who have given birth to healthy infants, spend one or two days in hospital. Women who had difficult birthing processes or a caesarean section may have a slightly longer hospital stay. The challenge for the midwife during the short stay is to teach the woman, her partner and family the essential aspects of postpartum care.

protect the body against infection and to aid in the healing processes of the postnatal period.

The reproductive system

The involution of the uterus occurs rapidly after birth. Two major changes occur, namely, the placental site is sealed off and the uterus returns to its non-pregnant state.

Bleeding from the placental site is controlled by compression of the vessels by the contracted uterine fibres (figure of eight effect). The sinuses at the site become thrombosed and the area is sealed off. Healing takes place by exfoliation, which entails the undermining of the site by the growth of endometrial tissue. This process does not cause fibrous scarring of the endometrium, so future implantation sites are not compromised. Failure of the placental site to heal completely results in persistent lochia and episodes of brisk, painless bleeding. This is referred to as *subinvolution*.

Following the separation and expulsion of the placenta, the fundus of the uterus may be palpated midway between the umbilicus and the symphysis pubis. An hour later it rises to the level of the umbilicus where it remains for 12 to 24 hours. From then on it will decrease by one fingerbreadth (1 cm) per day and this should be monitored. Within two weeks the uterus resumes its position as a pelvic organ and cannot be palpated abdominally. In a breastfeeding woman involution is hastened due to the release of oxytocin from the posterior lobe of the pituitary gland, in response to the sucking stimulus of the newborn infant. By six weeks the uterus has almost returned to its non-gravid size. The term involution describes the reduction in the size of the uterus to non-pregnant state.

Lochia

The uterus cleanses itself of debris after childbirth by a vaginal discharge known as lochia. Table 17.1 illustrates the characteristics of lochia.

The normal progression of changes in the lochia reflect the re-establishment of the endometrium and the healing of the placental site. The midwife must educate the woman to report on any deviation from the norm.

The cervix

Following the birth, the cervix is spongy and flabby. The internal os closes. Following a vaginal birth, the external os remains slightly open and star-shaped. Observing this change during a cervical examination suggests that childbirth has occurred.

The vagina

During the early postnatal period, the vaginal walls have few rugae and appear oedematous, bruised and small lacerations may be visible. The hymen is torn and the edges form small tags. The distended vaginal canal and outlet gradually contract. The woman can increase the strength and tone of the perineum by doing Kegel's exercises. The vaginal rugae return by three weeks and the vaginal mucosa remains fragile and thin walled until the hormonal cycle regulating the menstrual cycle is resumed.

The perineum

The pressure and distension that the perineum is exposed to during a vaginal delivery results in a reduction of its muscle tone. The perineum may also be bruised and tender. The midwife should encourage the woman to do regular exercises to strengthen the tone of the pelvic floor muscles.

The urinary system

The descent of the fetal head during labour, particularly during prolonged labour, causes a transient loss of muscle tone of the bladder and bruising/oedema of the urethra. This may result in overdistension and incomplete emptying of the bladder.

Table 17.1 Characteristics of lochia

Name	Duration	Normal discharge	Abnormal discharge
Lochia rubra	Day 1 to day 3	Bloody, small particles of decidua and mucus.	Blood clots, foul smell, copious.
Lochia serosa	Day 4 to day 9	Pink or brown with a serosanguinous consistency.	Foul smell, saturated perineal pad.
Lochia alba	Day 10 day to 21	White or colourless. Odour similar to menstrual flow.	Foul smell, saturated pad. Return to pink or red colour. Persists for more than three weeks.

The increased diameter of the ureters until the fourth postpartum week increases the likelihood of urinary stasis and subsequent urinary infection. Excess fluid that accumulated in the tissues during pregnancy is eliminated by diuresis. The catabolic processes that occur in the uterus during involution may result in proteinuria. Routine assessment of the bladder is crucial in assuring early detection of complications.

The gastrointestinal system

Most women are hungry after delivery and enjoy a light meal and something to drink. They may be thirsty for the first two to three days, as a result of perspiration, diuresis, and the reduced fluid intake during labour. Women who had a caesarean section may be offered clear fluids after the first post-operative day, light solids introduced shortly after and solid foods when the bowel sounds return.

During the puerperium the gastrointestinal organs are restored to their pre-gravid state and the normal motility of the gastrointestinal tract improves within two weeks. During the second stage of labour, considerable pressure is exerted on the pelvic floor, resulting in decreased tone of the anal sphincter. The mother needs to be given the assurance that she will gradually regain tonicity of the anal sphincter.

Constipation is common during the first three to four days post-delivery. The main contributory factors are dehydration associated with loss of fluids and low fluid intake during labour, lack of tone of the gastrointestinal tract, and reflex inhibition of defaecation arising from a painful episiotomy, perineal lacerations, or from haemorrhoids. Analgesic drugs may also cause constipation. Stool softeners or suppositories may be used to promote elimination. Early ambulation following delivery aids in preventing and correcting constipation. A diet with plenty of roughage, increased fluid intake, daily exercise and an attempt to establish a regular time for bowel movement, will be helpful.

Principles of postnatal care

Assessment

History

On admission to the postnatal ward, the midwife makes the woman comfortable and responds to her immediate needs. A complete report on the woman and her baby is received from the midwife transferring the woman from the labour ward to the postnatal ward. Any complications, such as postpartum haemorrhage, perineal tears, or a depressed emotional state should be reported on, as well as the relevant interventions. The postnatal midwife needs to know how the baby is doing in the case where he does not accompany the mother to the ward.

Observations

On admission to the postnatal ward the temperature, pulse, blood pressure, uterine contraction and blood loss are assessed. Check the last Hb level as it may decrease after the intrapartum and postpartum blood loss. The frequency of observations is guided by the condition of the patient.

Vital signs

▶ *Temperature.* Usually elevated to 38 °C during the first 24 hours post-delivery. It may increase beyond 38 °C after 24 hours. If it persists beyond 48 hours it suggests infection and calls for action. Exclude other causes and/or symptoms such as pain in the calf, foul odour of lochia, infection or dehydration.
▶ *Pulse.* Ranges between 50 to 90 bpm. Tachycardia may result following haemorrhage, or a difficult labour and birth.
▶ *Blood pressure.* An elevated BP may suggest pre-eclampsia, chronic hypertension, renal disease, or anxiety. A drop in BP may be normal for the mother, or it may indicate postpartum haemorrhage.
▶ *Respiration.* This should remain within normal range of 16 to 24 breaths per minute.

General assessment

Enquire whether the woman is experiencing pain or discomfort. Ask specifically about her emotional state, lochia, micturition, defaecation, breastfeeding and infant care, mobilisation, exercise, sleep and diet. Examine the perineum for signs of infection. Educate the woman about vulval and perineal hygiene.

Assessment and management of specific health problems

Uterine atony

Uterine atony accounts for 80 to 90% of post-partum haemorrhage in the first 24 hours of the postnatal period. It occurs when the uterus does not contract effectively after childbirth and bleeding persists from the placental site (see Chapter 21). The midwife should educate the woman to look out for the following signs:

▶ The uterus is not palpable as a hard mass.
▶ Vaginal bleeding persists.
▶ Full bladder (a full bladder will prevent the uterus from contracting).

Educate the woman on simple methods to assist micturition such as a nearby running tap. Should this fail then she should seek appropriate assistance. The cause of retention of urine, such as a painful episiotomy site or vulval haematoma, should be established and the condition managed.

The midwife should be on the alert for the following instances where there is an increased susceptibility to develop an atonic uterus.

▶ Multiparous women.
▶ Overdistension of the uterus during pregnancy (multiple pregnancy, large baby, polyhydramnios).
▶ History of PPH with previous delivery.
▶ Prolonged labour.
▶ Precipitous labour and delivery.
▶ *Oxytocin* induction during labour.

Health education should be given to the woman to encourage regular checks that the uterine contraction is sustained, that vaginal bleeding is average, and that the bladder is emptied regularly. Rubbing up the uterine fundus should be demonstrated to the woman and she should be encouraged to report odd or abnormal findings promptly.

Abnormal findings must be documented and reported to the doctor immediately. Exploration of the uterus under general anaesthesia and removal of the retained placental products may be necessary. If an antibiotic is prescribed, the midwife should advise on the significance of compliance and the importance of completing the prescribed course of antibiotics.

Subinvolution

Subinvolution is a term used to describe a uterus that remains large and fails to reduce in size and mass. It may result from retained placental fragments, infection and myoma. Appropriate health education is essential and subinvolution should be suspected if the following are evident:

▶ The lochia fails to progress from rubra to serosa.
▶ The woman gives a history of excessive bleeding.
▶ The uterus is tender to palpation (which suggests endometritis).
▶ There is leucorrhoea and back pain.
▶ There is an accompanying infection.
▶ An enlarged uterus is palpated.

Painful episiotomy or perineal laceration site

Haematomata are formed when a blood vessel is injured without any noticeable trauma or laceration to the overlying tissues. This is associated with forceps deliveries, inadequate repairs of episiotomies or pressure necrosis following spontaneous vaginal deliveries. Haematomata occur along the birth canal, more commonly at the perineal or vaginal sites and less frequently as retroperineal and broad ligament sites. When haematomata occur in the latter sites it is dangerous because bleeding can cantinue unnoticed for a prolonged period of time. These sites are more susceptible to infection.

One of the symptoms of a haematoma is that the woman may complain of an excruciating pain in the vagina, perineum or rectum that may radiate down to the leg. Initial examination may not confirm diagnosis, since external swelling may not be evident. Examination, under sedation, in the theatre may be required to assess and treat the haematoma. Small vulval haematomata may be managed with ice packs, pressure to the area and analgesics. The size of the haematoma and signs of shock should be monitored.

Thrombophlebitis, thrombosis and deep vein thrombosis (DVT)

Thrombophlebitis is an inflammation of a blood vessel with a possible concurrent development of a thrombus. Thrombus formation may result from an injury to a vessel wall, diminished vascular flow and/or changes in clotting factors. Women who are at risk and who should be promptly identified and optimally managed are those with increased parity, varicosities and anaemia and those who have had caesarean births or forceps deliveries.

The most common superficial site for thrombophlebitis is the saphenous vein of the leg. Symptoms include mild calf pain, tenderness and induration along the vein. The midwife's responsibilities include vigilant monitoring of the vital signs and checking the legs for signs of inflammation, swelling and pain in the calf on passive dorsiflexion of the foot (Homan's sign). This is indicative of DVT.

All women during the postnatal period should be well informed about the following preventive measures:

▶ Maintaining an adequate fluid intake.
▶ Avoiding constriction to the popliteal area.
▶ Walking regularly during the day.
▶ Elevating the feet while sitting.

Treatment for DVT consists of an increase in fluids, the use of support stockings, anti-inflammatory and analgesic medications. In addition to this DVT requires anticoagulant therapy. Midwives are reminded to review their responsibilities and precautionary measures for a woman receiving anticoagulant therapy.

Infection of the breast (mastitis)

Injury to the lactating breast and poor drainage of milk are the primary predisposing factors to infection in the breast. Overdistension, stasis or cracking of the nipple may result in breast infection.

Symptoms of mastitis include a rapid rise in temperature up to 40 °C, rigors, tachycardia, reddened, tender breast tissue, and palpable hard masses in the breast.

Conservative treatment consists of monitoring the temperature four-hourly and when necessary using measures to reduce the pyrexia. The woman should increase the fluid intake to 8 to 10 glasses of water daily, use heat or ice packs to promote circulation to the area and analgesia to relieve pain. It is essential that the woman continues to breastfeed. Frequent feeding will prevent mastitis from worsening and aid in its treatment. Gentle massage may also offer relief. A breast abscess could be suspected if a lump does not respond to the usual treatment within a few days. This is serious and should be treated with antibiotics and possible surgical drainage. A culture and sensitivity test of the breast milk should be done for a definitive diagnosis of the causative organism so that an appropriate antibiotic is prescribed.

> ### Measures to guard against the development of mastitis
>
> ▶ Adequate non-restrictive support of the breasts at all times.
> ▶ Regular and thorough hand-washing.
> ▶ Breast cleanliness and avoidance of abrasive cleansing agents.
> ▶ Keep the nipple soft and lubricated and avoid bruising by using the correct latching and releasing techniques.
> ▶ Frequent changing of breast pads.
> ▶ Intermittent exposure of the nipples to air.
> ▶ Avoidance of known sources of infection.

Postpartum blues, depression and psychosis

Assessment of the psychological wellbeing of the woman post-delivery does not always receive the vigilant monitoring that it deserves. Midwives must be able to implement preventive measures; differentiate one condition from the other; identify the early signs and symptoms of each condition; and report promptly to the doctor when warning signs of puerperal depression or psychosis set in (refer to Chapter 23).

Education about psychological care and support must be emphasised during antenatal parenting sessions which couples participate in jointly. Student midwives should engage in self-directed learning and undertake projects to empower them to adopt a comprehensive and holistic approach when caring for the woman and her family during the postnatal period. Promotion of rest and sleep is critical in helping the mother to adapt.

CRITICAL THINKING EXERCISES

1. Design brochures on various postnatal education topics.
2. Where possible translate them into the languages commonly used by the community that is served by the local maternity unit/midwifery obstetrical unit.
3. Do a follow-up survey to determine the effectiveness of the brochures.
4. Use the findings to effect the necessary changes.

Breastfeeding

The woman who chooses to breastfeed her baby needs all the support she can get. Breastfeeding is discussed in depth in Chapter 30.

General support and education

Early discharge within six hours of the birthing process is the norm in public sector maternity units and midwife obstetrical units in South Africa. Antenatal preparation of preg-nant women to cope with postnatal demands is essential. Comprehensive health education that encompasses psychological, social, and physical aspects of the postnatal period and care of the newborn should be provided during the antenatal period. Reinforcement of these aspects should occur prior to discharge.

Postnatal district services are not always available. For that reason midwives in South Africa should investigate the possibility of encouraging community participation by introducing a Postpartum Doula System. Midwives should set up meetings with relevant community structures to effect the existence of doulas either on a voluntary basis or for a nominal hourly rate depending on the community's circumstances.

Doulas nurture the mother so that she in turn can nurture her newborn baby. First and foremost they assist with breastfeeding. In addition they assist with other tasks such as demonstrating and helping with baby baths, advice on cord care, sleeping issues for mother and baby, general household support, practical help with multiple births and more, depending on the individual's circumstances.

In the presence of brief stays in hospital, discharge planning is crucial to ensure that the woman and her baby are safe. The extent of the health education given by the midwife depends on whether the woman received comprehensive education during the antenatal period or received little or none. The woman

Advantages gained by the use of postpartum doulas

- Less maternal exhaustion, frustration and apprehension during the early weeks.
- Increased maternal physical wellbeing.
- Earlier bonding due to more confidence.
- Increased incidence of successful breastfeeding.
- Informed care reduces chances of infant dehydration and hospitalisation.
- Greater understanding of the newborn's emotional and physical needs.

should be given instruction on self-care and baby care before she leaves the hospital. She should be counselled with regard to family planning (fertility control) and signs of illness in both herself and the baby.

A range of well-designed pamphlets that cater for the health education needs of literate and illiterate groups are always of value. These should include the telephone numbers of the nearest clinic and ambulance services.

Conclusion

The support of the midwife, partner and family is essential for a positive postnatal experience for the woman and her newborn baby.

References

Bobak, I. M. & Jensen, M. D. 1993. *Maternity and gynaecologic care: The nurse and the family*. Fifth edition. St Louis: Mosby.

Cronje, H. S., Grobler, C. J. F. & Visser, A. A. 1996. *Obstetrics in Southern Africa*. Pretoria: Academica.

Ladewig, P. W., London, M. L. & Olds, S. B. 1994. *Maternal–newborn nursing*. Third edition. Redwood City: Addison-Wesley Nursing.

May, K. A. & Malmeister, L. R. 1994. *Maternal and neonatal nursing: Family-centred care*. Third edition. Philadelphia: J. B. Lippincott.

Pillitteri, A. 1999. *Maternal and child health nursing*. Third edition. Philadelphia: Lippincott.

Sellers, P. M. 1993. *Midwifery. Volume 1*. Cape Town: Juta.

CRITICAL THINKING EXERCISES

1. Conduct a needs assessment at your local well-baby clinic, review available educational material and design flip charts, z cards and pamphlets based on the needs identified.
2. Conduct peer group assessments.
3. Conduct a survey on the admission of women with postnatal complications.
4. Brainstorm the key components of a module for the education and training of postpartum doulas.
5. You have been asked to coordinate a few training workshops for postpartum doulas in your local community. Give a systematic description of your implementation of this project.

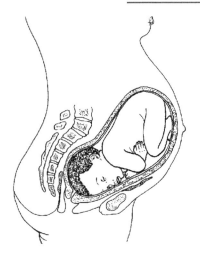

High-risk
pregnancy,
labour and
puerperium

Chapter *18*

Assessment and risk screening

Joan Dippenaar

Introduction

In this chapter the focus moves to the high-risk pregnancy, labour and puerperium. Although this period is viewed as normal in the life of most women, it carries risks, some of which are life threatening in nature. A high-risk pregnancy, labour, birth or puerperium occur when factors are present which add an increased risk of adverse outcome on the woman or the fetus. One of the primary objectives of midwifery care during pregnancy, labour and puerperium is to identify those women and fetuses who have a high-risk status. It is important that they are identified early so that appropriate and timely interventions or referrals can be made to promote and ensure optimal health for the woman, the fetus, the newborn infant and the family.

A high-risk pregnancy does not necessarily end in a poor outcome, while at the same time a healthy pregnancy with low risk may cause unexpected complications. The predictability of outcomes in the presence of known identifiable factors remains problematic and no single instrument has proven effective to predict outcomes thus far.

The emphasis of this chapter is to provide the midwife with a conceptual framework to evaluate thinking processes and practices in the identification of high-risk pregnancies. This chapter should be studied in conjunction with Chapters 5, 9 to 11, and Chapters 20 to 24.

The scope of practice for the midwife and the high-risk pregnant woman

The WHO acknowledges midwives as the most cost-effective caregivers in pregnancy and childbirth. Midwives care for 77% of pregnant women in South Africa, making midwifery practice integral to healthcare delivery. Provided that a high standard of care and best practice principles are maintained, low-risk pregnancies and births are safe in the hands of midwives.

It is important for the midwife to know whether the woman and unborn baby in her care are at risk from complications. Should any risk factors be present, the woman should be referred for medical help (SANC, 1990). Regulation 2488 (SANC, 1990) provides guidelines of illnesses, abnormalities and complications during pregnancy, labour and the puerperium which, when identified, should be referred for medical assistance. The application of this regulation will differ depending on the situation midwives practise in, whether it be rural or urban, level 1, 2 or 3 facilities, private or public health, or as independent private practitioners. In addition, the resources available, protocols of institutions and the quality and availability of the medical team or back-up system for the midwife all influence the application of the regulation. This regulation serves to protect the public. Midwives need evidence-based guidelines to identify risk and protocols for referral.

The philosophy of risk screening

Screening for disease could be very costly and the cost could outweigh the risk. It has been demonstrated that routine fetal monitoring, for example, leads to an increase in operative deliveries without showing any benefit, while practices known to be beneficial are not adopted as clinical standards.

Screening programmes are useful only where:
▶ The outcome in question is an important public health problem in the population.
▶ There is a detectable pre-clinical phase or high-risk state preceding this outcome.
▶ Screening tests have useful likelihood ratios (positive and negative) to permit identification of those at risk and those who are not.
▶ There is an effective treatment available for this early stage of disease.

▶ Early intervention is more effective than waiting and treating the overt disease.

'Sensitivity' of a screening test refers to its ability to correctly determine the proportion of women with the disease (true positives). The 'specificity' of a test refers to its ability to correctly identify the proportion of those women who are disease-free (true negatives). The 'predictive value' relates to the matter of false positive tests and false negative tests in estimating the test's overall effectiveness in predicting the presence or absence of disease. The 'efficiency' of a test is the combination of both positive and negative predictive values. For a screening test this may be defined as its ability to discriminate between those with and without the condition in question. In contrast, a treatment's effectiveness may be judged by its ability to prevent, cure or prevent progression of a condition or reduce case fatality.

Risk scoring as a screening test

The central issue in monitoring women and fetuses during pregnancy and labour is to determine which women and/or fetuses are at risk of developing complications, so as to increase their surveillance, refer them for appropriate care and to intervene where possible. Over the years a number of scoring systems have been developed and tested. The limitation of these formal scoring systems is that none have proven to be accurate in predicting the outcome of pregnancy. It may also 'label' a woman as high risk and expose her to more interventions than may have been necessary, as well as to a high level of anxiety. Another problem is that most of these scoring systems are based on previous pregnancies, rendering them of no value to the primigravida.

Asking the right questions depends on the knowledge, skills and experience of the midwife, and the philosophy of care. The basic knowledge required in order to ask the right questions includes:

▶ The community's risks and profiles, expectations, resources and outcomes.
▶ Evidence-based maternity care.
▶ Best practice obstetrical protocols.
▶ Diseases and conditions affecting pregnancy outcomes.
▶ The cost of care.
▶ Psychosocial aspects and their effect on pregnancy.

History taking is an essential screening tool that recognises the features that may negatively affect the course of pregnancy, labour and birth. Midwives should keep accurate records, which include noting the risks, interventions and actions taken in relation to the risk. *Accurate and complete records* are crucial to the defensibility of professional care.

The Department of Health prescribes standard records for care, including the antenatal card and the partogram for labour (DoH Guidelines for maternity care in South Africa, 2001). It calls for complete medical, surgical, gynaecological and obstetrical history, a physical examination (with urine test) and basic essential screening investigations, including:
▶ VDRL rapid card test.
▶ Rh grouping rapid card test.
▶ Haemoglobin test using a portable haemoglobin meter.
▶ Voluntary counselling and testing for HIV.
▶ Urine dipstick for glucose and protein.

All women should have these basic screenings done on the first contact. It is required that women keep the record with them at all times to present to whoever is taking care of them in order to provide continuity of care (see Chapter 9).

The early evaluation of women will affect the outcome of pregnancy as certain preventive interventions will be effective only if instituted before conception or early in pregnancy like the detection of abnormalities through the triple test, and sonar between 16 to 20 weeks of pregnancy (see Chapter 10). Most risk factors can be identified at the initial first visit. Other risk factors may be detected only during subsequent visits because a low-risk pregnancy may change to a high-risk pregnancy due to complications that may occur. Some problems and infections are without symptoms and need to be detected by blood tests like TORCH (infections known to cause congenital abnormalities). The standard assessment protocol of the DoH requires midwives to do a speculum examination to determine vaginal infections, followed by standard treatment. Further risks should also be assessed continuously on admission for labour, during labour and after birth.

Once risk factors have been identified they can be categorised as:
▶ *Obstetrical*. Age, size of pelvis, number of fetuses, abnormalities of the uterus, placental function and implantation.
▶ *Pre-existing or medical conditions*. Abnormalities and diseases, known or unknown, present, which can be aggravated by the pregnancy or affect the pregnancy, such as infections, diabetes, anaemia, renal and cardiac conditions. It needs to be noted that some conditions during pregnancy are asymptomatic with no signs or symptoms or are masked by the pregnancy. Taking a structured, comprehensive history should reveal women prone to such conditions.

A word of warning

Enkin, et al (2000:51) warn us that risk factors are only markers, associations with possible adverse outcomes and not causes thereof. Very often these factors cannot be changed, for example, poor pre-pregnancy weight, high parity, height and past reproductive history. At the same time, coming to the conclusion that a particular pregnancy is 'low risk' may lower our watchfulness and complications may arise without proper surveillance and action.

Screening and diagnostic tests

All women have the right to be tested if the possibility of an abnormality of a fetus is in question. Diagnostic tests of value include histology, blood and urine tests, cytogenic analysis, blood glucose, thyroid function tests, and microbiological growth and sensitivity. It is the task of the midwife to identify potential problems and advise women of available tests or alternatives.

More sophisticated tests and investigations might not be freely available at public facilities as a routine screening protocol, however at relatively lower cost, women may be able to afford a 20 weeks ultrasound scan at a nearby private doctor's rooms or private hospital (BHF, 2001). Midwives should explore alternative resources in the community for the support of pregnant women.

Tests that are only available on indication

for high-risk cases in the public health sector are indicated in Table 18.1. Since these tests are not generic in the care of pregnant women midwives should have guidelines to indicate when the tests are required.

Due to the high cost of generic screening care must be taken when routine screening is instituted for healthcare. Table 10.2 (Chapter 10) indicates the essential investigations to determine risks and optimal times to do them during the pregnancy. Once the risk has been identified a more specific test can be done to verify and confirm the risk. Cost incurred in screening programmes must be weighed up against the cost of abnormal infants and death. Two screening tests not included in the generic

Table 18.1 Specific tests needing an indication

Tests	Indication
ABO blood grouping	Previous APH and PPH or risk for bleeding. Previous babies with high bilirubin.
Triple test for Down's syndrome	History of previous abnormalities. Diabetic women. Infections, such as rubella. Age more than 35 years. Black women.
Rubella	Rubella contact in family or community in early pregnancy (less than 20 weeks).
Blood glucose screening	Previous abortions. Previous abnormal babies. Previous IUD. Previous baby weighing more than 4 kg. Glucose and ketones on two consecutive visits.
Pap smear	All women should be advised to have a Pap smear in pregnancy before 28 weeks.
Urine culture	Women with a history of preterm labour. History of UTI. Vaginal infections.
Mid-trimester ultrasound	All women should have at least one ultrasound at 16–22 weeks to detect abnormalities (see Chapter 10).

Source: Department of Health, Guidelines for maternity care in South Africa, 2002.

screening of antenatal patients in the South African National Programme are a Pap smear and the alphafeto-protein blood test. The costs of fetal abnormalities, PROM, bacteriuria and preterm births need to be weighed up against the cost of generic screening protocols.

The impact of a high-risk pregnancy on the woman and her family

Although it is important for the midwife to know whether the woman under her care is at risk from complications, it may add a lot of stress on the woman and her family, not only during the time of waiting for the results, but also when getting the diagnosis of a pregnancy at risk. More often these women have to attend antenatal care more often, undergo more tests and interventions, all with their own risks, and even spend time in hospital. Support in the form of listening to concerns, possible guilt feelings and practical problems is important. Accurate information on their progress and future care is necessary.

Conclusion

The *skill of the clinician* is an important factor in the positive outcomes of pregnancy and birth, even in the use of high technology and interpretation of such. The *process* and *style of care* are also crucial factors identified for outcome evaluation. In addition, midwives have other tools beside the generic assessment of the DoH available to assist with the identification of problems during pregnancy and labour. The nutritional and body mass evaluation including weight monitoring and evaluation, birth plans, the postnatal depression indicator scale, high blood pressure evaluation, deep tendon reflexes, side room HB, urine test and microscopic evaluation, and the partogram are structured ways of evaluating women during pregnancy and birth. Midwives in South Africa also need to be involved in decision-making and research to develop tools suitable for the South African practice.

CRITICAL THINKING EXERCISES

1. Perform a retrospective risk evaluation of a 21 year old woman who presented with unknown diabetes and was admitted to an intensive care unit with a blood sugar of 24mm/l, and was diagnosed 24 weeks pregnant after the second admission. The woman had a retrospective score of 32 on a risk score. Outcome: The baby died after 32 weeks IUD and had congenital abnormalities.
2. Develop an algorithm for the detection of Down's syndrome in pregnancy. Utilise the Cochrane Library to obtain the latest evidence.
3. Perform a retrospective risk assessment and outcome of your 15 deliveries during your training and consider:
   ▶ The outcomes of events.
   ▶ Potential alternative interventions that could be considered.
   ▶ Constraints hampering best practices.

References

Bates, S. M., Ginsberg, J. S. 1997. *Thrombosis in pregnancy*. Rapid Science Publishers.

Beck, C. T. 1998. A checklist to identify women at risk for developing post partum depression. Principles and practice. *Journal of Obstetric Gynecologic and Neonatyal Nursing*, January/February 39–45.

Christiani, K. 1996. Women's health: Effects on mortality and morbidity in pregnancy and birth. *Midwifery*, 12:113–116.

Corry, M. P. & Rooks, J.1999. Promoting the midwifery model of care in partnership with the maternity center association. *Journal of Nurse Midwifery*, 44(1) January/February 47–56.

Dawson, E., Gauld, R. & Ridler, J. 1993. Empowering mothers. *Nursing RSA*, 8(4):10.

Department of Health (DoH). 2002. *Guidelines for maternity care in South Africa*. Pretoria: DoH.

Department of Health (DoH). 2002. *Human*

genetic policy guidelines. For the management and prevention of fenetic disorders, birth defects and disabilities. www.DOH.gov.za. 27 May 2003.

Department of Health (DoH). 2003. *Saving mothers. Second report on confidential enquiries into maternal deaths in South Africa.* 1999–2001. Pretoria.

Editorial. 1991. Midwives and the empowerment of women. An international perspective. *Journal of Nurse-Midwifery*, 36(2):85.

Enkin, M., Keirse, M. J. N., Neilson G. et al. 2000. A guide to effective care in pregnancy and childbirth. Third edition. London: Oxford University Press.

Gunnar, T. & Bungum, L. 1987. The grand multipara. Maternal and neonatal complications. *Acta Obstetrics Gynecology Scandinavia*, 66:53–56

Mathai, Matthews. 1999. Routine antenatal care for low risk pregnancy in under-resourced settings. *Cochrane*. WHO Reproductive health library. Issue 2:1–3.

Midmer, D. K. 1992. Does family centred maternity care empower women? The development of the women centred childbirth model. *Family Medicine*, April 24(3):216–221.

Moore, M. L. & Freda, M. C. 1998. Reducing preterm and low birth weight babies. *Maternal Child Nursing*, July/August 23:4.

Murphy, P. A. & Fullerton J. T. 2001. Measuring outcomes of midwifery care: Development of an instrument to assess optimality. *Journal of Midwifery & Women's Health*, September/October 46(5).

Muller, M. 1990. Navorsingsmetodologie vir formulering van verpleegstandaarde. *Curationis*, December 13(3 & 4).

Nielsen, N. P. 1998. Routine ultrasound in early pregnancy. *Cochrane*, WHO Reproductive Health library. Issue 2:1–7.

Oates, J. K. 1993. Genital herpes in pregnancy and its management. *Obstetrics Update*, September 37–45.

Phillips, C.1999. Family-centred maternity care. Past, present and future. *International Journal of Childbirth Education*, 14:3–5.

Robertson, A. 2000. Models of midwifery across Australia. January. Andrea@ace-graphics.com.au.

SANC (South African Nursing Council). 1990. Regulation relating to the conditions under which registered midwives and enrolled midwives may carry on their profession (Regulation 2488 of October 1990.) Pretoria: SANC.

Stagiannis, K., Bower, S. & Fisk, N. 1994. The twin fetus. *British Journal of Midwifery*, 2(10):469–73.

Strategies for improved evidenced based practices. 2001. The Better birth initiative. gulmezoglum@who.int. 15 November 2002. The Cochrane Collaboration. *The Cochrane Library*. Oxford 2002.

Theron, G. B. 1999. Effects of the maternal care manual from the Perinatal Education Programme on the quality of antenatal and intrapartum care rendered by midwives. *South African Medical Journal*, March 89(3):33–39.

Van Dongen, P. W. J. 1998. Editorial. Preconception care. *Obstetric and Gynecologic Forum*, February.

Villar, J. & Gulmezoglo, A. M. 1998. Maternal health. Annual technical WHO report:172–181

WHO (World Health Organisation). 2002. Strengthening midwifery. Making pregnancy safer. http:// www.who.int/reproductive-health/rtis/inex.htm. 15 November 2002.

WHO (World Health Organisation). 2001. WHO consultation on integrated management of pregnancy and childbirth. 9 July 2002.

WHO (World Health Organisation). 1987. The hypertensive disorders of pregnancy. Technical report series 758. WHO: Geneva.

WHO (World Health Organisation). 1992. ICD 10. *International statistical classification of diseases and related problems.* Tenth revision. WHO: Geneva.

WHO (World Health Organisation). 1998. Why are women dying. www.who.int. 27 May 2003.

Chapter *19*

Infections

Karin Minnie and Antoinette du Preez

Introduction

Although pregnant and puerperal women and neonates have always been vulnerable to infections, the incidence and effects of these conditions have increased since the impact of HIV/AIDS has become clear. Non-pregnancy-related infections, of which AIDS contributes the largest portion, are the most common causes of maternal death in South Africa (31.4%). Pregnancy-related sepsis, mainly septic abortion and puerperal sepsis, is the fourth most common cause of maternal deaths (Second Report on Confidential Enquiries into Maternal Deaths in South Africa, 1999–2001). AIDS and other non-pregnancy-related infections are considered indirect causes of maternal deaths, since these deaths are not directly caused by obstetric complications, but by septic shock or multi-organ failure.

There is a relationship between perinatal deaths and HIV/AIDS. Although a direct cause–effect relationship has not yet been proven, there have been concurrent increases in the occurrence of unexplained macerated intra-uterine deaths (probably because of chorio-amnionitis/amniotic fluid infection syndrome) and the occurrence of HIV/AIDS. Even babies who survive the pregnancy are at risk of being infected by their HIV-positive mothers and they then die at a later stage because of AIDS. As HIV/AIDS has such a large impact on both maternal and perinatal mortality and morbidity, it is fitting to start with a discussion of this condition.

HIV/AIDS

AIDS is the acronym for Acquired Immunodeficiency Syndrome. The virus that causes this condition is the Human Immunodeficiency Virus (HIV). Because the virus mainly targets the immune system, especially the T-helper cells and the CD4 lymphocytes, the body's defence mechanisms are suppressed and other infections occur more frequently and more severely. Infection with HIV is associated with an increased risk of opportunistic diseases that will eventually lead to death.

Effect of pregnancy on HIV/AIDS

While the infection is still at an early stage, pregnancy does not usually influence the progress of the disease. The physiologically suppressed resistance during pregnancy and the added burden on the body may, however, accelerate the progress to full-blown AIDS or quicker deterioration if the woman is already in the final stage of AIDS.

Effect of HIV/AIDS on the pregnancy and birth

Pregnancy complications occur more frequently, especially if there are clinical signs of AIDS. The following conditions are more common:
- spontaneous abortion
- ectopic pregnancy
- other sexually transmitted diseases
- urinary tract infection
- pneumonia
- severe varicella (chicken pox)

- anaemia
- intra-uterine growth restriction
- chorio-amnionitis/amniotic fluid infection syndrome
- preterm prelabour rupture of membranes (pPROM)
- spontaneous preterm labour
- intra-uterine death.

Because of the risk of these conditions, HIV-infected women are considered high-risk patients and must be closely monitored during pregnancy, labour and birth.

Effect of HIV/AIDS on the fetus/neonate

Perinatal death

Due to the effects on the pregnancy and birth, the risk of stillbirth is increased fourfold. Many unexplained intra-uterine deaths resulting in macerated stillborns can be associated with chorio-amnionitis/amniotic fluid infection syndrome occurring in women with HIV/AIDS. As HIV-positive women have double the risk of spontaneous preterm labour compared to HIV-negative women, many babies die as a result of the complications of prematurity.

Mother-to-child transmission (MTCT) of HIV

There are different opinions on the actual risk of MTCT (or vertical transmission) if the mother is HIV positive. In the absence of interventions to prevent MTCT, approximately 30% of HIV-infected untreated mothers will pass the infection to their infants. This 30% consists of the following:
- 5% will be infected during pregnancy
- 15% will be infected during labour and delivery
- while 10% will be infected through the transmission of the virus in breast milk.

HIV/AIDS infection of the baby

Absolute neonatal HIV infection can only be positively diagnosed by tests that identify the virus itself and not the antibodies, such as the p24 antigen test or the RNA PCR (polymerase

Table 19.1 Factors that influence the risk of MTCT

Maternal factors	Obstetrical factors	Infant factors
▶ *Immune status.* The risk is increased with the severity of the immune deficiency. Women with low CD4 counts (<200 cells/µL) are more likely to transmit HIV to their infants. ▶ *Maternal viral load.* The higher the viral load in the maternal blood, the higher the risk of MTCT. The risk is especially high during the period just after infection, re-infection, when the woman has progressed to AIDS or has a documented high viral load (more than 50 000 HIV particles per ml). ▶ *Nutritional factors.* If a woman is generally malnourished, the maternal disease will progress more rapidly and thus the risk for MTCT will also increase. A multivitamin supplement may improve the woman's general health and raise her resistance to infection. ▶ *Behavioural factors.* Cigarette smoking, alcohol and drug use, as well as unprotected sexual intercourse during pregnancy, have been associated with an increased risk of MTCT.	▶ *Placental infection.* Chorion-amnionitis/amniotic fluid infection syndrome increases the risk of MTCT and can be caused by genital infections, sexually transmitted infections or prolonged rupture of membranes. The risk increases significantly if the membranes were ruptured for more than four hours. The first born baby of a multiple pregnancy has a higher risk of being infected during the birth process than the second baby. ▶ *Mode of delivery.* Because of the presence of the HI virus in blood and secretions in the birth canal, vaginal birth carries a higher risk of MTCT when compared to elective caesarean sections.	▶ *Gestational period at birth.* Preterm birth places the infant at a higher risk for MTCT compared to full-term births. ▶ *Fetal trauma.* Traumatic births and births where the skin was traumatised during obstetrical procedures increase the risk of MTCT. ▶ *Feeding method.* HIV can be transmitted through breast milk. However, exclusive breastfeeding carries a lower risk of MTCT than mixed feeding where breast milk is given with other fluids or food. If trauma or infection of the maternal breast, nipple, mouth or gastrointestinal tract of the baby is present, the risk of MTCT is higher.

chain reaction) test. These tests are more expensive than the screening tests (Elisa, Western blot or rapid tests) that are commonly used to screen for the presence of antibodies of the HI virus in adults. Because the HIV antibodies are transmitted through the placental barrier, all babies born to HIV-positive women will test positive when tested for the HIV antibodies. The maternal antibodies will disappear from the infant's blood by the time that trhe baby is 9 to 18 months old.

Babies who are infected in the first half of pregnancy usually present with signs of AIDS in the first weeks after birth and deteriorate rapidly. Without treatment with antiretroviral drugs, these babies usually die within the first three months. If the infection occurred during the last months of pregnancy the baby usually becomes ill in the first three months after birth and dies before six months. Babies infected during labour and delivery, or via breast milk, usually present much later with AIDS and have a slower progression in their illness. Signs of AIDS present between six months and five years. If the signs of AIDS are only present after three months, the child may survive beyond five years.

Management during the antenatal period

Health education

The first line of intervention in preventing maternal infection and MTCT is health education to the community, especially to the youth before they become sexually active and to partners before they conceive a child. Pregnant women must be encouraged and assisted to maintain a healthy lifestyle. This will prevent primary infection of HIV before and during pregnancy, as well as during the breastfeeding period. All pregnant women should be advised on safer sexual practices (Abstinence, Be faithful, Condom use). Even women already HIV positive must practice safer sex, as it is possible to be re-infected with a different strain of HIV. It causes the viral load in the blood to increase, and consequently progress to AIDS and the risk of MTCT also increase.

Voluntary HIV counselling and testing

Voluntary counselling and testing (VCT) must be available to all pregnant women (and their partners). The benefits for a pregnant woman of knowing her HIV status include:
▶ The ability to access the best care available for both mother and child.
▶ The opportunity to make use of safe termination of pregnancy, if desired.

▶ The ability to make an informed choice regarding infant feeding options.
▶ The ability to make an informed choice regarding future family planning (fertility control).

In addition to the matters that are usually discussed during post-test counselling, the following must be added when counselling a HIV-positive pregnant woman:
▶ The effect of pregnancy on HIV and the effect of HIV infection on pregnancy.
▶ The option of termination of pregnancy.
▶ The treatment options in pregnancy.
▶ The advantages and disadvantages of the different baby feeding options.
▶ The need for follow-up of mother and baby, as well as future family planning (fertility control).

Confidentially is important, but women should be encouraged to share this confidentiality with their loved ones and the health professionals directly involved with their care. The woman will be able to be supported by her loved ones and health professionals will be able to render appropriate care.

Prevention and treatment of genital infections

The prevention and treatment of genital infections will reduce the likelihood of placental infection (chorio-amnionitis/amniotic fluid infection syndrome) and the risk of MTCT.

Nutritional supplementation

Multivitamins, iron and folic acid should be given from the first antenatal care visit. These supplements result in improved pregnancy outcomes and may reduce the incidence of stillbirth, prematurity and low birth weight. Studies in South Africa, Malawi and Tanzania, however, have failed to prove that Vitamin A supplementation reduces MTCT (Dabis et al, 2000).

Antiretroviral therapy

HIV-positive women in developed countries usually receive a combination of antiretroviral drugs during pregnancy. These are given to reduce the viral load, thus prolongs the period before AIDS develops and enables the mother to raise her child for a longer period than would otherwise have been possible. As an additional effect it also reduces the risk of MTCT of HIV. The option of antiviral drugs given as treatment for the mother is often not affordable in the developing world, but it should be discussed. The financial implications must be considered and the woman can be referred to the private sector, if appropriate. Current recommendations for the use of antiretroviral therapy is a treatment combining two antiretroviral drugs with the addition of a protease inhibitor. The protocol that is followed depends on the CD4 count of the woman.

Additional antenatal care

HIV-positive women should not have invasive interventions like amniocentesis or an external cephalic version, as these may cause the fetus to come in contact with infected blood or body fluids.

Due to the increased risk of complications and even maternal death, HIV-positive women should receive optimal care in order to identify and treat any complications as soon as possible. Women must be asked about symptoms like weight loss, coughing and diarrhoea. When performing a complete physical examination at the first visit, the midwife must look for evidence of opportunistic infections like oral candidiasis, herpes zoster, tuberculosis and enlarged lymph nodes. If evidence of these infections is found, the woman should be referred for appropriate treatment. She can also receive prophylaxis for opportunistic infections. Prophylaxis for *Pneumocystis carinii pneumonia* (PCP) is given if there is a history of previous PCP, a CD4 count of 200 cells/µl and when AIDS-defining conditions, such as tuberculosis or oesophageal candidiasis occur. The protocol for PCP treatment is two *co-trimoxazole* tablets daily. The prophylaxis for tuberculosis is 300 mg *isoniazid* daily with 25 mg *pyridoxine* daily – both for six months. This regime lasts for two years.

If there are signs of sexually transmitted infections, urinary tract infections or anaemia, these must be treated appropriately. There must be careful fetal growth monitoring.

Pregnant women who are HIV-positive must receive health education on how to keep healthy as long as possible. Apart from vitamin supplementation, they must eat as healthy as possible, for example, by drinking lots of fluids, especially soup and fruit juices. Coffee, tea, cola, chocolate and alcohol must be avoided if diarrhoea is experienced. Lots of vegetables and fruits should be eaten and meals should be frequent, small and rich in energy and protein, rather than large meals consisting of fast foods. Dairy products may make the woman feel ill, but she can still take sour milk, buttermilk or yoghurt. It is important that she avoid smoking or visiting a malaria-prevalent area, as she could be more vulnerable to infection.

Management during the intrapartum period

Infection control

As vaginal and cervical secretions, blood and amniotic fluid may contain the virus, midwives are at risk when assisting HIV-positive women during birth. Women are at risk from HIV-positive healthcare workers if there is an exchange of blood during procedures like perineal suturing or slash injuries during caesarean section. Because the HIV status of all the women and healthcare workers are not known, universal precautions must be followed in the delivery or operating room during management of all women.

Immunodeficiant women should not be put in situations where they could easily become infected with other infections like tuberculosis.

Antiretroviral therapy

While a complete regimen to treat HIV/AIDS in the mother is the ideal, it may not be a feasible option in developing countries. This can be an ethical dilemma, as the mother will probably die before the child is a teenager, who would then be left as an orphan.

> ## Universal precautions to protect women and health-care workers from infection
>
> ▶ After contact with body fluids hands should be washed with antiseptic soap and running water, and dried with paper towels.
> ▶ During all procedures where hands may come into contact with body fluids new latex gloves should be worn.
> ▶ If there is a risk of fluid splashing in the eyes, glasses, goggles or a mask with a visor should be worn.
> ▶ A plastic apron should be worn to prevent the soiling of clothes.
> ▶ Foot protection such as rubber boots should be worn during delivery and operations.
> ▶ A sharps container should be used to discard used needles or lancets.
> ▶ When creating a sterile area, on a tray for example, sharp instruments should be kept in a separate container.
> ▶ It is best to suture perineal lacerations with a needle holder and dissecting forceps rather than using fingers.
> ▶ Take special care when handling soiled linen, as well as when disposing of blood and placentas.
> ▶ Avoid the need for mouth-to-mouth resuscitation and use an ambubag and mask instead.

Even a short course of antiretroviral therapy during labour reduces MTCT risk by up to 50%. Even if the life of the mother cannot be saved, every effort must be taken to spare the child.

The easiest and most cost-effective short course regime is a single dose of 200 mg *nevirapine* taken during labour by the mother and a single dose of *nevirapine* paediatric suspension (2 mg per kg) for the baby. HIV-positive women should receive an intra-partum pack at 28 weeks gestation and self-administer the medication at the onset of labour or the rupture of membranes. In the case of prolonged labour, the 200 mg *nevirapine* is repeated 24 hours after the first dose. All infants born to HIV-infected women should receive a single dose of *nevirapine* paediatric suspension (2 mg per kg) between 12 and 72 hours after birth. All the *nevirapine* dispensed must be entered into the appropriate *nevirapine* registers. The World Health Organisation recommends use of the short course prophylactic treatment with *nevirapine* as the advantages of it far outweigh the possible disadvantages (*nevirapine*-resistant virus traits after treatment or a very small chance of toxicity).

Caesarean section

Elective, not emergency caesarean section within four hours of rupture of the membranes is of value in significantly reducing the risk of MTCT. If the prevalence of HIV-infection is high and the conditions not ideal, the universal use of caesarean section is not only costly, but may lead to increased maternal morbidity and mortality. Caesarean sections must only be done for obstetrical reasons.

Vaginal cleansing

Vaginal cleansing with an antiseptic solution (0,25% *chlorhexidene* or *povidone iodine*) prior to vaginal examination in labour is associated with reduced MTCT and improved perinatal outcome. This cleaning can be done by douching or wiping the vagina with a dripping wet swab soaked in the antiseptic solution.

Prevention of prolonged rupture of membranes

There should be no routine artificial rupture of membranes. The perceived benefit of rupturing membranes should be weighed up against the benefits of leaving them intact. This procedure should only be done for a specific obstetric indication and then as late as possible. If membranes have ruptured spontaneously, labour must be augmented if there is evidence of slow progress and there are no contraindications.

Prevention of maternal trauma

Episiotomies should be avoided, if possible, as MTCT is increased by exposure of the fetus to maternal blood. It should only be used for obstetric indications such as fetal distress, medical indications to shorten the second stage and assisted delivery.

Prevention of trauma to the fetus/neonate

Trauma to the fetus/neonate caused by interventions like using scalp electrodes, or scalp blood sampling for pH determination, increase the risk of MTCT by opening a pathway for the virus when coming into contact with the maternal blood and secretions. Assisted instrumental delivery with both vacuum extraction and forceps delivery may damage the neonate's scalp or skin and increase the risk of HIV transmission during delivery. No oropharyngeal suctioning should be done routinely at birth because of the danger of injuring the delicate mucosa and giving the virus an entry point to the baby's circulation. Controlled gentle suctioning with a wide bore catheter and appropriately reduced negative pressure is only indicated in the presence of meconium-stained liquor or asphyxia neonatorum. The neonate must be wiped after delivery to remove all maternal body fluids.

Prophylactic antibiotics

Prophylactic antibiotics must be given before an elective or emergency caesarean section, in case of rupture of the membranes for more than four hours, or other interventions like assisted deliveries, as well as for HIV-positive women with CD4 counts of less than 200 cells/µl or where there are signs of AIDS.

Active management of the third stage

The third stage of labour must be managed actively as described in Chapter 14. Because of the higher incidence of anaemia in HIV-positive women, postpartum haemorrhage can have catastrophic consequences.

Management during the postpartum period

Infection control

All women should receive health education to safely used shared toilets and showers, to conduct personal hygiene, manage lochia discharge and appropriately discard used sanitary towels. The woman must be closely observed for signs of infections, especially after a caesarean section.

Choice of infant feeding

The woman should receive enough information during pregnancy to make an informed decision of the best baby-feeding option in her circumstances.

The choice of a feeding method for the baby of an HIV-positive woman is a complicated and emotional issue. It is often difficult for the midwife and the woman to be entirely objective and rational in decision-making. In a society where breastfeeding is the norm, a deviation from this may lead to victimisation and stigmatisation. In unfavourable socioeconomic circumstances, the risk of infant death from complications of feeding with a breast milk substitute can be up to 15 times more than the risk of possible HIV transmission by exclusive breastfeeding. The midwife should have the correct knowledge to give accurate health education that would enable the woman to make an informed and suitable choice.

As MTCT through breastfeeding can occur at any time during the period that the HIV-positive mother is breastfeeding, the only way to totally avoid this is to use a breast milk substitute. It must, however, only be used by mothers who can use it safely and where the benefits of using it outweigh the risk of possible complications.

Feeding with a breast milk substitute is a better feeding option if:
- The woman knows she is HIV-infected.
- A sustained supply of breast milk substitute is available (she can afford it

herself or it is supplied by health services or an NGO).

▶ The breast milk substitute can be prepared safely, with clean water and equipment.

▶ There is no history of a previous child dying of gastroenteritis or malnutrition.

▶ Not to breastfeed is accepted in the community and household.

▶ The woman is already ill because of AIDS or its complications.

As the practice of formula feeding is associated with a high infant mortality rate, especially in non-hygienic conditions, women who select this option must receive additional health education. Instructions on the correct and safe way to prepare, store and give formula feeding must only be given to HIV-positive mothers who have chosen this infant feeding method. Cup feeding instead of bottle feeding is advised, as it is easier to keep clean, and less expensive.

In the following circumstances breastfeeding is a better option:

▶ The HIV status of the woman is unknown or she is HIV-negative.

▶ Hygiene, sanitation and access to clean water are poor.

▶ There are many infectious diseases such as gastroenteritis in the community.

▶ The woman has already lost a baby to an infectious disease or to malnutrition.

▶ There is no sustained supply of breast milk substitute.

▶ Breastfeeding exclusively is accepted in the community and household.

If feeding with a breast milk substitute is not a safe option, absolutely exclusive breastfeeding with no additional water, glucose, gripe water, cereals or food with the breast milk is relatively safe ('safer breastfeeding'). Exclusive breastfeeding carries a reduced risk of MTCT because of the following reasons:

▶ Exclusive breastfeeding ensures protection against the permeability of the intestinal mucosa because of the high concentration of growth factor that promotes the development of the epithelial barrier of the gut.

▶ With exclusive breastfeeding there is less exposure to antigens that cause inflammation and thus increased permeability of the mucosa.

▶ With exclusive breastfeeding there is less exposure to pathological organisms.

▶ Exclusive breastfeeding stimulates advantageous intestinal micro flora like *Lactobacillus bifidus* that lowers the intestinal pH and thus destroys pathogens.

Early introduction of solids is very common. In a study done in KwaZulu-Natal, it was found that the average period of exclusive breastfeeding of participants was one month, and the average age of introducing solids three months (Coutsoudis et al, 1999). To get the maximum benefit of exclusive breastfeeding it is preferable to postpone the introduction of solids to as near as possible to six months after birth. After the age of six months breast milk alone cannot sufficiently supply all the nutritional needs of a baby. When the mother starts to give solid food, she must abruptly wean the baby from the breast, as prolonged weaning will involve a period of mixed feeding with all the danger that it holds.

The following conditions must be prevented through health education and other treatment

---

Research highlights

Until 1999 all research to calculate the risk of HIV transmission through breast milk compared the risk of babies who have never been breastfed with those who have ever taken breast milk (not exclusively breastfeeding, but most often mixed feeding). In 1999 a study done in KwaZulu-Natal showed that exclusive breastfeeding carried a significantly lower risk of transmission than mixed feeding and a similar risk to no breastfeeding. This research influenced policies around the world.

Source: *Coutsoudis et al, 1999:471–476.*

Procedure for heat treatment through pasteurisation

Requirements:
- One-litre aluminium pot.
- 410 g size peanut butter glass jar. Plastic lids must be used or metal lids must be replaced as soon as they begin to rust.
- Electric kettle or other means of boiling water.
- Water, soap and a cloth or brush for washing the jar.
- Sterilising equipment (solution and container).

Method:
- Mother to wash hands with soap and water.
- Express milk in clean dry glass jar and cover with lid.
- Place the jar in the aluminium pot.
- Pour boiling water in the aluminium pot until it reaches 1 cm from the top of the pot (700 ml).
- Leave the jar in the hot water until it is a comfortable temperature to touch (about 25 to 30 minutes).
- Remove the jar from the pot and spoon feed the baby directly from the jar, or use a sterilised cup.

Source: Jeffery & Mercer, 2000.

as they increase the possibility of HIV transmission:
- Mastitis, breast abscess, bleeding or cracked nipples.
- Candida infection on the nipples or in the baby's mouth.
- If the baby is born preterm or develops other oral lesions or gastrointestinal infection.

If one of these conditions does occur it must be treated and the mother must stop breastfeeding or express the milk and heat-treat it with pasteurisation before giving it to the baby. Normal breastfeeding can be resumed after the complication has cleared up.

A HIV-positive mother can choose between the following:
- Exclusive feeding with a breast milk substitute like milk formula.
- Exclusive breastfeeding until the age of four to six months, with abrupt weaning as soon as solid food is introduced.
- Heat treatment of breast milk with pasteurisation when high-risk conditions occur.
- After six months the babies of all HIV-infected mothers should receive family foods with breast milk substitute, cow's or goat's milk.

Prevention of sexually transmitted infections and fertility control

It is recommended to use barrier methods, either male or female condoms, for the

CRITICAL THINKING EXERCISE

Maria Swart, a 26-year-old G3 P2 visits the antenatal clinic for the first time and she is currently 20 weeks pregnant. When motivated to have herself tested for HIV (VCT) she says that she does not have to be tested as she does not have any symptoms of HIV. She will encourage her husband to come for testing as he is a truck driver and she suspects he may have been unfaithful on some of his long trips.
1. What are the benefits of testing for Maria and her baby?

Maria requests testing and is tested with a rapid test and the result is positive. She is very upset. After some more counselling, she asks you what she can do to keep as healthy as possible.

2. What information would you include in your health education to Maria?
3. How can the usual procedures during labour and birth be modified to limit the risk of MTCT?
4. Explain the advantages and disadvantages of the different feeding options that Maria can use.

prevention of genital infections and re-infection of HIV. Effective methods of contraception, including sterilisation, must be discussed as each pregnancy places an additional burden on the body. If the health of the mother deteriorates, she may die and her children will be motherless.

Genital lesions

Syphilis

This common, preventable and treatable sexually transmitted infection is caused by the spirochate of the *Treponema pallidum* bacterium. Both the woman and neonate can be cured successfully if diagnosed early and treated appropriately. It is characterised by genital ulcers and progresses through different stages.

During the early stage of the infection the painless ulcer (chancre) may be intra-vaginal and the woman may not even be aware of its presence. The chancre is teeming with spirochaetes and is very infectious.

Treponema pallidum spirochaetes are capable of infecting any organ of the body and it is possible to become re-infected after treatment, since there is little immunity development. During the later stages the symptoms are of a non-specific, general nature, and the condition is then usually diagnosed by serology testing rather than by clinical features.

Effect of syphilis on the fetus/neonate

The spirochaete crosses the placenta and infects the fetus from the sixteenth week of pregnancy. This leads to a high incidence of perinatal deaths – especially macerated stillbirths. More recent maternal infection will affect the fetus/neonate more severely.

The symptoms of congenital syphilis are a copper-coloured maculopapular or pustular rash on the palms, soles and perianal regions, peeling of skin from hands, cracks around the mouth or anus, jaundice, oedema, hepato-splenomegaly, swollen glands and serous nasal discharge and failure-to-thrive. Babies born with congenital syphilis are ten times more likely to die in the perinatal period. Some of the symptoms of late congenital syphilis is Hutchinson's teeth (notched incisors), deafness, saddle-shaped nose and bone deformities (sabre-shaped tibia).

Diagnosis

All pregnant women should undergo syphilis serology screening at the first antenatal clinic visit and ideally receive the results before she goes home so that treatment can be started without delay. Because impairment of the fetus can occur early in pregnancy, it is important that pregnant women initiate antenatal care early in pregnancy in order that syphilis testing and treatment, if necessary, can be done in time. If the incidence of syphilis is high in the community being served, the test should be repeated in the third trimester.

The RPR (Rapid Plasma Reagin) or VDRL (Venereal Disease Research Laboratory) tests are non-specific tests because they can give false positive results in the presence of other conditions. High antibody levels are strongly indicative of syphilis infection but the result may also be as a result of a previously treated infection or caused by pregnancy, collagen diseases, measles, vaccinations or liver diseases. It is therefore advisable that a positive RPR test be followed by a specific syphilis test such as the Treponema Pallidum Haemo-glutination (TPHA) or FTA-Abs (Fluorescent Treponemal Antibody Absorption) tests.

Table 19.2 The effect of untreated syphilis on the fetus/neonate

Duration of infection	Effect on pregnancy or neonate
Primary early infection	Intra-uterine death or preterm labour
Secondary early infection	Intra-uterine death or congenital syphilis
Latent infections	Late congenital syphilis or no infection

Treatment

Intense and active community health educa-tion should take place to prevent this disease, especially since it predisposes to infection with HIV, which is fatal. Although a positive RPR antibody-screening test may be caused by conditions other than active syphilis infection, it is recommended that all women with a pos-itive RPR should be treated as though infect-ed. If the woman presents with a genital ulcer or has chancre-like lesions, an RPR test must be done and treatment be commenced as though it is a primary syphilitic chancre.

The usual treatment is *benzathine penicillin* 2.4 million units administered deep intramus-cularly, weekly for three doses. Provided the *penicillin* treatment had been completed more than four weeks prior to delivery, there is little risk of transmission to the fetus/neonate. As *penicillin* can cause anaphylactic shock to sensi-tive persons, care must be taken to exclude *penicillin* allergy before injecting the woman.

Penicillin-sensitive women should be treat-ed for syphilis with *erythromycin* 500 mg oral-ly six hourly for 28 days. The baby must then be treated with *penicillin* after delivery, as *erythromycin* does not treat the fetus as effec-tively as *benzathine penicillin*. *Penicillin* sensi-tivity is often familial and special care should be taken when treating the baby of a *penicillin*-sensitive woman. The woman's sexual part-ner(s) must also be tested and treated to pre-vent re-infection.

Management of the neonate

If the woman had a positive RPR test, the neonate must be examined at birth for evi-dence of congenital syphilis. This is especially important if the woman was treated with *erythromycin*, or she has shown evidence of syphilis in pregnancy or was unbooked. If evi-dence of congenital syphilis is found, the infant must be referred for full examination and treatment. The postnatal follow-up visit is an important time to check for congenital syphilis, as physical signs are not always pres-ent at birth. Note that congenital syphilis is a notifiable disease.

Herpes genitalis

This sexually transmitted infection is caused by *Herpes simplex virus type 2*. The main symp-tom is pruritic vesicles on the genitals that rupture after two to three days to form painful shallow ulcers. Inflammatory changes, sys-temic infection and secondary infection can occur. The signs disappear spontaneously within two weeks, with re-occurrence during times of increased stress or illness.

Effect of herpes genitalis on the fetus/neonate

The amniotic membranes do not give protec-tion against this infection and spontaneous abortions, preterm birth and fetal growth restriction can occur, especially with a pri-mary infection. However, the risk of perinatal transmission is highest during delivery. If the infection is diagnosed for the first time during pregnancy and there are active lesions, there is a 30 to 50% risk that the neonate will be infected while passing through the birth canal. Fifty percent of infected babies will not sur-vive or will have serious abnormalities of the central nervous system. Recurrent maternal genital herpes simplex infections carry a 1 to 3% risk of neonatal infection if the recurrence occurs around the time of a vaginal delivery. If the woman's infection is latent, the risk of infection of the baby is minimal.

Most of the infants infected by perinatal transmission are born to mothers without a history of herpes infection or any evidence of lesions, since the primary infection had not been diagnosed yet. With the primary infec-tion, there are insufficient maternal antibodies available for transport via the placenta to help protect the infant from infection. Congenital herpes infection is evident from the character-istic localised skin vesicles and/or the systemic symptoms with involvement of the lungs, liver and brain. The neonate may have symptoms like irritability, seizures, respiratory distress, jaundice and shock. Diagnosis of the neonate is difficult if there is not a clear history of exposure to herpes. Infants with early treat-ment have better outcomes than infants with late diagnosis and delayed treatment with intravenous *acyclovir*.

Management

Treatment (*acyclovir*) for this condition is not very effective as it is treated symptomatically. Pregnant women with a history of genital herpes should be carefully monitored during their pregnancy for evidence of active disease. Affected women should have annual PAP smears taken until at least the age of 50 years. Contacts must be examined for evidence of genital ulceration.

A caesarean section must be done electively or as soon as labour starts. If spontaneous labour occurs, caesarean section within four hours of rupture of membranes will prevent infection of the fetus/neonate. If there is an indication that the amniotic fluid is infected with the virus or if the membranes have been ruptured for longer than four hours, the woman can deliver vaginally. Both the mother and baby are then infectious and must be treated with *acyclovir*.

Genital warts/condylomata accuminata

Genital warts is a sexually transmitted infection which is caused by the human papilloma virus (HPV). Pregnancy seems to have a stimulating effect on this condition, and warts generally grow larger during pregnancy. The lesions start as red-pink and pinhead in size. As they enlarge they become penduculated and coalesce to form firstly mulberry-like growths in single or multiple clusters and eventually large cauliflower-like masses. The lesions may become septic or malignant. Large warts can obstruct vaginal delivery and there is a risk of transmission to the infant and it may cause juvenile laryngeal papillomatosis. Women are often co-infected with candidiasis and trichomoniasis as well.

Health education on good hygiene should be given. The usual treatment for warts (*podophyllum resin*) is contraindicated in pregnancy. If the lesions become septic or enlarge enormously during pregnancy then cryosurgery, electro-cauterisation or laser therapy can be performed. An elective caesarean section may be considered when the warts are too large and can obstruct vaginal delivery. Although the wart will decrease in size the woman still needs to be treated after pregnancy. If vaginal delivery is chosen, an episiotomy should not be performed through the infected area, but the perineum should rather be allowed to tear. As there is an association with cancer of the cervix, women with a history of genital warts are advised to have regular PAP smears (six-monthly or annually).

Vaginal discharges

Increased physiological vaginal discharge (leucorrhoea) of white mucus is present during pregnancy. If a discharge causes pruritis or smells offensive it is probably pathological.

Gonorrhoea

This disease is caused by the *Neisseria gonorrhoeae* organism and is also transmitted during sexual contact. There may be a mucopurulent discharge but up to 80% of women do not have clear clinical pictures. If signs like an abnormal discharge, infection of the urethra, infection of the Bartholin's glands or a strong history of likely contact with an infected person exists, then the woman should have swabs taken from the endocervix, the urethra and the anus for microscopy, and treated accordingly.

Effect of gonorrhoea on pregnancy and the fetus/neonate

The condition can cause pPROM, preterm labour and chorio-amnionitis/amniotic fluid infection syndrome. The infection is not transmitted to the baby during the pregnancy, but it can cause blindness by infecting the baby's eyes (ophthalmia neonatorum) during the birth process.

Treatment of the mother

The South African Department of Health recommends the following treatment if a mucopurulent discharge from the cervical os can be observed. *Clotrimazole* pessary 500 g (first trimester) or *metronidazole* 2 g orally as a single dose (second and third trimester only) together with *ceftriaxone* 250 mg (or *spectinomycin* 2 g) intramuscularly as a single dose and *erythromycin* 500 mg orally every six hours for seven days. The sexual partner must also be treated and condoms used during sexual intercourse.

Treatment of the neonate
Ophthalmia neonatorum can be prevented with prophylactic eye drops or ointment. *Chloramphenicol* eye ointment must be used, as it is also effective against chlamydia infection. The symptoms of ophthalmia neonatorum are red puffy eyes with a greenish purulent discharge. It appears two to five days after birth. An eye swab must be taken for cultivation and identification, but treatment must not be postponed to wait for the laboratory results. The eyes must be swabbed with sodium chloride 0.9% and antibiotics (ointment and intravenously) should be administered as prescribed. Careful hand-washing before and after touching the baby and correct use of protective gloves are important. Both caregivers and the mother should be aware of infection control measures and practise them. Note that ophthalmia neonatorum is a notifiable disease.

Chlamydial infection
This condition caused by *Chlamydia trachomatis*, can cause a mild vaginal discharge or slight reddening of the vaginal walls but it is often asymptomatic. Some infected women may have a mucopurulent cervicitis, salpingitis or urethral syndrome. It is also associated with pelvic inflammatory disease, infertility and ectopic pregnancy.

Effect of chlamydial infection on the fetus/neonate
It may be responsible for preterm labour and intra-uterine death. The infant of a woman with untreated chlamydia is at risk of developing ophthalmia neonatorum. The neonate may also develop chlamydial pneumonia.

Management
As some of the symptoms of gonorrhoea and chlamydia are similar, it is difficult to differentiate between the two in a clinical situation. In practice any mucopurulent discharge can be treated as discussed with gonorrhoea. The prevention and treatment of ophthalmia neonatorum, caused by chlamydia, is also the same as with gonorrhoea.

Candidiasis
Candidiasis or thrush is a fungus infection caused by *Candida albicans*. Although it can be spread through sexual contact it also occurs very commonly from other causes – especially in diabetics and when using antibiotics. There is an increased incidence of thrush in pregnancy and diabetes mellitus because of the change in vaginal pH balance. Antibiotics disturb the normal vaginal flora and the woman is more vulnerable for fungus infections like candidiasis. The discharge is thick and has a cottage-cheese appearance and causes intense pruritis of the vulva and vagina. It may be adherent to the vaginal wall and leave raw areas when dislodged. The introitus is swollen, red and painful. Oral candidiasis in an adult is often a sign of HIV infection.

Effect of candida on the fetus/neonate
The fetus is not affected in-utero but after birth the infected baby can have thrush in the mouth or as diaper-rash on the buttocks and genitalia. The infection can also be transmitted to the mother during breastfeeding and can cause infection of her nipples. Both must be treated.

Management
The recommended treatment is *clotrimazole* single-dose 500 g pessary. If treatment is unsuccessful, the woman must be referred to a medical practitioner. Other treatment methods that can be used are *fluconazole*, *nystatin* or *miconazole* (Daktarin®) ointment or cream. The sexual partner must also be treated to prevent re-infection and condoms must be used during sexual intercourse.

Other causes of vaginitis

Other pathological vaginal discharges are caused by *Trichomonas vaginalis* and *Gardnerella vaginalis*. These infections cause infection of the vagina with a yellow-greenish, frothy or a grey-whitish watery discharge that may have an offensive or fishy smell. It also causes pruritis and dyspareunia.

Effect of vaginitis on pregnancy

All the causes of vaginitis may contribute to preterm prelabour rupture of membranes (pPROM) and possibly preterm labour.

Management

The recommended treatment for these discharges is *metronidazole* 2 g orally as a single dose. As *metronidazole* is tetratogenic in the first trimester, *clotrimazole* pessary 500 g is then recommended. The sexual partner must also be treated and condoms used when engaging in sexual intercourse.

Antenatal infections that mainly affect the fetus

Any condition that is accompanied by a high temperature or serious systematic impairment may result in abortion, preterm labour or intra-uterine death. If a woman had an abnormal baby, abortion or stillbirth from an unknown cause, she can be tested for the TORCH infections to find out if one or more of these infections could be the cause.

The TORCH infections is an acronym for: T – toxoplasmosis, O – others like syphilis, R – rubella, C – cytomegalovirus or H – herpes simplex.

Toxoplasmosis

This multisystem disease is caused by the protozoa *Toxoplasma gondii*. It is capable of infecting all mammals but is most commonly found in cats. Touching cat faeces, eating undercooked meat or working with raw meat from an infected animal, can infect humans. In the adult the symptoms are fever, headache, malaise and lymphadenopathy. The fetus can only be infected during the acute maternal infection, and antibodies from a previous infection protect against re-infection. Repeated early abortions are common. If the infection occurs late in pregnancy it may be asymptomatic or cause anaemia, jaundice, bleeding or intra-uterine death. The principal locus of the infection is the central nervous system. Ten to 15% of babies born with congenital toxoplasmosis will die. Symptoms present in the neonate may be convulsions, hydrocephaly, microcephaly, mental retardation or blindness. Women at risk must be made aware of the dangers of toxoplasmosis and receive health education regarding taking precautions, for example, not to touch cat litter with bare hands or work with raw meat. The treatment is with long-term antibiotics.

Rubella

This condition is caused by the Rubella virus. It does not cause serious symptoms for the mother (rash and muscle pains), but the fetus may be damaged in 50 to 70% of cases where the woman contracted this disease during the period of organogenesis. The specific organs affected and the level of risk of the impairment that occurs depends on the gestational age at the time of infection. If the woman was in the first four weeks of pregnancy at the time of infection, the eyes will be affected. At five to eight weeks cardiovascular abnormalities are common and if the infection occurs at between 9 and 12 weeks of pregnancy, the ears may be affected and macrocephalus and mental retardation could occur. The triad of eye, ear and cardiovascular abnormalities is known as the congenital rubella syndrome. There is a 10 to 20% risk of the fetus being affected if the infection occurs between 13 and 16 weeks of pregnancy. Abnormalities are thrombocytopaenia, purpura, microcephaly, pneumonia, meningitis, myocarditis, restricted growth and failure-to-thrive. Abortions and intra-uterine deaths are doubly more likely to occur than in an uninfected pregnancy. The baby excretes the virus in the urine for months after the birth and any person taking care of the baby or his urine-soaked diaper is at risk of contracting rubella infection. Women who are unsure of their own immunisation or had a previous infection, should be tested before pregnancy. If unprotected, they can be immunised but must wait three months before falling pregnant. If infected before 16 weeks of pregnancy, the woman can receive gamma globulin but it will not necessarily protect the fetus. The woman may consider termination of pregnancy after counselling (see Chapter 27).

Cytomegalovirus disease

This condition is caused by a virus from the herpes family and it is often asymptomatic in the adult who has contracted it. Symptoms that may occur are an erythematous maculopapular skin rash, malaise, sore throat and coughing, nausea and lymphadenopathy. The condition can be sexually transmitted or spread through other routes. Those most at risk for symptomatic infection are people immunocompromised by certain drugs, diseases such as AIDS, or an immature immune system such as in fetuses or neonates. The condition may lie dormant indefinitely in host tissue and be periodically reactivated, particularly during pregnancy. It is the most common cause of congenital infection. Following primary infection during pregnancy, approximately 40 to 50% of fetuses will become infected, although transmission to the fetus/neonate is most commonly caused by the reactivated virus that causes a milder infection. The infection can occur any time during the antenatal period, during birth or after the birth via breast milk. Congenital cytomegalovirus infection carries a 20 to 30% mortality rate. There may be congenital malformations like microcephaly, hydrocephaly, cystic brain lesions, hydrops or stillbirth. However, the majority of the infected infants are asymptomatic at birth and symptoms only become evident months or years later. This condition is the leading infectious cause of deafness, learning disabilities and mental retardation in children.

Serum antibody tests can be done to diagnose the condition in the mother. A high level of IgG antibodies but a low level of IgM indicates that antibodies are present from a past infection, but a high level of IgM antibodies indicates an acute primary infection. Treat with antiviral medication, but viral shedding may occur again at times after cessation of therapy. Health education for hand-washing and good hygiene practices can help reduce the number of women who contract this infection as the virus is found in all body fluids.

Neonatal diagnoses are made with laboratory tests. Early detection will enable the early institution of antiviral therapy, parental counselling and early screening and treatment of neurodevelopmental disorders. Support and health education are important for the families of infants with symptomatic cytomegalovirus disease. There needs to be referral as well as follow-up for developmental and hearing assessment and therapy, if necessary.

Malaria

This condition is caused by a *Plasmodium* (*P. malariae, P. ovale, P. vivax* or *P. falciparum*). People living in an endemic area usually acquire some immunity and the clinical picture may be mild. If the general immunity of a member of the endemic population is deficient (because of AIDS or other reasons), malaria attacks during pregnancy may be very serious and occur more often. Visitors to an endemic area have no immunity and will be worse affected. The symptoms are pyrexia, anorexia, headaches, vomiting and diarrhoea. The *Plasmodium* parasites attack the red blood cells, causing haemolysis and eventually anaemia.

Malaria in pregnancy is associated with serious complications, such as cerebral malaria, hypoglycaemia, pulmonary oedema and death. Because of the haemolysis caused by the disease, serious folic acid deficiency and iron deficiency may occur. The anaemia increases the risk and severity of ante- and postpartum haemorrhage as well as infection.

Because of the hyperpyrexia and poor general health, abortion and preterm labour occur more frequently. The placental intervillous space is filled with parasites and macrophages that disturb the placental circulation and result in intra-uterine growth restriction and fetal distress. Stillbirth and serious jaundice can also occur. Breastfeeding is safe when using *chloroquine* and *proguanil*, but the baby needs to receive his own prophylaxis.

Prevention

It is advisable that pregnant women without immunity do not enter an endemic area. Otherwise they should take precautions against mosquito bites, like wearing light-coloured clothing which covers the legs, arms and body, applying insect repellents and using mosquito nets treated with insecticide. Although antimalaria drugs are associated with fetal abnormalities like retinopathy, nerve deafness and other neural abnormalities, the World Health Organisation advises that susceptible women should receive prophylactic treatment prescribed by a physician.

Treatment

If a pyrexial illness with headache and nausea occurs up to six weeks after returning from an endemic area, the woman must be referred for diagnosis and treatment. All pregnant women with malaria must be admitted to hospital. Blood must be tested for full blood count, urea and creatinine levels and parasite count. In uncomplicated malaria where the Hb is more than or equal to 6 g/dl, the parasitaemia count less than 5% and there is no organ dysfunction, the woman can be admitted to a level 1 hospital. She should be treated with *quinine/sulfadoxine-pyrimethamine* orally but if she is vomiting and unable to tolerate it, the medication must be given intravenously. The blood glucose level must be monitored and CTG must be done daily after 28 weeks. After discharge, she must be followed up at a high-risk antenatal clinic, since there is a risk of intra-uterine growth restriction.

If a woman has severe malaria with one of the following symptoms: parasitaemia count equal to or more than 5%, a Hb of less than 6 g/dl, coma or depressed consciousness, renal dysfunction, jaundice or severe thrombocytopaenia (less than 50 000 per mm^3), she should be transferred to a level 2 or level 3 hospital. Because the clinical cause of severe malaria is unpredictable and deterioration may be rapid, the woman must receive a loading dose of intravenous *quinine* before transferral to a centre with an intensive care unit. Note that malaria is a notifiable disease.

Tuberculosis

Tuberculosis (TB) is caused by *Mycobacterium tuberculosis bacillus*. The primary lesion may occur in different organs but the most common is pulmonary TB. The AIDS epidemic which has increased the susceptibility of people to infectious diseases has caused a rise in the TB epidemic. Approximately 50 to 60% of people living with HIV/AIDS will develop active TB disease at some stage of their infection. TB is often the final cause of death in patients with HIV/AIDS. An HIV-infected woman must be asked about the classic TB symptoms, and if some are present she should be further investigated and treated, if necessary.

The normal clinical course of the condition is not affected by pregnancy, but a woman with active TB should delay her pregnancy until her treatment is completed. The increased physical and emotional demands of the puerperium may lead to a deterioration of her condition. Pregnancy is not directly affected by TB, unless the woman is terminally ill and very weak. The neonate can be infected by the mother after birth but can be protected through the administration of prophylactic medication.

After diagnosis of TB (with sputum culture), it is usually not necessary to admit the woman to hospital. She is only infectious for 24 hours after she has begun treatment. Referral to social workers, home-based carers, friends and family should be done to ensure that she is able to take adequate rest and eat a nourishing diet. With her drug therapy and follow-up at the TB clinic she can be

completely cured. The treatment is usually administered through DOTS (Directly Observed Treatment Short Course), where community support is used to ensure that the medication is taken. Newly diagnosed women are started on the standard regime of treatment. Medications that are contraindicated during pregnancy are:
- *Streptomycin* as this may cause deafness in the neonate.
- *Ethionamide* and *prothionamide* that are used to treat multiple drug resistant (MDR) TB, because they can cause developmental abnormalities of the fetus.

Most of the drugs have side-effects but these can usually be controlled.

Breastfeeding is encouraged and the neonate must not be separated from the mother, except for the period when the mother has active unmedicated TB. The baby must be protected by the administration of *isoniazid* (INH) syrup (8 mg/kg per day) for as long as the mother's sputum is positive and for six months thereafter. The baby should be immunised with BCG. Note that tuberculosis is a notifiable disease.

Urinary tract infections

Urinary tract infections are common in pregnancy, because progesterone causes dilatation of the ureters and the immune system is depressed during pregnancy. The growth of the uterus and the displacement of the bladder lead to difficulty in complete emptying of the bladder, stasis of urine and subsequent infection.

Asymptomatic bacteriuria

With this condition the woman does not experience any urinary symptoms, but a clean catch specimen of urine shows a bacterial count of more than 100 000 per ml. The most causative organism is *Escherichia coli* (*E. coli*). This condition is often associated with pyelonephritis. If it were possible to diagnose all affected women, the incidence of acute pyelonephritis would

decrease by 70%. Ideally, a urine culture from a clean catch specimen should be done during a woman's first antenatal visit and treatment instituted as for cystitis. Financial constraints limit universal testing.

Cystitis

This is the most common complication of pregnancy. The infection is limited to the bladder, but because of the physiological changes during pregnancy, there is a risk of ascending infection. It is diagnosed by symptoms of dysuria, frequency of micturition, and nocturia in the absence of systemic signs, like fever. There may be tenderness over the bladder area. The dipstick urine-screening test may indicate leukocytes, nitrites, protein and blood and must be followed by a midstream urine specimen sent for examination by microscopy, as well as culture and sensitivity. A definite diagnosis can only be made after laboratory results are indicative of infection. Due to the cost of laboratory tests and the delay before results are available, treatment is often started without an initial positive diagnosis.

In the clinic situation, the usual treatment is *amoxycillin* 3 g in one dose orally or for *penicillin*-sensitive women, *co-trimoxazole* four tablets orally. High fluid intake must be encouraged. Alternative antibiotics will be ordered according to the sensitivity results if necessary.

Pyelonephritis

Pyelonephritis is a common and serious cause of pyrexia in pregnancy. The pelvis, calyces and parenchyma of the kidney are affected. It usually begins after 16 to 20 weeks of pregnancy. Contributing factors are cystitis and previous urinary tract surgery, physiological changes in the urogenital tract of the pregnant woman, incomplete emptying of the bladder, catheterisation or atony of the bladder, underlying renal lesions or coitus. During the acute phase of the condition it may cause abortion, preterm labour and intra-uterine death, probably because of the high fever. Septic shock, anaemia or a perinephrenic abscess can also occur. The woman appears acutely ill. Positive signs and symptoms are dysuria, frequency of micturition, abdominal pain, suprapubic tenderness, fever (38° C or more), rigors, anorexia and nausea.

The woman requires hospitalisation for the management of pyelonephritis. A midstream urine specimen must be sent to the laboratory for microscopic examination, culture and sensitivity. A blood specimen for urea and creatinine, full blood count and smear as well as a blood culture can also be done. The woman must be hydrated intravenously with an infusion of one litre Plasmalyte B® or Ringer's lactate over two hours, followed by one litre Maintelyte every eight hours. Until laboratory results have been received she must be treated with antibiotics like *ampicillin* 2 g intravenously bolus followed by *ampicillin* 1 g intravenously six-hourly or a first generation cephalosporin in a similar dose regime. The antibiotics must be administered intravenously until the woman's temperature has been normal for 24 hours, after which they can be given orally and continued for a total of ten days. Suitable antipyretics like *paracetamol* and sponging can be used to control the pyrexia, while pain can be controlled by analgesics. The intake and output as well as blood pressure must be closely monitored. If signs of septic shock are observed, the woman must be admitted to an intensive care unit for monitoring and treatment. The fetus must be monitored with a CTG if the woman is more than 28 weeks pregnant and the woman monitored for signs of preterm labour. Her urine should be cultured regularly throughout the rest of the pregnancy, and her haemoglobin should be monitored, as there is an increased risk of anaemia. In cases of repeated infections an intravenous pyelogram should be performed in the puerperium.

Pregnancy-related infections

Septic abortion

This complication of infection of the uterus and reproductive organs may occur after any incomplete abortion (spontaneous or induced) although it is more commonly associated with unsafe abortions. Despite the choice contained in the Choice on Termination of Pregnancy Act (No 92 of 1996) women are still using unsafe abortion agents. This leads to an increase in maternal mortality and morbidity. Septic abortions may arise from a number of causes and each has different clinical patterns and presentations. The possibilities are as follows:

▶ An ordinary infection restricted to the uterus and adnexae.
▶ Gangrene of the organs which could have been caused by a chemical substance that was used to initiate the abortion.
▶ Septic shock because of toxins.
▶ Septic thrombo-embolism from the pelvic vessels.
▶ Acidosis.
▶ Multi-organ failure.

Septic shock affects the cardiovascular system, the haemopoietic system, the kidneys and the lungs. It can initiate Disseminated Intravascular Coagulation (DIC) leading to death. If a woman with an abortion has signs of peritonitis, or the uterus is more than 16 weeks in size, she has a high risk of organ failure or death.

Clinical signs

The diagnosis of septic abortion is made in a woman who has had a spontaneous or induced abortion and presents with:

▶ A temperature of 38 °C or more.
▶ An offensive, profuse cervical discharge.
▶ A tender and enlarged uterus.
▶ A white blood cell count of 15 000 per mm^3 or more.
▶ Signs of peritonitis may also be present.

Management

To prevent infection in incomplete abortions, prophylactic antibiotics against the most common organisms, preferably *doxycycline*, should be administered. The uterus must be emptied within six hours with suction curettage under local anaesthetic.

If there are signs of possible septic abortion, the woman must be referred to a level 1 or 2 hospital and if there is organ failure she must be referred to a level 3 hospital. There the infection must be controlled, by removing the septic focus (by curettage or hysterectomy if necessary) and treatment with high doses of antibiotics. The function of all the vital organs must be assessed and supportive treatment given, as needed.

Chorio-amnionitis

Chorio-amnionitis is also known as amniotic fluid infection syndrome and it is associated with prelabour rupture of the membranes, pPROM (infection causes the membranes to weaken) and preterm labour (prostaglandins stimulate uterine contractions). This condition may be the reason for the high rate of preterm labour seen with HIV-positive women. Chorio-amnionitis/amniotic fluid infection syndrome may also be the result of prolonged ruptured membranes when vaginal infection ascends and invades the membranes and amniotic fluids.

Clinical signs

The following clinical signs may indicate infection:

▶ Maternal pyrexia of the same and more than 37.5 °C.
▶ Maternal pulse rate more than 100 beats per minute.
▶ Uterine tenderness and/or irritability.
▶ Fetal heart rate of more than 160 beats per minute.
▶ Offensive or meconium-stained liquor.

Often the only indication of a possible infection is a fetal tachycardia and it is often only diagnosed after birth when the amniotic liquor is found to have an offensive smell. Chorio-amnionitis can precede puerperal sepsis.

Management

Prophylactic antibiotics for HIV-positive pregnant women may prevent chorio-amnionitis/-amniotic fluid infection syndrome with its complications. Women with pPROM or prolonged rupture of membranes must receive prophylactic antibiotics against the most common organisms. After prelabour rupture of membranes and pPROM only a sterile speculum examination should be done to confirm the diagnosis, and no digital examinations are to be performed until the woman is in active labour. After diagnosis the woman must be transferred to a hospital. Treatment is with wide-spectrum antibiotics like *ampicillin* 1 g six-hourly orally, with *metronidazole* 400 mg orally three times daily. Monitoring is essential during labour and delivery. The *ampicillin* and *metronidazole* must be continued for five full days after delivery.

Puerperal infection

Infection in the postpartum period may involve various organs and systems. The time of onset of fever helps in differentiating the source of the infection: pneumonia or urinary tract infection occurs within 72 hours of birth, wound infection or septic trombophlebitis occurs three to seven days postpartum and wound abscess formation is common after one or two weeks. Mastitis can occur 72 hours or more after birth but frequently develops at about two weeks postpartum. Puerperal infection of the reproductive tract occurs at any time up to six weeks postpartum.

The trend in modern care of the woman is early discharge, for some women four to six hours after delivery if all appears well. Because of this, a woman may be discharged before the clinical signs of puerperal infection are evident. Therefore midwives need to carefully screen each woman's history for signs of impending puerperal infection and inform them that they must return to the clinic or hospital for treatment. Community-based midwives should always be alert for signs of infection in the postpartum women they meet in the community, because the symptoms are often of a general nature and can be quite obscure. It is imperative that any abnormal observation in a postpartum woman should be reported to a medical practitioner for further investigation and an evaluation of organ dysfunction.

Postnatal uterine infection

The most common postnatal infection is uterine endometritis that is limited to the uterus, but can spread by means of the lymphatic and circulatory systems and result in pelvic cellulitis and peritonitis. The prognosis is directly related to the stage to which the infection has progressed at the time of diagnosis, the virulence of the causing organism and the general state of the woman's health and immunity.

The causative organisms can be divided into endogenous and exogenous organisms. Endogenous organisms are those that are naturally resident in regions such as the lower intestine, the vagina and the perineum where they do no harm but play a role in the normal ecology of the region. Examples of endogenous organisms are *Eschericia coli* and *Streptococcus faecalis*. Exogenous organisms come from sources outside the body and are usually transmitted by another person. Examples of exogenous organisms are Group A *Streptococcus, Staphylococcus aureus* or anaerobic organisms.

The risk factors for uterine infection are:
▶ Caesarean section.
▶ Prolonged rupture of membranes.
▶ Multiple vaginal examinations.
▶ Compromised resistance against infection (HIV/AIDS, low socioeconomic status, anaemia, obesity etc.).
▶ Chorio-amnionitis.
▶ Vaginitis.
▶ Obstetric trauma (episiotomy, lacerations of the perineum, vagina or cervix).
▶ Prolonged labour.
▶ Assisted birth (vacuum or forceps).
▶ Badly torn placenta or membranes.
▶ Placenta accreta.
▶ Manual removal of the placenta.
▶ Lapses in aseptic technique.

Clinical signs

The woman with endometritis presents with general malaise and lower abdominal pain.

There is subinvolution of the uterus, tenderness in the lower abdomen (but not classical acute abdomen as abdominal muscles have not regained their pre-pregnancy tone). The lochia may be scant, profuse, bloody and foul smelling. It is possible that there is little sign of external infection and indeed the woman may develop serious pelvic infection or septicaemia whilst the perineum continues to heal.

Pelvic cellulitis involves the connective tissue of the broad ligament. A pelvic abscess may form in the uterine ligaments or pouch of Douglas. The symptoms of pelvic cellulitis are marked by high temperature, chills, malaise, abdominal pain and tachycardia.

If the infection has spread to involve the peritoneal cavity (peritonitis) the woman will be acutely ill with severe pain, marked anxiety, high fever, rapid, shallow respiration, pronounced tachycardia, excessive thirst, abdominal distension, nausea and vomiting. Any pyrexia following birth or abortion, which persists for 24 hours, should be regarded as an infection of the genital tract until proven otherwise.

Prevention

Antenatal care should ensure that the woman is as free from infections as possible before she enters labour, especially sexually transmitted infections. Strict aseptic technique must be used during labour. Vaginal examinations must be restricted to the absolute minimum but be preformed if indicated to do so safely, and trauma during labour prevented. Women with obvious infections should be nursed separately from others in order to prevent cross-infection. As anaemic women are more prone to infections, the haemoglobin concentration must be checked within 24 hours of delivery, and anaemia appropriately treated before discharge. All women should have health education on hygiene, coitus and wound care. Women should know the danger signs (fever, foul-smelling lochia, etc.) and they should also know where to go for immediate assistance.

Treatment

Women who had a caesarean section, retained placenta or prolonged rupture of membranes should receive prophylactic antibiotics. If the woman's temperature is 37.7 °C or lower and involution of the uterus occurs as normal, she can be treated as an outpatient with oral antibiotics, with follow-up checking after 24 hours. Suitable antibiotics are *ampicillin/-erythromycin* or *co-trimoxazole* for aerobic organisms, taken together with *metronidazole* for anaerobic organisms.

If offensive lochia and subinvolution of the uterus are present, the woman must be hospitalised, as these are indications of retained products of conception. These must be removed surgically under general anaesthetic. A cervical smear should be sent to the laboratory for microscopic examination, culture and sensitivity, as well as a blood specimen for full blood count and smear, urea and creatinine, blood culture and HIV serology. Treatment with widespectrum intravenous antibiotics like *ampicillin* and *gentamicin* together with *metronidazole* suppositories should also be started as soon as possible. In severe cases, observation of vital signs must be done hourly for the first 24 to 48 hours. Pyrexia should be controlled and analgesics given as needed. An intravenous infusion should be in situ, fluids must be encouraged and intake and output monitored. An indwelling urinary catheter must be inserted to measure output accurately. If a woman who is acutely ill does not improve within 24 hours while on conservative treatment, a laparotomy for drainage of an abscess must be performed. Prior to this procedure the possibility of a hysterectomy being necessary needs to be discussed with the woman and her informed consent obtained for this life-saving operation. While recuperating, the woman needs a diet rich in protein and vitamin C, which promotes healing and combats further infection. Health education needs to include specific advice about wound care and hygiene. While the mother is ill, special arrangements may need to be made for baby care and every effort made not to disrupt bonding and breastfeeding.

Perineal wound infection

Infection of a perineal wound (episiotomy or lacerations) is recognised by redness, warmth, oedema, local pain, purulent drainage or gaping of the wound coupled with the signs of sepsis (pyrexia, rigor, tachycardia and tachypnoea).

Broad-spectrum antibiotics and analgesics should be given. The sutures must be removed so that the puss can drain freely. Sitz baths are advised with a dilution of *chlorhexidine* or coarse salt solution two to three times daily for approximately 20 minutes. When granulation has taken place a localised infrared lamp may be used to assist with reduction of swelling, drying and healing of the area. When the surface of the wound is free of infectious exudate and tissue granulation is evident, secondary surgical repair is recommended.

Caesarean wound infection

The infection rate following caesarean section can be up to 12%, with the highest rate occurring after an emergency caesarean section where there have been many vaginal examinations, as well as manipulations, which have traumatised tissue. The symptoms usually become apparent three to ten days after the operation. Together with the general signs of sepsis (fever, pain, malodourous lochia, etc.) the following may be observed: erythema, warmth, oedema, purulent drainage and gaping of the wound edges.

Antibiotic prophylaxis must be administered prior to all elective and emergency caesarean sections. Where there is a high risk for sepsis, antibiotics must be continued for three days postpartum. If the diagnosis of a septic caesarean wound is made, the woman must be re-admitted to hospital. All stitches must be removed and the wound irrigated and dressed. The advice of a midwife skilled in wound care is invaluable in caring for these women. Secondary wound closure can be done when the wound is clean. Intravenous or oral antibiotics are indicated.

> ## In a nutshell
>
> ▶ Infections during pregnancy and the puerperium can cause morbidity as well as contribute to the maternal and perinatal mortality. Some of the conditions cause long-term suffering.
> ▶ It is a matter of great concern that a large number of women, even in areas with a high incidence of unexplained stillbirths, are not thoroughly tested during pregnancy for conditions that contribute to perinatal mortality and morbidity. The midwife can make a valuable contribution in identifying infectious conditions.
> ▶ Ensuring that the correct treatment is both administered and completed is a vital part of the independent midwifery practice and is especially important in community settings.
> ▶ Adherence to national, provincial and local guidelines has been shown to improve maternal and neonatal outcomes and should be followed.
> ▶ The midwife should always apply universal precaution and infection control measures.

Postpartum urinary tract infection

Urinary tract infection is the second most common postpartum infection. The woman in her puerperium is at increased risk to develop urinary tract infections because of:

▶ The increased bladder capacity.
▶ Decreased bladder sensitivity from stretching or trauma.
▶ The effects of normal postpartum diuresis.
▶ Possible inhibited neural control following the use of general or regional anaesthesia.
▶ Contamination from catheterisation.

Cystitis is most common, but pyelonephritis can also develop. If untreated, the renal cortex may be damaged and kidney function impaired.

Prevent infection by effectively treating urinary tract infection during pregnancy. Frequent emptying of the bladder throughout labour and the postnatal period should be encouraged to prevent overdistention and trauma. Bladder catheterisation should be done only if necessary and then with strict aseptic technique.

Treat the infection as in urinaty tract infection. Once sexual intercourse is resumed, the woman should void before (to prevent bladder trauma) and following intercourse (to wash contaminants from the vicinity of the urinary meatus). Wearing cotton crotch underwear to facilitate air circulation reduces the risk of urinary tract infection.

References

Bennett, V. R. & Brown, L. K. (Eds.) 2000. *Myles textbook for midwives*. Thirteenth edition. London: Churchill Livingstone.

Coutsoudis, A., Pillay, K., Spooner, E., Kuhn, L. & Coovadia, H. M. 1999. Influence of infant-feeding patterns on early mother-to-child transmission of HIV-1 in Durban, South Africa: A prospective cohort study. *Lancet*, August 354(7):471–476.

Cronje, H. S., Grobler, C. J. F. & Visser, A. A. 1996. *Obstetrics in Southern Africa*. Pretoria: JL van Schaik.

Dabis, F., Leroy, V., Castetbon, K., et al. 2000. Preventing mother-to-child transmission of HIV-1 in Africa in the year 2000. *AIDS*, 14(8):1017–1026.

Damato, E. G. & Winnen, C. W. 2002. Cytomegalovirus infection: Perinatal implications. *Journal of Obstetric, Gynecologic and Neonatal Nursing*, 31(1):86–92.

DoH (Department of Health). 2000. *Breastfeeding and HIV. An information booklet for health workers in South Africa*. Cape Town: Provincial Administration of the Western Cape.

DoH (Department of Health). 1998. *Standard treatment guidelines and essential druglist for South Africa: Primary health care*. Pretoria: Department of Health.

DoH (Department of Health). 2002. *Guidelines for maternity care in South Africa. A manual for clinics, community health centres and district hospitals.* Pretoria: Department of Health.

DoH (Department of Health). 2002. *Saving Mothers. Second report on confidential enquiries into maternal deaths in South Africa 1999–2001.* Pretoria: Department of Health.

DoH (Department of Health). 2000. *The South African tuberculosis control programme. Practical guidelines.* Pretoria: Department of Health.

DoH (Department of Health). 2001. *Saving mothers. Policy and management guidelines for common causes of maternal deaths.* Pretoria: Department of Health.

Donahue, D. B. 2002. Diagnosis and treatment of herpes simplex infection during pregnancy. *Journal of Obstetric, Gynecologic and Neonatal Nursing*, 31(1):99–106.

Enkin, M., Keirse, M. J. N. C., Neilson, J., Crowther, C., Duley, L., Hodnett, E. & Hofmeyer, J. 2000. *A guide to effective care in pregnancy and childbirth.* Third edition. New York: Oxford University Press.

Evian, C. 2000. *Primary AIDS care.* Third edition. Houghton: Jacana Education.

Jeffery, B. S. & Mercer, K. G. 2000. Pretoria pasteurisation: A potential method for the reduction of postnatal mother-to-child transmission of the Human Immunodeficiency Virus. *Journal of Tropical Pediatrics*, August 46:219–223.

Jeffery, B. S., Webber, L., Mokhondo, K. R. & Erasmus, D. 2001. Determination of the effectiveness of inactivation of Human Immunodeficiency Virus by Pretoria pasteurisation. *Journal of Tropical Pediatrics*, December 47:345–349.

Nolte, A. G. W. (Ed.) 1998. *A textbook for midwives.* Pretoria: JL van Schaik Publishers.

MRC Research Unit for Maternal and Infant Health Care Strategies. 2002. *Guidelines for the implementation of pasteurisation in health care institutions – a feeding method for low birth weight infants born to HIV infected women using their own pasteurised breast milk.* Pretoria: MRC.

MRC Research Unit for Maternal and Infant Health Care Strategies. 2002. *Saving babies 2001. Second perinatal care survey of South Africa.* Pretoria: Department of Health.

Olds, S. B., London, M. L. & Ladewig, P. A. W. 2000. *Maternal–newborn nursing.* Sixth edition. Upper Saddle River, New Jersey: Prentice-Hall.

Sellers, P. M. 1993. *Midwifery. Volume 2.* Kenwyn: Juta.

Van Dyk, A. 2001. *HIV/AIDS care and counselling. A multidisciplinary approach.* Second edition. Cape Town: Pearson Education.

Walker, G. J. A. 2002. Antibiotics for syphilis diagnosed during pregnancy (Cochrane Review). *The Cochrane Library, Issue 4.* Oxford: Update Software.

Woods, D. L. (Ed.) 1999. *Perinatal Education Programme. Manual 1. Maternity care.* Observatory: PEP.

Woods, D. L. (Ed.) 1999. *Perinatal Education Programme. Manual 3. Perinatal HIV/AIDS.* Observatory: PEP.

World Health Organisation (WHO). 2001. Fact Sheets on HIV/AIDS for nurses and midwives. *African Journal of Nursing and Midwifery*, 3(1) Supplement.

Chapter 20

Hypertensive conditions

Dr Lou Pistorius

Introduction

Physiologically, blood pressure drops in the middle of pregnancy, and rises towards the end of pregnancy. To diagnose hypertension in pregnancy, this should be understood, and the blood pressure reading should be taken accurately. It is important to understand the differences between chronic hypertension in pregnancy and hypertension that was induced by pregnancy. Chronic hypertension generally has a favourable outcome, whereas hypertension that was induced in pregnancy has a higher risk of maternal and fetal complications.

Understanding blood pressure

Physiological changes in pregnancy

The cardiac output rises by 40% in pregnancy. Most of this increase occurs in the first trimester of pregnancy and anticipates the demands of the growing pregnancy. At the end of the pregnancy the cardiac output possibly decreases slightly. The rise in cardiac output is the result of an increase in both cardiac stroke volume and heart rate. Despite the rise in cardiac output, there is a decrease in vascular resistance which results in a decreased blood pressure. This decrease starts in the first trimester, and reaches the lowest point in the middle of pregnancy. During the third trimester, the blood pressure rises again to the pre-pregnancy levels.

Standardisation of blood pressure reading

Blood pressure should be taken in a standardised way, to minimise possible technical errors of measurement. The woman should lie in a semi-recumbent position leaning slightly to the side in order to avoid supine hypotension, or sit down with her feet supported for two minutes before taking the blood pressure. The blood pressure cuff should be applied snugly to her arm. If the woman is obese, and her upper arm is more than 33 cm in circumference, a wide blood pressure cuff should be used. Keep her arm at the level of her heart. Palpate her radial pulse while inflating the cuff until the pulse is not palpable any more, and inflate the cuff 20 mmHg above this level. Place the stethoscope on the brachial pulse and listen while slowly deflating the pressure in the cuff. The systolic blood pressure is equivalent to the cuff pressure when you start hearing the pulse. This is also called Korotkoff phase I. Note the diastolic blood pressure as the pressure when the sounds disappear (Korotkoff phase V). If the pulse sounds do not disappear, use Korotkoff phase IV (muffling of the pulse sounds) to denote the diastolic blood pressure. Use a mercury sphygmomanometer, as automated blood pressure monitors are more unreliable and can yield significantly different values.

Definitions

A single blood pressure reading cannot be used to diagnose a woman as hypertensive. Because of the many fluctuations of blood pressure levels within a 24-hour period, sampling errors can cause a woman to be classified falsely as being normotensive or hypertensive.

Hypertension is not a disease entity, but simply reflects the higher end of the distribution curve of individuals' blood pressures. As

---

Classification of hypertension in pregnancy

Gestational hypertension:
▶ Hypertension arising in pregnancy after 20 weeks gestation.
▶ Without any other feature of pre-eclampsia present.
▶ It resolves within three months postpartum.

Pre-eclampsia: Hypertension arising in pregnancy after 20 weeks, with one or more of the following (also arising for the first time after 20 weeks):
▶ Proteinuria (300 mg or more per 24 hours).
▶ Renal insufficiency (oliguria or serum creatinine above 90 µmol/l).
▶ Liver disease (raised transaminases and/or epigastric pain).
▶ Neurological problems (convulsions, hyperreflexia, severe headaches or persistent visual disturbances).
▶ Haematological problems (low platelet count, haemolysis or disseminated intravascular coagulation).
▶ Fetal growth restriction.

Chronic hypertension:
▶ *Essential hypertension:* Hypertension noted before 20 weeks without any apparent cause.
▶ *Secondary hypertension:* Hypertension noted before 20 weeks associated with renal, renovascular, or endocrine disorders or aortic coarctation.

Superimposed pre-eclampsia: A woman with chronic hypertension that developed pre-eclampsia.

Eclampsia: Convulsions in a woman with hypertension and proteinuria after 20 weeks gestation and before 7 days postpartum, in the absence of other causes of convulsions.

HELLP syndrome: Haemolysis, elevated liver enzymes and low platelets associated with hypertension and proteinuria.

such, any cut-off point is arbitrary. However, a blood pressure of 140/90 mmHg is the dividing line conventionally used to denote hypertension. Because of the fluctuation in blood pressure readings over time, two measurements of a diastolic blood pressure of 90 mmHg at least four hours apart is needed to classify a woman as hypertensive. A single measurement of a diastolic blood pressure of 110 mmHg or higher is sufficient to classify a woman as hypertensive.

Hypertension is also present when the diastolic blood pressure increases by 10 to 15 mmHg above the previous baseline even if the reading is still below 90 mmHg. Many women attend the antenatal clinic for the first time during the second trimester, during which a physiological lowering of the blood pressure takes place. If that second trimester blood pressure reading is taken as baseline, the normal rising of blood pressure during the third trimester will give a false pathological appearance. Therefore this parameter can only be used if the baseline blood pressure was taken before or during the first trimester of pregnancy.

Proteinuria can be defined as 2+ proteinuria detected on a dipstick on two occasions taken at least four hours apart. Clean catch urine specimens should be used. Proteinuria can also be defined as 300 mg protein in a 24-hour urine specimen.

Chronic hypertension

Preconception care

Prior to pregnancy, the use of medication should be reconsidered. The woman with mild hypertension might not need antihypertensive therapy if she exercises moderately, reduces her weight to ideal levels, stops smoking, and uses less than 2 g dietary sodium and less than one unit of alcohol daily. Reduction in salt intake does not, however, reduce the chances of developing pre-eclampsia.

If medication is still required to control hypertension this should be changed prior to conception or as soon as possible after the

pregnancy is diagnosed. Medication should be changed to achieve optimal control of the blood pressure and changed to medication which is safe in pregnancy.

Angiotensin-converting enzyme inhibitors (such as *captopril*, *enalapril* or *ramipril*) should not be used in pregnancy, because of severe fetal side-effects. The preferred drug is *methyldopa* because its fetal effects have been studied well. Infants exposed to *methyldopa* in utero have been followed up in detail to the age of seven years, with no significant adverse effects noted. The usual dose of *methyldopa* is 1 g to 4 g daily in divided doses. If a woman complains of unacceptable drowsiness, an unequal dose can be given, with a higher dose at night. Therapeutic levels are reached within two and a half hours after an oral dose.

The use of beta-adrenergic blockers (*propanolol* and *oxprenolol*) in pregnancy has been associated with intra-uterine growth restriction, neonatal bradycardia and hypoglycaemia. These effects appear to have been overstated and it appears that the beta-adrenergic blockers are generally safe, but they should not be used indiscriminately in pregnancy.

Hydralazine, prazosine and *nifedipine* have all been used with relative safety, but their effects on the fetus have not been fully studied. These drugs are usually used as 'second line drugs', which means that they are added if the blood pressure cannot be controlled satisfactorily with another drug (such as *methyldopa*).

In a woman with superimposed pre-eclampsia, the plasma volume is reduced. Diuretics have an additional negative impact on the plasma volume, and should only be used if they are essential for blood pressure control.

Prior to pregnancy, the possibility of a secondary cause for the chronic hypertension should be excluded. The renal function should be evaluated to obtain a baseline. This is done by assessing serum urea, creatinine and electrolytes, the creatinine clearance and 24-hour urinary excretion of protein.

The aim of preconception care is to achieve optimal blood pressure control with drugs that are safe in pregnancy. The evidence that this will result in an improved pregnancy outcome is not as convincing as that of the effects of preconception care for diabetics, where optimal control reduces the risk of diabetes-related effects on the pregnancy.

Pregnancy care

During pregnancy, medication use should be adapted to the maternal blood pressure. There is no clear-cut advantage of antihypertensives to prevent superimposed pre-eclampsia.

Unless severe hypertension develops, or there is end organ damage (such as renal damage secondary to chronic hypertension), or superimposed pre-eclampsia develops, a good perinatal outcome is anticipated. Conversely, if proteinuria develops, intra-uterine growth restriction is almost inevitable.

It is uncertain whether the use of low-dose *aspirin* and/or calcium supplementation helps to prevent the development of superimposed pre-eclampsia, unless there is an underlying connective tissue disease or thrombophilia.

If no superimposed pre-eclampsia or other complication develops, the pregnancy can continue to term. The woman does not need to be managed in a high-risk obstetric unit but should be followed up by an advanced midwife or medical practitioner. Labour can be induced at 38 to 40 weeks gestation. The route of delivery would depend on the normal obstetric factors, and a caesarean section is not indicated purely because of hypertension.

Pre-eclampsia

Pre-eclampsia is a condition in pregnancy where hypertension and proteinuria develop after 20 weeks gestation. Although hypertension is an essential part of the definition, it is a consequence, and not a cause of the primary pathophysiology of pre-eclampsia. The underlying pathology is probably a defect in the development of the placenta. As the placenta develops during the late first and early second trimester, there is an invasion of trophoblast (originating from the implanting embryo) into

the spiral arterioles in the uterine wall. This invasion changes the reactive arterioles into funnel-shaped vessels that are unresponsive to vasoconstrictive substances. If this process occurs incompletely, the placenta would be insufficiently perfused later on in pregnancy. This leads to an increased production of thromboxane, which increases platelet aggregation and causes vasoconstriction (and therefore hypertension), and an increased capillary permeability (which contributes to oedema and a reduced plasma volume). The production of prostacyclin, which has the opposite effects to thromboxane, is decreased. There is an increase in capillary permeability, which can lead to proteinuria and oedema.

Although hypertension can be treated, this does not change the underlying pathophysiology, and the only cure is to deliver the fetus and placenta. Because of the underlying placental pathology, the fetus is always involved to some extent. On the maternal side, any organ can be affected, with the cardiovascular, renal, coagulation, hepatic and central nervous systems at special risk.

Maternal risk factors

The following are risk factors for the development of pre-eclampsia:

- First pregnancy.
- Multigravida but with a new partner.
- A history of pre-eclampsia (especially which had developed in the second trimester).
- A positive family history of pre-eclampsia.
- Thrombophilia (for example protein C or anti-thrombin III deficiency).
- Auto-immune disease, especially SLE and antiphospholipid syndrome.

> Hypertensive conditions (eclampsia, pre-eclampsia, HELLP syndrome, chronic hypertension and liver rupture) caused 20.7% (507 women) of all maternal deaths in South Africa for the period 1999–2001. It is therefore the second biggest contributor to primary causes of maternal deaths.
> *Source*: DoH, Saving Mothers, 2002:38.

> ### Severe pre-eclampsia
>
> Severe pre-eclampsia is defined as follows:
> ▶ Two readings at least four hours apart of a systolic blood pressure of 160 mmHg or higher, or a diastolic blood pressure of 110 mmHg or higher, or at least one reading 120 mmHg.
> ▶ Persistent 3+ proteinuria irrespective of blood pressure.
> ▶ Organ dysfunction.
> ▶ Signs of imminent eclampsia.
> ▶ Complications such as elevated liver enzymes or thrombocytopenia.

▶ Multiple pregnancies.
▶ Molar pregnancies.
▶ Chronic hypertension.
▶ Diabetes mellitus.
▶ Hydrops fetalis.
▶ Fetal triploidy.

Maternal complications

Any organ system can be affected by pre-eclampsia. The most commonly affected organs are the kidneys, lungs, coagulation system, liver and brain.

Renal complications

The kidneys are directly and indirectly affected by pre-eclampsia. The decrease in plasma volume causes a decrease in glomerular filtration. There is also swelling of the glomerular endothelial cells. Tubular function is first affected, leading to an increase in serum urate levels. Glomerular function is later affected, with an increase in proteinuria, a decrease in creatinine clearance and finally an increase in serum creatinine levels. Fluid retention is caused by renal retention of sodium and potassium due to reduced glomerular blood flow. In severe pre-eclampsia, this can lead to ascites, pulmonary oedema and laryngeal oedema. Acute renal failure is a terminal complication and is more common where an abruptio placentae adds extra stress on the already compromised renal function. Too much intravenous fluid might precipitate pulmonary oedema due to endothelial damage. However, too little intravenous fluid may precipitate renal failure.

Pulmonary complications

An increased capillary permeability (caused by increased thromboxane and platelet factors) causes peripheral oedema. The lungs are relatively protected against the development of oedema by the intravascular fluid depletion typical of pre-eclampsia. If the woman receives too much fluid intravenously, there is a high risk of pulmonary oedema. This is a life-threatening complication. It is therefore of paramount importance to ensure the woman is not overloaded with intravenous fluid. Colloids given intravenously can aggravate pulmonary oedema, as the colloids leak through the pulmonary capillaries to cause lung oedema, which is worsened by the hygroscopic action of the colloids, which would draw further fluid into the intercellular space of the lungs.

Complications of the coagulation system

In pregnancy, there is an exaggerated effect of the coagulation system to stimuli of clotting. The normal coagulation-thrombolysis-turnover therefore occurs more rapidly. In pre-eclampsia, this is more obvious. Because of the damaged endothelium, collagen in the basal membrane of the capillaries comes into contact with the elements of the coagulation system, which triggers coagulation. This causes small blood clots and platelet aggregation. The blood clots are dissolved by the thrombolytic system. Initially, the coagulation-thrombolysis system can compensate for the more rapid turnover, with only a mild to moderate decrease in platelet count. Eventually, however, the system decompensates, and thrombocytopenia and coagulopathy result because the blood platelets and coagulation factors are used up by this continuous cycle of thrombosis and thrombolysis. This can result in a full-blown diffuse intravascular coagulopathy (DIC), which is also a life-threatening condition.

Hepatic complications

The liver, as a reticulo-endothelial organ, is affected by the platelet coagulation in an advanced stage of coagulopathy. A micro-angiopathic haemolysis can result. Petecheal bleeding under the hepatic capsule results from a coagulopathy, and causes clinically apparent epigastric pain. Damage to hepatocytes causes the release of liver enzymes into the circulation. HELLP syndrome is a feared complication of pre-eclampsia, with the following features:

▶ H = haemolysis
▶ EL = elevated liver enzymes
▶ LP = low platelets

HELLP syndrome can develop in a woman without severe hypertension or proteinuria. In any pregnant woman with epigastric pain, HELLP syndrome should be excluded with the following special investigations:

▶ A blood smear and/or serum haptoglobin level to exclude haemolysis.
▶ Liver functions: serum AST (aspartate aminotransferase) and ALT (alanine amino-transferase).
▶ Full blood count to evaluate the platelet count and a dropping haemoglobin or haematocrit level.

In earlier stages of pre-eclampsia, the haematocrit is usually high due to haemoconcentration. If haemolysis ensues, this causes a drop in haemoglobin level. Therefore, normalisation of the haematocrit can be a sign of haemolysis. In severe cases, a liver haematoma can form by bleeding under the liver capsule. This may rupture (especially if handled during a caesarean section), resulting in catastrophic bleeding and even death.

Complications of the nervous system

Although eclampsia was seen as an 'end-point' of pre-eclampsia, a woman does not need to have very severe pre-eclampsia to develop eclampsia. In hypertension, there is vasospasm of the arterioles of the brain. This prevents damage to the microcirculation of the brain by overperfusion. However, it can cause local ischaemia in the brain, with resulting convulsions. The opposite can also occur, with pressure-forced loss of tone in the arteriole, with the development of hyper-perfusion of the brain and hypertensive encephalopathy. In the woman with eclampsia, there are also areas of thrombosis and necrosis in the arterioles, as well as micro-infarcts and small petecheal haemorrhages. Cerebral oedema, cerebrovascular incidents and cerebral haemorrhage are common features of eclampsia.

> Although the premonitory signs of eclampsia (including persistent severe headache, visual disturbances, mental confusion, epigastric pain and hyperreflexia) can alert the midwife that eclampsia is imminent, 20% of women develop eclampsia without any imminent symptoms, 40% of women with eclampsia have little or no proteinuria, and 40% have very little oedema. Only 30% are thrombocytopenic.

Eye complications can occur primarily, or secondary to eclampsia. Retinal artery vasoconstriction can lead to retinal oedema with blurred vision and transient or permanent retinal detachment with visual impairment. Transient cortical blindness, due to cerebral oedema in the visual centre in the brain, can be distinguished from retinal detachment by the presence of the pupillary light reflex.

Fetal and placental complications

The underlying placental pathology is the formation of fibrin and platelet aggregates in the uterine spiral arterioles. This reduces the blood flow through the placenta, and causes placental hypoxia and infarcts. This in turn reduces the amount of oxygen available to the fetus. Chronically, the fetus compensates for the hypoxia and decreased availability of nutrients by redistributing blood flow away from the non-essential organs to the heart, adrenal glands and brain (see Chapter 24). As the condition progresses, the fetus would decompensate, become acidotic and die.

Abruptio placentae, separation of the placenta from the uterine wall, can develop in an otherwise healthy pregnancy, but is much more common in pre-eclampsia and hypertension. In a small abruption, the fetus can survive and significant maternal coagulation problems do not develop. The rule, however, is that fetal demise and maternal diffuse intravascular coagulopathy would develop unless the fetus is delivered as soon as the signs of abruptio placentae develop (see Chapter 21).

Management

The cure for pre-eclampsia is to deliver the fetus and placenta. If pre-eclampsia develops at term, this is the obvious answer. If pre-eclampsia develops preterm, there is a place for expectant management to improve the fetal maturity before the fetus is delivered. This has an obvious risk of increasing the risk of maternal complications and stillbirth, and should be undertaken only with appropriate monitoring at a tertiary level of care or special hypertension unit at a secondary hospital.

Mild pre-eclampsia

The woman with mild pre-eclampsia (with a diastolic blood pressure below 100 mmHg, and no significant proteinuria) can be treated on an outpatient basis. She should be admitted if proteinuria develops (which she can monitor herself with urine dipsticks), if there are reduced fetal movements, or if symptoms of imminent eclampsia develop. Her blood pressure should be monitored weekly, and her urine checked weekly for proteinuria. Daily fetal movement monitoring as well as weekly CTG monitoring should be done. She should be delivered at 38 weeks because of suboptimal uteroplacental circulation.

Indications for hospitalisation

If the woman's diastolic blood pressure is above 100 mmHg, or if there is significant proteinuria, she should be admitted. Baseline investigations include a full blood count, liver transaminases, serum urea, uric acid, creati-nine and electrolyte levels and an umbilical artery Doppler ultrasound.

Indications for delivery

Once the woman has stabilised, delivery should be expedited in case of the following:

Fetal compromise:
▶ Reversed end diastolic flow in the umbilical cord (see Doppler ultrasound in Chapter 24).
▶ Cardiotocographic signs of fetal compromise (poor variability and/or decelerations).

Maternal compromise:
▶ Uncontrolled severe hypertension (persistent systolic blood pressure above 160 mmHg or diastolic blood pressure above 110 mmHg despite maximum doses of two antihypertensive medications).
▶ Renal complications:
  ✦ Oliguria (less than 0.5 ml per kg per hour), which does not resolve.
  ✦ Serum urea 8 mmol/l.
  ✦ Serum creatinine above 100 μmol/l.
▶ Pulmonary oedema.
▶ Thrombocytopenia (platelet count below 100 000 per mm^3).
▶ AST or ALT of more than two times upper limit of normal, with epigastric or right quadrant pain or tenderness.
▶ Eclampsia.
▶ HELLP syndrome.

Gestational age:
▶ Pregnancy duration 38 weeks.
▶ In severe pre-eclampsia pregnancy duration of 32 weeks; or estimated fetal weight of 1.5 kg; or less than 26 weeks gestation.
▶ Signs of abruptio placentae.
▶ Dead fetus.

Stabilisation and delivery

If a woman with severe pre-eclampsia stabilises (with no sign of the complications noted above), it might be in the interest of the baby to manage the woman conservatively in hospital and to allow the pregnancy to continue. The woman should be admitted to a hospital experienced in managing severe pre-eclampsia with a unit that can cater for very low birth weight infants. The management should be as follows:

▶ A cardiotocograph should be done six- to eight-hourly, mainly to detect a poor variability, which can be the first sign of an abruptio placentae.
▶ Umbilical artery Doppler should be done weekly.
▶ Blood pressure should be measured four-hourly.
▶ The platelet count should be measured daily and serum AST on alternate days.
▶ The urine output should be measured daily.
▶ Proteinuria should be monitored weekly on a 24-hour urine sample.

Delivery is indicated when the pregnancy reaches a favourable gestational age or the maternal condition indicates delivery (as above). Delivery can be by induction of vaginal delivery if the cervix is favourable, or by caesarean section. If there are signs of fetal compromise, delivery should be by caesarean section. Epidural or spinal analgesia is contraindicated in case of thrombocytopenia. The woman with severe pre-eclampsia is at high risk of hypotension and decreased cerebral perfusion. Careful preloading with intravenous fluid is therefore necessary before an epidural or spinal block. An epidural block can be preferable because it is possible to titrate more carefully than a spinal block. The woman might need admission to an intensive care unit pre- and postoperatively.

During labour the fetus is monitored with continuous CTG, where available, because the fetus has a high risk of developing fetal distress due to placental insufficiency. The midwifery monitoring of the woman continues as indicated in the box on page 20-9. A vacuum extraction should be performed if the blood pressure is at or above 160/110 mmHg.

Ergometrine is absolutely contraindicated during the third stage of labour because it causes vasoconstriction and thus raises the blood pressure further.

Magnesium sulphate should be considered for a woman with severe pre-eclampsia as part of her stabilisation prior to delivery to prevent eclampsia. This has been the topic of a recent randomised trial (The Magpie Trial Collaboration, 2002). The use of *magnesium sulphate* does reduce the risk of eclampsia by half, and probably reduces the risk of maternal death and abruptio placentae, with no apparent increase in maternal or neonatal morbidity. However, 90 women need to be treated with *magnesium sulphate* to prevent one case of eclampsia, and the benefits should be weighed up against the side-effects.

Corticosteroid administration (two doses of 12 mg *betamethasone* or three doses of *dexamethasone* 8 mg eight hourly) should be considered to improve the fetal lung maturity where delivery is planned prior to 34 weeks (or estimated fetal weight of 2kg). Intravenous fluid therapy should be restricted to 80 to 120 ml per hour of a balanced solution such as Ringer's lactate. Maintenance solutions should be avoided, as these solutions have a high potassium content which might be dangerous in a woman with renal compromise. Colloid solutions should also be avoided, as these solutions might aggravate pulmonary oedema.

Antihypertensive therapy

In the woman with mild pre-eclampsia antihypertensive therapy should be used as for a woman with essential hypertension (as previously described). In the woman with severe pre-eclampsia, the objective is to reduce the hypertension to reduce the risk of maternal cerebrovascular incidents, while not reducing the blood pressure so much that there is a reduction in the fetoplacental perfusion. The blood pressure should be maintained below 160 mmHg systolic and below 110 mmHg diastolic.

To reduce the blood pressure acutely,

<table>
<tr><td>

Midwifery care of women with severe pre-eclampsia

▶ Manage at or transfer to a level 2 or 3 hospital.
▶ Blood pressure should be recorded at least hourly.
▶ After the initial 300 ml Ringer's IV pre-load, ensure IV intake of 80 to 120 ml per hour.
▶ Insert indwelling urinary catheter and strictly record the urine output hourly.
▶ Test for proteinuria four times daily.
▶ Monitor for signs of imminent eclampsia.
▶ Monitor fetal wellbeing by listening to the fetal heart four hourly and CTG monitoring six to eight hourly.
▶ Explain to the mother what is happening with her and the importance of hospitalisation and treatment.

</td></tr>
</table>

hydralazine (Nepresol®) should be used after an intravenous fluid bolus of 300 ml Ringer's lactate. The *hydralazine* should be given by an intravenous injection of 1.25 mg (1 ml of a dilution of 25 mg ampoule into 20 ml normal saline) intravenously every 20 to 30 minutes until the target blood pressure is obtained.

Intramuscular administration of *hydralazine* should be avoided. The initial absorption is decreased due to peripheral vasoconstriction. When the vasoconstriction improves, there can be absorption of repeated doses of *hydralazine*, with severe hypotension. This can lead to fetal distress and maternal brain infarcts.

To maintain the blood pressure, *methyldopa* (Aldomet®) can be used to a maximum of 4 g daily (in divided doses). *Nifedipine* (Adalat®), *hydralazine* (Apresoline®) or *labetalol* (Trandate®) can be added as a second drug.

Management of eclampsia

Eclampsia is a sign of multi-organ involvement in pre-eclampsia. The first priority is to maintain the woman's airway and to administer oxygen by facemask. Turn her on her left side. Prevent injuries by removing objects that can harm her and use cot sides on the bed. *Magnesium sulphate* (MgSO⁴) is given as anti-convulsant; 4 g MgSO⁴ is given slowly intravenously, followed by 5 g as a deep intramuscular injection in each gluteal area. The total dose of *magnesium sulphate* is therefore 14 g. Most eclamptic convulsions resolve in less than two minutes. If another convulsion occurs after the loading dose has been given, another 2 g MgSO⁴ can be given intravenously over three to five minutes. An intramuscular dose of 5 g should be repeated every four hours, provided that the patellar (knee) reflex is present, the respiratory rate is at least 16 per minute, and that there was a normal urine output (of at least 0.5 ml per kg body weight per hour). Alternatively, a maintenance dose of 1 g hourly can be given as an alternative to the intramuscular dose.

<table>
<tr><td>

Research highlight

A large multinational randomised trial confirmed the superiority of *magnesium sulphate* over *diazepam* and *phenytoin* to prevent further eclamptic fits. It was also associated with less respiratory depression, and possibly fewer maternal deaths. *Diazepam* should therefore not be used to stop convulsions.

Source: *The Magpie Trial Collaboration, 2002:1877–90.*

</td></tr>
</table>

The woman who has received *magnesium sulphate* should be stabilised, as other women with severe pre-eclampsia, and delivery expedited. Only once the woman is stabilised, should the fetus be monitored, as the safety of the woman herself is the first priority. If there is a favourable cervix, labour can be induced; otherwise a caesarean section is preferable. *Magnesium sulphate* should be continued for 24 hours after delivery. Eclampsia can occur postpartum, and *magnesium sulphate* should then be continued for 24 hours after the last convulsion. The woman should not be transferred to a lower level hospital and should not be discharged for at least three days. Inform the neonatal unit when the mother of the baby received *magnesium sulphate*.

Magnesium sulphate overdose

An overdose of *magnesium sulphate* would result in the loss of patellar reflexes, nausea, slurred speech, muscular paralysis, respiratory arrest and cardiac arrest. If a woman does not regain consciousness after eclampsia, *magnesium sulphate* toxicity is one of the possible causes. Serum magnesium levels should be maintained between 4 to 8 mg/dl, and can be monitored in case of a confusing clinical picture. In case of magnesium toxicity, 10 ml of a 10% *calcium gluconate* solution can be given slowly intravenously. If respiratory failure develops, the woman should be intubated and ventilated.

CRITICAL THINKING EXERCISES

Thandi, a G1P0, is transferred to a level 3 hospital where you are working with severe pre-eclampsia and pulmonary oedema.
1. On what grounds can severe pre-eclampsia be diagnosed?
2. What signs and symptoms can you expect to be present as a result of the pulmonary oedema?
3. If convulsions develop, what is Thandi's new diagnosis and what is the most effective way to manage this condition?

In a nutshell

▶ Blood pressure drops in the middle of pregnancy, and rises in the third trimester.
▶ Chronic high blood pressure is associated with a favourable pregnancy outcome, unless it is severe, long-standing, and associated with end organ damage.
▶ Pre-eclampsia is treated by delivering the baby.
▶ If remote from term, pre-eclampsia can be managed expectantly, with good monitoring of the mother and fetus, and delivery expedited in case of complications.
▶ *Magnesium* sulphate is the anticonvulsant of choice in the woman with eclampsia

Management of other complications

The pre-eclamptic woman with complications is by definition a critically ill patient. Whether the complication is oliguria, DIC or pulmonary oedema or any other, the woman should be managed in a unit with the necessary facilities and expertise to care for such a patient. If she was managed in a unit without these facilities, the midwife managing the patient should discuss her with the referral unit to determine what should be done prior to transfer. For example, a woman with pre-eclampsia with a decreased urinary output after delivery, might benefit from an increased bolus of fluid intravenously as she may be in a negative fluid balance. However, such a fluid bolus would only put her at higher risk of developing pulmonary oedema if she is in a positive fluid balance.

References

Brown, M. A., Hague, W. M. et al. 2000. Consensus statement: The detection, investigation and management of hypertension in pregnancy. Australasian Society for the Study of Hypertension in Pregnancy.

Department of Health (DoH) . 2002. *Guidelines for maternity care in South Africa.* Second edition. Pretoria: Department of Health.

DoH (Department of Health). 2002. *Saving Mothers: Second Report of Confidential Enquiries into Maternal Deaths in South Africa 1999–2001.* Pretoria: Department of Health.

Duley, L. & Gulmezoglu, A.M. 2001. *Magnesium sulphate versus lytic cocktail for eclampsia.* Cochrane Database Systematic Review: CD002960.

Enkin, M., Keirse, M. J. N. C, Renfrew, M., Neilson, J. 1995. *A guide to effective care in pregnancy and childbirth.* Second edition. Oxford: Oxford University Press.

Enkin, M., Keirse, M. J. N. C, Neilson, J., Crowther, C., Duley, L. & Hofmeyr, J. 2000. *A guide to effective care in pregnancy and childbirth.* Third edition. Oxford: Oxford University Press.

Redman, C. & De Swiet, M. (Ed.) 1989. Hypertension in pregnancy. In: *Medical disorders in obstetric practice.* Second edition. Oxford: Blackwell Scientific.

The Magpie Trial Collaboration. 2002. Do women with pre-eclampsia, and their babies, benefit from magnesium sulphate? The Magpie Trial: a randomised placebo-controlled trial, *Lancet* 359:1877–90.

Whitlin, A. G. & Sibai, B. M. 1999. *Hypertensive diseases in pregnancy, in medicine of the fetus and mother.* Philadelphia: Lippincott-Raven.

Woods, D. L. & Theron, G. B. *Perinatale onderrigprogram. Handleiding 1, Verloskunde.* Cape Town: Perinatal Education Trust.

Chapter 21

Haemorrhage

Dolly Nontuthuzelo Nyasulu

Introduction

Haemorrhage in pregnancy refers to bleeding that can occur from the start of pregnancy until the end of the postnatal period, 42 days after delivery. This involves bleeding that occurs before or after viability, with or without pain, and occurs before, during or after delivery of the baby. Haemorrhage in pregnancy is one of the major contributory causes of maternal mortality and morbidity in developing countries. In South Africa, the National Committee on Confidential Enquiries into Maternal Deaths (NCCEMD) report for 1999 to 2001 indicates that obstetric haemorrhage (antepartum and postpartum haemorrhage) accounts for 13.9% of all maternal deaths.

However, this figure does not include the haemorrhage associated with other primary causes of maternal death such as abortion and ectopic pregnancy; therefore the problem is much bigger than the figure indicates. Of all the causes of maternal deaths haemorrhage is believed to be the easiest to reduce; possibly by as much as 10%.

In South Africa, the midwife is the major role-player in maternal and neonatal care. Therefore, midwives have to be skilled practitioners who are able to appropriately assess a woman with haemorrhage, plan specific nursing interventions and re-evaluate the effect of the interventions. Only then will maternal deaths due to haemorrhage decrease.

Management of haemorrhage during pregnancy

General preventive measures

Anticipation is the key to prevention of antepartum haemorrhage (APH). Prevention should begin in the antenatal period when women can be screened and high-risk cases referred to high-risk clinics for specialised care throughout the pregnancy and delivery. Midwives should ensure that they inform women about the danger signs and what actions should be taken.

Women with hypertensive disorders should be referred to the obstetrician for full assessment, investigation and treatment. Routine iron supplementation should be provided to prevent anaemia. Pregnant women with haemoglobin levels of less than 8 g/dl, as well as those with a history of previous obstetric haemorrhage, should be treated only in health institutions that have facilities for blood transfusion and staff skilled to deal with complications of APH.

During labour the partogram should be utilised to enable early identification of obstructed labour. Active management of the third stage of labour should be practised as it significantly reduces the incidence of postpartum haemorrhage.

Pathogenesis of blood loss and its consequences

Hypovolaemic shock is caused by a reduction in blood volume and acute decrease in red blood cells, both of which reduce the oxygen-carrying capacity of the blood. Inadequate tissue perfusion, which results in cellular, metabolic and haemodynamic changes is therefore present. It is a widespread process and if not managed appropriately can result in a decreased oxygen utilisation by the tissues, organ dysfunction syndrome, multi-organ failure and eventually death.

The clinical manifestation of hypovolaemic shock varies, depending on the severity of blood loss and the woman's ability to compensate. There are four stages of shock:

1. *Initial stage*. During the initial stage (less than 15% or 750 ml blood loss) the compensatory mechanism is able to maintain the cardiac output and therefore the woman appears symptom-free.
2. *Compensatory stage*. As soon as the woman loses 15 to 30% (750 to 1 500 ml) of volume the cardiac output drops, resulting in various compensatory responses. These responses are designed to increase the circulatory volume initially, which aims to maintain tissue perfusion and therefore oxygen delivery to the vital organs. The first signs of shock are restlessness and anxiety. The woman could even appear to be scared. Other signs and symptoms include an increase in heart rate and vasoconstriction to non-vital organs, which then in turn cause a narrowing pulse pressure as the diastolic pressure increases, a decrease in urine output, nausea and vomiting.
3. *Progressive stage*. The progressive stage follows with a fluid loss of 30 to 40% (1 500 to 2 000 ml) and by this time the compensatory mechanism becomes overwhelmed and ineffective. The woman would now present with severe dysrhythmias due to myocardial ischaemia and hypotension. A falling blood pressure is therefore a late sign of shock. The midwife should therefore not wait for the blood pressure to drop before suspecting shock and beginning treatment.
4. *Refractory stage*. The fourth stage of shock occurs when the woman has lost more than 40% (more than 2 000 ml) of volume. The compensatory mechanism fails leading to irreversible shock and death.

Resuscitation of a woman with blood loss

Primary assessment and management

The initial management of the hypovolaemic woman will be the same as for the non-pregnant woman.

The 'ABC' of primary management is non-specific and should always be used during the resuscitation of women with hypovolaemic shock. Teamwork, speed, skill and effective resuscitation are essential aspects of the management.

The primary survey includes the 'ABC' (**A**irway, **B**reathing and **C**irculation) principle of resuscitation:

◗ *Airway.* Ensure that the woman can open, maintain and protect her own airway.
◗ *Breathing.* Administer the highest percentage oxygen via a face mask (60%).
◗ *Circulation:*
  ✦ Stop the source of bleeding if possible (this will be discussed further under each cause of haemorrhage).
  ✦ Turn the woman on to her left side.
  ✦ Insert two large-bore peripheral intravenous lines (14 to 16 G), including high-capacity sets and start administering crystalloid fluids (Ringer's lactate) as volume expanders, which should then be followed with colloids (such as Haemacell®). When inserting the intravenous line a blood sample can be obtained simultaneously for a full blood count and compact.
  ✦ Monitor the vital signs.
  ✦ Re-evaluate the woman's status continuously and make sure that your specific interventions have been adequate.

Secondary assessment and management
The initial survey should then be followed by a secondary survey or head-to-toe assessment of the woman, which includes:

◗ Assessment of the fetus.
◗ An indwelling catheter should be inserted to enable monitoring and recording of urinary output every 30 minutes. Urinary output of less than 30 ml per hour is a symptom of renal failure.
◗ If feasible, a CVP line can be inserted to accurately measure fluid intake and thus avoid overloading of the circulation. The CVP reading should be 6 cm H_2O.
◗ Blood transfusion should be commenced as soon as blood becomes available to prevent clotting defects. If blood is not readily available, fresh dried plasma (FDP) 2 to 4 units should be rapidly transfused.

The specific management of the different causes of hypovolaemic shock in the pregnant woman is discussed below.

Haemorrhage in early pregnancy

The major causes of bleeding in early pregnancy are:

◗ Abortion.
◗ Ectopic pregnancy.
◗ Cervical and vaginal lesions such as carcinoma of the cervix.
◗ Hydatidiform mole.
◗ Trauma of the genital tract.
◗ Implantation bleeding.

Types of abortion

Abortion is termination of the pregnancy before the fetus is viable. Defining the beginning of viability is difficult as it depends on the special care facilities available for the baby. There are two conventions in defining viability. The first convention is to define viability as occurring after 24 weeks gestation or when the baby has a birth weight of 500 g or more. This convention is used in developed countries because they have the facilities to deal with extremely small babies. In developing countries, which usually do not have the facilities needed to keep small babies alive, viability begins after 28 weeks gestation or if the baby has a birth weight of 1 000 g or more. There are currently no binding laws on this controversial issue in South Africa.

Abortion can either be spontaneous, induced for therapeutic reasons or it can be by choice on termination of pregnancy (CTOP). CTOP is a term used for the termination of pregnancy requested by the pregnant woman out of her own choice. 'Early pregnancy loss' or 'miscarriage' are terms often used when referring to abortion.

▶ *Spontaneous abortion/miscarriage.* This is the involuntary loss of a pregnancy prior to viability, which occurs without any medical or chemical interventions. It occurs in 15% of all pregnancies and 80% of them happen in the first trimester (see Table 21.1)

▶ *Therapeutic abortion.* Therapeutic abortion is the deliberate termination of pregnancy and evacuation of the uterus according to the terms of the Choice on Termination of Pregnancy Act (CTOP) of 1996 (see Chapter 27).

▶ *Safe abortion.* A safe abortion is where the temperature is 37.2 °C and less, pulse rate less than 90 bpm, respiration rate less than 20 per minute, size of the uterus is less than 12 weeks, and the haemoglobin concentration is more than 10 g/dl. There should also be no clinical signs of infection, organ failure, system failure and suspicious findings should be absent when evacuation of the uterus is performed.

▶ *Unsafe abortion.* The WHO defines unsafe abortion as abortion not provided through approved facilities and/or persons. The procedure is usually conducted under unhygienic conditions and most of the time dangerous instruments and poisonous substances are used to evacuate the uterus.

▶ *Recurrent spontaneous or habitual abortion.* This is defined as three or more consecutive pregnancies that ended in spontaneous abortion.

Predisposing causes of abortion

A large number of abortions are due to chromosomal abnormalities (50% of first trimester spontaneous abortions), impaired development of the ovum and abnormalities of the placenta. Maternal diseases, such as poorly controlled diabetes mellitus, hypertensive disorders, renal disease and anaemia, ABO and Rhesus allo-immunisation are predisposing factors of abortion, as are multiple pregnancy and maternal age of more than 35 years. Acute infections resulting in hyperpyrexia such as malaria, as well as systemic and chronic infections such as pneumonia, tuberculosis (TB) and TORCH can also result in early pregnancy loss. The major cause of second trimester habitual abortions is cervical incompetence. Abnormalities of the uterus, trauma, and teratogenic drugs such as chemicals used in industry and anaesthetic gases also predispose to abortion. Other causes are carcinoma of the cervix and fibroids.

Prevention of abortion

Women at risk of abortion should be identified and preventive measures should be initiated timeously. Chronic diseases, opportunistic infections such as TB and sexually transmitted

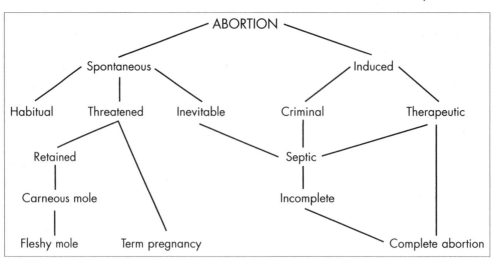

Figure 21.1 Classification of abortions

Table 21.1 Clinical picture of spontaneous abortion

Typical clinical symptoms and signs	Possible diagnosis
History: Light bleeding that persists for days, lower abdominal pains and backache. **Examination**: The size of the uterus corresponds to the dates and may be softer than normal. There is a history of spotting.	Threatened abortion
History: Light bleeding, abdominal pain or cramps and expulsion of products of conception. **Examination**: The cervix closed and the uterus softer and smaller than the dates.	Complete abortion
History: Heavy bleeding, no expulsion of the products of conception and severe abdominal pains and cramping. **Examination**: The cervix is dilated, a tender uterus and the size of the uterus corresponds to the dates.	Inevitable abortion
History: Heavy bleeding, cramping or lower abdominal pains and partial expulsion of products of conception. **Examination**: The cervix is dilated and the uterus smaller than the dates.	Incomplete abortion
History: Uterine growth ceases and the breast changes regress. **Examination**: The cervix is closed and there is a brownish vaginal discharge.	Missed abortion

infections (STI) can contribute to early pregnancy loss and therefore must be treated effectively to prevent complications. Unplanned and unwanted pregnancies should also be prevented. No medication or even bed-rest has been proven to prevent spontaneous abortions.

Management of abortion

The principles of management include:

- Effective resuscitation and physical care to preserve life and ensure continued fertility where possible.
- Adequate and effective psychological and emotional support to both the woman and her significant others to enable them to work through the grieving process (see Chapter 28).
- Adequate post-abortion follow-up care to ensure adequate recovery.

The observation and resuscitation of a woman with severe blood loss due to abortion will be conducted in the same manner as discussed on page 21-2 (Resuscitation of a woman with blood loss).

The type of abortion and the woman's condition usually determine the plan of management. It is important for the midwife to foster a relationship of trust in order to allay the woman's feelings of guilt and anxiety. Careful clinical examination and an accurate history must be obtained because death from haemorrhage associated with abortion tends to occur when the woman conceals her condition because of concerns about the nature of her actions. During history taking, the woman's general appearance must be observed for signs of distress, shock, dehydration and anaemia. From the history given, the period of gestation and blood loss must be estimated. Blood pressure, pulse, respiration and temperature must be monitored. An informed consent must be obtained in readiness for possible uterine evacuation and curettage or manual vaginal aspiration of the uterus. All observations and interventions should be entered in the woman's bed record. If the woman is seen in the residential clinic, she should be transferred to hospital with her records.

Specific aspects related to early pregnancy need to be kept in mind. Adequate sedation should be administered and *tetanus toxoid* given as a prophylactic measure for the possibility of inference with dirty instruments. Taking into consideration that many abortions can be unsafe abortions, the woman should be closely observed for signs of infection (see Chapter 19).

If abortion is incomplete, expulsion or evacuation of the retained products should be achieved by administering an infusion with 30 to 40 units *oxytocin* or alternatively prostaglandins. In addition, blood samples should be taken for full blood count and a vaginal swab must be sent to the laboratory for micro-culture and sensitivity. The woman is then prepared for evacuation, which may be done in theatre under general anaesthesia. If the woman is Rhesus negative, *Anti-D immunoglobulin* must be given.

In cases of habitual abortion cervical cerclage may be performed in the next pregnancy at 14 weeks gestation by inserting a suture to save the pregnancy where possible. The suture is removed at 38 weeks or when labour begins.

Post-abortion assessment

The main objective of post-abortion assessment is to prevent post-abortion infective morbidity and psychological pathology. Antibiotics should be continued for at least 7 to 14 days after the abortion. Any abnormal observation must prompt a systematic evaluation of the woman for any signs of organ dysfunction. Abnormal observations indicate pelvic sepsis, which needs to be referred and the symptoms include:
▶ Subinvolution of the uterus
▶ Tender abdomen
▶ Open cervical os
▶ Excessive foul-smelling lochia

During assessment, urinary tract infection, respiratory tract infection and breast engorgement must also be excluded and appropriate treatment commenced if necessary. Equal attention should be given to the woman's psychological and emotional needs at this distressing time, which will be discussed in detail in Chapter 28.

Antepartum haemorrhage (APH)

APH is defined as bleeding during pregnancy from the vagina after viability occurs and before the onset of labour. It is a major cause of mortality and morbidity in developing countries and according to the Confidential Enquiries into Maternal Deaths (1999–2001) the maternal deaths due to APH increased from 27 cases in 1998 to 37 in 2001. APH is a serious threat to the health of the woman and the fetus.

Causes of APH

The known causes of APH include:
▶ Premature separation of the placenta which includes placenta praevia and abruptio placentae. These conditions are responsible for the majority of haemorrhages in the last trimester.
▶ Extraplacental causes are local lesions of the lower genital tract, such as vaginal and cervical polyps. They are less frequent causes of APH.
▶ Ruptured uterus, partial or complete.
▶ Vasa praevia is one of the rare causes of APH whereby the fetal blood vessels happen to run across the cervical os. The clinical picture is similar to placenta praevia.
▶ Cancer of the cervix and fibroids.
▶ Trophoblastic diseases.
▶ Unknown causes.

Placenta praevia

Placenta praevia ('pre-via' means the placenta lies in front of the baby) is a condition in which the placenta is implanted either whole or partly in the lower uterine segment and therefore lies before the fetal presenting part. The implantation may be in a portion of the lower segment or over the internal cervical os.

Pathophysiology

In placenta praevia the fertilised ovum implants low in the uterine cavity, the cause of which is unknown. Placenta praevia is associated with high parity and is common among women of 35 years and older. Women who have undergone a low segment caesarean section appear to be at greater risk during the next pregnancy. A large placenta as in the case of multiple pregnancy is more likely to encroach on the lower segment. It is thought that when the endometrium and the decidua of the upper segment of the uterus are deficient, the placenta spreads over more of the uterine wall in an effort to obtain adequate supply of blood. This may occur in a scarred uterus where there is less blood circulation over the fibrosed areas. During formation of the lower segment, the placental villi are sheared from the uterine wall thus exposing the sinuses at the placental sites. The amount of bleeding is proportional to the extent to which the placenta encroaches on the lower segment. Because the endometrium in the lower uterine segment is not well developed, the placenta tends to become attached to the underlying muscle, developing to what is known as placenta accreta. Consequently, there is difficulty in expulsion and removal of the placenta in the third stage of labour.

Diagnosis of placenta praevia

A classic symptom of placenta praevia is painless vaginal bleeding with blood that is bright red in colour. In most cases the bleeding is unprovoked but trauma or coitus may precede it. The first haemorrhage is almost never catastrophic and may stop and start again. In such cases the next bleed may be catastrophic but it cannot be predicted. Sometimes there is a continuous trickle of blood which can result in anaemia.

On admission a detailed history should be obtained with regard to the bleeding, followed by a gentle speculum examination by a medical practitioner to exclude local lesions and to identify the source of bleeding. The diagnosis should be confirmed by ultrasonography. If placenta praevia is confirmed and the fetus is mature, the woman should be delivered. Almost 90% of symptomatic placenta praevia cases diagnosed by ultrasound in the early second trimester remain asymptomatic and become normally situated later. Women with low cervical placental implantation should be rescanned between the 30 and 32 week of pregnancy. In cases where, on ultrasound examination, the asymptomatic woman is found to still have a low-lying placenta that appears to be encroaching on the cervix after 32 weeks, she should be considered as having placenta praevia. Where there is a lesser degree of low-lying placenta, the possibility remains that placenta praevia will not be present at the time of labour. If ultrasound is not available, a digital vaginal examination can be done in theatre with everything ready so that,

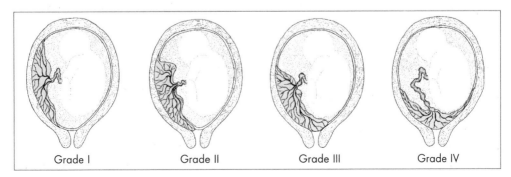

Figure 21.2 Degrees of placenta praevia

in the event of profuse bleeding, a caesarean section can be done immediately to save the woman's life.

Maternal, fetal and neonatal implications

There may be a delay in the engagement of the presenting part due to the placenta occupying this space. When heavy bleeding occurs in placenta praevia grades III and IV, the woman may go into shock and disseminated intravascular coagulopathy (DIC) may develop. Pulmonary embolism may occur due to patent venous sinuses in the placental site. During the third stage of labour the placenta may be retained due to abnormal attachment of the placenta. Women with placenta praevia are at risk of postpartum haemorrhage because the lower uterine segment does not have the same ability as the upper segment to contract and retract after delivery. Anaemia is another major complication.

Fetal prognosis depends on the extent of placenta praevia. If bleeding is profuse, the fetus becomes hypoxic and compromised. However, preterm delivery of the baby is associated with high perinatal mortality and morbidity.

> Management of placenta praevia may be either conservative or active depending on:
> ▶ The amount of bleeding and condition of the woman and the fetus.
> ▶ The location (degree) of the placenta.
> ▶ The period of gestation.

Conservative management of placenta praevia

Conservative or expectant management adopts the 'wait and see' approach which involves hospitalisation to ensure bed-rest, close observation of the woman's condition and delivery by caesarean section once the fetus reaches viability. Fetal and maternal condition is assessed and the vital signs are checked.

A blood sample should be sent to the laboratory for compatibility and grouping and a minimum of 2 units of blood should be kept in readiness because bleeding may occur without warning. A full blood count should be done to exclude anaemia. Iron supplements should be given and if anaemia is severe a blood transfusion may be commenced.

If the woman is sent home during this period, the family situation should be carefully assessed to determine whether she will be able to reach the hospital as soon as bleeding occurs. They should be warned that bleeding may occur without warning which is why the woman needs to be closely observed in hospital. The Saving Mothers report (1999–2001) shows that delay in seeking medical help and lack of transport are avoidable factors in maternal deaths. It is recommended that women who live far from the hospital be admitted in the antenatal care ward for close observation while waiting for confinement.

When a woman is less than 37 weeks pregnant and is being managed conservatively, the amount of bleeding will indicate when to deliver the baby. If the fetus is viable, but the period of gestation is less than 34 weeks, fetal lung maturity is stimulated by corticosteroids to improve chances of survival, as delivery may become necessary within a few days. The mode of delivery depends on the fetal and maternal condition. Should excessive bleeding occur, fetal maturity is ignored and the fetus/neonate delivered by caesarean section. Indications for caesarean section are:
▶ excessive bleeding
▶ fetal distress
▶ placenta praevia grade III or IV
▶ abnormal presentations of the fetus

Active management of placenta praevia

Profuse bleeding due to placenta praevia regardless of the grade necessitates an immediate delivery to save the woman's life. Resuscitation of the woman should be done as discussed on page 21-2 (Resuscitation of a woman with blood loss).

Subsequent care

The woman should be observed carefully for signs of postpartum haemorrhage and infection. Because her resistance against infection may be low as a result of the blood loss, the maternal temperature, pulse and respiration should be closely monitored and iron supplements given to correct anaemia. As long as shock and severe anaemia are prevented the prognosis is good. The following factors, however, may worsen the chances of fetal survival:

- Uncontrollable maternal haemorrhage and shock.
- Excessive placental separation.
- Anaesthesia.
- Preterm birth.

Abruptio placentae

Abruptio placentae means that part or the whole of a normally situated placenta has separated from the uterus before delivery of the fetus. It is the most common cause of antepartum haemorrhage leading to fetal distress.

Pathophysiology

Abruptio placentae is initiated by haemorrhage into the decidua basalis, which divides, leading to separation of part of the placenta. A haematoma forms between the placenta and the uterus. In most cases bleeding progresses to the edge of the placenta at which point it may break through the membranes and enter the amniotic cavity or, more often, the blood trickles down between the chorion and the decidua vera until it reaches the cervix, resulting in vaginal bleeding. In severe cases there is extensive infiltration of blood into the myometrium, causing a condition called Couvelaire uterus. Such a uterus will appear bruised and oedematous.

Concealed haemorrhage leads to enlargement of the uterus in excess of the gestation. Uterine hypertonus is a common sign of severe abruptio placentae, especially after the death of the fetus. Severe pain and shock may be present as a result of hypovolaemia. Abruptio placentae often results in fetal distress and intra-uterine death.

In certain instances a small abruption occurs with no clinical symptoms and signs. Diagnosis in these cases is made in retrospect.

Presence of a retro-placental clot seen at delivery confirms the diagnosis.

Complications of abruptio placentae

- Haemorrhage with complications and possibility of hypovolaemic shock.
- Renal failure due to renal vasoconstriction and renal hypoperfusion, which leads to a fall in urinary output.
- Coagulation defects. The complex maternal coagulation disturbances triggered by severe abruptio placentae may culminate in thrombocytopenia, hypofibrinogenaemia and high levels of fibrin degradation products. Increased fibrinolysis results in disseminated intravascular coagulation (DIC), a serious complication indicated by prolonged thrombin time.
- Shock is often out of proportion to the amount of visible blood loss.
- Total separation or separation of more than 50% of the placenta is incompatible with fetal survival.

Active management

The principles of management of severe abruptio placentae are:

- Intensive correction of hypovolaemia.
- Prevention/early detection of DIC.
- Prevention of acute renal failure.
- Expeditious vaginal delivery whenever possible.
- Prevention of postpartum haemorrhage.

Abruptio placentae is an obstetric emergency and resuscitation is done as discussed on page 21-2 (Resuscitation of a woman with blood loss). If the fetus is alive and the expected weight is 1 kg or more, a caesarean section should be performed as soon as the woman is resuscitated and any clotting defect corrected. A vaginal delivery may be considered when the cervix is 9 cm or more dilated, fetal weight is estimated at less than 1 kg or where the fetus is dead. The membranes are then ruptured and labour is augmented with *oxytocin*, however, membranes should not be ruptured until the woman has been fully

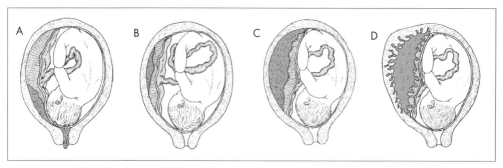

Figure 21.3 Abruptio placentae
A: Marginal separation with revealed haemorrhage, B: Central separation with concealed haemorrhage, C: Complete separation, D: Couvelaire uterus

Risk factors

Pregnant women with the following conditions or a history thereof are at risk of abruptio placentae:
▶ Abruptio placentae in a previous pregnancy.
▶ Pre-eclampsia in the current pregnancy. In pre-eclampsia the blood pressure can even be normal in the presence of clinical shock.
▶ Proteinuria suggests underlying pre-eclampsia with abruptio placentae.
▶ Intra-uterine growth restriction.
▶ Smoking during pregnancy.
▶ Poor socioeconomic conditions.
▶ Abdominal trauma, such as a fall or violence-related injuries.
▶ A short umbilical cord.
▶ Placental separation after the birth of a first twin or loss of a tremendous amount of fluid, such as rupture of membranes in a pregnancy with polihydramnios.

resuscitated. The blood loss should be carefully monitored and a caesarean section performed if the following conditions are present:
▶ No cervical dilatation is present and the membranes cannot be ruptured.
▶ The woman does not progress to the active phase of labour within 6 hours after rupture of membranes.
▶ There is life-threatening haemorrhage when the cervix is not fully dilated.

Active management of the third stage is necessary to prevent postpartum haemorrhage. After birth, 20 to 40 IU of *oxytocin* in Ringer's lactate should be administered rapidly by intravenous infusion to ensure sustained contraction of the uterus. Close observation for

bleeding is necessary and the woman should be kept warm and provided with psychological support and analgesia for any pain and anxiety. *Morphine* 15 mg IM four-hourly can be administered in cases where the fetus has died. In cases where bleeding does not respond to *oxytocin*, the obstetrician may prescribe 600 µg *misoprostol* or prostaglandins (*dinoprostone*) to control bleeding.

Subsequent care
The woman should be observed closely for the next 24 hours and during this time intravenous *oxytocin* should be continued to prevent an atonic uterus. Fluid intake and output should also be monitored and recorded. Vital signs must be checked and the woman monitored for any signs of infection. The Hb,

platelet count, and serum urea and creatinine should all be checked within the first 24 hours. Physical and emotional support must be provided for the woman and the family, especially if the baby has died as the result of the antepartum haemorrhage (see Chapter 28).

Postpartum haemorrhage (PPH)

Bleeding from the genital tract in excess of 500 ml after delivery of the baby is defined as postpartum haemorrhage. The amount of blood loss stated in this definition may, however, be misleading because fluid loss is difficult to measure with any degree of accuracy. There is usually an underestimation of actual blood loss because the blood is often mixed with amniotic fluid and sometimes urine. Blood is dispersed on dressing towels, linen savers and swabs and some spills on the floor, as a result it becomes difficult to estimate the actual blood loss. Measurable solidified clots represent only about half the total fluid loss. Furthermore, the importance

of a given volume of blood loss varies with the woman's haemoglobin level. In women who already had low haemoglobin levels, the blood loss can be fatal regardless of the amount lost. What is of importance is that bleeding that occurs at a slow rate over several hours may not be recognised until the woman suddenly enters into shock. Bearing these factors in mind, it is therefore crucial to realise that any blood loss that adversely affects the woman's condition should be regarded as postpartum haemorrhage. A blood loss of 500 ml therefore must be treated as an emergency situation irrespective of the woman's condition. The woman should be observed closely for signs of shock.

Postpartum haemorrhage is the most common direct cause of maternal deaths in developing countries and it is often an associated complication in other direct causes such as obstructed labour and HIV/AIDS-related sepsis. In South Africa available data shows that of the 13.9% deaths caused by obstetric haemorrhage, 9.8% are due to postpartum haemorrhage (DoH, *Saving Mothers*, 1999–2001).

Table 21.2 Differential diagnosis of placenta praevia and abruptio placentae

Typical clinical symptoms and signs	Possible diagnosis
▶ Vaginal bleeding after viability. ▶ Bleeding is concealed, intermittent or constant. ▶ The abdomen is tense and tender and hard if the bleeding is concealed. ▶ Uterine size is bigger than expected for gestational age. ▶ Possible signs of shock. ▶ Fetal distress or intra-uterine death. ▶ Dark red blood with clots.	*Abruptio placentae*
▶ Painless vaginal bleeding after viability. ▶ Constant bleeding or episodes of bleeds. ▶ Bright red blood. ▶ Effects on blood pressure and pulse proportionate to blood loss that can be seen. ▶ Bleeding may be precipitated by sexual intercourse. ▶ Abdomen: The uterus is relaxed and soft, fetal parts are easy to palpate, usually normal fetal condition, fetal presentation not in pelvis or abnormal lie.	*Placenta praevia*

Pathophysiology

Bleeding from the genital tract in excess of 500 ml which occurs during the third stage or within the first 24 hours of delivery is known as primary postpartum haemorrhage.

The uterine muscle fibres are arranged in an interlacing network through which the blood vessels pass. After placental separation, retraction results in permanent shortening of the uterine muscle fibres. This compresses, kinks, twists and closes the sinuses resulting in the cutting off of blood supply to the placental site, and bleeding is thus controlled. If the uterus fails to retract properly after separation of the placenta, the blood vessels remain open and severe bleeding will take place.

Symptoms of postpartum haemorrhage vary according to the quantity and the rate of blood loss, as well as the general condition of the woman. A woman who starts labour already anaemic may have far more serious symptoms, characterised by an initial tachycardia, and later a bradycardia and hypotension.

Management of PPH

Preventive measures

Postpartum haemorrhage is almost always preventable through anticipation, effective antenatal care and proper management of labour. All women attending antenatal care should be screened for risk factors and referred for high-risk care if necessary. Prophylactic iron supplements should be provided to prevent anaemia and further investigation should be conducted for women who have a haemoglobin level of less than 8 g/dl.

The partogram should be utilised to enable prompt recognition of obstructed labour. Prevention of prolonged labour and maternal exhaustion, as well as prevention of premature

---

Contributory factors to PPH

PPH should be anticipated in women who have a history of PPH in their previous pregnancy. Contributory factors in the current pregnancy are:

▶ *Uterine atony*. Uterine atony means failure of the uterus to contract as a result of hypotonic myometrium. The common causes of myometrium hypotonicity include:
  ✦ Retained placental tissue, including a morbidly adherent placenta, placenta accreta, placenta increta and a succenturiata lobe.
  ✦ Overdistension of the uterus as seen in multiple pregnancy, hydramnios, macrosomia and uterine fibroid.
  ✦ Uterine muscle exhaustion as seen in prolonged labour, precipitate labour, abruptio placentae and vigorous use of *oxytocin* to stimulate contractions.
  ✦ Uterine muscle relaxation as seen in high parity. In grande multiparous women, a large proportion of the uterine muscle is replaced by connective tissue, which does not allow for optimal contraction of the uterus.
  ✦ A full bladder prevents the uterus from contracting optimally.
  ✦ Carcinoma of the cervix and fibroids.
  ✦ Drugs such as anaesthetic drugs (*halothane*) and some chemicals used in industry such as mercury.
▶ *Trauma to the genital tract*. Trauma as a result of vaginal lacerations, cervical lacerations, instrumental delivery, uterine rupture associated with previous uterine surgery and intra-uterine manipulations, such as breech extraction, internal version and, in some cases, of uterine inversion.
▶ *Coagulation defects*. These may result from abruptio placentae, amniotic fluid embolism, sepsis, severe eclampsia and inherited coagulation disorders such as von Willebrand's disease.

bearing down is of vital importance in prevention of PPH. Injudicious use of *oxytocin* should also be avoided. Full dilatation of the cervix should be ensured before delivery by vacuum extraction or forceps application to avoid cervical tears and rupture of the uterus. Active management of the third stage of labour should be practised. Women at risk of postpartum haemorrhage must not be discharged early and iron supplements must be continued for at least a month post delivery. PPH should be anticipated in all grandmultiparous women.

Anaemic pregnant women have a lower tolerance to bleeding during delivery than non-anaemic women. For these women excessive bleeding should be anticipated and preventive measures included in their management plan. In pre-eclamptic women hypovolaemia is common, therefore the reduced blood volume makes such women particularly vulnerable to blood loss. Availability and access to efficient healthcare services are important measures in the prevention of deaths and disability due to obstetric haemorrhage. The role of HIV/AIDS as a contributory factor of early and/or late pregnancy bleeding should not be underestimated.

Active management

The main objective is to save the woman's life by controlling the haemorrhage. The first step involves rapid and effective resuscitation and restoration of blood volume as discussed on page 21-2 (Resuscitation of a woman with blood loss). Specific measures related to postpartum bleeding are as follows:

▶ Rubbing up the uterus to obtain and maintain it in a state of contraction.
▶ The bladder should be empty as a full bladder causes uterine relaxation.
▶ Rapid infusion of 20 to 40 IU *oxytocin* in Ringer's lactate to control bleeding by uterine contraction.
▶ Quick assessment of the amount of blood loss and whether the uterus is atonic or not.
▶ The placenta should be evaluated for completeness.

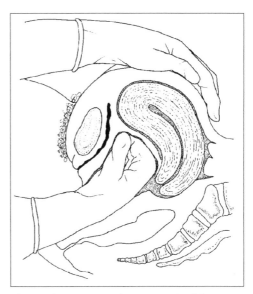

Figure 21.4 Bimanual compression of the uterus

▶ Should there be lacerations or trauma to the cervix or lower genital tract, compression or surgical suturing should arrest haemorrhage. It is important to check if *oxytocin* 10 IU was given at delivery of the baby and the dose repeated before compression can be done in order to aid effective uterine contraction.
▶ Bimanual compression should be applied by placing the clenched fist of one hand into the anterior fornix and applying pressure against the anterior uterine wall. The other hand exerts external pressure on the abdominal wall, causing pressure on the posterior uterine wall (see Figure 21.4).
▶ Manual compression of the abdominal aorta can be performed by applying downwards pressure through the abdominal wall on the abdominal aorta. The pressure is applied with a fist just above the umbilicus and slightly to the left. If the femoral pulse is not palpable with the other hand, the pressure exerted is adequate.

Secondary postpartum haemorrhage

Secondary postpartum haemorrhage is defined as fresh bleeding from the genital tract during the puerperium after the first 24 hours. The retention in the uterus of blood clots, pieces of membrane and placental tissue is the most common cause but the bleeding may also be from infected wounds, fibroids or, in rare cases, malignant trophoblastic disease.

The earlier bleeding in the puerperium occurs, the more likely it is to be caused by retained products of conception. If signs of shock are present, resuscitation is done as described previously. If bleeding is severe, add 40 IU *oxytocin* per litre of intravenous fluid and run it at 40 drops per minute. Broad-spectrum antibiotics in high doses may be prescribed. Exploration of the uterus under general anaesthesia to remove the retained products should be done. Digital evacuation of the uterus can be undertaken provided it is still within seven days after delivery. Beyond seven days, when the cervical os is already closed, instrumental cervical dilatation and light curettage will be necessary. The infected lacerations in the genital tract become septic and sometimes bleed when the sloughs separate. Clinical signs of infection are fever, excessive localised pain, tenderness and an offensive discharge. If bleeding is from the infected uterine wound, the bleeding is typically recurrent and heavy, especially following complication of a repaired ruptured uterus. In such cases hysterectomy is done to control bleeding. Iron supplements should be given to treat anaemia and the general condition of the woman must be monitored closely. Vital signs, blood loss, fluid intake and output, and level of consciousness should be checked and the findings recorded.

CRITICAL THINKING EXERCISE

A woman presents with severe haemorrhage during the fourth stage of labour. Of the bloodclots 800 ml has already been collected and the woman is still bleeding. The woman looks scared and has a tachycardia.
▶ Is the woman in hypovolaemic shock?
▶ How should this woman be managed?

Injuries to the genital tract and uterus

Cervical tears

Small, superficial cervical lacerations are common during a vaginal delivery. They are responsible for the 'bloody show' during labour and heal spontaneously without treatment. Deep lacerations, however, can cause severe haemorrhage and lead to hypovolaemic shock. The uterus is usually well contracted. The bleeding is bright red with a continuous flow and differs from bleeding due to atony of the uterus, which is dark red with blood clots. If the laceration extends into the lower segment, it should be regarded as uterine rupture.

Excessive bleeding after a delivery requires a complete examination of the cervix and vaginal passage. A medical practitioner must do the exploration. While preparing for the exploration the midwife should do the following:
▶ Treat the woman for shock as discussed on page 21-2 (Resuscitation of a woman with blood loss).
▶ Perform bimanual compression.
▶ Arrange for urgent transport, accompanied by a midwife, to a hospital or medical practitioner, if not already available.

Uterine rupture

There are two types of uterine ruptures, namely complete (the serosa is also torn) and incomplete rupture (the serosa covering the uterine wall remains intact). An incomplete rupture is more dangerous and is frequently accompanied by more severe haemorrhage. Rupture of the uterus can occur before, during and after delivery.

Silent or quiet rupture

In cases of a silent or quiet rupture the woman may experience some pain. A rising pulse rate, pallor and perhaps slight vaginal bleeding, usually accompanied by signs of severe fetal distress, may be present. The contractions fade away and the cervix fails to dilate. This type of rupture may be associated with the scar of a previous caesarean section.

Causes of uterine rupture

The causes of uterine rupture include:

▶ The careless use of oxytocic drugs such as *oxytocin, misoprostol* and *dinoprostone*, which will cause tetanic contractions that may cause rupture.
▶ Previous classical caesarean section scars are particularly prone to uterine rupture.
▶ Cephalopelvic disproportion (CPD).
▶ Multigravity.
▶ Use of fundal pressure.
▶ Difficult forceps delivery.
▶ Manual dilatation of the cervix.
▶ Manual removal of an adherent placenta.
▶ Version.
▶ Craniotomy.

Usual rupture

The clinical picture of a usual uterine rupture develops over a few hours. The woman may present with abdominal pain, vomiting, faintness, vaginal bleeding, rapid pulse rate, pallor, tenderness on palpation and the absence of the fetal heart. If undiagnosed, hypotension and shock will follow.

Violent rupture

This is a dramatic rupture, which is noticed almost immediately, especially following obstructed labour. Severe pain due to tetanic contractions are present just prior to the rupture, followed by a feeling of something given way and a sharp continuous pain in the lower abdomen. The multiparous woman may note that the baby seems to be rising towards the fundus instead of descending towards the pelvis. Labour ends immediately and shock develops quickly with the possibility of complete maternal collapse.

Diagnosis and management

The diagnosis of uterine rupture is made on a clinical basis and the following clinical manifestations may be present:

▶ Intra-abdominal and/or vaginal bleeding.
▶ Concealed or revealed bleeding.
▶ Abdominal distension.
▶ Tender abdomen.
▶ Rapid maternal pulse.
▶ Signs of shock.
▶ Abnormal uterine contour.
▶ Easily palpable fetal parts.
▶ Absent fetal movements and fetal heart sounds, or signs of fetal distress.

With a ruptured uterus vaginal bleeding is present unless the fetal head blocks the pelvis. Rupture that occurs during the second stage causes bright red vaginal bleeding as the baby is born (unlike postpartum bleeding due to uterine atony, which usually occurs a little later with separation of the placenta). Bleeding may also occur intra-abdominally.

The presence of pain may differ between no abdominal pains or severe abdominal pains, and may decrease as time goes on. The woman who is in labour with a previous caesarean section should be closely monitored for possible uterine rupture.

After rupture is diagnosed, the woman is resuscitated as discussed on page 21-2 (Resuscitation of a woman with blood loss) and transferred to a level 2 or 3 hospital. The baby and placenta should be delivered after the woman has been stabilised. If the baby is delivered completely either into the woman's abdomen or externally, bimanual compression should be applied to reduce blood loss. Repair should be considered only if the woman wants to have more children, but a hysterectomy is sometimes indicated.

Uterine inversion

Inversion of the uterus means that the uterus has turned inside out. Although it is rare, it remains an obstetric emergency. If neglected, the cervical ring around the uterus contracts causing oedema, a decrease in blood supply, and eventually necrosis and gangrene of the uterus takes place. Inversion may occur as a result of:

▶ Excessive cord traction in the presence of a relaxed uterus.
▶ Inappropriate cord traction without counterpressure to prevent fundal descent.

▶ Vigorous fundal pressure.
▶ Exceptionally high intra-abdominal pressure as a result of coughing or vomiting.

The woman presents with shock accompanied by severe pain due to the traction on the ovaries by the inverted uterus. On abdominal palpation a concave shape will be felt and, if there is complete inversion, the uterus will not be palpable.

Haemorrhage occurs in most cases. Resuscitation should not be delayed as the shock is out of all proportion to the amount of blood loss. Except for resuscitation (see page 21-2) the management consists of immediate replacement of the inversion, pain relief and prophylactic antibiotic therapy. An oxytocic agent must be put up to aid contraction of the uterus. Sometimes replacement is done under general anaesthesia. If necrosis is suspected a vaginal hysterectomy may be performed.

Genital tract haematomata

Haematomata may develop due to blood vessel trauma during spontaneous or operative deliveries. The blood vessel trauma is caused by the pressure from the presenting part, forceps delivery or inadequate homeostasis during a repair of an episiotomy or laceration.

Clinical manifestations

▶ A *vulvar haematoma* presents as a painful swelling on one side of the vulva. The skin over the area often appears bluish purple in colour and may feel fluctuant on palpation. After continuous bleeding, the perineum becomes tense and distended. Bruising and swelling may extend into the adjacent buttock.
▶ A *vaginal haematoma* causes persistent pain, a feeling of pressure in the vaginal and rectal area (the woman may indicate the need to pass a stool but is not able to void). On vaginal examination soft masses may be found protruding into the vagina.
▶ *Broad ligament haematomata* are often less obvious and may go undetected until they are very large. Further investigation is

indicated with persistent, unexplained, lower abdominal or lower back pain and a persistent deviation of a contracted uterus.

Management

Most haematomata are small and require no interventions as they resolve spontaneously. Some may continue to enlarge, necessitating incision, drainage and ligation of blood vessels. If neglected, blood loss into these haematomata may lead to hypovolaemic shock, anaemia, infection and possible maternal death. If it becomes infected, extensive sloughing may result.

Further management includes:
▶ Ice to the perineum can promote comfort, decrease swelling and may limit bleeding into the tissues.
▶ Observe for signs of continued bleeding such as rising pulse rate, persistent or increasing pain, fatigue and pallor or a drop in blood pressure.
▶ Reassure the woman that a small haematoma will reabsorb over 4 to 6 weeks and should cause no difficulty unless the area becomes infected. Explain which signs and symptoms of infection she should be aware of.
▶ Broad-spectrum antibiotics are usually used as prophylaxis against infection.
▶ Hypovolaemia and anaemia should be treated if present.

> **In a nutshell**
> ▶ Hypovolaemic shock can initially be symptom free, but will later present with restlessness, anxiousness, tachycardia, slight increase in diastolic pressurre, decreased urine output, and also nausea and vomiting.
> ▶ Hypotension is a late sign of hypovolaemic shock and will develop if the woman's compensatory mechanism starts to fail. Treatment should not be delayed until hypotension develops.

> ▶ Although the initial management of any type of haemorrhage will be based on the ABC principle, the specific management of the different causes should follow thereafter.

References

Bennett, V. R. & Brown, L. K. (Eds.) 1999. *Myles textbook for midwives*. Thirteenth edition. Edinburgh: Churchill Livingstone.

De Brouwere, V. & Van Lerberghe, W. (Eds.) 2001. *Safe motherhood strategies: A review of the evidence*. Antwerp: ITG Press.

Enkin, M., Keirse M. J. N. C., Renfrew, M. & Neilson, J. 1995. *A guide to effective care in pregnancy and childbirth*. Oxford: Oxford University Press.

Enkin, M., Keirse, M. J .N. C., Neilson, J., Crowther, C., Duley, L. & Hofmeyr, J. 2000. *A guide to effective care in pregnancy and childbirth*. Third edition. Oxford: Oxford University Press.

DoH (Department of Health). 2002. *Confidential enquiries into maternal deaths in South Africa*. Triennial Report 1999–2001.

DoH (Department of Health). 2002. *Guidelines for maternity care in South Africa*. Second edition. Pretoria: Department of Health.

DoH (Department of Health). 2002. *Saving mothers: Second report on confidential enquiries into maternal deaths in South Africa 1999–2001*. Pretoria: Department of Health.

Larsen, J. 2001. *Obstetrics in peripheral hospitals*. Third edition. Durban: Pricewaterhouse.

Lawson, J. B., Harrison, K. A. & Bergstrom, S. (Eds.) 2001. *Maternity care in developing countries*. London: RCOG Press.

Marivate, M. 1996. Maternal injuries. In: *Topics in obstetrics and gynaecology*, Bassin J. (Ed.). Johannesburg: Julmar Communications.

Nolte, A. G. W. (Ed.) 1998. *A textbook for midwives*. Pretoria: J.L. van Schaik.

WHO (World Health Organisation). 1996. Maternal health and safe motherhood programme. *Midwifery education*. Geneva: WHO.

WHO (World Health Organisation). 2000. *Managing complications in pregnancy and childbirth: A guide for midwives and doctors*. WHO/RHT/00.7. Geneva: WHO.

Woods, D. L. (Ed.) 1993. *Perinatal education programme: Maternal care manual*. Observatory: Perinatal Education Trust.

Chapter 22

Medical and surgical conditions during the perinatal period

Dr Patricia McInerney

Introduction

Pregnancy, labour and the puerperium are all marked by physiological changes in the woman's body. This means that for the woman who already has an alteration in the physiological functioning of a body system, the strain on that system is compounded by the additional demands made during childbirth. Whilst some of these alterations are not life-threatening to the woman and fetus, others are. This chapter will deal with the most common medical and surgical conditions found in South African women during pregnancy and childbirth.

The cardiovascular system

During pregnancy the cardiovascular system has to cope with an increase in the blood volume. This amount is variable but it is usually about 1 500 to 2 000 ml. The maximum increase occurs around the 34th week of pregnancy and this volume is then maintained until term. Both the red blood cells and plasma volume increase but the total red blood cell increase is less than that of the plasma. This results in a relative dilution of the red blood cells and gives rise to a physiological anaemia of pregnancy. The white blood cell count and platelets are also increased in pregnancy.

In order to cope with the increased cardiac workload, the heart increases both its rate and its stroke volume. For the normal heart, this does not pose a problem. However, for the heart that is damaged it is problematic. During a three year period (1999–2001) cardiac disease accounted for an average of 3.7% of maternal deaths in South Africa. The main contributory causes of death are cardiac failure and respiratory failure where the majority of women die because of pulmonary oedema.

It is generally accepted that a woman who has a cardiac problem will experience deterioration in her cardiac function during pregnancy, so a woman who shows no signs or symptoms of disease in the non-pregnant state may begin to show symptoms during pregnancy. A deterioration of one grade of functional capacity is usually expected during pregnancy (see Table 22.1). The New York Classification of Functional Capacity, which is universally accepted, is used to grade cardiac disease.

Management of the woman with a cardiac problem during pregnancy

A woman with a known cardiac problem should be examined both by a cardiologist and obstetrician before careful planning of the conception of a child at the time at which she is the healthiest. She should be encouraged to book into the high-risk antenatal clinic as early as possible in the pregnancy. This is to obtain early baseline data of her haemodynamic status from which the remainder of her pregnancy can be monitored. A thorough history must be taken of the woman's cardiac status in previous pregnancies and of her condition in the non-pregnant state. Important factors such as age, parity, socioeconomic status and occupation that may adversely affect her condition must be noted. Medication that could be teratogenic (such as *warfarin*) should be changed before conception (see Table 22.2).

Physical examination

A full physical examination must be conducted and a cardiologist must auscultate the heart and lungs. In the absence of a cardiologist the midwife should suspect a cardiac condition when observing some of the symptoms as indicated below. Clinical manifestations of the cardiac status such as the following should be noted:

▶ *Pulse*: Pulse rate and rhythm (100 bpm or irregular) and the fullness of the pulse (feeble or bounding).
▶ *Symptoms*: Oedema, breathlessness, dyspnoea on exertion, paroxysmal noc-turnal dyspnoea, fatigue or dizziness, hae-moptysis, palpitations, cyanosis, chest pain and clubbing of the fingers.

During pregnancy the woman should be carefully monitored for obstetric complications

Table 22.1 Grades of cardiac disease

Grade 1	Although cardiac damage is present the woman does not present with any symptoms. This means that her physical activity is not limited.
Grade 2	Ordinary daily activities begin to cause symptoms such as palpitations, dyspnoea and fatigue. The woman is usually comfortable, i.e. she has no symptoms when she is at rest.
Grade 3	Whilst comfortable at rest, the woman experiences symptoms on slight exertion. The symptoms are dyspnoea, palpitations and anginal pain.
Grade 4	Even at rest, the woman experiences symptoms such as dyspnoea and cardiac insufficiency.

Table 22.2 Medications that may need to be considered

Medication	Indications
Iron supplementation	If the woman is anaemic.
Digoxin	May be considered for the woman who has mitral valve disease.
Diuretics	If indicated, for instance if there is evidence of congestive cardiac failure or pulmonary oedema.
Beta-blockers	May sometimes be prescribed by the cardiologist to reduce the cardiac output.
Anticoagulants	Where there is a history of prosthetic valves, thrombosis or emboli, atrial fibrillation and mitral stenosis.

Specific investigations

Specific investigations that should be carried out include:
▶ Monitoring with ECG.
▶ Regular monitoring of haemoglobin levels.
▶ Monitoring of prothrombin index if the woman is on anticoagulant therapy.

such as anaemia, multiple pregnancy, hypertension and infection. These conditions place an added strain even on the normal heart, which means the woman with a cardiac problem should attend antenatal clinic (at a level 2 or 3 hospital) more frequently, preferably fortnightly instead of monthly. This is particularly important if she is on medication for her cardiac condition.

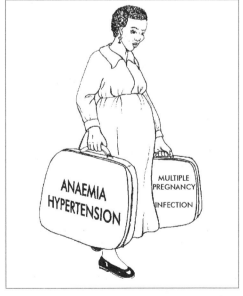

Figure 22.1 Additional factors that place a burden on the compromised heart

> **Note**
>
> It is important to consider the period of gestation when administering anticoagulant therapy. *Warfarin* is of small molecular weight and can easily cross the placenta. It has been shown to be teratogenic before 12 weeks gestation and to be associated with periventricular haemorrhage infarction and intra-uterine death. Thus *warfarin* should be discontinued during the first trimester of pregnancy and replaced with *heparin*. From 12 to 36 weeks gestation, *heparin* is discontinued and replaced by *warfarin*. Then from 36 weeks to the onset of labour *heparin* is recommended. *Heparin* does not cross the placenta and therefore does not expose the fetus to the danger of haemorrhage during labour and delivery. However, *heparin* has a shorter half-life than *warfarin* and therefore the advantage to the mother at this stage is that maternal haemorrhage can also be prevented.

Indications for admission to hospital include the following:
▶ Deterioration in cardiac function.
▶ Grade 4 women should be kept in hospital. Although the ideal situation is to deliver a viable baby and not to endanger the health of the woman, it may be necessary to terminate the pregnancy if the woman's life is in danger, for example, if she has pulmonary hypertension or if she presents with cyanosis and congestive cardiac failure.
▶ Ideally, grade 2 and 3 women should be admitted at 36 to 37 weeks gestation to await the onset of labour.

Intrapartum management of the woman with a cardiac problem

These women usually have quick labours and therefore the midwife needs to be alert to this possibility. Anticoagulant therapy must be discontinued when labour commences.

Specific measures for the first stage of labour

The following specific measures should be instituted when caring for a cardiac woman during the first stage of labour:
▶ Stabilise, transfer and/or admit to the labour ward of a level 3 hospital.
▶ Treat the woman as a high-risk case.
▶ The woman should be nursed in a high-Fowler's position.
▶ Ensure that oxygen is available and used when necessary.
▶ To prevent fluid overload, make use of 200 ml vacolitres or use paediatric volume controllers (not 60 drop drip sets, but buretrols that allow preset volumes of fluid to flow into a second controlled chamber). It is suggested that Ringer's lactate be commenced with the onset of labour so that a line is functional should the need arise. The intravenous fluids should not exceed 70 ml per hour.
▶ Administer other medications as prescribed. In some instances antibiotics are administered prophylactically to prevent infection and the possible development of bacterial endocarditis. *Gentamicin* and *ampicillin* (*vancomycin* if allergic to penicillin) are commonly used.
▶ Administer analgesia. *Pethidine* 100 mg intramuscularly is the drug of choice. Spinal anaesthesia is only advocated when there is expert supervision as fluid overload and hypotension must be avoided.
▶ It is important to prevent infection in these women and therefore vaginal examinations should be kept to a minimum. In addition, artificial rupture of the membranes should be avoided, as should the use of fetal scalp electrodes.
▶ Observe for signs of cyanosis and monitor the respiratory rate hourly.
▶ Auscultate the lung bases every two hours for possible pulmonary oedema.
▶ Great care should be taken when labour is augmented. *Oxytocin* 2 IU is administered in 200 ml Ringer's lactate or normal saline,

starting at 12 ml per hour. This should be increased to 24, 36 and 46 ml per hour every 30 minutes until adequate contractions are present.

Source: *DoH, 2002:118.*

Specific measures for the second stage of labour

Do not use the lithotomy position. The woman's legs must always be kept below the level of her heart to prevent extra workload being put on her heart. The second stage of labour should be kept as short as possible with the minimum amount of effort spent on bearing down. For this reason, it may be necessary to perform an episiotomy. When local anaesthetic is used for an episiotomy it should not contain *adrenaline*. An assisted delivery (a low-outlet forceps) may be performed by an obstetrician or by an advanced midwife in an emergency.

Specific measures for the third stage of labour

Never administer *ergometrine* for the active management of the third stage of labour. It causes a prolonged vasoconstriction and hypertension, thus placing an increase on the workload of the heart. *Oxytocin* 10 IU intra-

Antibiotics
If antibiotics were not used prophylactically, they should be considered if: ▶ There was a prolonged labour. ▶ The woman is HIV positive. ▶ A manual removal of the placenta was necessary. ▶ Delivery ended in a caesarean section.

muscularly may be used instead. *Furosemide* 20 mg IV should be administered after the delivery of the baby.

Postpartum management of the woman with a cardiac condition

Blood volume returns to normal after delivery through diuresis. As fluid is lost there is a tendency for the development of deep vein thrombosis and the woman must be observed carefully for signs of this condition. For the cardiac woman this aspect is particularly important and therefore *heparin* is usually recommenced after delivery. The woman's haemodynamic status needs to be carefully monitored during the first 48 hours after delivery. Her pulse, blood pressure and hydration status should be monitored hourly for the

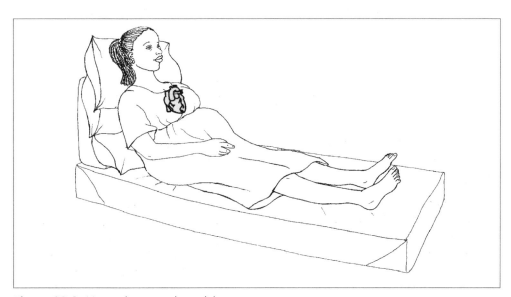

Figure 22.2 Maternal position during labour

first 24 hours. Any cyanosis, cough and dyspnoea or any other sign of pulmonary oedema should be reported. The midwife must also observe the woman for episodes of dizziness and fainting. Careful attention must be given to hygiene and the prevention of infection and therefore four-hourly pad checks of the lochia are suggested. The woman should be taught how to care for the episiotomy.

Cardiac disease is not a contraindication to breastfeeding. The stage of the cardiac disease and prescribed medications are the main factors that need to be considered when deciding on whether a woman can breastfeed. If a woman does wish to breastfeed she must be given assistance and the midwife must take note of the baby's feeding patterns in order to prevent the woman becoming exhausted.

Family planning methods should be discussed with the woman prior to her discharge from hospital. Women with a history of cardiac disease are usually advised to limit the size of their families and to complete their childbearing at an early stage. Sterilisation is the method of choice in women whose cardiac status is severely compromised. This is best done six to eight weeks after the delivery. Intra-uterine contraceptive devices are contraindicated

---

CRITICAL THINKING EXERCISE

Thandi Nkosi is a 31-year-old G3 P0. She has a history of a previous miscarriage at 12 weeks gestation and an ectopic pregnancy at 8 weeks.

Thandi had rheumatic mitral valve disease as a child. She cannot remember exactly how old she was when she became ill. This has left her with mitral stenosis. She had a balloon valvotomy just prior to becoming pregnant and she is currently on the following medication:

- *Hydralazine* 10 mg twice daily.
- *Isosorbide mononitrate* 10 mg twice daily.
- *Furosemide* 40 mg daily.
- *Potassium chloride* two tablets twice daily.
- *Ferrous fumarate* two tablets daily.

Thandi has no allergies and does not smoke or drink alcohol. Her HIV status is positive. She is now 27 weeks pregnant according to dates. When Thandi attended the antenatal clinic for a routine visit she said that she had been coughing for the last two weeks and she is short of breath. She experiences dyspnoea when she walks a short distance (500 m), even when the surface is flat. She also reported that she has a sharp pain in the chest. This has been present for the last two weeks.

On examination she is found to have pretibial oedema. Thandi is not experiencing palpitations. Her blood pressure is 100/65 mmHg and her heart rate 80 bpm. Her liver and spleen are not enlarged. Breath sounds are equal. Cardiac auscultation reveals S1   S2   with a systolic murmur. Abdominal palpation reveals a pregnancy that is consistent with the period of gestation.

1. What other information would you need to fully understand Thandi's condition and to be able to care for her appropriately?
2. What is your immediate management of Thandi's condition?
3. Discuss the ethical issues that you can identify in her history and in her future management.
4. How would you plan Thandi's care for the rest of her pregnancy?
5. Identify members of the health team who may be significant in the management of Thandi's pregnancy.

because of the risk of infection. Low dose oral contraceptives may be used, as may the progesterone-only oral preparations. The depot progestogens may also be used.

The baby of the woman with a cardiac condition

Typically these babies are small for gestational age and therefore need to be carefully monitored in the first 24 to 48 hours after birth for hypothermia and hypoglycaemia (see Chapter 31).

The haematological system

By far the most common haematological condition that the midwife has to manage during pregnancy is that of anaemia. Thromboembolic disease may occur during pregnancy but it is more common during the puerperium.

Physiological anaemia of pregnancy

During pregnancy there is an increase in the blood volume. Whilst there is an increase in all the constituents of the blood, the increase in the red blood cell count is lower than that of the plasma volume. This means that there is a relative dilution of the red blood cells and this is known as the physiological anaemia of pregnancy. The normal range of haemoglobin (Hb) in the non-pregnant woman is 12–16 g/dl. This may fall to 12 g/dl in the pregnant state.

Iron deficiency anaemia

All pregnant women must have their haemoglobin estimation done at the booking visit and again at 28 and 36 weeks. When a low Hb is detected with an on-site test, it should be confirmed with a full blood count. Iron deficiency anaemia is common amongst South African women because the majority of the population are of low socioeconomic status. This means that a woman's store and/or intake of iron in her diet may be low. In addition, HIV-immunosuppressed women are prone to anaemia. However, depending on the geographical area in which the midwife is practicing, she must also be alert to the possible causes of parasite infections such as hookworm and whipworm, infections such as malaria, which cause haemolysis of the red blood cells, and bilharzia that causes bleeding. Urinary tract infection and tuberculosis can also be possible causes of anaemia.

Manifestations of anaemia

A diagnosis of anaemia is made on the haemoglobin estimation. A normal haemoglobin level is 12–16 g/dl. Therapeutic treatment is usually commenced when the level is less than 10 g/dl. Other manifestations of anaemia include:

◗ Pallor, especially of the sclera, nail beds and mucous membranes.
◗ Tiredness and lethargy.
◗ Dizziness and fainting.

Many anaemic women do not present with these symptoms because their bodies have compensated for the reduction in the haemoglobin level. The midwife must be alert to this possibility and remember that a clinical assessment of anaemia may not always be accurate.

Management of anaemia

Women should be empowered to prevent this condition by educating them about the condition and its prevention. The cause of the anaemia should be sought and treated accordingly. The body is dependent on dietary intake of iron to maintain its stores and therefore it is important to provide women with a list of cheap but good sources of dietary iron. These include green herbs, imifino, dark green spinach, beetroot, eggs, legumes and dried fruit. Women should be encouraged to try and eat red meat at least once a week and to have fish or poultry on the remaining days. Liver is a very good source of iron. Second class proteins such as legumes and soya are good alternatives for the woman when her socioeconomic status is poor.

When her haemoglobin level is less than

10 g/dl the woman should be given iron salts in the form of *ferrous sulphate, gluconate* or *fumarate*. These preparations are taken orally and the dose depends on the haemoglobin estimation. It is better to prescribe one tablet twice or three times a day than two or three tablets daily as there is better absorption of the iron when it is taken in separate doses. Women should be advised to take these tablets with meals to avoid side-effects such as nausea, even though there is maximum effect when the preparations are taken on an empty stomach. However, they should not be taken with tea or coffee. The vitamin C in orange juice may enhance the absorption of the iron. In some health centres, ascorbic acid is administered together with the iron preparation.

The haemoglobin estimation should be repeated two to three weeks after treatment commenced. If there is no improvement in the haemoglobin level, or when the haemoglobin

---

Specific tests

The following tests should be administered when there has been no response to oral iron supplementation:

▶ MCHC – Mean corpuscular haemoglobin concentration (normal 34 g/dl).
▶ PCV – Pact cell volume (normal 39 to 42%).
▶ Serum iron (normal 6 to 30 mmol/l).
▶ Total iron binding capacity (normal 45 to 72 mmol/l).
▶ Percentage saturation (normal 30%).
▶ FBC and smear.
▶ HIV serology.
▶ Urine for microscopy and culture.
▶ Chest X-ray and stool for occult blood and parasites if indicated.

It is important for the midwife to consider the individual woman's blood results in the light of her existing state of health, e.g. pre-eclampsia and HELLP syndrome (haemolysis, elevated liver enzymes and low platelets).

---

level is less than 7 g/dl, further specific tests should be carried out.

According to the Department of Health a blood transfusion is indicated in the following situations:

▶ Anaemia together with cardiac failure.
▶ Woman experiences severe symptoms of anaemia.
▶ Anaemia in women before delivery or caesarean section where there is not enough time for *ferrous sulphate* to have an effect (Hb <7–8 g/dl).
▶ Presence of severe haemorrhage.
▶ Anaemia present in a woman at increased risk of haemorrhage, e.g. placenta praevia.

Source: Guidelines for maternity care in South Africa, 2002:115.

Thromboembolic disease

This may present as either a superficial thrombosis or as a deep vein thrombosis. The former is more common. A superficial thrombosis occurs when a thrombus forms in a varicose vein and inflammation of the vein wall develops due to a primary infection. A deep vein thrombosis is more serious because there is obstruction of a vein by a blood clot, without prior inflammation of the vein wall. It is caused by initial minor trauma to the vessels and is aggravated by circulatory stasis and sepsis.

Prevention and management of thromboembolism during pregnancy

Risk factors should be identified at history taking. Anaemia and infections must be treated promptly in women who have a predisposition to thromboembolism. The woman who has varicose veins must be encouraged to wear elastic support stockings from toe to groin. These must be put on before she gets up in the morning and must be worn at all times. Encourage her to perform passive leg exercises such as flexion and extension of the feet and rotation of the feet in both directions. The woman should be advised to avoid stasis of blood in the legs, which means avoiding standing for long periods of time and crossing her legs whilst sitting. If her job requires that

Predisposing factors to thromboembolic disease

▶ Progesterone causes relaxation of the smooth muscles. This leads to stasis of blood and a slower venous return.

▶ There is alteration in the constituents of the blood during the puerperium. The excess plasma volume is excreted from the body through diuresis, which results in an increased viscosity of the blood during this period until the cell and platelet counts return to the non-pregnant state.

▶ Varicose veins predispose to stasis.

▶ A history of previous thromboembolism: A recurrence rate of 12% is reported.

▶ Poor ambulation of the woman after delivery, for instance post-caesarean section.

▶ Older women are more predisposed to the development of thrombi than younger women.

▶ Pre-existing medical conditions such as cardiac disease and diabetes mellitus.

▶ Poor management of labour where the woman has been allowed to become dehydrated.

▶ Assisted deliveries where the woman has been placed in the lithotomy position. Trauma to the saphenous vein may occur if the woman is left in this position for a prolonged period of time.

▶ Preconception history, such as the use of oestrogen in a combination contraceptive pill and heavy smoking.

she sits for long periods of time then she should be encouraged to walk around her desk every one to two hours. Any leg tenderness or pain must be reported immediately. When these symptoms of deep vein thrombosis (DVT) or pulmonary embolism (acute shortness of breath, chest pain, haemoptysis, cyanosis and tachycardia) exist, the woman should be transferred to a level 2 or 3 hospital by ambulance for anticoagulant therapy.

Prevention and management of thromboembolism during labour

If the woman presented with a thrombosis during her pregnancy, she is a candidate for a hospital birth. Dehydration and haemorrhage must be prevented. Supine hypotensive syndrome results in a decreased venous return and therefore it must be avoided, as well as any trauma to the legs when the lithotomy position is used.

Prevention and management of thromboembolism during the puerperium

Early ambulation and postnatal exercises are encouraged and dehydration must be avoided. The legs should be examined daily for evidence of swelling or tenderness and it should include

Further investigations

▶ *Doppler ultrasound.* This is done to detect the flow of blood through the underlying vein. It allows normal blood flow to be distinguished from a vein that is occluded by a thrombosis.

▶ *Ultrasound.* This will show the thrombosis.

dorsiflexion of the foot, which should not cause any pain. When pain is evident it will typically be a sharp pain behind the knee, which is known as a positive Homan's sign. If a positive Homan's sign is present, then referral and further investigations should be carried out.

If the woman presents with a thrombosis the foot of the bed must be elevated. Anticoagulant therapy will depend on the medical team. Where prescribed, it must be carefully monitored and clotting times must be done on a regular basis. Use should be made of a bed cradle and analgesia prescribed for pain.

The respiratory system

Pregnancy does not cause any respiratory problems but it may aggravate an existing condition, such as asthma, or develop secondary to conditions such as pre-eclampsia or cardiac conditions.

Asthma

The effects of pregnancy on asthma are not consistent but asthma does tend to have effects on both pregnancy and labour. In asthmatic women there is an increased incidence of hyperemesis, pre-eclampsia and antepartum haemorrhage. An increased incidence of spontaneous preterm labour, low birth weight, perinatal mortality and late neonatal deaths has also been reported. Fortunately, most of the medications used in the treatment of asthma in the non-pregnant state (steroids and *theophylline*) can safely be used during pregnancy and labour.

Pulmonary oedema

Pulmonary oedema may occur as a result of left-sided heart failure. However, in the absence of cardiac disease the causative factor may be pre-eclampsia, the side-effects of betamimetic drugs or an amniotic fluid embolism. In cases of the latter, the onset of pulmonary oedema is rapid.

Immediate management of pulmonary oedema

▶ The woman should be nursed in semi-Fowler's position.
▶ Administer oxygen by mask.
▶ Restrict intravenous fluid.
▶ Administer *furosemide* 20–40 mg IV and repeat if necessary.
▶ Monitor with ECG.
▶ Use a pulse oximeter where available.
▶ Transfer to a level 2 or level 3 hospital for further management.
Source: *Guidelines for maternity care in South Africa, 2002:119.*

Clinical manifestations of pulmonary oedema

▶ cyanosis
▶ dyspnoea and orthopnoea
▶ frothy sputum
▶ haemoptysis
▶ tachycardia
▶ grunting and wheezing
▶ paroxysmal nocturnal dyspnoea

The endocrine system

By far the most common disorder of the endocrine system during pregnancy is that of gestational diabetes. The midwife should be careful to distinguish between the gestational diabetic (that is the woman who presents with glycosuria for the first time during pregnancy) and the pregnant diabetic (that is the woman who is a known diabetic). However, pregnancy also has an influence on the thyroid gland and therefore the midwife must be alert to possible alterations in thyroid activity.

Gestational diabetes

This is a condition that occurs during pregnancy in women who are not known diabetics. Carbohydrate metabolism is altered during pregnancy. The normal fasting blood sugar is lower than in the non-pregnant state. This, together with the anti-insulin effects of a number of hormones and the alteration in renal physiology, may account for glycosuria. The increased levels of oestrogen, progesterone and human placental lactogen create a resistance to insulin and as a result blood sugar levels remain raised longer than in the non-pregnant state. During pregnancy the glomerular filtration rate and renal blood flow increase because of the increase in the blood volume. The tubular cells of the kidney have a decreased capacity to reabsorb certain substances due to an increased workload, and amongst these is glucose. Thus a lowered renal threshold may account for glycosuria. This phenomenon commonly occurs early in the third trimester of pregnancy. When the woman attends her antenatal follow-up visit she will present with 2+ or 3+ of glucose in her urine.

Screening for diabetes

A woman with glycosuria should be screened for possible gestational diabetes with a random blood glucose (RBG) measurement. The outcome will determine whether the woman is a gestational diabetic, unlikely to be a diabetic or whether further investigation is needed in the form of a fasting blood glucose (FBG) measurement before a diagnosis can be made. The woman should fast from 10 pm the night before the test. Test results for RBG and FBG are indicated in Table 22.3 below.

If the woman's FBG is 6.0 to 7.9 mmol/l a glucose tolerance test (GTT) should be arranged. A glucose tolerance test should also be performed when there is a history of the following, irrespective of whether there is glycosuria or not:

- Obesity – if the woman weighs 80 kg or more.
- Previous unexplained stillbirth late in pregnancy.
- Evidence of hydramnios.
- A previous baby weighing more than 4 kg.
- Poor obstetric history – two or more miscarriages or unexplained stillbirths.
- Family history of diabetes and certain races, such as the Asian population.

A glucose tolerance test requires that the woman arrives at the antenatal clinic early the next morning, a fasting blood sugar is taken and the urine tested for glucose. The woman is then given a glucose load to drink – this is usually 50 g of glucose mixed in a glass of ice-cold water. It is unpleasant to drink and the woman should be advised not to sip it over a long period of time, as this will alter the results. Blood samples are repeated at half-hourly intervals for the next two hours. The diagnosis of gestational diabetes is based on the result of the glucose tolerance test. The results should be as follows:

- *Fasting blood glucose*: less than 5 mmol/l.
- *At one hour*: less than 9 mmol/l.
- *At two hours*: less than 8 mmol/l.

If one or more of these results are raised then the woman should be treated as a diabetic and in most cases insulin should be commenced.

Table 22.3 Guidelines on random blood glucose (RBG) and fasting blood glucose (FBG) interpretations

RGB values	Implications
<8 mmol/l	Most probably not a diabetic. Repeat RGB if glycosuria recurs.
11 mmol/l	Gestational diabetes present. Refer to specialist clinic at a level 2 or level 3 hospital. Follow-up care can continue at a level 1 hospital according to their guidelines.
8.0–10.9 mmol/l	Requires further testing in the form of FBG.
FGB values	**Implications**
<6 mmol/l	Most probably not a diabetic. Repeat RGB if glycosuria recurs.
8 mmol/l	Gestational diabetes present. Refer to specialist clinic at a level 2 or level 3 hospital. Follow-up care can continue at a level 1 hospital according to their guidelines.
6.0–7.9 mmol/l	Admission is required for a glucose tolerance test (GTT).

Source: Adapted from Guidelines for maternity care in South Africa, 2002:116.

Reasons for commencing insulin

▶ Fetal complications such as macrosomia are associated with high glucose levels.

▶ Dietary control is not always sufficient.

▶ Oral hypoglycaemic agents do not allow for precise control and they may be teratogenic. If given shortly before delivery, they cross the placenta and can have long-term effects on the fetus.

It is important to review the woman's history for any evidence or incidences of infection, such as *Candida albicans*, thus far in the pregnancy. After delivery the woman with gestational diabetes will not require insulin, but a repeat glucose tolerance test should be done on the third day postpartum.

The pregnant woman with diabetes

Preconception care

Ideally a woman with diabetes who is planning a pregnancy should consult with her midwife, family physician, obstetrician and endocrinologist prior to conceiving.

This preconception planning means that her blood sugar is controlled at the time of conception and so congenital abnormalities can be avoided.

Once the woman suspects that she is pregnant she should have the pregnancy confirmed as soon as possible and be seen by an obstetrician. The reason for this urgency is that pregnancy is a diabetogenic state. The diabetogenic state results from the alteration in carbohydrate metabolism in pregnancy and the increased hormone levels that have an anti-insulin effect. These hormones are human placental lactogen, cortisol, adrenalin and noradrenalin, oestrogen and progesterone and the thyroid hormones. This results in hyperglycaemia in the woman and as a result her body produces more insulin than is required. Blood glucose readily crosses the placenta resulting in fetal hyperglycaemia. Maternal insulin does not cross the placenta, however, and the fetus responds by producing excessive amounts of insulin. These two factors, hyperglycaemia and hyperinsulinaemia, result in a macrosomic infant.

The demand for insulin increases as the pregnancy progresses and so the woman's blood sugar levels should be reviewed at regular intervals. The frequency with which this needs to be done is determined by the daily monitoring of her blood glucose levels. However, this is usually necessary at two-weekly intervals. The review of her insulin needs is usually done in the form of a glucose profile. Venous blood for glucose levels is taken at 06:00, 10:00, 14:00 and 18:00. A combination of a long-acting and a short-acting insulin is usually prescribed and the decision to alter either one or both of these amounts is influenced by the results obtained in the profile. Insulin is usually administered in the morning and again in the evening.

Antenatal period

Women with diabetes should be referred to a clinic that specialises in the care of women with diabetes in pregnancy, usually at a level 2 or 3 hospital but follow-up management can take place at a level 1 institution.

In addition to monitoring insulin needs carefully during the antenatal period, the woman should also be continually monitored for hydramnios, which may occur in the second half of pregnancy. It is thought to be caused by the high glucose levels which cross the placenta and which stimulate the trophoblast to produce excess liquor. Excessive amounts of liquor are produced when diabetes is not well controlled and it predisposes the woman to preterm labour. The woman is also at greater risk to develop hypertension during the pregnancy and is more prone to infections. Moniliasis and bacteriuria, which lead to urinary tract infections, are twice as common in diabetic women.

The fetal status and fetal growth need to be carefully monitored throughout the pregnancy. Regular abdominal palpations for the estimation of the fetal size and the amount of liquor are essential. The fetus of a diabetic woman is prone to macrosomia because of the excessive amount of glucose, which crosses the placenta. This increased fetal growth may result in problems during the labour such as cephalopelvic disproportion, shoulder dystocia and/or dystocia which require operative delivery. The possibility of intra-uterine growth restriction (IUGR) and intra-uterine death (IUD) during the last four to six weeks of pregnancy due to maternal acidosis and placental insufficiency requires that the fetal status be carefully monitored. The woman should be encouraged to keep a record of the fetal movements. In addition, these women should be seen more frequently during the antenatal period, preferably two weekly up to 32 weeks and then weekly. Where such facilities exist, regular monitoring of fetal growth by means of ultrasound should be undertaken.

Intrapartum period

The decision of when to deliver depends on how well controlled her diabetes has been during the pregnancy. If the blood glucose levels have not been well controlled then delivery should not be delayed beyond 36 weeks. Prior to delivery an amniocentesis is performed to determine the fetal lung maturity. If the lecithin:sphingomyelin (L:S) ratio is 2:1 or greater, then delivery may be pursued. If the fetal lungs are not sufficiently mature and delivery is necessary, then the intramuscular administration of *betamethasone* may be prescribed. In this case delivery may be achieved through a caesarean section. If the condition has been well controlled throughout the pregnancy, then it is possible to allow the woman to go to term and to allow her a trial of labour if the fetus is considered to be of normal size. Should the woman be allowed a trial of labour, insulin will be administered according to a sliding scale. An intravenous infusion of 5% dextrose water is to be administered during the labour. The labour must be carefully monitored for progress. Her blood sugar level must be monitored hourly. The aim is to keep the blood sugar level between 4.4 and 5.5 mmol/l. If after eight hours there is no progress or delivery is not likely within the next three to four hours, a caesarean sec-

> ### Research highlight
>
> A review of the literature found that there is little evidence to support either elective delivery or spontaneous labour in women with insulin-dependent diabetes. Only one randomised controlled study was identified and the findings from this study suggested that induction of labour in women with gestational diabetes treated with insulin reduced the risk of macrosomia. This was probably related to the fact that early delivery of the fetus reduced the risk of shoulder dystocia that may be a problem with a large fetus.
>
> *Source*: Boulvain, Stan & Iron, 2002.

tion should be considered. If delivery is to take place by means of an elective caesarean section, the woman is to fast from 10 pm the night before. It is important that the midwife remember to monitor the woman for hypoglycaemia during this period of fasting. On the morning of delivery, an intravenous infusion of 5% dextrose water is commenced and half to one third of the normal dose of the short-acting insulin is administered.

Postpartum period

After delivery the need for insulin decreases because the levels of human placental lactogen, oestrogen and progesterone will have decreased. The woman may not require insulin for the first two to three days after delivery. During this period blood glucose is monitored three hourly and insulin is given according to a sliding scale. Thereafter, the woman usually returns to her preconception insulin requirements.

During the postpartum period the woman should be carefully monitored for signs of infection. Breastfeeding is not contraindicated in the woman with diabetes, but is often difficult due to inadequate lactation. Therefore the woman may need assistance and the neonate's nutritional requirements need to be monitored.

(Please note that the baby of a diabetic mother has special needs. Refer to Chapter 31).

Family planning should be discussed with the woman because pregnancy aggravates diabetes. Sterilisation may be suggested when the woman has two children. Alternative methods each have their disadvantages. The pill increases insulin requirements and intra-uterine contraceptive devices predispose the woman to infection. Therefore a suitable method should be decided on after taking the individual woman's situation and her choice into consideration.

Disorders of the thyroid gland

The thyroid gland enlarges and becomes more vascular during pregnancy as a result of the increased secretion of thyroid stimulating hormone by the anterior pituitary gland. Whilst the level of protein-bound thyroxine is raised, the level of free thyroxine (T_4) is normal.

Hyperthyroidism

In hyperthyroidism the gland is enlarged and is overactive with increased levels of T_4. Mild hyperthyroidism is not uncommon during pregnancy and is not harmful to either the woman or the fetus. If the overactivity of the thyroid gland is caused by a long-acting thyroid stimulator (LATS), this will cross the placenta and neonatal hyperthyroidism may develop but it will subside within three weeks after birth.

The decision to treat with antithyroid drugs such as *carbimazole* or *propylthiouracil* should be carefully assessed by means of a thorough clinical assessment and an assay of T_4. These drugs cross the placenta and may cause fetal hypothyroidism. This risk can be reduced by keeping the woman euthyroid by giving her a small dose, 0.2 mg per day of T_4 during the last trimester of pregnancy. If the condition is not treated, the rates of abortion, intra-uterine death and stillbirth increase. Breastfeeding is contraindicated because antithyroid drugs are excreted in breast milk.

Hypothyroidism

This condition is characterised by decreased levels of T_4 and protein-bound thyroxine. The level of thyroid-stimulating hormone is raised and the thyroid gland may be enlarged. These women usually have excessive weight gain, a lack of energy, an intolerance to cold, dry skin and may suffer from constipation. Severe hypothyroidism causes infertility. Pregnancy

---

CRITICAL THINKING EXERCISE

Jessica Long is a known diabetic. She is referred to the hospital for a cervical cerclage. Her history is as follows: Jessica is a G5 P1 and has had three miscarriages – all in the first trimester of pregnancy. After each miscarriage she had a dilatation and curettage (D&C). Jessica has had one normal vaginal delivery nine years ago. She has no known allergies.

Her current health status is as follows: Jessica is on 16 IU of fast-acting insulin three times a day and 26 IU of long-acting insulin at night. For the last three weeks she has had a chronic cough. The physician saw her and no abnormalities were found on physical examination. However, she was given a course of antibiotics.

Auscultation of her heart and lungs revealed no abnormalities. There was no hepatosplenomegaly. On abdominal examination no abnormalities were felt but her period of amenorrhoea was equivalent to 13 weeks.

Jessica is booked for surgery. Prior to surgery, she is seen by the endocrinologist, who states that her insulin requirements are to be met according to a sliding scale post-surgery.

Suggested approach:
1. Identify further information that you may need.
2. Develop a plan of care for the remainder of Jessica's pregnancy.

may occur in mild cases, but there is an increased risk of abortion. Women who are on treatment for myxoedema may require an increased dose of T_4 during pregnancy. The newborn infant's thyroid profile should be assessed at birth.

The gastrointestinal system: Hyperemesis gravidarum

The majority of conditions of the gastro-intestinal system are seen as normal and common in pregnancy and are discussed in Chapter 11. These include nausea and vomit-ing, constipation and haemorrhoids.

If nausea and vomiting are excessive and the woman is unable to eat, she will become ketoacidotic. Ketosis triggers the chemorecep-tor zone and hence causes more vomiting. If the woman is unable to tolerate food, there is weight loss and ketonuria and then the condi-tion is known as *hyperemesis gravidarum*, meaning excessive vomiting in pregnancy. This condition may occur in early pregnancy when morning sickness is excessive. It often occurs after 12 weeks of pregnancy when the morning sickness should have subsided.

Management of hyperemesis gravidarum

- Admission to hospital is preferable.
- On admission the woman's vital signs must be noted and recorded. The skin and mucous membranes should be checked for evidence of dehydration and the urine tested for ketones.
- Intravenous therapy should be commenced to replace fluids and to provide glucose.
- Antiemetics should be prescribed with caution (e.g. *prochlorperazine* or *meto-clopramide*).
- The fetal status must be noted by estimating the size of the fetus on abdominal palpation. In later pregnancy, the fetal heart rate should be auscultated, at least twice a day, and note taken of fetal movement. If possible, fetal heart rate monitoring should be done.

- The woman's psychological and emotional wellbeing should be assessed and if necessary she should be referred to a psychologist.
- As the nausea subsides the woman should be encouraged to take small frequent meals. It is the midwife's responsibility to support the woman while she eats and to note how she tolerates the meals.
- Once meals are tolerated, hydration is restored and the urine is free of ketones, the intravenous therapy may be discontinued.
- The woman should be weighed daily.
- Once the woman tolerates food and gains weight she may be discharged. It is important to advise her that, should the nausea and vomiting recur, she must seek help immediately.

Differential diagnosis

The midwife should consider the differential diagnosis of anorexia nervosa, if the pregnancy was unwanted or if the condition existed prior to the pregnancy. This requires skilful and tact-ful history-taking by the midwife.

Autoimmune diseases during pregnancy

The autoimmune diseases include systemic lupus erythematosus (SLE) and rheumatoid arthritis.

Systemic lupus erythematosus (SLE)

SLE is an autoimmune condition that presents with a range of inflammatory conditions, including nephritis, joint inflammation and neuropathies. It may also present with depression. The influence of pregnancy on the disease is variable. Should the joint inflamma-tions and neuropathies be exacerbated by the pregnancy, they are treated with *prednisone* and low-dose *acetylsalicylic acid* may be prescribed.

Effective care of this woman requires a multidisciplinary team. The midwife will need to coordinate the care prescribed by the

Implications of SLE

Fetal/neonatal:
- Increased risk of abortion, stillbirth, preterm labour and low birth weight.
- Neonatal lupus and congenital heart abnormalities are rare but may occur in severe cases.

Maternal:
Increased risk of exacerbation of the disease in the postnatal period.

Implications of rheumatoid arthritis

Fetal/neonatal:
The continued use of salicylates in pregnancy is associated with a low risk of fetal abnormalities.

Maternal:
- There may be remission of the symptoms in pregnancy with a relapse postpartum.
- Extra rest is needed to relieve the weight-bearing joints but exercise remains important.
- The exercises should be of a non-weight-bearing nature and include a range of motion exercises.

obstetrician and specialist in the immune system disorders. The woman will also need to be educated about the need to avoid exposure to infection, stress and fatigue. In addition, she should be informed of the signs of preterm labour and urinary tract infection and the need for prompt assessment and treatment, should these occur.

Rheumatoid arthritis

In this autoimmune condition the joints become inflamed, causing fatigue, pain, low-grade fever and swelling with progressive loss of joint function. There is usually morning stiffness with pain on movement. It is believed to be caused by a genetically influenced antigen–antibody reaction. Treatment of the condition with salicylates and other non-steroidal anti-inflammatory drugs (NSAIDs) usually remains unchanged in pregnancy, although the woman may choose to reduce the amount of salicylates if the pain and inflammation are reduced during the pregnancy.

The midwife should encourage the use of non-pharmacological self-care measures, such as cold compresses applied to the affected joint, rest and flexibility exercise. She should advise the woman to use salicylates only when needed.

The central nervous system

Neurological conditions that may present in pregnant women are epilepsy, myasthenia gravis and multiple sclerosis.

Epilepsy

This is a chronic disorder characterised by seizures. The cause of the epilepsy may be idiopathic or be secondary to other conditions such as a head injury or encephalitis. It is

Implications of epilepsy

Fetal/neonatal:
- There is no increased risk of abortion or preterm labour.
- Anticonvulsant therapy is associated with an increased risk of congenital abnormalities such as cleft lip and heart defects, although the incidences of these defects have decreased over the years.

Maternal:
- The effect of the pregnancy on epilepsy is variable.
- Anti-epileptic treatment is continued during pregnancy. Prior to conception, known teratogenic drugs may be replaced with others or the lowest effective dose prescribed.
- Vitamin K deficiency may be present in both mother and baby.
- Folic acid supplementation should also be commenced prior to conception.

usually treated with anticonvulsants. Epilepsy has no significant effect on pregnancy, even in women in whom the fits have been difficult to control.

The midwife needs to encourage the woman to attend preconception counselling to change therapy if needed, to maximise control and to motivate compliance. The woman should rest as much as possible and be seen more frequently at clinic. A careful record should be maintained of seizure incidents. In this way any needed alteration to the medication can be made without unnecessary delays. If facilities permit, second trimester screening of the fetus for abnormalities should be done by means of ultrasound. Folic acid 5 mg daily should be supplemented throughout the pregnancy.

Myasthenia gravis

Myasthenia gravis is a chronic disease characterised by variable degrees of muscular weakness, which may progress to paralysis. The disease attacks the point at which the

---

Implications of myasthenia gravis

Fetal/neonatal:
▶ The newborn infant may be temporarily affected after birth. The infant may be hypotonic and motionless after birth but this usually passes within ten days after birth. Treatment is only necessary if there is difficulty in breathing, sucking and swallowing.

Maternal:
▶ Uterine action is unaffected, but assisted delivery may be necessary due to weak voluntary bearing-down effort.
▶ These women are very sensitive to general anaesthesia and therefore local analgesia should rather be used when necessary.
▶ Postpartum exacerbation of the disease is common and the necessary assessment should be done.

---

nerve meets the muscle, interfering with the normal release of acetylcholine (ACh) and subsequent depolarisation of the end plate and excitement of the muscle fibre. It may be caused by circulating antibodies to the ACh receptor. Pregnancy has a variable effect on the disease, but pregnancy and labour are usually uneventful.

Multiple sclerosis

Multiple sclerosis is a condition in which the myelin sheath of the nerve fibres is destroyed. It results in muscle weakness, neurological changes, fatigue with marked loss of sensation and muscle strength during exacerbations. The current view is that pregnancy has no effect on the disease progression and that any changes that occur with pregnancy would have taken place in any case.

Implications of multiple sclerosis

Fetal/neonatal:
Termination of pregnancy is sometimes considered depending on the degree to which the woman in incapacitated.

Maternal:
Spinal analgesia must be avoided at delivery.

Dermatological conditions

Skin changes during pregnancy are not uncommon. Some women report that their skin has never been better, whilst others complain of a very dry skin during pregnancy. Rashes are not uncommon but they are usually more irritating than anything else. However, measles, chicken pox and rubella must be ruled out before reassuring the woman that the rash is of no consequence. If the rash causes an itch then the use of a mild, non-perfumed lotion, such as calamine lotion, may be prescribed. *Striae gravidarum* (stretch marks) may become itchy and the woman should be advised to rub a mild body lotion on the affected area.

Surgical conditions: Cervical incompetence

The most common surgical complications, apart from caesarean sections, associated with pregnancy are ectopic pregnancies (see Chapter 27) and cervical incompetence.

Cervical incompetence gives rise to repeated mid-trimester abortions. The problem is related to the internal os of the cervix. The os is not able to remain closed with the increasing weight of the pregnancy. An incompetent cervix may be due to previous obstetric trauma, injudicious surgical dilatation, cone biopsy or cervical amputation.

Manifestation of the problem

The woman presents with a history of repeated, almost painless abortions after the 16th week of pregnancy. It may be possible to observe the membranes bulging through the partly dilated cervix.

Management of the problem

A purse-string suture of non-absorbable material is inserted in the thickness of the wall of the cervix before the 14th week of pregnancy. The suture is removed around the 38th week of pregnancy. The midwife must inform the woman that should contractions commence before the suture has been removed, she must return to the hospital immediately. This is important because contractions result in dilatation of the internal os and if the suture is still in situ, tearing of the cervix may occur.

Trauma

Possible causes of trauma to the pregnant woman are motor vehicle accidents (either as an occupant of a car or as a pedestrian) or some form of violence. When a pregnant woman is injured the midwife and healthcare professional have to remember that two lives are at risk and that the survival of the fetus is dependent on the survival of the mother. Prioritisation of the management of the pregnant woman remains the same as in the non-pregnant state, although resuscitation

and stabilisation should be modified to allow for the anatomical and physiological changes that have taken place during the pregnancy. If the woman is conscious the midwife must remember that she will be very anxious and must take steps to reassure her.

Anatomical changes

As pregnancy progresses, the uterus moves out of the protection of the pelvis, the uterine wall becomes thinner and the amniotic fluid volume is reduced with a decreased cushioning effect of the liquor. It is therefore more exposed to injury. Furthermore, the placenta does not have any elastic tissue and so shearing forces to the abdomen may result in abruptio placentae.

Management of trauma in the pregnant woman

Initial assessment

Life-threatening conditions or injuries should be assessed first:

- *Airway*. Assess the airway first, stabilise the neck, determine ventilation and, if possible, administer oxygen. Keep in mind that there is an increased risk of regurgitation and aspiration during pregnancy due to physiologic ileus or diminished emptying time of the bowel.
- *Breathing*. Assess for increased tidal volume and/or respiratory rate. As pregnancy progresses, the diaphragm becomes elevated, with a decreased functional residual capacity. This decreases the pregnant woman's oxygen reserve and therefore the airway and breathing must be monitored carefully and supplemental oxygen administered.
- *Circulation*. The pulse and blood pressure may be difficult to interpret because blood will be shunted away from the uteroplacental site to the woman's vital organs. This means that the fetus may be in shock before the woman develops a tachycardia, tachypnoea or hypotension. Furthermore, the midwife must remember that the supine position compresses the

large vessels. If a spinal board is available, the woman can be immobilised and then be turned on her left side and kept in place by a wedge. Once a spinal injury has been excluded the woman should be nursed in a left lateral position for increased venous return.

▶ *Drugs.* Drug administration is the same as in a non-pregnant woman.

The next important step is to establish two large-bore catheters for aggressive fluid resuscitation. Maternal hypovolaemia can mask 15 to 30% blood loss as a result of normal haemodynamic changes in pregnancy. Early aggressive fluid resuscitation is recommended to prevent maternal hypovolaemia (see Chapter 21).

Lastly, a rapid neurological assessment should be made according to the Glasgow coma scale or any other reliable scale.

Secondary assessment

This assessment includes a thorough assessment of the woman and the fetus.

The woman must be assessed from head to toe. Whilst it is recognised that radiation is harmful to the fetus up until 36 weeks gestation, radiography must not be withheld if it is necessary to exclude life-threatening injuries to the woman. When possible the uterus should be shielded with a lead apron during these examinations. Appropriate coverage of the abdomen may be achieved with lead blankets. Thereafter the treatment of injuries should proceed as for a woman in the non-pregnant state.

An obstetrician should make the assessment of the fetus. The examination must include the fundal height, uterine tenderness, contractions and fetal position. A vaginal examination should be carried out for cervical dilatation, effacement and the drainage of amniotic fluid. The fetal heart rate should be auscultated and fetal wellbeing determined.

If the woman is known to be Rh-negative and does not have antibodies, then *anti-D immunoglobuline* at the time of the injury protects against rhesus allo-immunisation as a result of a possible feto-maternal haemorrhage.

Maternal cardiac arrest

Maternal cardiac arrest may occur in the presence of an amniotic fluid embolism, eclampsia or drug toxicity. It may also occur during a motor vehicle accident, assault or when there has been a penetrating injury.

Immediate management of a cardiac arrest

▶ Place the woman in the left lateral position.

▶ Administer 100% oxygen by face mask.

▶ Administer a fluid bolus commencing with a crystalloid infusion such as Ringer's lactate and then change to a colloid infusion (Haemacell®). However, this does depend on the preference of the medical team and the possibility of underlying pregnancy-related diseases such as pre-eclampsia.

▶ Re-evaluate the need for any drugs being administered.

When performing cardiopulmonary resuscitation (CPR) on a pregnant woman, consideration must be given to her period of gestation because during the third trimester chest compressions are ineffective when the woman lies on her back. This is because the gravid uterus blocks the return of blood from the inferior vena cava. In order to overcome this problem, a wedge can be placed under her right side to tilt her right buttock and decrease the pressure on the inferior vena cava. The standard procedures of CPR should be performed and advanced cardiac life support measures instituted to ensure survival of both the woman and her fetus.

When the woman is in irreversible cardiac arrest, the decision to perform a postmortem caesarean section (PCS) must be made. The caesarean section should be performed while CPR is in progress and as soon after maternal death as possible.

Abnormalities of the genital tract: Cervical intraepithelial neoplasia

Cervical intraepithelial neoplasia (CIN) is probably the most commonly diagnosed abnormality of the cervix during pregnancy. CIN is the pre-invasive stage of carcinoma of the cervix, sometimes referred to as stage 0. At this stage the condition may either regress or progress.

CIN is usually diagnosed in a younger age group of women than invasive carcinoma – women who are usually of childbearing age. Whilst pregnancy does have an effect on the cellular structure of the cervix, this alteration in the cell structure can be differentiated from the abnormal cellular structure of CIN.

CIN is usually diagnosed during pregnancy when the woman has a routine Papanicolaou's smear taken at her booking or first visit. When the results of the smear reveal CIN, it is not treated during pregnancy. Instead, the woman is alerted to the findings but she should be made aware that it is not an indication for a caesarean section. What is important for her to understand is that she must have a repeat Papanicolaou's smear six weeks after the delivery. Explain that after delivery her condition may have regressed and a negative result is possible. However, it may also have progressed and further treatment will depend on the result of the postnatal smear. It is also important to reassure her that pregnancy does not affect the condition.

Classification of CIN

The condition is classified as follows:

▶ *Mild dysplasia:* Immature cells are present in the deep zone.
▶ *Moderate dysplasia:* Immature cells are present both in the deep zone and in part of or throughout the intermediate zone.
▶ *Severe dysplasia:* Immature cells are present in the deep and intermediate zones and in the deeper half of the superficial zone.
▶ *Carcinoma in situ:* Immature cells and mitotic figures are found in all layers of the epithelium and the architecture of the epithelium is totally disrupted. There is no sign of invasion of the underlying stroma.

In a nutshell

▶ Some medical or surgical conditions may be aggravated by the pregnancy, such as cardiac disease and diabetes mellitus. Others, such as epilepsy, may actually appear to improve, whilst others remain unaffected.
▶ It is the responsibility of the midwife to take a careful and thorough antenatal history and to be alert to the influence that the physiological changes of pregnancy may have on the condition. In this regard the midwife must in particular be aware of her Scope of Practice, and sources of referral.
▶ The management of these women calls for team management, in which the midwife will frequently play the role of the primary caregiver.
▶ These women all require additional support and encouragement during their pregnancy, labour and puerperium.

References

American Heart Association. 2000. Guidelines for Cardiopulmonary Resuscitation and Emergency Cardiovascular Care. *Circulation*, supplement 102(8): I 247–I 249.

Bassin, J. (Ed.) 1994. *Topics in obstetrics and gynaecology*. Johannesburg: Julmar Communications.

Boulvain, M., Stan, C. & Irion, O. 2002. Elective delivery in diabetic pregnant women. *Cochrane Review*. http://www.updatesoftware.com/ccweb/cochrane/revabstr.

Clayton, S. G., Lewis, T. L. T. & Pinker, G.

1980. *Obstetrics by ten teachers*. London: Edward Arnold Publishers.

Cronjé, H. S., Grobler, C. J. F. & Visser, A. A. 1996. *Obstetrics in Southern Africa*. Pretoria: J.L. van Schaik Publishers.

DoH (Department of Health). 2002. *Guidelines for maternity care in South Africa*. Second edition. Pretoria: DoH.

DoH (Department of Health). 2002. *Saving mothers: Second report on confidential enquiries into maternal deaths in South Africa 1999–2001*. Pretoria: DoH.

Dox, I. G., Melloni, B. J. & Eisner, G. M. 1985. *The Harper Collins illustrated medical dictionary*. New York: Harper Collins Publishers.

Jewell, D. & Young, G. 2002 Interventions for nausea and vomiting in early pregnancy. *Cochrane Review*. http://www.update-software.com/ccweb/cochrane.revabstr.

Jewell, D. & Young, G. 2002. Interventions for treating constipation in pregnancy. *Cochrane Review*. http://www.updatesoftware.com/abstracts.

Ladewig, P. A., London, M. L. & Olds, S. B. 1998. *Maternal–Newborn nursing care*. Menlo Park California: Addison-Wesley Publishers.

Mahomed, K. 2002. Iron supplementation in pregnancy. *Cochrane Review*.

http://www.update-software.com/abstracts.

May, K. A. & Mahlmeister, L. R. 1994. *Maternal and neonatal nursing: Family-centred care*. Third edition. Philadelphia: J.B. Lippincott.

McQuillan, K. A., Von Ruenden, K. T., Flynn, M. B. & Whalen, E. 2002. *Trauma nursing: From resuscitation through rehabilitation*. Third edition. Philadelphia: W.B. Saunders.

Nash, P. & Driscoll, P. 2000. Trauma in Pregnancy. In: Driscoll, P., Skinner, D. & Earlam, R. (Eds.) *ABC of major trauma*. Third edition. London: BMJ Books.

National Committee on Confidential Enquiries into Maternal Deaths. 2000. Third Interim Report on Confidential Enquiries into Maternal Deaths in South Africa. Pretoria: Department of Health.

Oxorn, H. 1986. *Human labor and birth*. Fifth edition. London: Appleton-Century-Crofts.

Sellers, P. M. 1993. *Midwifery*. Volume 2. Kenwyn: Juta & Co.

Young, G. L. & Jewell, D. 2002. Creams for preventing stretch marks in pregnancy. *Cochrane Library*. http://www.updatesoftware.com/ccweb/cochrane/revabstr.

Chapter 23

Women and families with special needs in pregnancy

Joan Dippenaar

Introduction

The developed and developing worlds meet in South Africa, and create a multicultural society with a kaleidoscope of lifestyles, beliefs and practices. Concepts of sexuality, pregnancy and childbirth within these societies differ, as do healthcare practices. Religious and cultural beliefs in combination with demographic, economic, and political factors create the determinants for outcomes of health in all societies. As poverty levels in South Africa as a developing country remain high in spite of a stable economy, the health of the largest portion of the population will be affected.

The White Paper (Notice 667, 1997) states that 35 to 55% of the South African population lives in poverty. Of these 73% are women and children, and 75% live in rural areas. The infant mortality rate (IMR) and maternal mortality rate (MMR) are associated with these factors. In this complex situation the South African midwife will encounter women and families with special needs in different societies. Special needs arise from risk factors, which may be due to personal lifestyle or community circumstances and they can have an adverse effect on health outcomes. The aim of this chapter is to create awareness of the

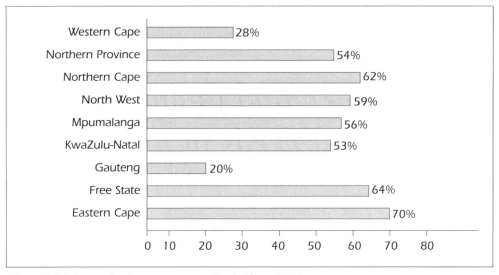

Figure 23.1 Poverty levels per province in South Africa, 2001

categories of special needs most commonly encountered in South Africa in the pregnant population. These cases require early identification and appropriate effective intervention to ensure the best possible outcomes. Women presenting with special needs are at risk and should be referred to level 2 or 3 hospitals or to specialised private care.

Needs related to maternal age

The ideal biological time for childbirth is when the woman is between 19 to 35 years of age. In our postmodern society pregnancy often occurs outside these time periods due to a variety of factors.

Early motherhood

Early motherhood, which is also referred to as 'adolescent pregnancy', is pregnancy at any time before 18 complete years of age, which means between 10 to 19 years of age. The age at which young people become sexually active varies between societies and countries. In both developed and developing countries the incidence of adolescent pregnancies is mainly determined by the availability and effective use of contraceptives. Socioeconomic factors

and cultural behaviour also play an important part in determining the rate of adolescent pregnancies. The United States of America (USA) has the highest incidence of adolescent pregnancy in the developed world while Japan has the lowest. The USA reports an inconsistent use of contraceptives by young women as the causal factor.

Although the use of contraceptives among women aged 15 to 19 years in South Africa is high for a developing country, the incidence of adolescent pregnancy is still, however, as high as 35% (350 per 1 000), as reported by the South African Demographic and Health Survey (SADHS, 1998). This is believed to be due to low levels of education and the socio-economic factors caused by urban and rural living. The risks for adolescent pregnancy are aggravated by poverty. Sexually active adolescents in this survey reported a 75% use of a modern family planning method (injection method 50%) and also demonstrated a 95% awareness of HIV/AIDS.

Obstetric risks associated with early motherhood

The birth rate for adolescents aged 18 to 19 years is more than twice that for 15 to 16 year olds, indicating that most young women are likely to fall pregnant after age 16. In pregnant women of 15 years and younger only two complications are common, namely hypertensive disease and contracted pelvic inlet (resulting in cephalopelvic disproportion). One in eight deliveries in this group is by caesarean section (12.5 per 100 deliveries).

Nutritional risks

In young women under 18 years with incomplete physiological development, pregnancy adds a nutritional burden on the growth and development of the adolescent as well as the unborn baby. Due to poverty and the poor eating habits of young people, malnutrition develops which results in complications such as abortions, haemorrhage, preterm birth, anaemia, infections and hypertensive disorders.

Economic risks

Adolescents are generally not yet economically independent, well established or self-sufficient. If education is interrupted the adolescent mother may not have the economic ability to care for herself and her baby and this may lead to poor physical and psychological development of the child, or may even result in abuse or abandonment. Furthermore, adolescent mothers tend to have more children during their lifespan and their daughters subsequently also have early pregnancies. Early

> ### Research highlight
>
> The 1998 SADH survey report on adolescent health in South Africa states that:
> - Only 3% of pregnant adolescents indicated that they were married.
> - 60% were sexually active in the last year prior to this survey.
> - Most women experience their first sexual intercourse at the age of 18 years.
> - 35% have been or were pregnant at the age of 19 years.
> - The incidence of adolescent pregnancy is highest among girls of colour from disadvantaged rural communities with lower education levels.

motherhood thus poses risks for the adolescent, her partner, family, child and the community and it has a negative impact on their education opportunities, economic potential and social development. South African society found to be burdened by early motherhood, as it is a developing country with high poverty and unemployment rates. It is also a strain on the country's healthcare resources and the growing economy. However, in societies with a negative population growth like Norway and Australia, early motherhood is now encouraged.

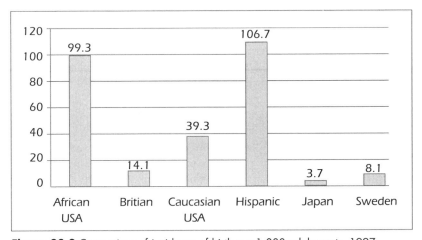

Figure 23.2 Comparison of incidence of birth per 1 000 adolescents, 1997

Risks for impaired social development

The social development and the transition to adulthood of young women are found to be adversely affected by early motherhood as it forces them into the development tasks of early adulthood, often resulting in social and psychological strains. Researchers have described a 10-year delay in maturity and readiness for parenthood in countries of the developed world. Such a development delay would also be applicable to a percentage of the South African adolescents. The underprivileged and poor communities are even more disadvantaged due to other reasons. There is a high percentage of abandoned babies in South Africa, despite legalised abortion, and abandoned street children remain a constant social concern.

Advanced maternal age (AMA)

In certain sectors of society demographic changes have resulted in a decrease in early motherhood and an increase in the incidence of late in life first-time pregnancies. This contemporary trend, where women become pregnant in their twenties to fourties, is more prevalent in sectors of society that are developed, and where higher education levels are found. The term 'elderly primigravida' refers to a first-time pregnancy after the age of 35 years.

AMA for a first time pregnancy is associated with special risks for the woman and the fetus. A woman's entire lifetime supply of ova is completely developed at eight weeks in utero and held in a suspended state. Ovulation at 45 years of age means that the ova were dormant for 45 years, leading to a higher incidence of chromosomal abnormalities. Other factors such as nutrition, drugs, smoking, alcohol and radiation, however, are also contributing factors for mutations.

Other risk factors to be considered for this age group are the increased chronic diseases associated with age, such as diabetes, hypertension and fibroids. However, older women seem better equipped for the tasks of motherhood both socially and economically. The Second Report on Confidential Enquiries into Maternal Deaths in South Africa found an increased risk for maternal death after the age of 35 (1999–2001:5).

Needs related to infertility

Artificial Reproductive Technology (ART)

Infertility is the failure to fall pregnant after one year of coitus. Delayed pregnancy can be caused by infertility or sterility. Couples may resort to technological medical advances (ART) to conceive their own genetic child or a child genetically related to one of them. A third party may be added to the equation and an egg or sperm donation or surrogacy is available at special centres. The midwife should be informed about the special emotional and psychological needs associated with infertility and the options available to provide the necessary support and guidance for these couples. The emotional strain that infertility causes can have a profoundly negative effect on both the mental health and personal relationships of couples trying to conceive.

Adoption and surrogacy

Adoption and surrogacy are other options available to childless couples. However, there has been a decline in availability of babies for adoption in South Africa. Legal adoption is not yet practiced in all South African cultures and the illegal stealing of babies does occur (Child Care Amendment Act No. 13 of 1999

The risk of Down's syndrome

The risk of giving birth to a child with Down's syndrome increases with maternal age. Women aged 45 are 100 times more likely than women under 19 years to give birth to babies with mutations and abnormal development. The global incidence of having a child with Down's syndrome is 1 per 800 births, yet the incidence in an African rural population was found to be 16,8 per 800 births.

Source: Pistorius, Pelser & Christianson, 1999.

Section 18). Giving up a baby for legal adoption requires the involvement of a social worker and it is a decision that has a lifelong effect on all those involved. 'Open adoption' arrangements allow the mother some information and contact with the child. Adopting parents are often desperate and unfortunately they can easily be exploited. Adoptions are legal procedures and parents go through a selection process.

Surrogacy is when a women bears a child which is not genetically her own through ART. Currently there are two types of surrogacy, namely partial and full surrogacy. In partial surrogacy the mother shares the genetic code of the child. The issues of adoption, ART, and surrogacy and their occurance in society are ethical, legal and highly emotional. Midwives who practise in this field are usually specially trained for this purpose and have a thorough knowledge of these issues and their legal aspects.

A first for South Africa

South Africa had the world's first surrogate grandmother. On 1 Oct 1987 Pat Anthony became the first woman to give birth to her daughter's children, the Karen Ferreira-Jorge's triplets.

Source: Editors Inc., 2001.

Needs related to parity

Primigravida (Nullipara)

First-time pregnancies are always considered to be at risk, regardless of maternal age or other contributing factors. All primigravidae should be encouraged to deliver in a hospital because of the lack of previous obstetrical history. In such cases the outcomes for labour are often unsure and are usually predicted within the parameters of age, nutrition, habits, socioeconomic background and the clinical information gathered during pregnancy. Primigravidae often have longer labours with an increased need for pain relief and there is a tendency for a higher incidence of abnormal

---

Record number of children

The greatest official record of number of children produced by one woman is 69 (Moscow). In 27 deliveries she bore 16 sets of twins, seven sets of triplets and four sets of quadruplets. Of the 69 children 67 survived infancy.

Source: Guinness Book of Records, 1988:13.

---

uterine action with increased surgical interventions. The Second Report on Confidential Enquiries into Maternal Deaths in South Africa found an increased risk for maternal deaths in primigravidae (1999–2001:5). This does not mean that the primigravida's pregnancy and childbirth should not be approached in a natural way.

Grande multiparity

The grande multipara is a woman who has given birth to five or more viable children. Risks for the grande multipara in pregnancy are associated with age, socioeconomic factors, nutrition and the availability of healthcare. The maternal mortality is twice as high as that of the lower parity population and increases with each consecutive pregnancy.

Risk factors more common in the grande multipara

▶ Multiple pregnancies.
▶ Obesity.
▶ Hypertensive condition.
▶ Diabetes mellitus.
▶ Anaemia.
▶ Preterm labour.
▶ Antepartum haemorrhage and placenta praevia.
▶ Abnormal lie and presentation (e.g. breech presentation and transverse lie) with increased cord prolapse.
▶ Increased mean birth weight with increased operative interventions.
▶ Postpartum haemorrhage, uterus rupture and retained placenta.

Due to the increased risk of perinatal mortality and morbidity the woman should deliver in a level 2 or 3 hospital with neonatal intensive care facilities.

Needs related to nutrition

Pregnancy is a unique period in life and the nutritional status prior to and during pregnancy significantly influences the wellbeing and outcome for both woman and fetus. Aaronson and Macnee describe a correlation between fetal mass and maternal weight gain independent of the level of nutrition as recalled by mothers (1989:223). The assessment of pre-pregnancy weight, weight gain and nutrition during pregnancy is essential. A pre-pregnancy weight that is less than 85% of the standard weight for height should be considered a risk during pregnancy. Without complications the pattern of weight gain on the antenatal chart is a good indicator of the growth and wellbeing of the fetus.

Underweight

The history of the pre-pregnancy weight of the woman should be determined at the first antenatal clinic visit. For this reason, visiting the clinic for the first time late in pregnancy can have a negative impact on a woman's healthcare. If a woman has limited physical resources and reserves prior to pregnancy, her health and that of the fetus may be at risk. Particularly in the third trimester, problems such as intra-uterine growth restriction (IUGR), fetal distress with meconium, stillbirth and fetal abnormalities may occur. A complete history which includes nutritional information may reveal any nutritional shortcomings. It is uncertain whether calcium supplementation prevents pre-eclampsia. The World Health Organisation recommends vitamin A supplementation to prevent anaemia during pregnancy (Villkar & Gulmezoglu, 1998).

Obesity

Obesity is defined as 120% weight for standard height or a maternal weight of 90 kg or more. This is the upper normal limit (not considering the height) during pregnancy. Women presenting with obesity in pregnancy are usually older and they are at increased risk of hypertension and diabetes mellitus. In the absence of such complicating factors, there is no evidence of a higher incidence of maternal or perinatal mortality or morbidity due to obesity. Major surgery for obese pregnant women has been associated with an increased risk of intra- and post-operative morbidity and complications. In particular the risk of infection, thrombosis or problems related to anaesthesia may be further complicated by existing medical problems, and, if present, the woman should be delivered in a specialised maternity unit. Babies born to obese women are usually large for gestational age but healthy unless complicating factors were present.

Needs related to mental health and social behaviour

Substance abuse or dependence

Regardless of the type of drug used in pregnancy the health of the woman and the fetus will be at risk in drug-dependant women. The degree of placental permeability depends on the chemical properties and molecular weight of the drug and whether it is used alone or in combination with other drugs. Commonly used substances are alcohol, cocaine, crack, marijuana, amphetamines, barbiturates, hallucinogens, heroin, caffeine and nicotine. Marijuana contains 400 complex chemicals and it interferes with the production of hormones which are critical for sexual and reproductive development. Drugs used during pregnancy are found in the same concentration in the baby's blood stream as in the mother's blood stream and they cause respiratory and cardiovascular suppression in the baby. Hallucinogens like LSD are known to be teratogenic.

A comprehensive team approach is needed to secure the safe outcome for both the woman and the fetus. It is the task of the midwife to identify these cases early during antenatal care and to evaluate all the medical, socioeconomic and legal aspects involved. The fetus is at great risk and should be monitored throughout the pregnancy, and the baby should be delivered in a maternity unit with neonatal intensive care facilities.

Alcohol in pregnancy

The abuse of alcohol is the most common drug problem in society, also among women. There are no determined safe levels of alcohol intake during conception and pregnancy, therefore women should avoid consuming alcohol when pregnant or during conception. Fetal alcohol syndrome (FAS) is therefore a preventable condition and caregivers should educate women to avoid the use of alcohol to prevent the adverse fetal alcohol effects (FAE).

The term FAS has been applied to a variety of problems exhibited by neonates after birth due to the use of alcohol during pregnancy. The quantity and frequency of alcohol intake appears to be an important factor, however, research has documented cases where despite equal alcohol consumption by women, some babies develop FAS while others do not.

Mental retardation is the single most serious problem associated with alcohol use in pregnancy and although babies may not present with full-blown FAS other FAE may be present that adversely affect the child for life.

Research highlight

It was reported that the highest incidence of FAS in the world occurs in the Western Cape and 7.5% (75 per 1 000 births) of the children born in this community are affected. Women between the ages of 21–29 seem to be mostly affected. The incidence in four other high-risk areas in Gauteng are:

▶ Soweto 2.2%
▶ Lenasia 1.2%
▶ Westbury 3.7%

Source: DoH survey for birth defects and disability (Viljoen et al, 2001)

The potential effects of alcohol use

▶ Two or more drinks per day: An increased risk for intra-uterine growth restriction (IUGR), decreased placental weight, immature motor activity/tone, poor sucking and stillbirth.

▶ Four or more drinks per day: An increased risk for structural brain abnormalities.

▶ Six or more drinks per day: An increased risk for FAS.

▶ Women who do not usually use alcohol on a regular basis but who binge occasionally in early pregnancy, or while not knowing that they are pregnant, are at high risk for FAS.

Nicotine (Tobacco)

More women than men now smoke. Smoking is also found to be more addictive in women. Most smokers start the habit between the ages of 14 and 19 years and 10% of adolescents in South Africa are smoking. A written health warning on all cigarette products in South Africa alerts the population to the dangers of smoking in pregnancy.

Domestic violence

The first global report on violence and health was released by the WHO on 2 October 2002 and it recognises violence as a global health problem. Violence occurs in all professional, occupational, ethnic and socioeconomic groups. Community, cultural and other external factors create a situation in which violence can occur but it can be prevented. It is women who face the highest risk for domestic violence and abuse. In South Africa 25% of women suffer sexual violence from a partner. Furthermore, every six days a woman is murdered by her husband or boyfriend in South Africa. According to the Act on Domestic Violence (1999) all women and children in South Africa must be protected against all forms of violence.

Effects of nicotine in pregnancy

When smoking a cigarette the levels of nicotine in the blood peak at 14 to 41 ng/ml depending on the way in which the woman smokes. Depth and length of inhalation will also affect nicotine blood levels. The nicotine is then reabsorbed in the fetus and this results in an increase in fetal heart rate. Nicotine is also secreted in the breast milk for a period of 7 to 8 hours after smoking the last cigarette.

The most common effect of regular smoking on the fetus is IUGR with the average reduction of weight for a baby of a regular smoker being at 200 g. There is a relation between the number of cigarettes smoked and the severity of IUGR. Smoking 11 or more cigarettes per day also increases the risk for spontaneous abortion by 16.7%. The greatest risk for abortion of the fetus is during the first trimester but the effects are most potent in the last trimester when the CNS (central nervous system) develops. Midwives should encourage pregnant women to stop smoking and use effective cessation of smoking programmes that do not include the use of nicotine patches.

Positive changes that occur when a woman stops smoking during pregnancy include improved fetal weight and improved placental function. There is also a lower risk of respiratory distress and sudden infant death syndrome (SIDS) after birth.

The underlying characteristics predisposing women to violence are identifiable. Injured women are often seen in obstetric units because violence frequently starts or occurs during pregnancy. It has been shown that women who have suffered physical violence during pregnancy have a three times greater chance of dying from future physical abuse than any other women. Clinics should have a policy and protocol in place for the recognition, counselling, referral and follow-up care for these women to prevent future deaths. Midwives can intervene in the cycle of violence by helping women to recognise their options and to take appropriate action. Parenting classes, conflict management and social programmes can all assist in combating violence in the family and community.

Psychiatric disorders

Midwives play an important role in the promotion of mental healthcare, whether it be through primary healthcare, problem identification, intervention and the coordination of care or through educating women in self-care. The development of a child can be seriously impaired if the mother suffers from depression in the first year of life. According to the WHO, the 10 to 15% incidence of depression during pregnancy is similar to that in the non-pregnant women population (WHO technical report, 1998). A normal pregnancy add 40 points on a scale of hundred stresses, as indicated on the 'Life event stressor scale', and under normal circumstances this stress may be tolerated. However, a compromised pregnancy will add to an already stressful situation and psychological problems such as depression are a common occurrence. Depression may already be identified in pregnancy but it often only presents in the postnatal period, when stress levels are increased, as postpartum depression. Postpartum depression is a classified mental health condition and 25% of

---

Risks indicators for mental disease

▶ A previous history of depression.
▶ Lack of support from the partner or family.
▶ Complications during the pregnancy.
▶ The loss of her own mother when she was a child.
▶ The accumulation of various misfortunes, bereavement, post-traumatic stress, job loss, housing and money problems can all predispose a woman to ill mental health.

---

pregnant women suffer from it to some degree. Symptoms may include insomnia, irritability, tearfulness, poor concentration, poor appetite, restlessness, being over-emotional, tearfulness, forgetfulness, emotional withdrawal, antisocial behaviour, tension, disorientation, anxiety, over-dependence and suicidal thoughts. Sometimes a person may lose the ability to take pleasure in things previously enjoyed.

Postpartum psychosis is a very serious condition that occurs in one in every 500 pregnancies. Women who harm their babies (referred to as non-accidental injury) have often been emotionally damaged or ill-treated themselves. Infanticide by a severely mentally disturbed mother due to this condition is very rare but it can be prevented through early recognition and treatment of women with psychiatric problems in pregnancy. Women suffering from puerperal psychosis lose contact with reality, which results in the neglect of their babies.

Women with a history of mental disease not related to pregnancy like schizophrenia, mental retardation, bipolar affective disorders or suicidal tendencies have special needs when pregnant. However, thorough antenatal history-taking and early identification with appropriate intervention can result in optimum outcomes for both mother and baby.

Needs related to physical disabilities

Female genital mutilation

Although female genital mutilation (FGM) is not practised in South Africa, midwives increasingly come into contact with refugees and migrating women from neighbouring African and some Asian countries. An estimated two million girls between the ages of five and eight years undergo the cultural ritual every year in Central and North Africa (26 countries). This practice is condemned and discouraged by the WHO in a joint statement with UNICEF, the International Association for Obstetricians and the International Confederation for Midwives as it

---

Classification of FGM

▶ *Type 1:* Excision of the prepuce with or without the excision of the clitoris.
▶ *Type 2:* Excision of the clitoris with partial or total excision of the labia minora.
▶ *Type 3:* Excision of part or all of the external genital organs and stitching or narrowing of the vaginal opening.
▶ *Type 4:* Unclassified – pricking, piercing, stretching, cauterising and scraping of tissue. The introduction of corrosive substances or herbs for tightening or narrowing of the vagina, or any other procedure.

---

impacts negatively on the physical and psychological wellbeing of women and girls. Several studies link FGM as a contributing or causal factor for maternal death, as well as stillbirths and neonatal deaths.

When FGM is encountered the midwife should note and determine the extent of the mutilation as early as possible. A vaginal delivery is possible if the woman has had a

---

Effects of FGM on pregnancy and childbirth

▶ A fear of labour.
▶ An inability to fall pregnant (surgical opening for sexual intercourse must take place).
▶ Spontaneous abortion.
▶ Products of conception may be retained.
▶ Vaginal and urinary tract infections.
▶ Problems in voiding.
▶ The constant contamination of urine with protein results in difficulty in diagnosing the degree of pre-eclampsia.
▶ Type 3 FGM will cause mechanical barrier, obstructed labour or severe perineal lacerations.
▶ Postpartum haemorrhage due to perineal and other trauma.
▶ Painful episiotomies.

good outcome in a previous delivery, the urinary orifice can be seen or if the vagina allows two fingers without discomfort. A vaginal opening of less than 1 cm poses a major risk for abnormal labour or perineal floor damage. Safe opening can be done at all levels by trained staff and the WHO suggests that enlargement should occur at 28 weeks of pregnancy if needed to allow enough time for healing before the delivery. It is also recommended that women with Type 3 FGM deliver in a hospital assisted by a doctor or competent midwife. Opening before birth and restoring after birth does take place in some communities, however, the WHO considers it unethical for a health professional to restore women to an unacceptable level of functionality after birth. The most important role of the midwife is that of educator regarding the physiological and psychosexual consequences of the practice.

Other physical disabilities

The midwife may care for women who have physical disabilities such as sight impairment and blindness, hearing impairment and deafness, paraplegia and physical deformity. Each disability will affect the needs of the woman and family differently in pregnancy and birth and will require special intervention from healthcare providers. For example, research has described that babies of mute and deaf mothers cry less due to less verbal stimulation. The physical care of the babies of mothers that are in wheelchairs needs to be planned and each case where there is disability has special considerations for safety measures, breastfeeding practices, mother-child bonding and care for normal development of the baby. For example, the mentally impaired woman would need constant supervision and support if the pregnancy is continued. The midwife as primary contact and caregiver should develop evidence-based protocols and standards for the care of each category of disabled pregnant women and involve the families and community resources where possible to ensure a positive outcome.

Needs related to life-threatening conditions and treatment

Prolonged hospitalisation during pregnancy negatively impacts on the mental and social lives of the families and it is very costly. Women with a history of habitual abortions, antepartum haemorrhage (placenta praevia), multiple pregnancy and preterm labour, as well as certain cardiac and renal conditions may be hospitalised for prolonged periods of time because of the health risks for themselves or their unborn babies. Special care plans and considerations should be developed for the physical and emotional care of the families involved.

The Department of Health has suggested the institution of special units in the rural areas for women who need hospitalisation in order to minimise perinatal mortality as specialised units (level 3) are not available in all provinces. Women with severe life-threatening conditions should be admitted to a level 2 or 3 hospital with specialised neonatal care facilities.

Prolonged bed rest with its associated physical health risks, financial constrains, boredom and the separation from and concern for the wellbeing of the family can cause anxiety and mental strain. Flexible visiting hours, including allowing children to visit, should be considered for these families.

Conclusion

The presence of special needs or risks does not necessarily predict adverse outcomes in childbirth. However, factors such as inequity in healthcare, accessibility of healthcare, poor nutrition and lack of transport are still problematic in South Africa and they create further health risks for pregnant women. More than 10% of reported births take place outside hospitals and it is unclear who attends these births. The goal of the Safe Motherhood Programme is to ensure that all pregnant women receive care from a trained caregiver. Since 77% of antenatal care in South Africa is provided by midwives and only 30% of women are assisted by a medical practitioner during labour, the midwife is not only the technical expert in pregnancy care and labour but she also acts as an important agent of social change.

The Guidelines for Maternity care in South Africa (2002) do not detail standards of care for all situations and needs. It is therefore the duty of midwives themselves to continually upgrade practices and develop the best possible practices for pregnant women, particularly in areas where risks are increased. The challenge remains for South African midwives to fulfil their important role in their communities and to make a difference.

References

Aaronson, L. S. & Macnee, C. L. 1989. The relationship between weight gain and nutrition in pregnancy. *Nursing Research, July/August,* 38 (4):223.

Banks, P. 1991. Community based primary prevention of adolescent pregnancy. *Birth Defects,* 27(1):200–205.

Beck, C. T. 1998. A checklist to identify women at risk for developing postpartum depression. Principles and Practice. *Journal of Gynecologic and Neonatal Nursing,* January/February, 27(1):39–46.

Coley, R. L. & Chase, L. 2002. *Adolescent pregnancy and parenthood. Recent evidence, future direction.* http://www.questia.com. 15/11/2002.

DoH (Department of Health). 1997. *White Paper for the transformation of the Healthcare System in South Africa.* Notice 667 of 1997. Department of Health. 16 April 1997. Vol. 382: No 17910. Pretoria: Government Gazette.

DoH (Department of Health). 2002. *Guidelines for maternity care in South Africa.* Second edition. Pretoria: DoH.

DoH (Department of Health). *Saving mothers: Second report on confidential enquiries into maternal deaths in South Africa 1999–2001.* Pretoria: DoH.

Dippenaar, J. M. 2001. Amniocentesis and foetal surveillance. Unpublished research, Johannesburg.

Gitlin, J. H. 1988. *Surrogacy is one answer – assisted reproductive technology is the other.* http://www.aml.org/ART.htm. 25/11/2002.

Gunnar, T. & Bungum, L. 1987. The grande multipara. Maternal and neonatal complications. *Acta Obstetricia et Gynecologica Scandinavia,* 66:53-56.

Mansfield, P. K. 1986. *Pregnancy for older women. Assessing the medical risk.* http://www.questia.com. New York: Preager Publishers. 25/11/2002.

May, P. A. Brooke, L. Gossage, J. P. Croxford, J. Adnams, C. Jones, K. L. Robinson, L. Viljoen, D. 2000. Epidemiology of fetal alcohol syndrome in a South African community in the Western Cape Province. *American Journal of Public Health,* December 90(12):1905.

McFarlane, D. 1988. *The Guinness Book of Records.* England: Guinness Book Publishers.

Mills, L. 2000. Depression, Anxiety and Childbirth. *PNDSA Research.* http://www.phdsa.co.za/research.htm. 26/11/2002.

Minirth, F. Meier, P. & Arterburn, S. 1995. The Holmes-Rahe social readjustment scale. In: *The Complete Life Encyclopedia.* Thomas Nelson Publishers. http://www.personal.psu.edu/. 21/4/2004.

Neeson, J. D. & May, K. A. 1986. *Comprehensive maternity nursing.* London: J. B. Lippincott.

Nieberg, P. Marks, J. McLaren, N. & Remington, P. 1985. The fetal tobacco syndrome. *The Journal of the American Medical Association*, May, 253(20):2998.

South Africa. 1998. *Domestic Violence Bill. No. 116 of 1998.* http://www.gov.za/bills/1998. 21/4/2004.

South Africa. 1998. *Tobacco Products Control Amendment Bill. No. 12 of 1998.* http://www.gov.za/bills/1998. 21/4/2004.

Olds, S. B. London, M. C. & Ladewig, P. W. 1992. *Maternal and newborn nursing.* Fourth edition. California: Mosby.

Oxorn, H. 1986 *Human labour and birth.* Fifth edition. Connecticut: Prentice-Hall International.

Pistorius, L. R. & Christianson, A. C. 1995. Screening for Down syndrome. *South African Medical Journal*, September 85(9):934.

Pistorius, L. R. Pelzer, J. & Christianson, A. C. 1999. Down's syndrome in the Black Population. Why so many? Why so old? Pretoria University, 13 May 1999. Research abstract presented at the Foetal Society meeting. Johannesburg.

SADHS (South African Demographic Health Survey). 1998. *Adolescent Health*, http://www.adolescent health. 14/11/2003.

Sheehy, G. 1997. *New Passages. Mapping your life across time.* London: Haper Collins.

South Africa at a glance. History, Politics, Economy, Trade, Tourism & Statistics. 2000–2001. Johannesburg: Editors Inc.

Stanford, D. 2002. Post-natal depression. *International Journal of Childbirth Education*, March, 17(1):10.

Statistics South Africa. 2002. *Recorded live births 2002.* Release P0305. Pretoria. http://www.statssa.gov.za. 30/7/2002.

The Royal College of Psychiatrists. 2002. *Postnatal depression: Help is at hand.* http://www.rxpsych.ac.uk/info/help/ pndep/. 4/10/2002.

Townsend, J. 2000. Impact of smoking on health. *Centre of Research in Primary and Community Care.* http://www.who/entity/tobacco/resources. 30/8/2000.

Villar, J. & Gulmezoglo, A. M. 1998. Maternal health. *Annual technical WHO report*, 172-181. Geneva. WHO.

Woller-Clear, K. 2002. *Surrogate mothers and the law.* http://www.hasa.co.za.issues_of_the_day.asp 15/11/ 2002.

WHO (World Health Organisation). 2002. *First Global report on violence and health release.* 3 October. Geneva. www.who.int/violence_injuryprevention. 15/11/2002.

WHO. (World Health Organisation). 1997. *Female genital mutilation.* A joint WHO/UNICEF/INFPA statement. http://www.who.int/docstore/frh-whd/pub-lication. Gender & Women's Health Department. 15/11/2002.

WHO (World Health Organisation). 2001. *Management of pregnancy, childbirth and the postpartum period in the presence of female genital mutilation.* Report of a WHO Technical Consultation. 15–17 October 1997. Gender & Women's Health Department. http://www.WHO/FCH/GWH/01.2 WHO/RHR/01.13.15/11/2002.

Chapter *24*

The compromised fetus

Dr Lou Pistorius

Introduction

Although pregnancy is usually a normal event, several problems can compromise the well-being of the fetus. It is important to be aware of these conditions and the specific medical and psychological needs of the pregnant woman with a compromised fetus.

The news that there is a potential problem with her expected baby (i.e. a compromised fetus) is emotionally traumatic for the pregnant woman. The degree of the reaction may differ but the normal grief reaction follows from news about fetal compromise, and not only from perinatal death. A grief reaction usually follows the sequence of shock and disbelief, anger, intense grief and guilt, equilibrium and depression, and finally reorganisation and acceptance. The psychological management will be discussed in more detail in Chapter 28 but the same basic principles apply.

Intra-uterine growth restriction (IUGR)

It is better to refer to 'growth restriction' rather than 'growth retardation', as many women make a subconscious connection between 'growth retardation' and 'mental retardation'. A small baby is not necessarily a growth restricted baby: a baby can be constitutionally small, and be perfectly healthy. Or a baby can be growth restricted and in potential danger, while its weight could still be within the normal range. Until growth restriction is firmly diagnosed, it is more accurate to refer to a 'small for dates' fetus.

Detection of small for dates fetuses

At the follow-up antenatal visits, fetal growth should be monitored routinely. This is ideally done through accurate and graphic assessment of the symphysis-fundal height, combined with careful history taking and a general and obstetrical examination. The use of landmarks like relating the uterine fundus to the maternal umbilicus and measuring the space between the uterine fundus and the maternal xiphisternum should not be used, as it is too inaccurate. A series of ultrasounds may be done, ideally commencing around the 16th to 22nd week of gestation. However, this is expensive and generally not available at the primary health level where the majority of South Africans receive antenatal care. The technique of symphysis-fundal height (SFH) measurement is discussed in Chapter 10.

A small for dates fetus would be suspected if:

▶ There is a plateau in SFH-growth (with three subsequent measurements on the same level).
▶ The SFH-measurements fall below the 10th centile.
▶ The SFH-measurement falls below the second last measurement.

Measuring the maternal weight does not aid the detection of small for dates fetus.

Causes of small for dates fetuses

A small for dates fetus is not necessarily a fetus with intra-uterine growth restriction. Once incorrect pregnancy dating has been excluded, the most common causes of small for dates fetus can be classified as shown in Table 24.1.

Investigation of the small for dates fetus

If a small for dates fetus is detected, whether by clinical examination, SFH measurement, or ultrasound examination, the management would depend on the underlying cause. The following factors would be important.

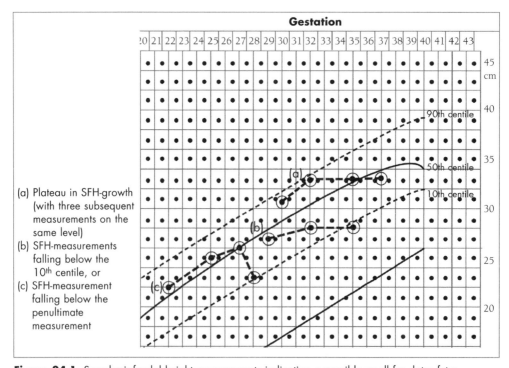

(a) Plateau in SFH-growth (with three subsequent measurements on the same level)
(b) SFH-measurements falling below the 10th centile, or
(c) SFH-measurement falling below the penultimate measurement

Figure 24.1 Symphysis-fundal height measurements indicating a possible small for dates fetus

Table 24.1 Causes of small for dates fetuses

Fetal causes	Placental causes	Maternal causes
▶ Constitutional (the normal small fetus). ▶ Congenital infection, e.g. syphilis and toxoplasmosis. ▶ Congenital abnormalities, e.g. chromosomal abnormalities such as Edward syndrome (trisomy 18).	▶ Maternal hypertension. ▶ Maternal auto-immune disease, e.g. lupus erythematosus. ▶ Maternal vascular disease, e.g. advanced diabetes mellitus.	▶ Smoking. ▶ Poor nutrition. ▶ Over-exercising and manual labour.

History and clinical examination

Look at the parents – if they are small boned or come from a cultural group which is characterised by short, fine-boned people then the intra-uterine growth of this fetus may be appropriate.

A history of smoking, heavy exercise, infections or medical problems should be sought. Try to find out whether the woman's diet is sufficient. Ask about a possible family history of congenital abnormalities. Check the blood pressure and urine (for protein and/or glucose).

Special investigations: General

Check the woman's syphilis, HIV and Rubella serology if it has not been done already, and consider checking serology for toxoplasmosis and cytomegalovirus. Findings on the history or clinical examination might warrant special investigations, such as serology for possible lupus, or fundoscopy in case of possible vascular disease.

Special investigations: Doppler and ultrasound

The single most important investigation is Doppler ultrasound of the umbilical artery (discussed later in this chapter). If the umbilical artery resistance index is normal (below the 95th centile), placental insufficiency is unlikely.

If the umbilical artery resistance index is increased, there is placental insufficiency. The fetus should be monitored more closely by

> **Research highlight**
>
> Meta-analysis of randomised controlled trials have confirmed that monitoring the small for dates fetus with Doppler ultrasound of the umbilical artery, with more intensive monitoring of the fetus with increased umbilical artery resistance index, has the following results:
> ▶ The perinatal mortality is reduced.
> ▶ There are fewer hospital admissions.
> ▶ There are less maternal interventions.
>
> *Source: Neilson & Alfirevic, 2001*

maternal monitoring of the fetal movements, and by means of fetal heart rate monitoring three times a week. If there is absent end diastolic flow in the umbilical artery, the woman must be admitted to hospital and the fetus should be monitored intensively by fetal heart rate monitoring three times a day. If persistent low variability is detected with fetal heart rate monitoring, the fetus should be delivered.

Ultrasound examination of the fetus can be useful to exclude congenital abnormalities, which can lead to fetal growth restriction. If there are ultrasound markers of fetal chromosomal abnormalities, an amniocentesis or fetal blood sample should be considered to exclude abnormalities such as Down's syndrome. Ultrasound markers of fetal chromosomal abnormalities include a thick fetal neck skin fold, short limbs and a single artery in the umbilical cord. The disadvantage of an amnio-centesis is the long time (up to three weeks) it takes to obtain the full chromosome report. A fetal blood sampling is more risky, but the results are available in a few days.

The ultrasound examination also helps to evaluate the fetal growth, and to confirm whether the fetus is really small for dates or not. Adjunctive signs of placental insufficiency would include oligohydramnios, asymmetric fetal growth (the abdominal size is relatively smaller than the skull size) and a calcified placenta. However, the Doppler assessment of the flow in the umbilical artery remains the most important way of excluding or confirming placental insufficiency. If placental insufficiency is diagnosed, the woman should be followed up as a high-risk pregnancy. If there is no placental insufficiency, the woman can be followed up routinely.

An inaccurate gestational age can lead to a false diagnosis of a small for dates fetus. If the woman presents late in her pregnancy, it can be difficult to determine the gestational age accurately. This, in turn, can make it difficult to determine whether a fetus is small for dates or not. The fetal growth can be followed up over time, which can help to determine whether the growth is normal or not. If there are risk factors (advanced maternal age, maternal hypertension, or a previous small for dates fetus or previous stillbirth) the woman should be referred for ultrasound and doppler ultrasound examination.

Up to date there is no good evidence that bed-rest during hospitalisation will promote fetal growth. High-protein supplementation is found to be harmful and should not be used.

Intra-uterine death (IUD)

IUD is defined as fetal death after fetal viability but the definition for viability can vary. In developing countries, viability is defined as 28 weeks of gestational age, or (where the gestational age is unknown or uncertain) a birth weight of more than 1 000 g. In developed countries, viability is defined as the 24th week of gestation, or a birth weight more than 500 g. In South Africa, the former definition is usually used, although the latter might be more appropriate in a setting with sufficient resources. Before viability, fetal death would be termed a missed abortion and a fetus born dead after viability is termed a stillbirth. It may be more appropriate to refer to first, second or third trimester fetal demise as this could be less distressing for the woman and her family than using the terms abortion or stillbirth.

Diagnosis of IUD

The pregnant woman might become aware of decreased or absent fetal movements, or the midwife might not find a fetal heart on auscultation or cardiotocograph (CTG) monitoring. If ultrasound is not available, clinical signs that are suggestive of fetal demise include:

- A symphysis-fundal height below the 5th centile.
- A boggy uterus where it is difficult to establish the fetal presentation.
- The fetal skull feels soft or demonstrates crepitus on palpation.

If it is available, it is important to do an ultrasound examination as soon as possible to confirm or exclude the possibility of an IUD.

CRITICAL THINKING EXERCISE

A pregnant woman visits the antenatal clinic for care of her third pregnancy. According to the history of her last normal menstruation, she is 28 weeks pregnant. On examination, the symphysis-fundal height (SFH) is 24 cm.

1. Where does the SFH fall on the SFH graph? What are the three main possibilities for this?
2. Which questions do you want to ask her?
3. Which other elements in the clinical examination are of importance?
4. Which special investigations would you like to suggest?

At ultrasound, the fetal heart should be checked quickly and efficiently, so as not to keep the woman in suspense. Ideally, the pregnant woman's partner should be present. If fetal death is confirmed, it should be communicated to the pregnant woman sympathetically and unambiguously. For example, tell her that the baby's heart has stopped beating, and that the baby has died. This is not the time to go into detail about possible causes, but the woman and her partner should have the chance to ask questions, and be reassured that it is not the result of anything she had done or not done. They should also be informed about what would happen next.

Care of the woman intrapartum

Not every woman with a fetal demise will want to terminate her pregnancy medically or surgically. Some will want to wait for spontaneous labour. If the woman prefers to await spontaneous labour, this is acceptable and she and her partner should be made aware that 80% of women with an IUD would go into labour spontaneously within three weeks. One third of women would, however, develop diffuse intravascular coagulopathy (DIC) if undelivered four to five weeks after the IUD. They should therefore be followed up with close attention to any laboratory signs of a coagulation problem. These laboratory signs include the platelet count, prothrombin time, partial thromboplastin time, fibrin split products and d-dimers. DIC is a potentially life-threatening condition and the woman will need intensive care and immediate delivery if DIC should develop.

Delivery

The baby can be delivered vaginally, or by means of a hysterotomy. A hysterotomy is an operation similar to a caesarean section, but to deliver a non-viable baby. If there is no contraindication to a vaginal delivery (such as previous uterine surgery), an induction and normal delivery is preferable. However, if the woman strongly prefers a hysterotomy, she should not be forced to go through a labour and delivery. Take time to ensure that she does not have an unrealistic fear of labour, as she does not need to have pain during the labour. An epidural block is an excellent form of pain relief but intravenous *morphine* (especially as an initial loading dose, followed by patient-controlled analgesia) is also a good option as there would be no concern (as in a normal labour) about the opiates causing neonatal respiratory depression. The woman should be managed in a ward separate from other pregnant women and newborn infants.

The woman's preference about the timing of the delivery should be taken into consideration as far as possible. Except for an IUD resulting from abruptio placentae, where the IUD would place the woman's health in jeopardy, there is no urgency to institute delivery. If she wishes to return home first, this is perfectly acceptable. However, she should not be left to go home alone. If her partner is not present at the time of the diagnosis of an IUD, he or a close friend or family member should be called to accompany her.

If the fetus has been dead for more than 24 hours in utero, it will show signs such as the skin peeling and softening of the organs due to autolysis. This is known as maceration.

Legal factors

After viability the birth has to be registered, a death certificate issued and a burial or cremation arranged by the family or by undertakers. If the pregnancy duration is unknown the birth weight should be used as indicator of viablility.

Causes of IUD

Some cases of IUD are unexplained but others can be categorised according to different causes as outlined in Table 24.2.

Investigating the possible causes of the intra-uterine death

The history is the most important aspect and the midwife should ask about previous miscarriages, stillbirths and other possible precipitating factors, such as bleeding, hypertension or infections.

Table 24.2 Causes of intra-uterine death (other than unexplained)

Fetal causes	Placental causes	Maternal causes	Obstetric causes
▶ Congenital abnormalities, e.g. chromosomal abnormalities and cardiac abnormalities. ▶ Congenital infection, e.g. syphilis or chorio-amnionitis. (HIV/AIDS can predispose to an infection but it does not cause an IUD directly.)	▶ Abruptio placentae. ▶ Cord accident, e.g. torsion or knotting of the umbilical cord. ▶ Chronic placental insufficiency, e.g. intra-uterine growth restriction or post-term pregnancy. ▶ Advanced extra-uterine pregnancy.	▶ Diabetes mellitus. ▶ Hypertension. ▶ Auto-immune diseases. ▶ Rhesus allo-immunisation.	▶ Birth trauma, e.g. breech or shoulder dystocia. ▶ Intrapartum hypoxia, e.g. cord prolapse.

Scrutinise the antenatal chart to look for missed clues, such as positive syphilis serology, increased or decreased fetal growth, hypertension, proteinuria or glucosuria, or post-term pregnancy.

Examine the woman for hypertension, hyperglycaemia (if the baby has been dead more than 24 hours, this should be done by obtaining glycosylated haemoglobin levels), feto-maternal bleeding (using a Kleihauer test) and infections such HIV. HIV/AIDS increases the risk of intra-uterine death fourfold. The maternal blood group should also be tested and an indirect Coombs done.

The baby should then be examined as follows:
▶ Measure the length, head circumference and weight.
▶ Look for signs of hydrops, or congenital abnormalities.
▶ Do an X-ray of the whole baby to look for abnormalities associated with congenital infections or skeletal dysplasia.
▶ Obtain the fetal kariotype by means of an axillary skin biopsy placed in a sterile container with normal saline.
▶ If possible, arrange a postmortem examination.

▶ Examine the placenta for signs of abruption (a blood clot indenting the maternal surface of the placenta) or dysmaturity (a small, calcified placenta).
▶ Examine the membranes for signs of meconium staining (indicating fetal hypoxia or post-term pregnancy) or infection (by taking a swab for bacteriological culture between the two layers of the membranes).
▶ Examine the umbilical cord for signs of cord entanglement: this can only be diagnosed as a cause of intra-uterine demise if there is venous engorgement on one side of a possible obstruction and a collapsed cord on the other side.
▶ Measure the length of the cord.
▶ Make sure there are three vessels in the cord as two vessels can be indicative of other congenital abnormalities.

Physical and psychological care of the woman after an IUD

The physical care of the woman will be the same as any other postnatal woman. Lactation may be suppressed with *bromocriptine* (2.5 mg twice daily for fourteen days) or *cabergoline* (1 mg stat). The latter is more expensive but it has fewer side effects. Some women require no medication at all to stop lactation.

The psychological wellbeing of the woman is an important aspect of the midwifery management and the emotional experience of the parents and the supporting role of the midwife are comprehensively discussed in Chapter 28. This includes showing the baby to the parents and collecting memory items.

Rhesus allo-immunisation and fetal anaemia

Rhesus allo-immunisation (also called iso-immunisation) develops where a Rhesus negative woman produces antibodies against the Rhesus positive red cells of her fetus. The immune response only develops when a sufficient amount of fetal cells appear in the woman's blood stream and trigger the response. The typical time when sufficient fetal red cells would appear in the maternal blood stream is at delivery. An increase in fetomaternal haemorrhage can occur with traumatic deliveries, abruptio placentae, manual delivery of the placenta, multiple pregnancies and caesarean sections.

An incompatible blood transfusion is a very potent stimulant of Rhesus antibodies. Other times of increased risk of fetomaternal haemorrhage associated with pregnancy include antepartum haemorrhage, miscarriages, physical trauma and interventions such as amniocentesis or external cephalic versions. The primary immune response is weak and leads mainly to IgM antibodies, which do not cross the placenta. It is therefore rare for fetal complications to develop from Rhesus allo-immunisation in a first pregnancy. The secondary immune response, however, is stronger and can be triggered by smaller amounts of antigen. In the secondary immune response mainly IgG antibodies are formed, which cross the placenta well.

In the fetus, these antibodies bind to the red cells and cause haemolysis in the reticuloendothelial system. The fetus compensates by increasing haemopoiesis (blood formation). If the haemolysis outstrips haemopoiesis, the fetus becomes anaemic and compensates by means of a hyperdynamic circulation. If this fails, the fetus goes into heart failure and becomes hydropic, eventually dying in utero.

Incompatibility of blood groups (such as Kell and Duffy) can also lead to allo-immunisation and fetal anaemia but they are less common.

Prevention of Rhesus allo-immunisation

Prevention of Rhesus allo-immunisation is more important than treatment. The Rhesus blood group should be checked in all pregnant women. If the woman is Rhesus negative an indirect Coombs test should be done. The indirect Coombs test detects antibodies which are present in blood but not bound to red cells. In contrast, the direct Coombs test detects antibodies which are present in blood and are bound to red cells. This test would be done on the baby's blood.

When the woman has a history of a previous blood transfusion or unexplained stillbirth, an indirect Coombs test should be done regardless of her Rhesus blood group to detect possible antibodies against other blood groups. If she is Rhesus negative and Coombs negative, the Coombs test should be repeated during her pregnancy at 28 and 34 weeks. At delivery, her baby's blood group should be checked. If it is Rhesus positive, she should receive 100 mg *anti-D immunoglobulin* intramuscularly within 72 hours after the delivery.

If possible, a Kleihauer test should be done to determine the amount of fetomaternal haemorrhage and to determine if the woman should receive a higher dose of *anti-D immunoglobulin*. If the Kleihauer test is not available, 300 mg *anti-D immunoglobulin* should be considered where the baby's ABO blood group is compatible with the mother's ABO blood group (such as baby's blood group is O and mother's blood group is A, B or AB), and there is a risk of an increased fetomaternal transfusion (such as a multiple pregnancy,

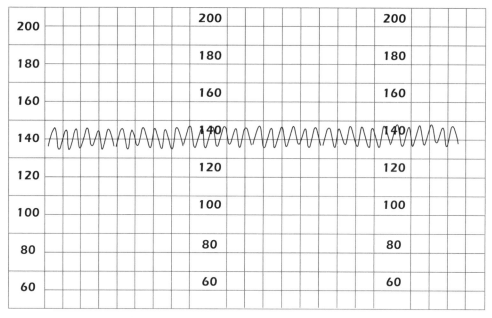

Figure 24.2 Sinusoidal fetal heart rate pattern

Note: Regular oscillations (2-5 cycles per minute) with amplitude 5-15 bpm above and below a normal baseline rate. Absent short-term variability and absence of accelerations.

caesarean delivery, maternal pre-eclampsia or a manual removal of the placenta). *Anti-D immunoglobulin* should also be administered for these conditions during pregnancy as they may lead to fetomaternal haemorrhage.

Management of established Rhesus allo-immunisation

Monitoring of the woman with Rhesus allo-immunisation

The woman with established allo-immunisation (a positive indirect Coombs test) has to be monitored carefully in (or in consultation with) a unit with experience in managing Rhesus allo-immunisation. Her Coombs titre should be monitored every two weeks. It is extremely rare for fetal hydrops or death to result from titres of 1:64 or lower. The woman with a titre of 1:128 or higher is at risk of fetal complications.

Traditionally, serial amniocentesis were performed to detect the DOD450nm to assess the severity of fetal haemolysis. The DOD450nm is a shift in light absorption caused by bilirubin and it is an indication of the amount of fetal haemolysis. However, amniocentesis can increase the severity of the allo-immunisation. Doppler ultrasound can detect the fetal hyperdynamic circulation by indicating an increased flow rate in the middle cerebral artery, the umbilical vein or the ductus venosus. Another approach is therefore not to do an amniocentesis, but to monitor the fetus by weekly Doppler ultrasound. In case of a high DOD450nm on amniocentesis or increased flow in the middle cerebral artery on Doppler ultrasound, an intra-uterine blood transfusion is done.

A hydropic fetus may present with a sinusoidal heart rate pattern. This is a preterminal pattern and the pregnancy should be managed in such a way that this finding is very rarely seen.

Intra-uterine transfusion (IUT)

A unit of O Rhesus negative, Kell negative, cytomegalovirus negative blood will be crossmatched with the maternal blood. The unit is filtered and irradiated to remove any inactive white cells (which may cause a graft versus host reaction) and packed tightly to a haematocrit of 85% or more.

The woman then receives sedation with a short-acting benzodiazepine such as *midazolam* (Dormicum®) if she prefers, and antibiotic prophylaxis with a cephalosporin like *cefuroxime* (Zinnat®). If the fetus is viable, the woman should be given two doses corticosteroids, *betamethasone* (Celestone Soluspan®) 12 mg or *dexamethasone* (Decadron®) 16 mg, prior to the IUT to enhance the fetal lung maturity in case of a complication of the IUT, which may necessitate urgent delivery.

The IUT is done under ultrasound guidance. First the maternal abdomen should be swabbed with antiseptic and draped. Local anaesthetic is then injected into the abdominal wall. A spinal needle is then inserted through the anaesthetised site into the umbilical vein at the placental insertion of the umbilical cord if possible, or otherwise into a free loop of umbilical cord, or the intrahepatic portion of the umbilical vein.

A sample of fetal blood is taken and the fetal haemoglobin must be tested immediately. The fetal blood sample should also be tested for the fetal blood group, direct Coombs, and if required, the fetal kariotype. Depending on the fetal haemoglobin, the gestational age, the estimated fetal weight and the haemotocrit of the donor blood, the transfusion volume is then calculated and given to the fetus as a direct transfusion, rather than as an exchange transfusion. After the transfusion the fetal haemoglobin should be tested again and more blood given if required. After the IUT, the fetal heart rate is monitored with electronic fetal monitoring if the fetus is viable. The transfusion would usually need to be repeated every two to three weeks until lung maturity is reached and the fetus can be safely delivered.

Neonatal care

The neonatal complications of the fetus that had been transfused differ from the complications of a Rhesus allo-immunised fetus that did not need transfusion. In the former, hyperbilirubinaemia is usually less severe because the repeated transfusions suppress the production of fetal red cells. The majority of the blood in the fetal circulation after three transfusions is donor, rather than fetal blood and the fetal blood group at delivery may test Rhesus negative. Neonatal anaemia is a bigger problem after repeated transfusions and also because of the bone marrow suppression.

Outcome

In cases of Rhesus allo-immunisation which require IUT, more than 90% of fetuses survive. However, in cases where the fetus was hydropic (in heart failure) prior to commencing IUT, only 70% would survive. In a subsequent pregnancy with a Rhesus positive fetus, the fetal involvement would be more severe.

Congenital fetal abnormalities

Two to four percent of babies have some form of congenital abnormality. Abnormalities are classified as minor or major abnormalities. Major abnormalities will impair the baby's functioning, have an adverse cosmetic impact or will need surgical correction.

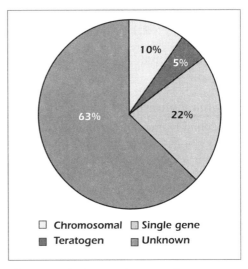

Figure 24.3 Causes of congenital abnormalities

In two thirds of babies with congenital abnormalities the cause cannot be determined.

With ultrasound, structural abnormalities of the fetus can be detected before delivery. In a similar fashion, chromosomal abnormalities of the fetus can be detected by an amniocentesis, chorionic villus sample or fetal blood sample. These forms of antenatal diagnosis are not a 'search-and-destroy' mission to eliminate babies with congenital abnormalities from society. Rather, the aim of antenatal diagnosis is to provide parents with accurate information in case of a congenital abnormality. This allows them the option of pregnancy termination if they wish, but otherwise allows them the time to come to terms with the anticipated abnormality.

Psychologically, it is also better to separate the moment of diagnosis from the moment of birth. In addition to the option of termination, there are other important differences between antenatal diagnosis and neonatal diagnosis. Firstly, the accuracy of diagnosis is less. Secondly, many fetuses with severe congenital abnormalities would die before birth due to the so-called 'intra-uterine lethality'. The spectrum of abnormalities which are seen antenatally, are therefore more severe than those seen after birth. Lastly, because of the less accurate diagnosis and intra-uterine lethality, there is a bigger risk of associated abnormalities. For example, in a fetus with a cleft lip and palate, there can be 194 other associated genetic syndromes.

Antenatal ultrasound

Ultrasound examination of the pregnancy is very useful in the first trimester of pregnancy to ensure an intra-uterine, viable pregnancy. Also, as mentioned previously, it is very useful to determine fetal growth, placental function and fetal wellbeing in the third trimester of pregnancy. However, in the context of congenital fetal abnormalities, the ultrasound examinations that are most useful are the late first trimester and mid second trimester examinations.

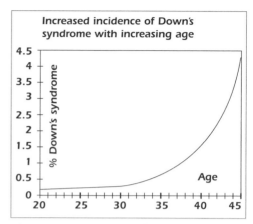

Figure 24.4 Prevalence of Down's syndrome relative to maternal age

Late first trimester ultrasound examination

Ultrasound is most useful between 11 and 13 weeks to detect fetal chromosomal abnormalities. It is well known that Down's syndrome becomes more common with increasing maternal age.

There is a rise in the prevalence of Down's syndrome in babies born to women aged 37 and older. Amniocentesis has therefore traditionally been offered to women aged 37 and above to exclude Down's syndrome. However, it detects only one third of babies with Down's syndrome. The rest is not tested for. Although the prevalence of Down's syndrome increases with advanced maternal age, there are so many more young women pregnant, that there are also more babies with Down's syndrome born to younger women.

A blood test (the triple test) has since been developed to improve screening for Down's syndrome. Although the test is an improvement, it still only detects two thirds of babies with Down's syndrome, while causing unnecessary distress in 5% of women with false positive results. A false positive result occurs where a screening test, such as the triple test, is positive, but the baby is normal. It has been discovered that the majority of babies with Down's syndrome have an increased amount of fluid behind the neck, which can be detected on ultrasound between 11 and 13 week as a nuchal translucency.

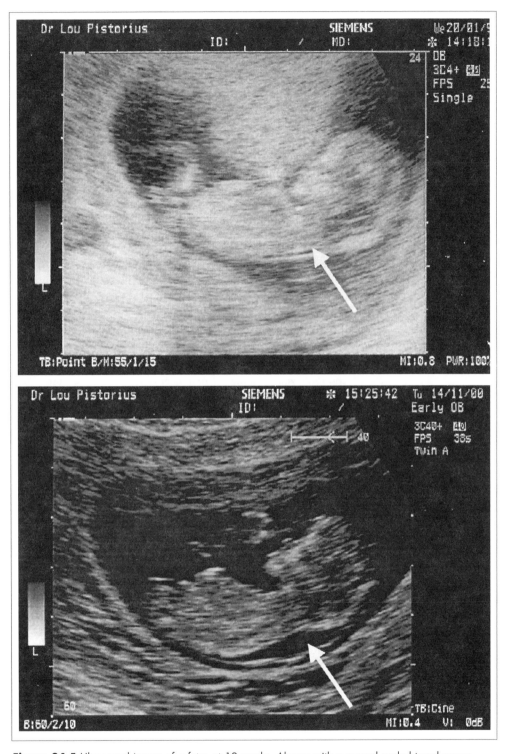

Figure 24.5 Ultrasound image of a fetus at 12 weeks, Above: with a normal nuchal translucency.
Below: With a thick nuchal translucency

Table 24.3 Usefulness of ultrasound at different gestational ages

Usefulness in determining:	6-8 weeks	11-13 weeks	20-22 weeks	>28 weeks
Whether pregnancy is in utero or ectopic	Good			
Gestational age	Good	Good	Good	
Fetal viability	Good	Good	Good	Good
Fetal chromosomal abnormalities		Good	Fair	
Structural fetal abnormalities		Fair	Good	
Intra-uterine growth restriction				Good
Placental function				Good

Table 24.4 Invasive antenatal tests

	Chorionic villus sample	Amniocentesis	Cordocentesis
Time in pregnancy	>10 weeks (usually 11–13 weeks)	>15 weeks (usually 16–18 weeks)	>20 weeks
Fetal target organ	Placenta	Amniotic cavity	Umbilical cord
Fetal cells obtained	Chorionic villi	Amniocytes	Fetal blood
Time until fetal chromosomes are available	2–3 weeks	2–3 weeks	2–3 days
Indications	▶ Fetal chromosomes (Usually if there was an abnormal first trimester ultrasound.) ▶ Fetal DNA analysis (for single gene defects.)	▶ Fetal chromosomes.	▶ Fetal chromosomes (Usually if structural abnormality is seen on second trimester ultrasound, or if there was a delay in performing amniocentesis.) ▶ Fetal blood group and haemoglobin.
Advantages	Early result, with easier termination if required.	Simplicity of technique.	Speed of results.

An increased nuchal translucency thickness is found in three quarters of babies with Down's syndrome. If a blood test is added to the risk estimate of Down's syndrome by nuchal translucency, 85% of babies with the condition would be detected, with still only a 5% false positive risk.

Other advantages of the 11 to 13 weeks ultrasound examination are that some structural fetal abnormalities can be detected and the duration of the pregnancy can be determined accurately.

Mid second trimester ultrasound examination

Between 20 and 22 weeks, ultrasound is most useful to detect structural fetal abnormalities. With ultrasound, a thorough examination of the fetus can be done and some abnormalities, such as spina bifida, can be detected very accurately. However, ultrasound is not a good screening test as probably less than 50% of fetal abnormalities would be detected on routine ultrasound examination. This can be improved somewhat by doing a blood test to detect the maternal serum alpha-feto protein (AFP) levels. The levels of this hormone are higher, usually more that twice the normal median levels, in case of spina bifida and other open neural tube defects. Ultrasound at 20 to 22 weeks can also detect some babies with chromosomal abnormalities but it is less effective than the earlier ultrasound examination.

Where a fetal chromosomal abnormality is suspected, either because of the maternal age, family history, blood tests or ultrasound findings, an amniocentesis, chorionic villus sample or cordocentesis can be done. All these are invasive tests, which means that a needle is inserted into the uterus, under ultrasound guidance, to obtain fetal cells. Due to the invasive nature of the tests there is a 1% risk of causing a miscarriage.

Management of the woman with a detected fetal abnormality

▶ The psychological management is the most important aspect. The woman will go through the different stages of a normal grief reaction. She will experience a sense of loss: she has lost the naïve enjoyment of pregnancy and anticipation of a normal baby. The woman needs support and empathy during her pregnancy and delivery, and especially after the baby is born (see Chapter 28).

▶ The woman deserves every effort to arrive at the most accurate possible diagnosis and prognosis. It might not be possible to arrive at a firm diagnosis antenatally but she will need guidance as to what the severity and implications of the most important abnormality and associated findings are. If an abnormality is detected on routine ultrasound, a detailed, high-resolution ultrasound should be performed.

▶ Amniocentesis or cordocentesis should be offered if applicable to exclude chromosomal abnormalities. Adjunctive imaging such as MRI scanning should be considered, especially in abnormalities of the fetal brain.

▶ The fetal prognosis should be discussed honestly but sympathetically. The woman should be made aware of the terms of the Choice on Termination of Pregnancy Act of 1996. It is her decision and she should not be coerced into a decision to continue or terminate the pregnancy according to the midwife's personal beliefs. Termination of pregnancy is discussed in Chapter 27.

▶ Once the baby is delivered, an examination should be performed by a dismorphologist (usually a clinical geneticist or paediatrician with an interest in congenital abnormalities), and the necessary tests should be done to arrive at a final diagnosis. Genetic counselling should be offered if at all applicable.

Fetal monitoring

Routine monitoring of the low-risk fetus during pregnancy and labour is discussed in Chapters 10, 13 and 14. This section deals specifically with monitoring of the compromised fetus. Doppler ultrasound, fetal heart rate monitoring, and the biophysical profile will be discussed.

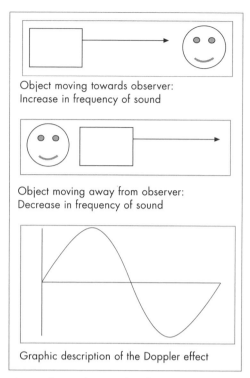

Object moving towards observer:
Increase in frequency of sound

Object moving away from observer:
Decrease in frequency of sound

Graphic description of the Doppler effect

Figure 24.6 The Doppler effect

Doppler ultrasound

Doppler is used to measure the rate of blood flow. The Doppler effect implies that moving objects reflect sound waves at a lower frequency if the object moves away from the observer or at a higher frequency if the object moves towards the observer. The speed at which the object moves causes a bigger or smaller shift in the frequency shift of the sound, which is reflected back to the observer.

In fetal monitoring, the red cells flowing in the specific blood vessel act as objects, which reflect ultrasound. The Doppler ultrasound can be done together with B-mode ultrasound (duplex Doppler), or 'blindly' with continuous wave Doppler. With duplex Doppler ultrasound, pulsed wave Doppler is used. The ultrasound waves used for the Doppler analysis are emitted in pulses, alternating with the pulses of ultrasound waves used to generate an ultrasound image. The flow can be measured in a specific vessel with duplex Doppler. Because the angle between the Doppler waves and the blood vessel can be measured, the absolute flow in the vessel can be measured, or Doppler indices can be calculated. With continuous wave Doppler, there is no image of the vessel, which is sampled. The specific 'footprint', or waveform pattern must be recognised to ensure that the right vessel is sampled. Because the blood vessel is not visualised, the absolute flow speed cannot be calculated but the different indices can be calculated. Continuous wave Doppler units are less expensive that ultrasound units with built-in pulsed wave Doppler.

The flow in any vessel, which can be visualised, can be investigated by Doppler

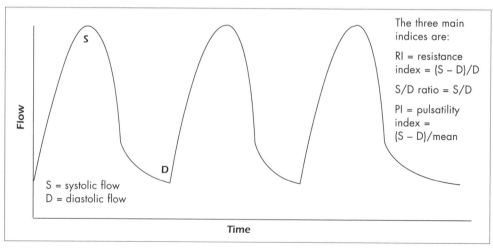

The three main indices are:

RI = resistance index = $(S - D)/D$

S/D ratio = S/D

PI = pulsatility index = $(S - D)/mean$

S = systolic flow
D = diastolic flow

Flow

Time

Figure 24.7 Doppler indices

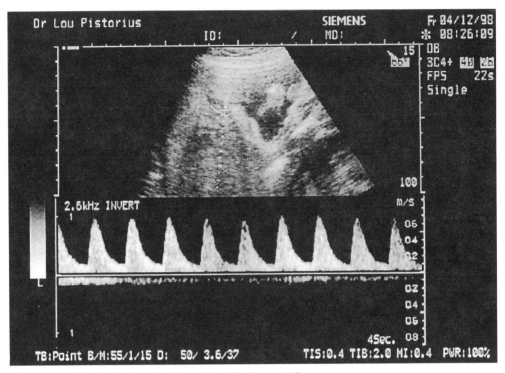

Figure 24.8 A: Duplex Doppler: Normal umbilical arterial flow

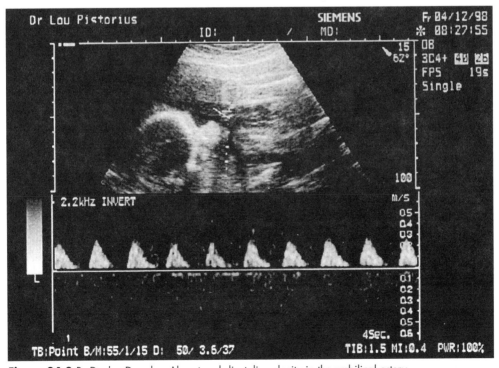

Figure 24.8 B: Duplex Doppler: Absent end diastolic velocity in the umbilical artery

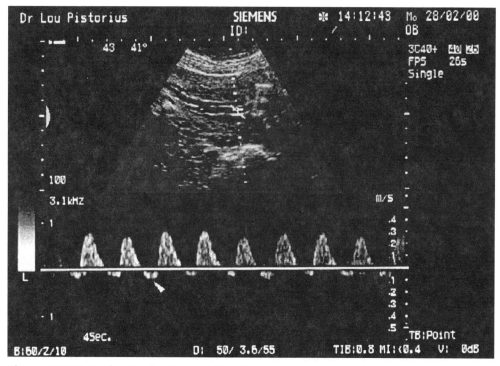

Figure 24.8 C: Duplex Doppler: Reversed diastolic velocity in the umbilical artery

ultrasound. However, the most important vessels in fetal monitoring are the umbilical artery and the middle cerebral artery. The examination of the flow in the ductus venosus or umbilical vein can also be of value but it is used less commonly.

Doppler ultrasound of the umbilical artery

In a normal placenta, the resistance to fetal

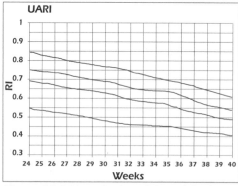

Figure 24.9 Normal values of the umbilical artery resistance index (UARI) during pregnancy (5th, 50th, 75th and 95th centiles)

blood flow through the placenta decreases with increasing gestational age. This is reflected in a decrease in the resistance index of blood flow in the umbilical artery.

In most cases of placenta insufficiency, there is an increase in the resistance to blood flow through the placenta. This causes a reduction in the diastolic blood flow in the umbilical artery and is reflected by an increase in resistance index above the 95th centile. In severe cases, the diastolic flow disappears which is called absent end diastolic velocity (AEDV). In even more severe cases there is reversed diastolic velocity (REDV).

If the umbilical artery resistance index is increased, there is placental insufficiency. The fetus should be monitored more closely by maternal monitoring of the fetal movements and by means of fetal heart rate monitoring three times a week. If there is absent end diastolic flow in the umbilical artery, the woman should be admitted to hospital and the fetus should be monitored intensively by fetal heart rate monitoring three times daily. If there is

Figure 24.10 Fetal heart rate monitoring: The development of hypoxia and acidosis (A, B, C, and D)

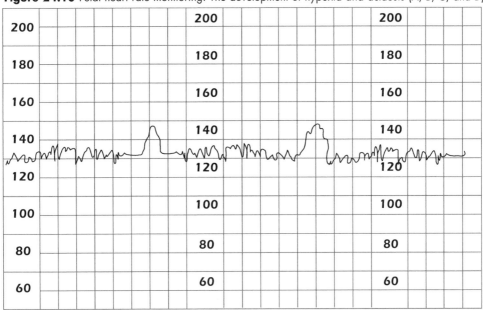

Figure 24.10 A: Normal fetal heart activity

Note: Baseline between 110 and 160 beats per minute (bpm). Fetal heart rate variability more than 5 bpm. Presence of accelerations (rising by at least 15 bpm; lasting at least 15 seconds). Absence of decelerations.

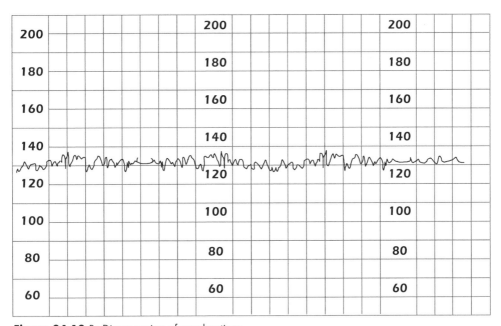

Figure 24.10 B: Disappearing of accelerations

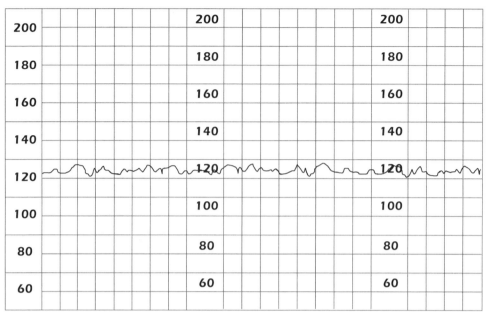

Figure 24.10 C: Reduced variability (below 10 bpm)

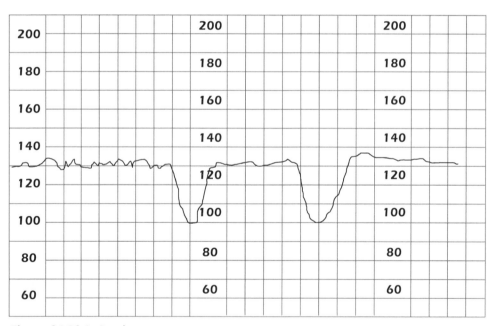

Figure 24.10 D: Decelerations

reversed diastolic flow in the umbilical artery, the fetus is severely compromised and should be delivered. The use of Doppler ultrasound of the umbilical artery is the only form of fetal monitoring which has been proven in randomised studies to improve fetal survival.

Doppler ultrasound of the middle cerebral artery

A normal reaction of a compromised fetus, especially in cases of placental insufficiency, is to redistribute the flow away from non-essential organs (such as limbs, gut and kidneys) towards the essential organs (heart and brain). An increased blood flow in the middle cerebral artery is therefore evidence of this redistribution. It confirms that the fetus is compensating for sub-optimal placental function but does not add much to the clinical management. Preterminally, the blood flow in the middle cerebral artery decreases again, however, the fetal heart rate monitoring would usually show ominous changes before the increase in the middle cerebral artery resistance index.

An increase in the absolute flow in the middle cerebral artery is useful to detect hyperdynamic fetal circulation. This helps to detect fetal anaemia in the fetus with Rhesus alloimmunisation without the risks of invasive tests like amniocentesis or cordocentesis.

Venous Doppler measurements

The flow in the ductus venosus is also sometimes used to evaluate the growth-restricted fetus. Absent or reversed flow in the ductus venosus are signs of decompensation and the fetus should be delivered if this develops. It can be very time consuming to obtain good Doppler ultrasound images of the ductus venosus and the majority of fetuses with placental insufficiency would develop signs of compromise on fetal heart rate monitoring before developing absent or reversed diastolic flow in the ductus venosus.

The flow in the umbilical vein can also be used to detect a hyperdynamic circulation, similar to the flow in the middle cerebral artery.

Fetal heart rate monitoring

The fetal heart rate is determined by the net effect of the output of the sympathetic and parasympathetic nervous system, with the sympathetic nervous system causing the fetal heart rate to increase and the parasympathetic nervous system causing the fetal heart rate to decrease. The fetal heart rate monitor is therefore an examination of the fetal central nervous system more than an examination of the fetal heart. The normal fetal heart rate characteristics for antenatal monitoring were discussed in Chapter 10 and those for intrapartum monitoring were discussed in Chapter 13. The characteristics of the fetal heart that are important are:

▶ baseline
▶ variability
▶ accelerations
▶ decelerations.

In a growth-restricted fetus, the first abnormality is the disappearance of accelerations. This correlates with reduced fetal movements and signifies a fetus which is cutting back on energy expenditure and is compensating for a reduced supply of nutrients and oxygen from the placenta. If the fetus starts decompensating, the variability reduces and it signifies a hypoxic fetus. This is the ideal time to deliver the fetus because if the fetus is not delivered, it will become acidotic and decelerations will ensue. If the fetus is left to become acidotic there is a higher risk of long-term neurological complications.

The fetal biophysical profile

The biophysical profile was developed as an intra-uterine Apgar score. This comprises evaluation of the following five fetal parameters:

▶ Fetal heart rate characteristics (as observed on fetal heart rate monitoring).
▶ The amniotic fluid volume.
▶ The fetal movements.
▶ The fetal muscle tone.
▶ The fetal breathing movements (as observed by ultrasound).

In a nutshell

▶ The psychological management of the woman with a compromised fetus is extremely important.

▶ In a suspected small for dates fetus, the umbilical artery Doppler resistance index is the single most important investigation.

▶ In Rhesus allo-immunisation prevention is better than cure.

▶ The psychological support of a woman after a pregnancy loss cannot be overemphasised.

A biophysical profile has the advantage of providing a more complete picture of the fetus but can be very time consuming. There is no advantage in clinical management of the biophysical profile over and above monitoring the fetus with umbilical artery Doppler and fetal heart rate monitoring. Therefore, the biophysical profile is not used routinely in monitoring the compromised fetus.

References

Enkin, M., Keirse, M. J. N. C., Neilson, J., Crowther, C., Duley, L., Hodnett, E. & Hofmeyr, J. 2000. *A guide to effective care in pregnancy and childbirth*. Third edition. Oxford: Oxford University Press.

Hadley, A. & Soothill, P. 2002. *Alloimmune disorders of pregnancy*. Cambridge: Cambridge University Press.

Ingemarsson, I., Ingemarsson. E., & Spencer, J. A. D. 1993. *Fetal heart rate monitoring: A practical guide*. Oxford: Oxford University Press.

Jones, K. L. 1997. *Smith's recognizable patterns of human malformation*. Philadelphia: WB Saunders Company.

Reece, E. A. & Hobbins, J. C. 1999. *Medicine of the fetus and mother*. Second edition. Philadelphia: Lippincott-Raven Publishers.

South Africa. 1996. Choice on the Termination of Pregnancy Act, 1996. Pretoria: Government Printer.

Neilson, J. & Alfirevic, Z. 2001. Doppler ultrasound for fetal assessment in high risk pregnancies. The database of abstracts of reviews of effectiveness. *The Cochrane Library*, issue 1. Oxford: Update Software.

Woods, D. L. (Ed.) Perinatale self-onderrig program. Handleiding 1. *Verloskunde*. Cape Town: Perinatal Education Trust.

Chapter 25

Multiple pregnancy

Dr Solina Richter

Introduction

Multiple pregnancy is when two or more fetuses develop simultaneously in the uterus. This represents a challenge for midwives and has significant psychological, social and economic effects on the parents. The possibility of a successful outcome is greater when there are appropriate preventive, diagnostic and management strategies in the hands of skilled and experienced midwives and physicians.

Types of twin

Monozygotic and dizygotic twins

Monozygotic and dizygotic twins are described in table 25.1 on page 25-2.

Conjoined twins

Conjoined twins arise when the separation in monozygotic twins is not complete. The degree of union between the twins can vary from the joining of the skin to a sharing of the thoracic cage and the internal viscera. The success of surgery to separate conjoined twins depends upon the degree of union and sharing of vital internal organs. Conjoined twins cannot be delivered vaginally and if the condition is suspected, the woman should be transferred to a high-risk unit.

Twin transfusion syndrome

This occurs in monozygotic twins, and is due to the anastomosis of the fetal circulations in a shared placenta. The recipient twin receives most of the blood and therefore most of the nourishment, while the donor twin is deprived of blood and nourishment. Twin transfusion syndrome is suspected when there is a big difference between the birth weight of the two infants. It is confirmed when the difference in the haemoglobin concentration is more than 5 g/dl between the two neonates.

Table 25.1 Differences between monozygotic and dizygotic twins

	Monozygotic (identical)	Dizygotic (fraternal)
Fetuses	Develop from one fertilised ovum. Identical.	Fertilisation of two ovums. Not identical.
Placenta	Division soon after fertilisation – two placentas. Division between 4 to 8 days after fertilisation – one placenta.	Always two placentas. Placental tissues may be fused but usually no vascular connection.
Chorion	Division soon after fertilisation – two chorions. Division between 4 to 8 days after fertilisation – one chorion.	Two chorions. May sometimes be partially fused.
Amnion	Division soon after fertilisation – two amnions. Division between 4 to 8 days after fertilisation – two amnions.	Two amnions.
Sex	Same sex; have the same genotype.	May be of the same sex or different sexes; genetically no more alike than siblings born at different times.

Incidence of multiple pregnancies

The incidence of twins occurs once in approximately 80 pregnancies. Triplets occur once in about 7 600 pregnancies. Naturally occurring quadruplets, sextuplets and septuplets are rare but when in vitro fertilisation was first introduced with no limit on the number of embryos that could be placed in the woman's uterus, the incidence increased. The survival rate in such multiple pregnancies is poor, because of the higher incidence of maternal and fetal complications.

The incidence of multiple births continues to rise. Various factors may contribute to this:
- *Induction of ovulation.* Increased incidence of multiple pregnancies is associated with fertility ovulation induction procedures such as the use of *clomiphene* and gonadotophins. Multiple births are also increasingly related to the use of in vitro fertilisation.
- *Population group.* The incidence of multiple pregnancies is higher among blacks, for example it is more or less 1:40 among the Zulu in South Africa.
- *Maternal age.* The incidence of multiple pregnancies increases with maternal age.
- *Parity.* The higher the parity the more likely it is that the woman will have a multiple pregnancy.
- *Hereditary tendency.* There is a strong hereditary tendency associated with a family history of multiple pregnancies and maternal history has the strongest influence. The incidence is especially high if the woman is herself one of twins.

Table 25.2 Characteristics of the recipient and donor twin in twin transfusion syndrome

The recipient twin	The donor twin
▶ Is the larger, heavier and plethoric twin.	▶ Is the smaller, lighter twin and small for the gestational age.
▶ Has polycythemia and often dies of cardiac failure.	▶ Has anaemia and is hypoglycaemic.
▶ May have respiratory distress.	▶ In severe cases the donor twin dies in utero and becomes amorphous and papery – the so-called *fetus papyraceus*.
▶ Has a higher chance of dying than the donor twin.	

Diagnosis of multiple pregnancy

The following factors are associated with an increased incidence of multiple pregnancy.

History:
▶ Mother is born as one of a multiple pregnancy.
▶ General family history of multiple pregnancies especially on maternal side.
▶ A pregnancy that has occurred after ovulation stimulation or in vitro fertilisation.
▶ Increased complains of minor disorders of pregnancy (for example severe nausea or vomiting in early pregnancy).
▶ Maternal weight gain more than expected.
▶ A report of increased fetal movements.
▶ If the woman develops pre-eclampsia before the 20th week of gestation.
▶ Polyhydramnios or unexpected anaemia develops.

Inspection:
▶ Uterine size is larger than expected for the gestational age (SFH above the 90th centile).
▶ Multiple fetal parts are felt on both sides of the uterine midline.
▶ A fetal head is felt that is smaller than expected for the size of the uterus.
▶ More than two fetal poles felt.
▶ The uterus is broad and round (rather than oval).

Auscultation:
Two or more fetal hearts heard at the same time that differ with more than 10 beats per minute.

Special investigation:
▶ Multiple pregnancy is confirmed by ultrasound which may reveal more than one fetal sac at 8 weeks gestation and more than one fetal head from 15 weeks onwards.
▶ Abdominal X-rays to confirm multiple pregnancies are rarely used and are contraindicated before 16 weeks gestational age because of the danger of radiation to the developing fetus.

The antenatal period
The effect of a multiple pregnancy during the antenatal period

There is a higher incidence of the following conditions in multiple pregnancies:
▶ *Exacerbation of minor disorders.* The presence of more than one fetus in utero and the subsequent higher levels of circulating hormones can cause an increase in the incidence and the severity of minor symptoms of pregnancy. Morning sickness, nausea and heartburn can be more troublesome than in a single pregnancy.
▶ *Pre-eclampsia.* The incidence of pre-eclampsia and eclampsia is greatly increased in multiple pregnancies and leads to an increase in abruptio placentae and antepartum haemorrhage.
▶ *Anaemia.* The increased demands of two or more developing fetuses may lead to maternal iron depletion and anaemia.
▶ *Polyhydramnios.* Both chronic and acute polyhydramnios are more likely to occur with a multiple pregnancy. The associated complication of polyhydramnios such as

malpresentations, cord prolapse, preterm labour and abruptio placentae also occur more commonly.

▶ *Pressure symptoms.* Symptoms like varicose veins, haemorrhoids, oedema of the lower limbs, difficulty in breathing and sleeplessness often increase in the third trimester.

▶ *Placenta praevia.* In multiple pregnancy the larger placental unit is more likely to be low lying in the uterus and therefore antepartum haemorrhage from placenta praevia is more likely.

▶ *Increased risks to the fetuses.* The increased risks to the fetuses include congenital malformations, monochorionicity (both fetuses sharing one placenta), poor fetal growth, preterm birth and perinatal death.

Nursing care during the antenatal period

During the antenatal period the midwife needs to pay special attention to the following:

▶ An early positive diagnosis of multiple pregnancy.

▶ Identification of women at risk (placenta praevia, antepartum haemorrhage, hypertension, polyhydramnios).

▶ Referral of all multiple pregnancies to a hospital for:
  ◆ Four-weekly antenatal visits up to 28 weeks, two weekly up to 36 weeks and weekly until delivery.
  ◆ Four-weekly ultrasound scan to monitor fetal growth.
  ◆ Cervical assessment at each visit for early detection of preterm labour.
  ◆ Prevent and/or treat anaemia, preeclampsia, polyhydramnios, fetal abnormalities, antepartum haemorrhage and the complications of these problems.

It is important to identify potential problems early in order to prevent them, to recognise existing problems and to participate in the management thereof or helping the woman to cope with her problems.

In the past, prolonged bed-rest in multiple

pregnancies was advocated and practised. The aim was to lengthen the duration of the pregnancy and thus improve the fetal growth, maturity and outcome. However, adequate research has not been done to prove the effectiveness of this practice.

The woman should be educated on the signs and symptoms of preterm labour, preeclampsia and other high-risk conditions, with specific steps she should take if symptoms develop. Parental education should also include counselling about diet, equipment and coping with newborn twins, their individuality and identity.

Counselling about diet

Fetal demands for iron and folate are increased in multiple pregnancies with an increased incidence of anaemia. Although it has not been proven to improve the clinical outcome of the pregnancy, routine iron and folate supplementation are still recommended (*ferrous sulphate* 200 mg orally three times a day). The midwife should also advise the pregnant woman on how to plan her meals to meet her increased needs. A higher intake of calcium and protein is recommended for optimal weight gain and fetal growth.

Coping with newborn twins, individuality and identity

Identical twins are often similar in temperament and tend to share a similar sleeping and eating pattern, which make life easier for the parents. Non-identical twins may be dissimilar in their demands for food and sleep and may be more challenging to care for. Parents are often given advice on how to manage 'the twin', or the triplets, when what they really need is individualised advice for each baby. They should be encouraged to develop individuality by calling each baby by his or her name, rather than as 'the twin' or 'the triplets'. It might also help to encourage the parents to spend time with each baby separately in order to become more sensitive to each child's personality.

The preterm birth rate is five to seven times

higher with multiple pregnancy than with singletons. Having two or more preterm babies can be a cause of great anxiety for the parents as they are concerned about their wellbeing. They may have to be separated from their infants until they are ready to be discharged home from hospital. It is not uncommon for the parents to experience feelings of loss and emptiness. Bonding between parents and two or more babies takes longer than in the case of only one baby. The mother may experience feelings of guilt because she sometimes forms a closer bond with one baby than with the other(s). This is a perfectly normal reaction and parents should be reassured about this.

Equipment (layette)

Advise the parents to prepare and budget for all the clothes, diapers and other items they will need for two or more babies. Borrowing cots, high chairs, strollers and other furniture may be helpful since they will most likely not need duplicates in the future.

Breastfeeding multiple babies

If the mother is choosing to breastfeed, she should be familiar with all the options and possibilities before delivery of the babies and supported after they are born. These options include:

▶ Feeding on demand or feeding according to a fixed schedule.
▶ Alternate breast feedings with formula milk feedings.
▶ Which positions are the most effective.
▶ Whether the babies should be fed together or separately.

The various options and possibilities will be discussed further in Chapter 30.

Labour

The effect of a multiple pregnancy on labour

There is a higher incidence of the following conditions in multiple pregnancies:

▶ *Malpresentation*. Although the uterus is large and distended, the fetuses are less mobile and their movement can be restricted, which may result in malpresentations such as breech or compound presentation.
▶ *Prolapse of the cord*. This is associated with malpresentation and polyhydramnios.
▶ *Intrapartum haemorrhage*. Intrapartum haemorrhage may occur when there is early separation of the placenta after the birth of the first baby but before the birth of the second or third.
▶ *Complicated deliveries*. There is a higher incidence of complicated deliveries due to malpresentation which may result in traumatic deliveries or caesarean sections, abruptio placentae and haemorrhage, preterm labour and postpartum haemorrhage.
▶ *Locked twins*. This is a rare complication of twin pregnancy where the presenting parts of the fetuses interlock while still in the uterus or birth canal. For example, the chin of the first baby in a breech presentation interlocks with the chin of the second baby in a cephalic presentation (see Figure 25.1). The management depends on when the diagnosis of a locked twin is made. If the diagnosis is made before one baby is born, an emergency caesarean section is the delivery mode of choice. If the diagnosis is made after one baby has partially been born an effort can be made under general anaesthesia to free the parts from each other and then to carry out an assisted delivery. If the diagnosis is made after one baby has been partially born and is locked behind the chin of the second baby, the first baby is often sacrificed and a decapitation may be performed to save the life of the second baby as it is unlikely that the first will survive.

Nursing care during the first stage of labour

Except for a few aspects, the monitoring and care of a woman with a multiple pregnancy is the same as any other high-risk woman in

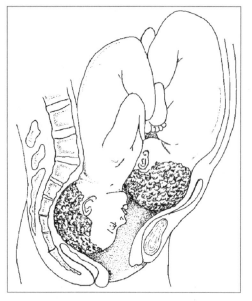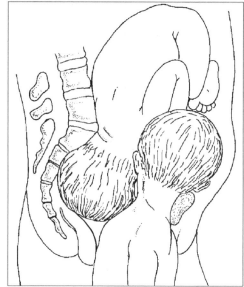

Figure 25.1 Locked twins

Factors affecting the mode of delivery

▶ *Gestational age of the fetuses at delivery*. An elective caesarean section for twin delivery is advocated by some obstetricians if the fetal weight is 1.5 kg or less. This is to reduce the incidence of periventricular haemorrhage infarction and possible damage to the preterm babies during difficult and manipulated vaginal deliveries.

▶ *Presence of pre-existing problems*. If severe intra-uterine growth restriction is suspected or oligohydramnios is present, a caesarean section is indicated to avoid asphyxia at birth.

▶ *Previous caesarean section* will lead to a follow-up caesarean section.

▶ *Presentation of twins*. A caesarean section is advocated if both twins are in non-vertex presentation or if the first twin is in a non-vertex presentation.

▶ *Number of fetuses*. Caesarean section is indicated if more than two fetuses are present in utero.

labour. Prescribed induction of labour and augmentation with *oxytocin* is not contraindicated in twin pregnancies. The partogram should be used to monitor the progress of labour and both fetal heart rates should be monitored, preferably by cardiotocograph monitoring. A vaginal examination should be performed immediately after the membranes have ruptured to exclude the possibility of a prolapsed cord.

Adequate sedation and analgesia must be provided and an epidural block is the method of choice. The midwife should explain that it provides excellent analgesia, if necessary, and allows easier management of a complicated delivery and also manipulation of the second twin. The midwife should be with the woman constantly to support her.

An intravenous infusion should be inserted to ensure an accessible line. This will enhance her labour but it is also needed for emergency surgery or for obstetric interventions, should they be required. An operating theatre should be available at all times for a possible emergency caesarean section. The delivery unit should be prepared in such a manner to safely receive two or more babies (skilled

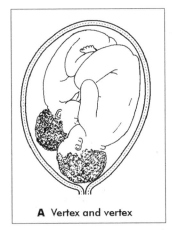

A Vertex and vertex

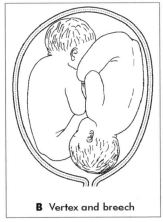

B Vertex and breech

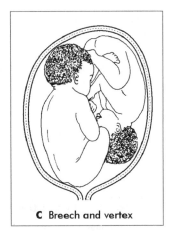

C Breech and vertex

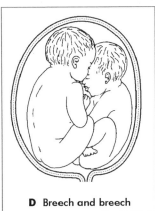

D Breech and breech

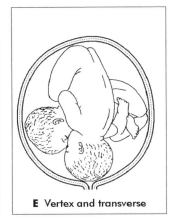

E Vertex and transverse

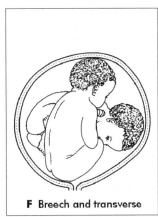

F Breech and transverse

Figure 25.2 Presentation of twins before delivery

midwives and physicians available at birth to resuscitate babies, two or more fetal overhead warmers, two or more incubators and two or more neonatal resuscitation sets should be available).

Nursing care during the second stage

The delivery should not be attempted without the assistance of an experienced physician or midwife at a hospital.

Delivery of the first twin

The first baby is delivered as in the case of a single pregnancy. The cord should be clamped immediately following delivery to prevent loss of blood from the fetal circulation and depriving the unborn twin should they be identical. The cord should be clamped with a cord

clamp or clearly identified artery forceps that indicates 'baby 1' as this will assist in identification of the cord and placenta after delivery of all the babies.

After the delivery of the first baby, the uterus is palpated to confirm the presence of another fetus and no Syntocinon® (*oxytocin*) or Syntometrine® must be administered at this stage. This may cause sudden forceful contractions of the uterus that can result in asphyxia and intra-uterine death of the second fetus.

Delivery of second twin

Ascertain the lie of the second twin by palpation and auscultation of the fetal heart. If uterine activity does not recommence, intravenous *oxytocin* may be used to stimulate the uterus. The fetal heart rate should still be monitored constantly. When the presenting part becomes visible, the mother should be encouraged to bear down to deliver the second twin. The membranes may be ruptured after engagement of the presenting part. In multiple pregnancies it is advisable to give the oxytocic drug after the delivery of the last baby's body and after ensuring that there is no unexpected fetus still in the uterus. Expected twins may in fact be triplets and triplets may be quadruplets.

Nursing care during the third stage

Active management of the third stage is imperative to prevent atonic postpartum haemorrhage. This is a critical stage because overdistension of the uterus results in poor uterine contraction and retraction. In addition, a large placental area has a higher incidence of retained placental tissue, which contributes to postpartum haemorrhage and increased maternal morbidity and mortality (see Chapter 21). Postpartum haemorrhage can be prevented by infusing 1 000 ml Ringer's lactate with 20 IU of *oxytocin* at a rate of 120 to 240 ml per hour.

Nursing care in the postnatal period

Although the parents may be excited about the delivery of their babies, the reality of caring for them may be overwhelming. It is not uncommon for these parents to feel overloaded and isolated from their friends and family. Sleep deprivation and a lack of personal time may lead to frustration and depression. The relationship between the parents may become strained which can compound the problems.

Planning for the care of the babies should ideally begin in the antenatal period and additional 'helpers' identified among family and friends. This is so that the almost constant attention required in caring for the infants can be synchronised in such a way that the parents are able to take some time for rest. Midwives can assist the parents in organising

and simplifying the daily care of the infants. In addition, there is a useful 'multiple birth association' support group that the parents can be referred to where they can exchange ideas and share problems.

In a nutshell

▶ Multiple pregnancies are high-risk pregnancies, which should be referred to a hospital for antenatal and intra-partum management.

▶ Careful antenatal, intrapartum and postnatal monitoring will decrease the risk of complications.

▶ *Ocytocin* should be administered only after confirmation that there are no fetuses left in the uterus.

References

Bennett, V. R. & Brown, L. K. 2000. *Myles textbook for midwives*. Edinburgh: Churchill Livingstone.

Bobak, I. M. & Jensen, M. D. 1993. *Maternity and gynecological care. The nurse and the family*. St. Louis: Mosby.

Bobak, I. M., Lowermilk, D. L., Jensen, M. D. & Penny, S. E. 1995. *Maternal nursing*. St. Louis: Mosby.

Crowther, C. A. 1999. Caesarean delivery for the second twin, (Cochrane Review). *The Cochrane Library*, issue 3. Oxford: Update Software.

DoH (Department of Health). 2002. *Guidelines for maternity care in South Africa*. Second edition. Pretoria: Department of Health.

Di Renzo, G. C., Luzietti, R., Gerli, S. & Clerici, G. 2001. The ten commandments in multiple pregnancies. *Twin Research*, 4(3):159–164.

Enkin, M. W., Keirse, M. J. N. C., Neilson, J. P., Crowther, C. A., Duley, L., Hodnett, E. D. & Hofmeyr, G. J. 2000. *A guide to effective care in pregnancy and childbirth*. Oxford: Oxford University Press.

Ladewig, P., London, M. & Olds, S. 1998. *Maternal–newborn nursing care.* California: Addison-Wesley.

Maxwell, C.V., Lieberman, E., Norton, M., Cohen, A., Seely, E. W. & Lee-Parritz, A. 2001. Relationship of twin zygotic and risk of pre-eclampsia. *American Journal of Obstetrics and Gynaecology,* 185(4):819–821.

May, K. A. & Mahlmeister, L. R. 1994. *Maternal and neonatal nursing. Family centered care.* Philadelphia: Lippincott.

Nel, J. T. 1995. *Core obstetrics and gynaecology.* Durban: Butterworth Publishers.

Nolte, A. G. W. (Ed.) 1998. *A textbook for midwives.* Pretoria: J.L. van Schaik Academica.

Novak, J. C. & Broom, B. L. 1995. *Maternal and child health nursing.* St. Louis: Mosby.

Reynolds, M. A, Schieve, L. A., Jeng, G., Peterson, H. B. & Wilcox, L. S. 2001. Risk of multiple birth associated with in vitro fertilization using donor eggs. *American Journal of Epidemiology,* 154(11):1043–1050.

Chapter **26**

Complicated labour and birth

Riana Hattingh

Introduction

The ability of maternity services and individual health workers to cope with complicated labour and birth is a good benchmark for measuring the efficiency of care. As individuals we are also concerned about how we will be able to cope with such an event.

The complications of labour and birth which will be discussed in this chapter are often not predictable and they may occur quite suddenly. For these reasons referenced and evidence-based guidelines or management protocols (that should be reviewed every one to two years) should be available to enable the attending care providers to act swiftly and as a team. According to Ball, 'expeditiously executed management drills are the key to a favourable outcome' (1996:67). If these guidelines and protocols are not in place, it can result in damage to or even the death of the woman and the baby.

Timely, discrete but frank discussion between the care providers and the family is critical if an injury to the woman or baby occurs. An explanation of the way the complication was dealt with reassures the woman and her relatives. This communication may also be an important factor in mitigating the litigation that may follow such an event. Another way to decrease liability is to provide comprehensive objective documentation of the events in the medical records.

Post-term pregnancy

Post-term pregnancy is defined as any pregnancy lasting 42 completed weeks or more. However, there are a number of confusing terms that are often used to describe a post-term pregnancy (see box).

Post-term pregnancy varies from 4 to 14%, depending on the population surveyed, how gestational age was assessed and the proportion of women who had an elective delivery. Preconception care, with emphasis on menstrual charting, may ensure that the woman is certain of her last normal menstrual period (LMP), however routine early ultrasound is more accurate in determining the duration of the pregnancy. An early ultrasound may reduce the frequency of induction of labour for what appears to be a post-term pregnancy.

In South Africa ultrasound is not available to all women. Women characteristically attend their first antenatal visit after the 16th to 22nd week of pregnancy when ultrasound is no longer accurate. Under these circumstances an experienced midwife or medical practitioner needs to establish the gestational age as accurately as possible by taking a complete history and performing a full abdominal examination (see Chapter 9).

The effects of post-term pregnancy

The increased incidence of perinatal mortality in post-term pregnancies is partly due to congenital malformations, which are more frequent among post-term births, than among births at term. Intrapartum-related birth asphyxia is the other main cause of death.

In a post-term pregnancy the fetus may continue to grow or may begin to lose weight. When fetal growth continues, ossification increases and the fetal head becomes harder and less able to mould during labour. Diminished placental perfusion causes poor nutritional status and leads to fetal weight

---

Confusing terms for post-term pregnancy

A post-term pregnancy is sometimes wrongly referred to as a *prolonged pregnancy* or a *post-dates* pregnancy. These terms refer to the time period after the woman's expected date of delivery (40 weeks and thereafter) and a pregnancy is only considered term at 42 weeks.

The term *post-mature* is also used in relation to the duration of pregnancy but is inappropriate because a *post-mature neonate* refers to a clinical syndrome of the neonate. These terms should therefore not be used to describe or define a post-term pregnancy.

loss. The placenta starts aging during the second trimester and compensates by developing new villi. In a post-term pregnancy, the placenta cannot keep up with the normal aging process and placental insufficiency may develop.

Other effects of post-term pregnancy may include the following:

◗ There is the obvious risk of a complicated birth, due to cephalopelvic disproportion or shoulder dystocia with subsequent neonatal injuries.

◗ The amniotic fluid volume is reduced because of diminished placental function, which may predispose to cord compression and subsequent fetal distress.

◗ The risk of perinatal death increases with the onset of labour.

◗ Meconium-stained amniotic fluid and meconium aspiration are common among the intrapartum and asphyxial neonatal deaths.

◗ The incidence of early neonatal seizures, which is an indication of perinatal asphyxia, is up to five times higher in infants born after 41 weeks.

Prevention of post-term pregnancy

Although women report increased discomfort during vaginal examination, which includes sweeping of the membranes (separation of the fetal membranes from the lower pole of the uterus), it does reduce both the need for formal induction of labour and the risk of the pregnancy continuing beyond 42 weeks. This procedure must be reconsidered when the HIV status of the woman is unknown or positive.

Routine induction of labour in post-term pregnancies reduces the risk of perinatal death in normally formed babies. However, there is no evidence of induction being of benefit when the pregnancy is considered to be less than 41 completed weeks gestation.

Diagnosis of post-term pregnancy

It is often difficult to make an accurate assessment of gestational age by questioning women about their menstrual history because they are seldom sure about the date of their last normal menstrual period (see Chapter 9).

There are several ways in which assessment can be done, but none are very accurate. Ultrasound is a useful tool but the earlier it is done the more accurate it will be. Between 12 to 24 weeks pregnancy the femur length is accurate to within 6 to 7 days. So even ultrasound carries a degree of inaccuracy, even when done early in pregnancy, although it is still the most reliable.

Surveillance of post-term pregnancy

Surveillance tests can detect pregnancies in which there is an abnormality but there is lack of evidence that their use improves the outcome or eliminates the additional risk of post-term pregnancy.

The surveillance tests commonly offered to women with post-term pregnancies are of poor quality. Obstetricians, midwives and women should be aware of the lack of evidence available to support the use of all methods of fetal surveillance for post-term pregnancies. (See Chapter 10 for monitoring of the fetus.)

Management of post-term pregnancies

There is a general trend towards conservative treatment of post-term pregnancies but after 41 weeks the monitoring of the fetus should be increased.

Low-risk women with reliable dates

The woman should be seen weekly from the calculated expected date of delivery. The woman should be referred to hospital if any risk factors develop, such as pre-eclampsia or decreased fetal movements, or when she reaches 42 weeks gestation.

Low-risk women with unreliable dates

The woman should be seen every week from the time she is considered to be approximately at term. Again she should be referred to hospital if any risk factors such as pre-eclampsia or decreased fetal movements develop. Fetal wellbeing should be monitored with cardiotocography and ultrasound measurement using maximum amniotic fluid pool depth. If there are no complications that would require earlier delivery, the spontaneous onset of labour should be awaited until she is considered to be 42 weeks. Induction of labour (IOL) should be performed at 42 weeks gestation.

Specific clinical scenarios

▶ At 41 weeks of pregnancy, if the cervix is favourable, IOL should be considered.
▶ If the estimated fetal weight exceeds 4 500 g, delivery by elective caesarean section should be the method of choice.
▶ If there is any deterioration in the maternal or fetal wellbeing, IOL should be performed.
▶ If oligohydramnios is present, amniotic fluid volume may be restored by doing an amnioinfusion after rupturing the membranes during labour. This will prevent or treat cord compression or a variable deceleration pattern. An amnioinfusion can prevent aspiration of meconium. This treatment, however, is only applicable when the woman is known to be HIV-negative.
▶ Dysfunctional labour patterns are common in post-term pregnancies, therefore an accurate assessment of the woman's labour is necessary.

Psychological effects on the woman

The psychological effects of post-term pregnancy are difficult to cope with. The woman will be worried about her own safety and that of her baby. Frustration due to the different opinions in the management of the condition, feelings of not being in control anymore and even depression are all commonly experienced. Due to the pregnancy being prolonged, social arrangements that were made to accommodate the birth of the baby will be interfered with.

Although a vaginal birth is anticipated, the woman should be prepared for the possibility of an assisted delivery or caesarean section.

Prelabour rupture of membranes

Prelabour rupture of the membranes is defined as the spontaneous rupture of the membranes before the onset of regular uterine contractions. When prelabour rupture of the membranes occurs before 37 weeks gestation, we refer to it as 'preterm prelabour rupture of the membranes' (pPROM). When occurring at or after 37 weeks, it is referred to as 'term prelabour rupture of the membranes'. This distinction is important both for prognosis and for care.

Prelabour rupture of membranes and preterm labour

Socioeconomic improvements and the development of therapeutic interventions have not reduced the incidence of preterm births in recent decades. In developed countries the proportion of births before 37 weeks remains 6 to 8%. A third of these are associated with preterm prelabour rupture of membranes (pPROM), which places both mother and child at risk of infection, preterm delivery and the complications of prematurity.

In South Africa, spontaneous preterm labour is the second most common cause of perinatal deaths and is by far the most common primary cause of perinatal death in the birth weight category 1 000 g to 2 000 g. Spontaneous preterm labour is an important problem for midwives as it was responsible for 49.7% of perinatal deaths in rural areas and for 22.2% in metropolitan areas in this birth weight category (Saving Babies, 2002:10).

Management and treatment will depend on the following factors:
▶ Whether the membranes are ruptured.
▶ Whether the woman is in labour or not.
▶ The presence of intra-uterine infection.
▶ The gestational age of the fetus.
▶ The circumstances, equipment and facilities available.

Diagnosis of prelabour rupture of membranes

In some women the diagnosis is obvious from the sudden flow of clear amniotic fluid from the vagina and dripping of fluid that continues thereafter. If the membranes ruptured some hours previously, much depends on taking a careful history from the woman since most of the amniotic fluid has drained from the vagina. It might be very difficult to establish or confirm the diagnosis with any degree of certainty.

Amniotic fluid is sometimes confused with leaks of other body fluid, such as urine or a vaginal discharge. It may be possible to confirm the diagnosis by asking the woman to sit on a clean container or obtaining a sample from a pool of amniotic fluid in the posterior fornix during a sterile speculum examination. This sample of fluid can be used for microscopic observation of ferning. There is a slight chance that the fern test may have false-negative results with the implication that the rupture of membranes may be undetected. Evaluation of constant draining (pad checks) may help to diagnose the undetected cases.

Phosphatidylglycerol determination can be performed by using the collected specimen of amniotic fluid to determine fetal lung maturity. Cultures can be grown from collected material or screening can be done for pathogens such as group B streptococci.

> ### Note
>
> A vaginal examination is never done on a woman with prelabour rupture of membranes, whether the gestational age is considered to be term or preterm, unless she is in active labour.

Assessment of women with prelabour rupture of membranes

The risk of infection. Women with prelabour rupture of the membranes should be assessed for signs of chorio-amnionitis, irrespective of the duration of pregnancy. Clinical features of chorio-amnionitis include:

> ### Taking a history from a woman with possible ruptured membranes
>
> The woman should be asked the following questions:
> - When and under what circumstances did you experience the flow of fluid?
> - Approximately how much fluid drained?
> - What was the colour of the fluid?
> - What did the fluid smell of? (The amniotic fluid does not smell of anything, unless the woman is suffering from chorio-amnionitis.)
> - Did anything like this happen before?
> - Did you see anything in the water? (Women may comment on the presence of white and/or greasy particles. This is a greasy substance called *vernix caseosa* that covers the body of a baby.)

- Fetal tachycardia.
- Maternal tachycardia and pyrexia.
- Uterine tenderness and/or irritability.
- Foul-smelling liquid or discharge from the vagina.

According to Enkin et al (2000:198) uterine tenderness and foul-smelling discharge are late signs of chorio-amnionitis. The earliest clinical signs of chorio-amnionitis are fetal tachycardia and a slight elevation of maternal temperature. Refer to Chapter 19 for the assessment and management of chorio-amnionitis/amniotic fluid infection syndrome.

The risk of fetal immaturity. Gestational age should be estimated carefully to determine the risk for fetal immaturity. Very immature or near to term fetuses are relatively easy to identify, but when a fetus is between 26 and 34 weeks of gestation, it becomes more difficult to determine the gestational age.

The more mature the fetal lungs are, the lower the risk of mortality and morbidity due to respiratory disorders. However, this does not imply that other complications associated with preterm birth, such as periventricular haemorrhage infarction, will be avoided.

Preterm prelabour rupture of membranes (pPROM)

A number of complications are associated with pPROM:

▶ Preterm birth is the most common serious complication of pPROM. The risk of morbidity and mortality is directly related to the gestational age and maturity of the fetus. Between 24 and 34 weeks it becomes very difficult to determine the risk of immaturity against that of infection.

▶ Infectious morbidity is the second most important complication for the baby. Observation for the clinical signs of chorioamnionitis is therefore of great importance. The causes of pPROM are multifactorial, but infection appears to have an important role, either as a cause or as a consequence of pPROM. Organisms produce enzymes that weaken the amnion and chorion and may lead to pPROM. Ascending infection may occur secondary to membrane rupture and lead to occult deciduitis or chorioamnionitis. A possible mechanism for the link between infection and preterm delivery is bacterial stimulation of the biosynthesis of prostaglandins.

▶ Prolapse of the umbilical cord may occur at the time of membrane rupture, with loss of amniotic fluid at a later stage, or with the onset of labour. Prolapse of the umbilical cord is frequently associated with a fetal head that has not yet engaged into the pelvis. Frequent assessment of the fetal heart rate is important under these circumstances.

▶ The amniotic fluid protects the umbilical cord against compression. The loss of a substantial amount of amniotic fluid may cause pressure on the umbilical cord. The incidence of fetal heart rate decelerations is directly related to the degree of oligohydramnios. Increase in pressure escalates with the onset of uterine contractions.

▶ When the membranes have been ruptured for a prolonged period of time, the result-

ing oligohydramnios may lead to fetal contractures and compression abnormalities.

▶ Normal amounts of amniotic fluid are necessary for normal fetal lung development. Oligohydramnios is related to underdevelopment of the lungs and may result in pulmonary lung hypoplasia which may be fatal (see Chapter 31).

▶ Whenever a woman with pPROM complains of abdominal pain and haemorrhage, abruptio placentae should be considered.

Care before the onset of labour

If the membranes rupture before 37 weeks gestation, most women will go into labour within hours or a few days. About 75% of all women with pPROM will give birth within one week. pPROM also accounts for about 25% of all preterm deliveries. The women should be transported to a maternity facility where intensive maternal and neonatal care is available. Timely transfer to an appropriate care facility seems to be the most effective form of care for women with pPROM.

Occasionally, women take longer than a week to go into labour. The following possibilities should be considered:

▶ A leak in the membranes in the fundal area of the uterus may seal off, so that the amniotic fluid volume returns to normal, but this very seldom happens. Under these circumstances it seems to be relatively safe for a woman to go home.

▶ The membranes might not have ruptured, therefore the diagnosis would have been wrong.

Care before the onset of labour should include the following:

Routine assessment. During the first few days the woman and fetus should be regularly assessed for signs of infection and/or uterine contractions. The following observations should be done:

▶ Maternal temperature and pulse.
▶ Fetal heart rate.
▶ Uterine contractions.
▶ Vaginal discharge and odour.

Prophylactic antibiotics. Prophylactic antibiotics following pPROM is associated with:
- A significant reduction in maternal infections and morbidity (including chorio-amnionitis).
- A reduction in neonatal infection.
- A reduction in the number of babies requiring neonatal intensive care and ventilation for over 28 days.
- A significant number of prolonged pregnancies.

Although one would expect an increase in neonatal survival because of these findings, controlled trials have failed to demonstrate this. According to Kenyon (2000) the cumulative evidence would be in favour of the antibiotic treatment but remains unproven. Furthermore, it is also not yet clear which antibiotics would be most effective, or what duration of therapy would be best. According to Enkin et al (2000:202) treatment probably should be guided by bacterial culture and continued until birth.

Prophylactic tocolytics. The use of prophylactic tocolytics before the onset of uterine contractions has not proven to be effective.

Corticosteroid administration. Corticosteroid administration is successful in reducing the incidence of respiratory distress syndrome. It is usually given over a period of 24 hours.

The concern that corticosteroid administration might both increase susceptibility to intra-uterine infection and mask early signs of infection in women with prelabour rupture of membranes seems to be unfounded. Maternal infection is not increased after corticosteroid administration, although maternal infection may be increased in women whose membranes have been ruptured for longer than 24 hours. Neonatal infection, however, remains a possible risk. Therefore the use of antibiotics with corticosteroids appears to be appropriate.

Emotional preparation of the woman. Preparing the woman for the birth of the preterm baby may help her to feel more in control of the situation. Whenever the situation allows she should be allowed to visit the neonatal intensive care unit and be introduced to its staff. The woman will need information on Kangeroo care and how to breastfeed a preterm baby. Information on developmental supportive care with all its advantages would be of great benefit (see Chapter 29). She could also be introduced to a support group for parents with preterm babies, which can provide reading material, as well as emotional support and encouragement.

The waiting period in the hospital due to this condition is often accompanied by increased anxiety for the woman and her partner. Relaxation activities (such as reading, hobbies, relaxation exercises) can help them to cope with the stress.

Management guidelines for preterm prelabour rupture of membranes (pPROM)
Refer to Table 26.1 for specific guidelines according to gestational age.

Care after the onset of labour
The onset of contractions, after the membranes have been ruptured for some time, may be the result of chorio-amnionitis. Under these circumstances labour should be allowed to proceed irrespective of the gestational age of the fetus. If extra-uterine survival of the fetus is unlikely due to severe immaturity, the following should be considered by everybody involved before any attempt is made to prolong the pregnancy:
- What might be gained in terms of infant outcome?
- What are the maternal risks?
- How do the parents feel?

The treatment would be as follows:
- Antibiotic treatment as soon as chorio-amnionitis is suspected.
- Tocolytic agents should only be used when the benefits of prolonging the pregnancy by a few days clearly outweigh the risk. Examples of this would be when the woman must be transferred to a centre with adequate facilities for care around preterm birth or to allow time for the administration of

Table 26.1 Management guidelines for pPROM	
Before 24 weeks gestation:	▶ Make sure that the membranes have definitely ruptured (reduced liquor volume on ultrasound). ▶ Transfer the woman to hospital. ▶ Termination of pregnancy is recommended (only 10% survival rate with a high risk of morbidity) if the parents agree. Counsel them appropriately. ▶ Induce labour with *oxytocin* 10 to 20 IU in 1 litre Ringer's lactate at 120 ml per hour. ▶ Antibiotics are administered as the risk of infection is high.
From 24 to 33 weeks gestation or estimated fetal weight 600 g to 1999 g (no chorio-amnionitis):	▶ Start antibiotics (*erythromycin* 250 mg orally four times daily and *metronidazole* 400 mg orally three times daily for seven days) and administer corticosteroids (*dexamethasone* 8 mg IM eight-hourly for three doses). ▶ Administer *hexoprenaline* or *nifidepine* regimen if contractions start in the first 24 hours after admission. ▶ Do observations four-hourly (pulse, temperature, fetal heart rate and pad checks). ▶ Daily cardiotocograph (CTG), if possible. ▶ Induce labour at 34 weeks or 2 kg, or if there are signs of chorio-amnionitis. ▶ Administer *ampicillin* 1 g IV six-hourly during labour.
From 24 to 33 weeks gestation (with chorio-amnionitis):	▶ If infection is mild: administer antibiotics and corticosteroids and deliver after 24 hours. ▶ If infection is severe: administer antibiotics and deliver immediately.
After 34 weeks gestation or estimated fetal weight more than 2 kg:	▶ Transfer from a community health centre to hospital. ▶ Administer *ampicillin* 1 g IV six-hourly and *metronidazole* 400 mg orally three times daily. ▶ Allow labour to proceed. ▶ If the woman is not in labour within 12 to 24 hours, induce labour with *oxytocin*, or ripen the cervix with prostaglandin.

Source: DoH, March 2002:102.

corticosteroids. Both these measures could improve the outcome for the preterm infant.
▶ The use of amnioinfusion reduces persistent variable decelerations of the fetal heart rate during the first stage of labour and increased umbilical artery pH.

Term prelabour rupture of the membranes

According to Enkin et al (2000:205) prelabour rupture of the membranes occurs in 6 to 19%

of all term births (at or after 37 weeks). Of these women statistics show that:

▶ Almost 70% will give birth within 24 hours.
▶ Almost 90% will give birth within 48 hours.
▶ A remarkably constant 2 to 5% will be undelivered after 72 hours.
▶ Almost the same proportion of 2 to 5% will be undelivered after 7 days.

A deficiency in prostaglandin production or in their prostanoid biosynthesis pathway is

---

Protocols and management guidelines for treatment

Whenever current available evidence from research is inconclusive or needs further evaluation, treatment of individual women will depend on the decisions taken by those who are responsible for the provision of care within a specific maternity service. It is therefore of the utmost importance that you, as midwife, are fully informed of the different protocols or management guidelines practised in your place of work. Should you be aware of new research or evidence that might change outdated practices, it is up to you to inform the relevant policy makers.

---

suspected because of the failure of these women to go into spontaneous labour, as well as poor cervical dilatation during induction.

Previously, infection has been associated with a high risk of maternal and perinatal mortality. Therefore immediate induction of labour was done to reduce the risk. According to Enkin et al (2000:206) a more expectant approach has recently become popular due to concern about the perceived increased risk of operative delivery after induction of labour.

Appropriate therapeutic antibiotics are required when there are signs of infection with prelabour rupture of membranes at term.

Preterm labour

Labour beginning before 37 completed weeks of gestation is considered as preterm labour. Preterm labour exists when the uterine contractions are accompanied by cervical change and descent of the presenting part. The more serious consequences of preterm labour occur before 34 weeks gestation.

Diagnosis and prediction of preterm labour

Early diagnosis and swift intervention are the keys to successful management of preterm labour. However, most of the early signs of preterm labour are both subtle and varied. None of the leading symptoms of preterm labour have an individual diagnostic sensitivity of more than 50%. In many cases, despite antenatal preparation, women do not notice contractions or other symptoms until the labour is quite advanced. Early diagnosis is

therefore generally not made because women do not recognise the features of preterm labour.

Midwives should be aware of the risk factors and clinical features of preterm labour:

Epidemiological factors. Although most epidemiological risk factors are related to poor socioeconomic conditions, the following factors may increase the risk of preterm labour:
- Poor socioeconomic, educational, hygiene or nutritional status.
- Very young or advanced maternal age.
- Nulliparity or grande multiparity.
- Coloured or black women.
- Women of short stature or low weight.
- Heavy or stressful work.
- Cigarette smoking.

Risk scoring. The most important factor for preterm delivery is a history of preterm delivery in a previous pregnancy, which will put the woman in a high-risk group, even in the absence of any other risks.

Preterm labour differs little from labour at term, except that it occurs too early. A woman who has more than one contraction in ten minutes with a history of ruptured membranes or dilatation and effacement of the cervix on vaginal examination, should be considered to be in preterm labour. Be careful not to observe the woman for too long for signs of progress because more advanced preterm labour is more difficult to stop.

It is difficult for a woman to distinguish between contractions of preterm labour and so-called normal Braxton Hicks contractions. To

Symptoms of preterm labour

▶ Uterine contractions every 10 minutes or less (with or without pain).
▶ Menstrual-like discomfort with cramps.
▶ A dull lower backache.
▶ Pelvic pressure.
▶ An increase in vaginal discharge which is thin, watery and greyish, white or yellow.
▶ Urinary frequency with pain in the groin.
▶ Intestinal cramping with or without diarrhoea.

minimise this problem any woman at 20 to 37 weeks should be instructed to contact her care provider or go to hospital if contractions (one every 10 minutes or less, with or without pain) do not stop after she has been lying down on her left side for an hour.

Women in preterm labour often experience one or more of the symptoms listed above (as well as the epidemiological factors described previously).

Prevention of preterm labour

Social interventions. The association between a woman's social and economic circumstances, and her risk of preterm birth, is strong. The high-risk woman should be discouraged from doing hard, manual labour or over-exerting herself during exercise. Cigarette smoking, the use of alcohol and/or the use of addictive drugs should be discouraged as it is implicated in preterm delivery and is a cause of low birth weight.

Infections and fever. Any sickness causing high fever may lead to preterm labour, and must be treated promptly and vigorously. The following infections are known to increase the incidence of preterm birth and should be prevented or treated as early as possible (see Chapter 19).
▶ Syphilis
▶ Bacteriuria and pyelonefritis
▶ *Gardnerella vaginalis*
▶ HIV infection

Physical measures. Bed-rest has *not* demonstrated to be effective in reducing the incidence of preterm birth although it is fequently prescribed. Moreover, bed-rest has significant physiological, psychosocial and economic costs.

Cervical cerclage. This seems to benefit women who have had two or more past pregnancies that ended preterm. Cervical cerclage carries the risk of infection and may stimulate uterine contractions. This surgical procedure should therefore be avoided in women who are unlikely to benefit from it. Vaginal examination or ultrasound measurement has been used to do cervical assessments, in the hope of recognising women who are likely to give birth prematurely. Although some of these approaches are promising, research is needed for proof. Both procedures are invasive and women might react negatively towards them.

Prophylactic pharmacological approaches. Betamimetic drugs prescribed to women who are considered to be at increased risk of preterm labour do not decrease the risk of preterm birth, low birth weight or perinatal mortality. *Magnesium sulphate* also does not decrease the risk of preterm labour.

Injections of *17-alpha-hydroxyprogesterone caproate* may reduce the incidence of preterm labour and preterm birth in women considered to be at high risk of preterm labour, although it does not reduce maternal mortality or morbidity.

Management of active preterm labour

Refer to Table 26.2 for the management of active preterm labour.

Tocolytic treatment for active preterm labour

Betamimetic drugs

Betamimetics are used more often than any of the other labour-inhibiting agents that are employed. According to Enkin et al (2000:214) available data from trials show

Table 26.2 Management of active preterm labour

Gestational age less than 26 weeks or estimated fetal weight less than 900 g:	▶ Transfer from a community health centre to hospital. ▶ Allow labour to proceed. ▶ If the baby is born alive, resuscitate actively and transfer the baby from a community health centre to hospital.
Gestational age 26 to 33 weeks or estimated fetal weight 900 g to 1999 g:	▶ Transfer from a community health centre to a hospital.* ▶ Administer *hexoprenaline* 10 micrograms IV to suppress contractions during transfer. ▶ Administer *ampicillin* 1 g IV six-hourly and *metronidazole* 400 mg orally three times daily until delivery (for *penicillin* allergy, substitute *erythromycin* 500 mg orally four times daily). ▶ Administer corticosteroids for 24 hours to improve lung maturity. ▶ Run a CTG tracing, if possible. ▶ If there is evidence of abruptio placentae or chorio-amnionitis, allow labour to proceed under close fetal monitoring with CTG, or consider caesarean section. ▶ If the cervix is 6 cm or more dilated, allow labour to proceed. ▶ If the cervix is less than 6 cm dilated, administer *hexoprenaline* or *nifedipine* regimen (see Table 26.3). ▶ If *hexoprenaline* or *nifedipine* fails to stop contractions, add *indomethacin* 100 mg suppository, followed by another dose after 12 hours if necessary. ▶ Deliver the baby in a slow and gentle fashion, with an episiotomy if the perineum is very tight 　　*If the estimated fetal weight is less than 1 500 g, transfer the woman to a hospital with neonatal intensive care facilities (level 2 or level 3).*
Gestational age of 34 weeks or more or estimated fetal weight of 2 kg or more:	▶ Exclude specific causes of preterm labour, such as chorio-amnionitis or other infections (with fever and tachycardia) and abruptio placentae. ▶ Manage labour as for term pregnancies. There is no need to transfer from a community health centre to a hospital.

Source: DoH, March 2002:99.

that betamimetic drugs reduce the proportion of births that occur within 48 hours after beginning treatment. The total incidence of preterm birth is also reduced in this way. The betamimetic of choice in South Africa is *hexoprenaline* (see Table 26.3 for *hexoprenaline* regimen).

Side effects
▶ Commonly observed symptoms are palpitations, tremors, nausea and vomiting, headaches, thirst, a feeling of nervousness and restlessness.
▶ Chest discomfort and shortness of breath should alert caregivers to the possibility of pulmonary congestion. Pulmonary oedema is a serious and common complication of betamimetics due to the use of aggressive intravenous therapy. This can be prevented mainly through administration of the drug in a small volume of fluid by using an infusion pump.

▶ Most women experience an increase in heart rate. The heart rate is usually kept between 110 to 120 bpm by adjusting the dose of betamimetic administration.

▶ Betamimetic agents do cross the placenta and cause fetal tachycardia, although this is usually less pronounced than in the woman.

▶ Women with pre-existing cardiac disease should not receive betamimetic drugs. The use of these drugs results in a marked increase in cardiac output. Myocardial ischaemia has been indicated as a complication of betamimetic treatment.

▶ Betamimetic agents show a clear tendency to lower diastolic blood pressure and increase the systolic blood pressure.

▶ All betamimetic agents influence carbohydrate metabolism as blood sugar and insulin secretion increase. The rise in blood glucose is more pronounced in women with diabetes, and in women with well-regulated blood sugar it will become unstable. This is even more applicable when betamimetics are combined with corticosteroids, which also have a diabetogenic effect.

According to Enkin et al (2000:216) the metabolic effects in the woman and fetus may result in hypoglycaemia and hyperinsulinism after birth. Assessment of blood sugar levels is therefore advisable in infants born when betamimetics were used to inhibit labour.

Inhibitors of prostaglandin synthesis

Prostaglandins are responsible for the initiation and maintenance of labour. Agents such as Naproxen®, *flufenamic acid*, *aspirin* and *sulindac*, as well as the most commonly used *indomethacin*, are prescribed to inhibit prostaglandin synthesis. *Indomethacin* causes a competitive and reversible inhibition of the enzyme, cyclooxygenase, that is necessary for the synthesis of prostaglandins. Contractions are effectively inhibited and as a result the incidence of preterm birth and low birth weight babies is reduced. There is also a trend towards a reduction in the incidence of perinatal mortality and respiratory distress syndrome. Treatment is started by inserting a rectal suppository containing 100 mg of the drug. If necessary, the dose may be repeated once after 12 hours.

Maternal side-effects

▶ Headaches, dizziness and gastrointestinal irritation may occur when treatment is initiated. More serious side-effects are peptic ulceration, gastrointestinal and other bleeding, thrombocytopenia and allergic reactions. With *indomethacin*, gastrointestinal irritation is less frequent with rectal rather than with oral administration.

▶ Signs of infection may be masked by prostaglandin synthesis inhibitors thereby delaying the diagnosis of chorio-amnionitis.

▶ Bleeding time will be prolonged and should be taken into consideration when performing any interventions.

Fetal side-effects

▶ Prostaglandin synthesis inhibitors cross the placenta and constriction of the fetal ductus arteriosus has been identified as a serious concern, especially when the gestational age is beyond 34 weeks. Prolonged treatment may result in changes similar to those seen in persistent pulmonary hypertension in the newborn.

▶ *Indomethacin* may reduce both fetal and neonatal renal function. The effect is dose related and appears to be transient. It does not lead to permanent impairment of renal function in the infant.

▶ Antenatal use of prostaglandin synthesis inhibitors may cause necrotizing enterocolitis. These drugs all inhibit platelet aggregation with prolonged bleeding time in the case of a woman, fetus and neonate at birth. Since neonates, and in particular preterm neonates, eliminate these drugs far less efficiently than their mothers, these effects will last longer in the baby than in the mother.

Magnesium sulphate

Magnesium sulphate has been used for inhibition of labour, particularly when medical conditions contraindicate the use of betamimetics and prostaglandin synthesis inhibitors.

Side effects
▶ Maternal pulmonary oedema has been reported when *magnesium sulphate* and corticosteroids are administered at the same time.
▶ Magnesium toxicity can occur if renal function is impaired. This may be evident as impaired reflexes, respiratory depression, alteration in myocardial conduction, cardiac arrest and death. Patellar reflexes must be examined regularly since these reflexes will disappear at lower magnesium levels than those that cause respiratory depression and cardiac conduction defects.
▶ Magnesium levels in the fetus closely parallel that in the woman. Infants born during or shortly after treatment are reported to be drowsy, with reduced muscle tone, low calcium levels and they may take three or four days to eliminate the excess magnesium.

Calcium antagonists (Calcium channel blockers)
Calcium antagonists, including *verapamil* and *nifedipine* (Adalat®), have been used in the treatment of ischaemic heart disease and arterial hypertension as well as for hypertension during pregnancy. They are also now used for preterm labour and seem to have fewer maternal side-effects, longer prolongment of pregnancy and fewer admissions to the neonatal intensive care unit. These agents act by inhibiting calcium influx across cell membranes, thereby decreasing tone in smooth muscles. They act as profound vasodilatory agents and have minimal effect on the cardiac conduction system (see Table 26.3 on page 26-14 for the *nifedipine* treatment regimen).

Maintenance of preterm labour inhibition
Preterm birth may recur before adequate fetal maturity has been achieved. Therefore treatment is directed at maintaining labour inhibition for as long as necessary.

Oral betamimetics administered after uterine contraction has been arrested by intravenous therapy, in order to maintain labour inhibition, does not reduce the incidence of preterm birth.

Other treatments for active preterm labour
Other treatments for active preterm labour include:
▶ *Hydration*. Hydration with intravenous fluid is not more useful than no treatment at all. There is an increased risk of pulmonary oedema if labour-inhibiting drugs are subsequently used.
▶ *Antibiotic treatment*. When membranes are intact, antibiotic treatment has no effect on the rate of preterm birth, prolonging of pregnancy, respiratory distress syndrome or neonatal sepsis. Antibiotic treatment reduces maternal infection (chorioamnionitis or endometritis) and neonatal necrotizing enterocolitis.

Preterm birth
Preterm birth is the most important single cause of adverse infant outcome, in terms of both survival and quality of life. Many of these small babies are already compromised by other factors such as inadequate fetal growth, pre-eclampsia, prelabour rupture of membranes, multiple pregnancy, placenta praevia, abruptio placentae, fetal congenital malformations, abnormal fetal lie and severe maternal disease – all of which add their own complications to the baby's wellbeing.

Place and preparation for birth
A very preterm infant should be born in a maternity centre with adequate intensive care facilities, equipment and efficient staff resources to ensure adequate medical and nursing care. According to Enkin et al (2000:31) misplaced self-confidence in your own and your hospital's abilities may result in failure of timely referral to those institutions where adequate facilities, equipment and experienced

Table 26.3 Hexoprenaline and nifedipine regimens in preterm labour	
Hexoprenaline regimen	**Nifedipine regimen**
▶ Administer *hexoprenaline* 10 micrograms IV slowly, then add 300 micrograms to 1 litre Ringer's lactate, to run at 60 ml/hour, increasing by 10 ml/hour every 30 minutes until contractions stop, or until the maternal pulse rate reaches 120 bpm, or the infusion rate reaches 120 ml/hour. ▶ Stop the *hexoprenaline* infusion after 24 hours and allow labour to proceed or discharge the woman if she is not in labour. No follow-up doses of *hexoprenaline* are required.	▶ Administer *nifedipine* 20 mg orally, followed by 10 mg orally after 30 minutes if the woman is experiencing painful contractions. ▶ Give *nifedipine* 10 mg orally after four hours and then four-hourly if there are painful contractions, up to a maximum of 24 hours. Then allow labour to proceed or discharge the woman if she is not in labour.

Precautions when using hexoprenaline or nifedipine:
▶ *Hexoprenaline* or *nifedipine* should not be used in women with cardiac disease or pre-eclampsia.
▶ The maternal pulse rate should never exceed 120 bpm. Observe the pulse rate half-hourly or connect to cardiac monitor if possible.
▶ Do not give *nifedipine* to women receiving *magnesium sulphate*.
▶ Admit the woman to a labour ward for close observation.
▶ Monitor the blood pressure hourly.
▶ Auscultate the woman's lungs every four hours to exclude pulmonary oedema.
▶ Do not allow the *hexoprenaline* infusion rate to exceed 120 ml/hour.

Source: DoH, March 2002:100.

professionals are readily available to treat these tiny babies, before and after birth.

The woman in strong preterm labour requires an immediate assessment as to whether transfer to a maternity centre would be appropriate. The decision will depend on:
▶ How advanced the labour is.
▶ The fetal presentation.
▶ Whether it is a single or multiple pregnancy.
▶ Whether the fetus is alive and well.
▶ Whether the fetus is normally formed or malformed.
▶ Gestational age of the fetus.
▶ The facilities that are available (which may, for example, be sufficient for a baby born at 36 weeks but not at 31 weeks).

Labour should be inhibited with drugs in order to postpone delivery until the woman arrives at the hospital. Corticosteroid therapy, to promote lung maturity in the neonate, should be administered before transfer, unless gestational age has advanced beyond 34 weeks gestation, at which stage respiratory distress is less likely to be a problem.

Resuscitation equipment, in proper working order, should be available in the labour ward. A midwife and/or paediatrician skilled in resuscitation and who can devote all her attention to the infant, should be in attendance at all preterm births.

Prevention of periventricular haemorrhage infarction

The very preterm infant is very vulnerable to periventricular haemorrhage infarction. It is an important cause of mortality and morbidity in these immature infants. As many as 90% of the haemorrhages occur in infants under 35 weeks gestation. By giving corticosteroids to these women, the risk of periventricular haemorrhage infarction is reduced.

Method of delivery

One of the most difficult decisions about care for preterm birth is the choice between vaginal birth and caesarean birth. Properly controlled studies are not available to guide this important decision. Caesarean birth seems to be the method of choice when preterm birth is complicated by fetal distress, abruptio placentae or chorio-amnionitis. In the event of an uncomplicated preterm birth the baby is usually born vaginally, whether the fetus is in a breech or vertex presentation. Caesarean birth is not the preferred method of delivery due to the many known risks to the woman.

The soft skull and wide sutures of the preterm baby is more vulnerable than that of the term baby to sudden decompression when the baby emerges from the birth canal. The baby should be delivered slowly and gently. An episiotomy should only be done if the perineum is very tight.

Vacuum extraction is not indicated due to the softness of the skull bones. Forceps delivery does not improve outcomes in the event of an uncomplicated preterm birth.

Immediate care at birth

An experienced paediatrician, neonatologist or midwife/neonatal nurse should be present at all preterm births. Decisions about resuscitation and ventilation should be taken preferably before the birth in consultation with the parents and the obstetrician.

Preparation and resuscitation of the baby will be discussed in Chapter 31. The woman who has given birth to a preterm infant should see and touch her baby and every possible step should be taken to facilitate mother-infant bonding, even when the baby must be admitted to the neonatal intensive care unit for further management.

Abnormalities of fetal lie, presentation and position

When the fetus is lying longitudinally in an occipitoanterior position, pregnancy and birth are associated with positive outcomes. However, when the fetus is in a breech, brow, face or shoulder presentation, lying transverse, or is in an occipitoposterior position, labour can be prolonged and difficult. In some situations these malpresentations can endanger the life of the fetus and possibly the woman.

The two abnormal fetal presentations and positions that are seen with some frequency in practice are the occipitoposterior position of a vertex presentation and the breech presentation. Fortunately, the other abnormal lies, presentations and positions are rarely seen.

Occipitoposterior position

The occipitoposterior position, such as ROP or LOP, is a common cause of prolonged labour as well as severe backache. The character of the labour, the abdominal shape and the position of the posterior and anterior fontanelles on vaginal examination help to establish the diagnosis. The woman often experiences a bearing-down feeling before her cervix is fully dilated. In the second stage, a gaping anus is common. Progress is slower than normal and the contractions are often of poor quality. Although this position is considered an abnormal position, it is quite common in black women.

When doing an abdominal examination, small fetal parts are felt in the anterior part of the uterus. When the woman is lying on her back the shape of the abdomen, from the umbilicus to the symphysis, has a depression at or immediately below the umbilicus. The cephalic prominence is not felt as easily as in anterior positions, because flexion is less marked.

On vaginal examination the posterior fontanelle will be in the left or right posterior position. Since flexion is less marked, the posterior fontanelle might be difficult to feel.

The diagnosis is confirmed when the

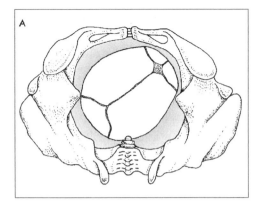

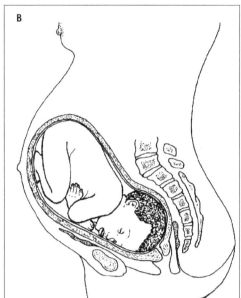

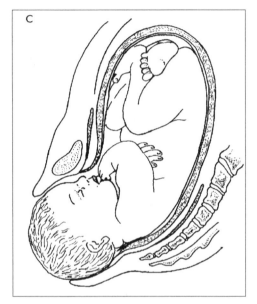

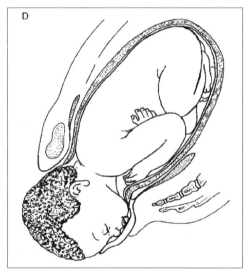

Figure 26.1 Occipitoposterior positions (A, B, C) and occipitoanterior position (D)

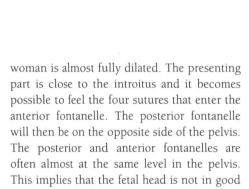

woman is almost fully dilated. The presenting part is close to the introitus and it becomes possible to feel the four sutures that enter the anterior fontanelle. The posterior fontanelle will then be on the opposite side of the pelvis. The posterior and anterior fontanelles are often almost at the same level in the pelvis. This implies that the fetal head is not in good flexion.

Given sufficient time, most posterior positions will rotate to the normal anterior position (long anterior rotation). As long as the fetus and the woman are in good condition and labour is progressing, there should be no interference. The woman will need considerable support and encouragement to cope with the discomfort and back pain of a slow labour. She will also need careful monitoring for fatigue, the judicious use of pain relief methods and adequate intake of fluids and nourishment. Labour may be augmented if the contractions are of poor quality and cephalopelvic disproportion has been excluded.

The following supportive measures will help the woman cope with the slow progress:

▶ A supportive labour companion.
▶ Using different massage and pressure techniques as well as superficial heat and cold.
▶ Encourage her to use different positions to help the baby to turn to an anterior position. The Sims' position on the side opposite to the side that the fetal head is directed, the hands and knees position or leaning forward over a bed are recommended. A birth ball, low stools and cushions will be of assistance to help the woman into different positions. Doing this may encourage anterior rotation by allowing the fetal spine to fall toward the anterior abdominal wall of the woman.

When the fetal head becomes arrested in a transverse position high in the pelvis, the situation is best managed by caesarean section. If the head is low into the pelvis, with no sign of cephalopelvic disproportion, vacuum extraction may rotate and flex the fetal head.

Delivery is the same as for any occipito-anterior position when the fetus rotates to an anterior position (long anterior rotation).

If short posterior rotation takes place and the occiput stays posterior, the baby will be delivered in the 'face to pubis' position. Others may be rotated by means of a vacuum extractor to an anterior position (this should be done only if the woman is HIV-negative).

When delivering the head in the posterior position, the larger posterior aspect of the head causes greater stretching and more lacerations of the perineum than the narrower anterior part of the head. Therefore the use of episiotomy is more common during this type of delivery. Slow progress during the second stage is more common (especially if the woman is pushing while lying on her back instead of using a squatting or hands and knees position) and low forceps or vacuum extraction is often the management of choice to save the mother and child from the effects of a prolonged period of bearing down.

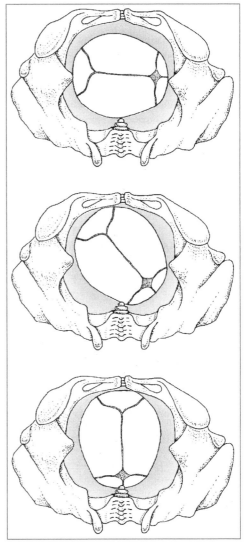

Figure 26.2 Occipitoposterior position: Long anterior rotation of the fetal head

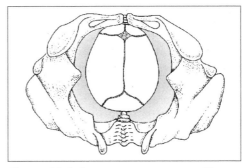

Figure 26.3 Occipitoposterior position: Short posterior rotation of the fetal head

26-17

Research highlight

A large international randomised trial of planned vaginal delivery versus elective caesarean section for term breech has shown that a planned caesarean section will lower the mortality and morbidity of these babies. Serious maternal complications are similar between the groups.

Source: Hannah, Hannah & Hodnett et al, 2002.

Breech presentation

In a breech presentation the baby's bottom, foot or feet present instead of the head. The denominator becomes the sacrum and the bitrochanteric diameter lies in the oblique diameter. The incidence of breech presentation decreases from about 15% at 29 to 32 weeks gestation to between 3 to 4% at term. In most cases the fetus converts to the cephalic presentation by 34 weeks gestation. Spontaneous changes from breech to cephalic presentation occur with decreasing frequency as gestational age advances in the third trimester.

The breech presentation is sometimes associated with uterine, placental or fetal abnormalities but it is often simply an orientation problem that places a healthy woman and her baby at risk. A breech presentation does not complicate the pregnancy, but during labour and birth the woman and fetus are at risk. Therefore breech presentations should be referred for follow-up care at a hospital from 36 weeks gestation. An ultrasound should be done to confirm the presentation and to exclude fetal abnormalities, placenta praevia, as well as multiple pregnancies. If an ultrasound is not available an abdominal X-ray may be of help.

Almost half of all breech presentations can be turned to a cephalic presentation by means of an external cephalic version, thereby reducing the caesarean section rate for breech presentations. External cephalic version will be discussed in Chapter 27.

Complications and dangers in breech presentations

Maternal complications and dangers	Fetal complications and dangers
▶ Infection is common, due to the high rate of interventions. ▶ Prolonged labour due to poor application of the presenting part. ▶ Maternal stress and post-traumatic stress disorder. ▶ Postpartum haemorrhage due to prolonged labour. ▶ Severe perineal lacerations as a result of poorly managed assisted deliveries. ▶ Obstructed labour of the after-coming head.	▶ Presentation and prolapse of the umbilical cord. ▶ Asphyxia neonatorum due to delay of delivering of the head and premature respiratory inspirations while the head is still in the pelvis. ▶ Neonatal birth injuries: fractures, damage to nerves, damage to abdominal viscera (the liver, spleen and adrenal glands) by incorrect handling of the baby during delivery, bruising of the buttocks and external genitalia. ▶ Periventricular haemorrhage infarction due to rapid and upward moulding. Excessive compression (as the head passes through the pelvis) is followed by rapid decompression when the head is allowed to deliver too quickly.

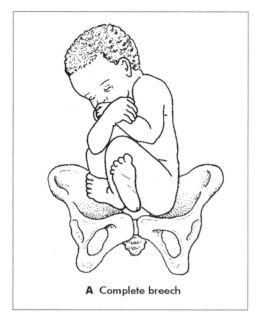

A Complete breech

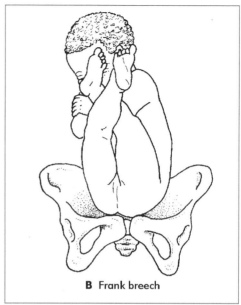

B Frank breech

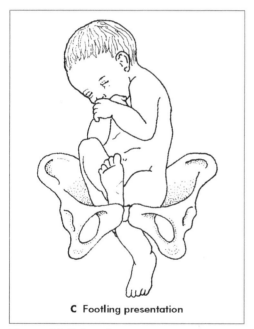

C Footling presentation

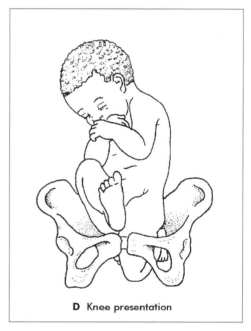

D Knee presentation

Figure 26.4 Breech presentations

At the time of admittance to the labour ward of a woman with a breech presentation, a decision should be made whether a trial of labour is indicated or whether a caesarean section is to be performed. The risk of a breech presentation to the woman is an increased likelihood of caesarean section or trauma to the birth passage during manipulative procedures of a breech delivery. The risks to the baby are possible cord prolapse and difficult vaginal or caesarean delivery. Caesarean is the chosen method of delivery.

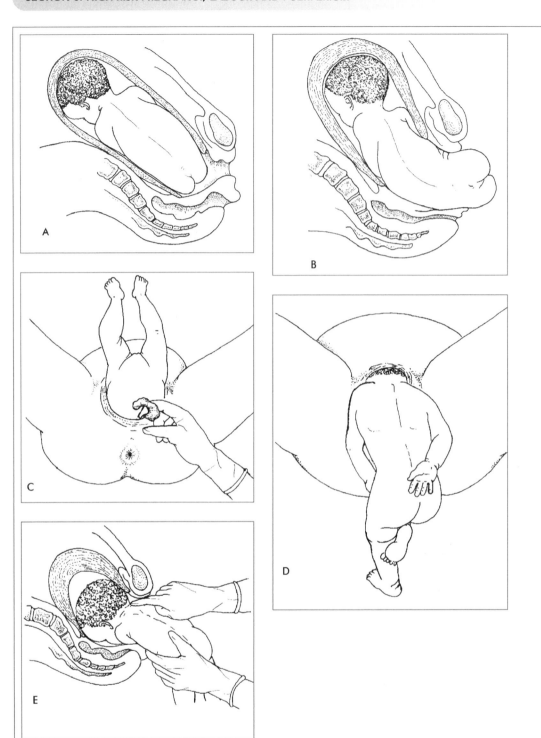

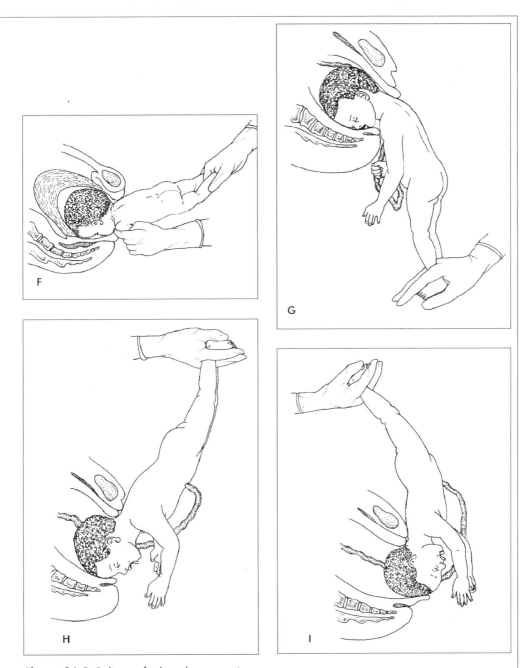

Figure 26.5 Delivery of a breech presentation

Delivery of a baby with a breech presentation

Preparing for delivery:	<ul><li>The woman must be fully dilated.</li><li>The bladder must be empty to aid descent of the breech and prevent bladder injuries.</li><li>Intravenous infusion must be prepared for possible augmentation of labour or management of postpartum haemorrhage.</li><li>Extra sterile, warm towels must be available to cover the baby's body during delivery to reduce spontaneous respiration from environmental cold before the birth of the head.</li><li>Piper forceps (forceps designed specifically for delivery of the after-coming head of a breech) are added to the normal delivery pack if a practitioner skilled in their use is available.</li><li>Resuscitation equipment and supplies are ready for use. A paediatrician and experienced midwife/neonatal nurse are notified and present at the birth.</li></ul>
Conducting the delivery:	<ul><li>When the baby's buttocks begin to distend the perineum, the woman is placed in the lithotomy position, with the legs in stirrups and the buttocks extending slightly past the end of the bed.</li><li>The fetal heart rate is checked frequently. As long as the baby is in good condition, spontaneous delivery is awaited.</li><li>The woman must be encouraged to bear down effectively during the contractions.</li><li>When the breech appears, the sacrum (usually anterior) eases upwards and is delivered spontaneously. This is followed by unassisted delivery of the legs.</li><li>Traction on the body of the baby must be avoided, since it can lead to deflexion of the head and extension of the arms above or behind the head.</li><li>As soon as the umbilicus comes into view, a short segment of cord is drawn down to avoid tension.</li><li>After the birth of the umbilicus the fetus should be born within three to five minutes in order to prevent hypoxic ischaemic damage to the fetus.</li><li>While the woman continues to use abdominal muscles to expel the fetus, an assistant applies gentle pressure over the suprapubic area, to maintain its flexion, and to avoid extension of the fetal arms above the head.</li><li>The baby's back must be kept anteriorly. Allow the body to hang down in an effort to encourage flexion and the scapulae and arm will deliver.</li><li>As soon as the posterior hairline (the nape of the neck) appears, the baby's ankles are grasped and the body held on the stretch to keep the spine in alignment and the legs and body are lifted in a wide arc of 180° up and over the woman's abdomen.</li><li>To encourage the head to descend in the birth canal, firm suprapubic pressure is continued. This will be followed by emergence of the nose, brow and the remainder of the head without traction.</li><li>There is now no urgency to deliver the vault of the head since the mouth and nose may be suctioned as soon as they appear, allowing time for slow and controlled delivery of the rest of the head.</li></ul>

$\Rightarrow$

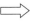

Alternative methods to deliver the head:	▶ *Wigand-Martin method.* The baby lies prone, straddling on the left hand of the person doing the delivery. The middle finger of that hand is placed in the baby's mouth with the index and ring fingers on the malar bones. The finger in the baby's mouth encourages and maintains flexion of the fetal head. With the other hand the operator exerts suprapubic pressure on the head through the woman's abdomen.
	▶ *Mauriceau-Smellie-Veit manoeuvre.* The position is the same as the Wigand-Martin, with one finger in the baby's mouth and two on the malar bones. The other hand is placed astride the baby's back and shoulders with the middle finger placed against the occiput in order to promote flexion of the head and produce traction in this way. Another person can apply suprapubic pressure on the fetal head.

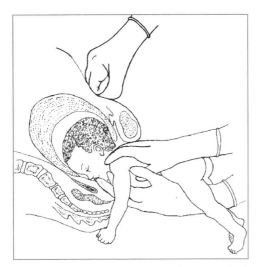

Figure 26.6 The Mauriceau-Smellie-Veit method for a breech presentation

Classification of breech presentations

There are four types of breech presentations (refer to page 26-19):

▶ *Complete.* Flexion at thighs and knees. The feet and bottom of the baby present.

▶ *Frank.* Flexion at thighs and extension at knees. This is the most common variety and includes almost two-thirds of breech presentations. Extended legs make it difficult for the fetus to turn spontaneously and may prevent a successful external cephalic version from being performed.

▶ *Footling.* Single or double, with extension at thighs and knees. The foot is the presenting part. This presentation is very rare.

▶ *Kneeling.* Single or double, with extension at thighs, flexion at knees. The knee is the presenting part. This presentation is also very rare.

Delivery of the fetus with a breech presentation

Although we now know that a planned caesarean section is better than a planned vaginal birth for a term fetus, it occasionally happens that a woman may arrive at a hospital or centre almost fully dilated. It is therefore of great importance that midwives should be able to assist the woman when a medical practitioner is not available. The delivery of the fetus with a breech presentation is discussed on page 26-22.

Transverse lie

When the long axis of the woman and fetus are at right angles to one another, a transverse lie is present. The denominator is the scapula (Sc); the situation of the head determines whether the position is left or right, and that of the back indicates whether it is anterior or posterior.

Transverse lie is associated with multiparity, uterine and fetal abnormalities, shortening of the longitudinal axis of the uterus by fundal or low-lying placenta, and conditions that prevent the engagement of the presenting part, such as pelvic tumours and a small pelvic inlet. Abnormal lie, particularly oblique lie, may be temporary and related to maternal position.

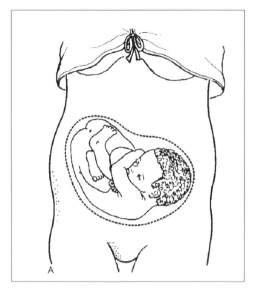

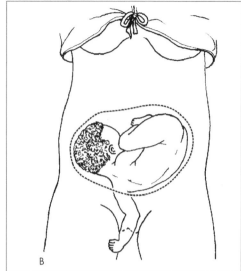

Figure 26.7 Transverse lie

External version to a cephalic presentation (see Chapter 27) may be attempted in a hospital from 37 weeks gestation. An ultrasound should be done to confirm the presentation and to exclude fetal abnormalities, placenta praevia as well as multiple pregnancies. If an ultrasound is not available an abdominal X-ray may be of help. Transverse lies at term, after failure of external version, are treated by caesarean section. They must never be neglected or left to nature. It is a dangerous situation near term or in labour, as there is a high risk for mother and fetus because of obstructed labour and cord/arm prolapse as the membranes tend to rupture early.

Face presentation

If the attitude is one of complete extension, the face is the presenting part; the chin (mentum – M) is the denominator and leading pole, and the presenting diameter is the submentobregmatic (9.5 cm). This is termed a face or chin presentation.

On abdominal examination of a face presentation where the head is in extension, the back and the cephalic prominence are on the same side of the abdomen. When the fetal head is well flexed, the back and the prominence are on opposite sides.

A face presentation is often difficult to diagnose on vaginal examination. The examiner is not usually expecting a face presentation, or on previous examination, the fetus was in an occipitoposterior position, which later extended and turned into a face presentation.

In most instances, a deflexed vertex presentation converts into a face presentation during labour. It must be kept in mind that in an anterior face presentation the baby's back and occiput are posterior. When the chin is posterior, on the other hand, the back and occiput are anterior.

In the anterior face presentation, extension of the fetal head must be maintained by holding back the sinciput, until the chin escapes under the symphysis pubis, before the occiput is allowed to sweep the perineum.

Whereas a baby with an anterior face presentation can deliver vaginally, a persistent posterior face presentation becomes arrested when the chin goes into the hollow of the sacrum. There is no further movement possible because the head and the neck are completely extended. Persistent posterior face presentations must be delivered by caesarean section.

If labour has been prolonged, marked oedema makes the face difficult to feel. The presenting part is soft and irregular. The mouth, with the gums, is diagnostic but might be confused with the anus. The mouth is open, whereas the anus grips the examining finger and stains it with meconium. The lips and labia majora might be confused. Care must be taken not to injure or infect the eyes during the vaginal examination.

Brow presentation

The brow presentation is midway between the vertex and the face presentation. The attitude is one of partial extension, in contrast to face presentation in which extension is complete. The presenting part is the area between the orbital ridges and the bregma. The denominator is the forehead (frontum – Fr). The mentovertical diameter is presenting, which at 13.5 cm is the longest presenting diameter of the fetal head.

During labour engagement takes place with extensive moulding, and when progress does occur, it is slow. Spontaneous delivery is rare, and can take place only when there is the combination of a large pelvis, strong contractions and a small baby or if flexion of the baby's head takes place.

Since brow presentation may be temporary, a trial of labour is permissible in the hope that flexion to an occiput presentation or complete extension to an anterior face presentation will take place. However it must be kept in mind that fetal mortality is high. The excessive moulding may cause irreparable damage to the brain. Mistakes in diagnosis and failure to respond to warning signs are causes of poor fetal prognosis.

Abnormal labour

Abnormal labour occurs as a result of:
▶ A labour which does not progress normally (referred to as poor progress or prolonged labour).
▶ Cephalopelvic disproportion (CPD), which is when the capacity of the woman's pelvis is insufficient (contracted, fractured or malformed) and/or the baby's head is too large

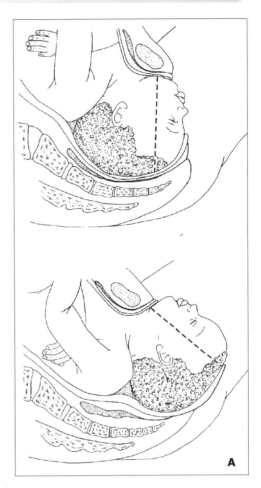

A

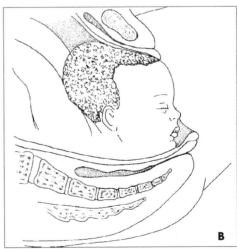

B

Figure 26.8 Face presentation A: Mechanism of birth in a mentoanterior position, B: Mechanism of birth in a mentoposterior position

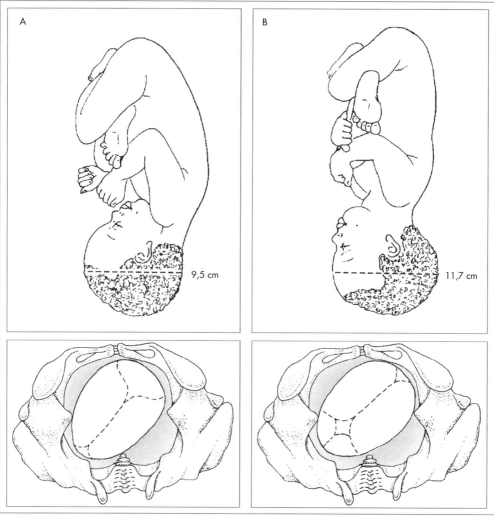

Figure 26.9 Types of cephalic presentations with their different diameters A: Head is flexed with occiput as denominator, B: Military presentation, C: Brow presentation, D: Face presentation with mentum as denominator

(malposition or malpresentation) for the safe vaginal delivery of the baby.

▶ Abnormal uterine contractions (referred to as dysfunctional uterine activity).

Poor progress or prolonged labour

Poor progress in labour can occur in either the first or second stage of labour. While there is certainly an association between prolonged labour and adverse outcomes, the extent to which this association indicates a problem is by no means certain. Deviation from the accepted defined normal rate of dilatation should be an indication for evaluation rather than for intervention.

When a midwife is observing and caring for a woman in labour, she must have a clear understanding of the different forces involved, as described in Table 26.4.

As many as eight other P's (physiology, preparations by the woman, professionals who provide care, place of birth, procedures, peoples – other than professionals, politics/-social context, pressure through decision-

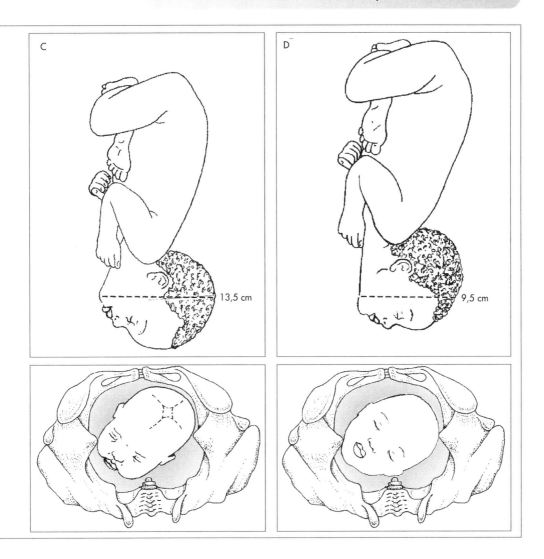

making) have been identified to ensure care that is holistic.

'Prolonged labour' must not be confused with 'cephalopelvic disproportion'. Cephalopelvic disproportion will cause the labour to be prolonged and will always require intervention, whereas prolonged labour may finally end with a normal unassisted delivery. Thorough observation and continual reassessment of the different P's are essential to identify prolonged labour. When prolonged labour does occur, the woman should be transferred to hospital or be seen by a medical practitioner.

Note
The diagnosis of slow progress depends on careful documentation of the labour progress, preferably by plotting changes in cervical dilation and descent of the head on a partogram.

Prolonged first stage of labour

Prolonged latent phase. This phase usually starts before the woman is admitted to a community health centre or hospital, therefore it is poorly understood since its precise time of onset is often difficult to determine. The

Table 26.4 The five P's of labour affecting labour progress

Powers	Definition:
	Powers are defined as uterine contractions as well as maternal voluntary pushing efforts during the second stage.
	Abnormalities in the powers:
	▶ Abnormal uterine action, such as hypertonic, hypotonic and incoordinated uterine action.
	▶ During induction with an unripe cervix (Refer to Bishop score in Chapter 13).
	▶ Inappropriate use of pharmacological and non-pharmacological methods for relief of pain.
	▶ Ineffective bearing-down efforts during second stage due to maternal exhaustion or epidural.
Passageway	Definition:
	Passageway is the maternal bony pelvis and related soft tissues, including the lower uterine segment, cervix, pelvic floor muscles, vaginal passage and introitus.
	Abnormalities in the passageway:
	▶ Placenta praevia.
	▶ A contracted, deformed or fractured pelvis.
	▶ Tumours of the bone or soft tissues of the pelvis.
	▶ Spondylolisthesis, which is the partial forward dislocation of one vertebra over the one below it. Most commonly it is the fifth lumbar vertebra over the first sacral vertebra.
	▶ Spinal malformation, such as kyphosis, lordosis and scoliosis.
	▶ Malformation of the uterus or cervix.
	▶ A full bladder can delay labour.
	▶ An anatomically rigid cervix, which may be due to scarring, or lack of nerve endings in the cervix.
	▶ An impacted or oedematous lip of cervix will not dilate properly.
Passenger	Definition:
	The passenger is the fetus.
	Abnormalities in the passenger:
	▶ Malposition, malpresentation and compound presentation.
	▶ A large baby or a large head.
	▶ A short umbilical cord causes traction.
	▶ Multiple pregnancy with locked twins.
	▶ Congenital abnormalities and fetal tumours.

Psyche	**Definition:**
	Psyche is defined as a woman's previous experiences, emotional readiness, cultural heritage, support network and aspects that contribute to her coping abilities and self-confidence.
	Abnormalities in psychological factors:
	▶ A woman suffering from post traumatic stress disorder after a previous birth, rape or physical abuse.
	▶ Unresolved anger and frustration, because she is not involved in choices about her care and treatment.
	▶ Feeling unsafe and scared during labour.
	▶ Her expectations of pain relief are not met.
	▶ No encouragement, praise and support from professionals or others (such as husband, friend or mother).
Position	**Definition:**
	Position refers to the spatial placement of the woman's body.
	Abnormalities in positioning:
	▶ Being forced to stay in the same uncomfortable position.
	▶ Lying on her back during labour and second stage or after an epidural.
	▶ The woman is not allowed to assume the position that makes her feel comfortable and in control.

accepted average length of the latent phase of labour is eight hours, thereafter the latent phase is considered to be prolonged.

If a woman still experiences pain after eight hours, with no progress, other reasons for abdominal pain should first be considered, such as urinary tract infection or abruptio placenta.

False labour should be excluded, which is characterised by no cervical changes and no increase in the intensity, duration and frequency of contractions. If the mother and fetus are not in danger, sedation and analgesia can be given and the situation reassessed in four to six hours. If cervical effacement has not improved the woman can be discharged.

Although routine rupture of membranes is not advised during labour, it is indicated where poor progress is present as long as cephalopelvic disproportion (CPD), HIV-positive status and fetal distress have been excluded. Evaluate the need for *oxytocin* infusion (as for the active phase of labour) if contractions are not effective.

Prolonged active phase. When active labour is mistakenly diagnosed and there is failure of the cervix to dilate within a prescribed period of time it may result in the incorrect diagnosis of dystocia (the term given to difficult, abnormal labour progress). It is very sobering to note that dystocia is the largest single cause of the increased caesarean birth rate in the United States. Thorough and complete assessment of the five P's (Table 26.4) is essential before such a diagnosis is made.

After 4 cm dilatation, a protracted or delayed active phase of labour is defined as a dilatation rate of less than 1 cm per hour. It is characterised by uterine dysfunction as well as occipitoposterior positions of the head, and occasionally CPD may be present.

In managing a prolonged active phase, CPD, malpresentation and fetal distress should be excluded. If one of them is present, a caesarean section should be performed.

Ensure that the woman has an empty bladder as well as adequate hydration (intravenous infusion of Ringer's lactate to run at 120 to 240 ml/h). Support and encourage the woman and do not leave her alone. Ensure that she has adequate pain relief. If there are no contraindications, rupture the membranes and start *oxytocin* infusion.

An arrest disorder is defined as no dilation for more than two hours and no descent for longer than an hour in a nullipara. In a multipara the same criteria is used. The 'two hour rule', however, is controversial and has been challenged by others.

Prolonged second stage of labour

If descent of the fetal head is slow and fails to reach the pelvic floor after two hours of full dilatation, the second stage is prolonged. A prolonged second stage should also be considered when effective maternal bearing-down efforts are present and the delivery has not occurred after 45 minutes in a nullipara, or 30 minutes in a multipara.

It may be more difficult to diagnose the prolonged second stage where arrest occurs late in the descent phase of the second stage. The head may be low (only one- to two-fifths palpable above the brim) and caput succedaneum will be present. The caput may give an erroneous impression that the head is on the perineum, and increasing caput may give a mistaken impression of progress, although slow. For these reasons it is advisable to assess the level of the head abdominally rather than vaginally.

A prolonged second stage of labour and obviously undesirable outcomes are closely associated. These outcomes are increased perinatal mortality, postpartum haemorrhage, puerperal febrile (infection) morbidity and neonatal seizures.

The duration of the second stage is not as important as the constant progress measured by descent of the presenting part. With continuous descent together with maternal and fetal wellbeing, putting a time limit on the second stage is unnecessary. However, if poor progress is suspected, a vaginal examination should be done after 15 minutes to assess for CPD or any abnormalities. The emphasis is rather on constant monitoring of maternal and fetal wellbeing and to identify poor progress and arrest than to intervene only after a pre-set period of time. There is, however, a much slimmer chance of spontaneous delivery after a second stage of more than two hours in nulliparous women and more than one hour in multiparous women.

If the woman is fully dilated but does not experience any pushing sensation (after having an epidural, this does not apply), the fetal head might still be high. If there is no fetal distress

The complications and dangers of prolonged labour	
Maternal dangers	**Fetal dangers**
▶ Maternal distress and exhaustion (keto-acidosis). ▶ Intra-uterine infection due to early rupture of membranes and/or from repeated vaginal examinations. ▶ Postpartum haemorrhage due to traumatic interventions or uterine atony as a result of prolonged labour. ▶ Psychological trauma (post-traumatic stress disorder) from pain and shock and the way the woman was treated by care providers during this ordeal.	The longer the labour, the higher the fetal and neonatal mortality and morbidity, and the more frequently the following conditions occur: ▶ Asphyxia from the prolonged labour itself. ▶ Cerebral damage caused by fetal hypoxia. ▶ Chorio-amnionitis of the fetus, leading to pneumonitis, meningitis, pyelonephritis and septicaemia. ▶ Fetal death.

and there are no signs of CPD, one hour should be allowed for descent of the fetal head, which will give the woman the urge to bear down. A more upright position should be considered to aid descent (refer to Chapter 14 for the different maternal positions that can be used). During this time the woman should not be lying on her back and observations should be carried out every 30 minutes until delivery. Continuous monitoring of the fetal heart rate would be the preferred method of observation. If not available, the fetal heart rate should be auscultated every five minutes directly after a contraction to rule out fetal distress.

If the woman is still not bearing down after the hour has past, confirm that the cervix is fully dilated and rupture membranes if still intact. The woman should be motivated to bear down in an upright position in an attempt to deliver the baby. If all attempts fail, she should be transferred to a level 2 or 3 hospital for re-evaluation. When CPD, fetal distress and breech presentation is ruled out, labour will be augmented with *oxytocin* infusion (see Chapter 13). If the delivery fails to take place in another hours' time, a caesarean section or vacuum extraction is indicated (see Chapter 27).

Prolonged third stage or retained placenta

If a placenta is not delivered within 30 minutes of delivery of the baby, the third stage is prolonged. A retained placenta is managed by emptying the bladder. If the woman cannot pass urine herself a urinary catheter should be used. An *oxytocin* infusion of 20 IU in 1 litre Ringer's lactate at 120 to 240 ml per hour should be started and she should be kept nil per os.

The woman should be observed closely for bleeding or placental delivery. If the placenta is not delivered after an hour of *oxytocin* or there is excessive bleeding she should be transferred to a hospital for manual removal of the placenta under general anaesthesia.

Cephalopelvic disproportion (CPD)

Cephalopelvic disproportion exists when the capacity of the woman's pelvis is insufficient for the safe vaginal delivery of the baby. In other words, the pelvis (passage) is too small (contracted, fractured or malformed) and/or the baby (passenger) too large (malposition or malpresentation). This will affect the course and possibly the eventual outcome of the labour.

Predisposing causes of CPD: The birth passage

Pelvic inlet contracture. Inlet contracture is present when the anteroposterior diameter is less than 10 cm or the transverse diameter is less than 12 cm. Inlet contraction may result from rickets and fractures, the specific type of pelvis and spinal deformities. When both diameters are contracted, dystocia is much greater than when only one is contracted.

Normally, cervical dilatation is facilitated by the pressure of the unruptured membranes or, after their rupture, by direct application of the presenting part against the cervix. When the head is arrested in the pelvic inlet, the entire force exerted by the uterus acts directly upon the portion of membranes that overlie the dilating cervix. Under these conditions early spontaneous rupture of membranes is more likely to result.

The better the application, the more efficient are the contractions. In the presence of a contracted pelvic inlet, application is poor and often results in prolonged labour. In women with contracted pelvises, shoulder and face presentations are seen three times more frequently. Cord prolapse, however, is four to six times more likely too.

The implication of non-engagement of the fetal head as an indicator of CPD is not well established. In black, primiparous women in whom such non-engagement commonly occurs, it is usually associated with longer labours, but not with an increased rate of operative delivery or increased maternal or fetal morbidity. In many cases the high station is related to the cervix and uterus being unprepared. The head cannot enter the pelvis until the lower segment is formed, which happens only in a term pregnancy.

Contracted midpelvis. Midpelvic contracture occurs when there is a reduction in the plane of least dimensions, the one that passes from the apex of the pubic arch, through the ischial spines, to meet the sacrum usually at the junction of the fourth and fifth segments. It is more difficult to recognise than the inlet and outlet contracture.

When the interspinous diameter is less than 9 cm and the distance between the ischial tuberosities is less than 8 cm the midpelvis is considered contracted. There is no accurate manual method of measuring midpelvic dimensions, but it is suspected when the ischial spines are prominent, the pelvic sidewalls converge or the sacrosciatic notch is narrow. Midpelvic contracture is a common cause of dystocia and caesarean section. These contractions may prevent anterior rotation of the occiput and may direct it into the hollow of the sacrum. Failure of rotation and deflection attitudes are frequently associated with a small pelvic cavity.

Outlet contraction. Most women with midpelvic contraction have outlet contraction as well. The best example being the android or funnel-shaped pelvis. A contracted pelvic outlet usually has a long, narrow pubic arch. Ideally the subpubic arch should be well rounded, low and wide (about 90°). A diminution of the intertuberous diameter and the subpubic angle forces the head backward, and so the prognosis depends on the capacity of the posterior segment, mobility of the sacrococcygeal joint and the ability of the soft tissues to accommodate the fetus.

Pelvic fractures and contractures. Automobile accidents are the most common cause of pelvic fractures. A history of pelvic fracture warrants careful review of previous X-rays. A caesarean birth is more commonly done under these circumstances.

Soft tissue obstructions. Myoma of the uterus occasionally develops in the lower segment of the uterus or in the cervix and may obstruct the birth passage. A caesarean birth is planned if the myoma becomes impacted in the pelvis and prevents descent of the fetus. Occasionally, an ovarian tumour gets incarcerated in the true pelvis. In such cases labour becomes obstructed and a caesarean birth is inevitable. Very rarely, a septum has been found in the vaginal passage, obstructing labour. It must be excised before the baby can be born.

Predisposing causes of CPD:
The passenger
Fetal size is important, but a fetus is rarely too large for any pelvis. The essential problem is the relationship of the fetus to the pelvis. The question that must be answered is: Can this fetus pass through this pelvis without physical or neurological damage? The problems may be classified according to the cause of the abnormality:
▶ *An oversized fetus.* Frequently as the result of diabetes, obesity, multiparity or large parents.
▶ *Fetal anatom.* Hydrocephalus, conjoined twins, gross ascites, abdominal tumour or myelomeningocele.
▶ *Fetal malpresentation or position.* Breech presentation, occiput posterior, transverse lie, brow presentation or shoulder presentation.
▶ *Inability of the fetal head to mould.* Face presentation, post-term pregnancy, hydrocephaly or craniostenosis.

The diagnosis of CPD
No reliable methods are available for accurate prediction of CPD before labour, however the following procedures and examinations should allow the woman to be placed into one of three categories:
▶ No disproportion is present. This fetus should go through this pelvis.
▶ There are definite signs of CPD.
▶ The fetopelvic relationship is borderline. A trial of labour is indicated.

Factors to consider in diagnosing CPD
History. It is the medical practitioner's responsibility to determine the amount of disproportion and to decide on the course of

action. Where a medical practitioner is not available the midwife or advanced midwife must be able to diagnose disproportion and recognise the degree of disproportion. If necessary, the woman must then be transferred for appropriate treatment.

Information from the woman's history will alert you to the possibility of CPD:
▶ The size and condition of previous babies at birth.
▶ Length of previous labour.
▶ Method of delivery.
▶ Maternal cervical or vaginal lacerations.

The most reliable predictor of pelvic adequacy remains the previous uncomplicated delivery of a baby of similar or greater birth weight than is estimated for the current pregnancy.

Abdominal palpation. The woman must be as relaxed as possible, and lying on her back. It may be helpful to ask the woman to raise herself up on her elbows during this procedure since it allows the head to enter the pelvic brim without so much manipulation on the part of the examiner.

A complete abdominal examination must be done. If the head is not engaged, the examiner presses the head gently but firmly into the pelvic brim. The fingers of the other hand are applied to the area of the abdomen above the pubic symphysis. If the head can be pushed into the pelvis it suggests that there is no disproportion at the inlet. If it does not go in, the following causes of failure to descend or override should be considered before a possible diagnosis of CPD can be made:
▶ Underdeveloped lower segment.
▶ Not close enough to term.
▶ Polyhydramnios.
▶ Full bladder or rectum.
▶ Placenta praevia.
▶ Soft tissue tumour.

The Munro (Muller) Kerr method:
▶ While doing a vaginal examination the inlet cavity and outlet of the pelvis are palpated

to estimate their capacities and to search for abnormalities.
▶ The position of the presenting part is noted, as well as its ability to flex.
▶ While the examining fingers are still inside the vagina, the thumb is placed on the outside of the pelvis on the upper, anterior border of the symphysis pubis. Care is taken not to exert pressure on the clitoris since this area is very sensitive.
▶ The left hand is placed on the abdomen over the fetal head and presses the head downwards and backwards, into the pelvic brim.
▶ The fingers inside the vagina assess the amount of descent of the presenting part, while the thumb determines the degree of overlap at the summit of the symphysis pubis.

Clinical pelvimetry. Clinical pelvimetry has not been evaluated by a randomised trial and therefore elective caesarean birth in a cephalic presentation is not justified on the basis of the findings of a clinical pelvimetry.

It is important to distinguish between the risk of disproportion to the presenting fetal part and that related to a non-leading part of the fetus. The dangers of obstructed labour to the partly born fetus, as in shoulder dystocia, or obstruction to the after-coming head in a breech presentation must be taken into consideration during examination.

X-ray pelvimetry. Since the reports of an association between antenatal irradiation (X-ray pelvimetry) and childhood leukaemia, irradiation that is not likely to benefit the woman or baby is now avoided. Its utility has been questioned because of its poor predictive value as a screening test for CPD. Management is also rarely influenced.

Trial of labour. CPD is best diagnosed by a carefully monitored trial of labour in cephalic presentations. With correct use and accurate monitoring on a partogram, any abnormality or delay can be recognised and acted upon immediately.

During the trial of labour the fetal heart

> ### The importance of doing abdominal palpations before vaginal examinations
>
> Before doing a vaginal examination it is of great importance to do an abdominal palpation to ascertain how many fifths of the fetal head are still above the symphysis pubis. Due to caput and excessive moulding the fetal head may appear lower on vaginal examination than it actually is. By doing the palpation this abnormality will be recognised.
>
> When three-fifths of the fetal head are still palpable above the pelvic brim and 3+ moulding of the fetal head is found on vaginal examination, it confirms the diagnosis of CPD.

rate and the uterine contractions are monitored. If the head does not descend well, and presents with excessive caput and moulding; if the rate of cervical dilation is less than 1 cm per hour; and if delivery does not take place within the allotted time, caesarean birth should be considered.

Women who do not make good progress due to inefficient uterine contractions are given a trial of augmentation of labour by an infusion of *oxytocin* (see Chapter 13).

Favourable progress of cervical effacement and dilatation, descent of the head into the pelvis, and the demonstration that the lower part of the pelvis is adequate are the criteria for continuing the trial of labour. The achievement of an easy vaginal delivery excludes disproportion and avoids caesarean birth.

Dysfunctional uterine activity

To understand dysfunctional uterine activity it is necessary to know and understand normal uterine function as described in Chapter 12. Dysfunctional uterine activity relates to the powers of labour.

Uterine overactivity

Hypertonic uterine action signifies an increase in the normal intensity, rate and duration of the uterine contractions. Often there is a raised resting tone, which means that the uterus does not relax completely between contractions.

Primary hypertonic uterine action. This results in precipitate labour. This means that the labour lasts less than three hours, from the beginning of contractions until the birth of the baby. This type of labour and birth may lead to uterine rupture or severe cervical, vaginal and perineal lacerations and trauma to the baby if the birth is unattended. The contractions are very strong and intense and therefore these women tend to push uncontrolled during the second stage of labour. Precipitate labour is associated with abruptio placentae, amniotic fluid embolism, meconium in the amniotic fluid, postpartum haemorrhage, cocaine abuse and low Apgar scores.

Secondary hypertonic uterine action:

▶ *Type 1.* In the multigravida, CPD may result in a tonic contraction of the uterus. Such a tonic contraction is strong and continuous and will cause the uterus to rupture if it is not treated and relieved. The clinical features of CPD will be present, with maternal and fetal distress and a pathological retraction ring (Bandl's ring). The management will be an emergency caesarean section.

▶ *Type 2.* The tonic contraction is caused by the misuse of *oxytocin* and/or prostaglandins. The *oxytocin* infusion must be stopped immediately and the medical practitioner informed. The medical practitioner may have to prescribe a beta 2 stimulant (*hexoprenaline*) to relax the uterus and intra-uterine resuscitation done if fetal distress is present.

Uterine inefficiency
Hypotonic uterine dysfunction

Hypotonic uterine action is observed when the contractions lessen in intensity, rate and duration. The slight rise in pressure during a contraction is not enough to dilate the cervix. The progress of labour will slow down and this will lead to prolonged labour.

- *Primary hypotonic uterine action.* When labour commences the contractions are already hypotonic, and if not managed the contractions will continue to be hypotonic into the active phase of labour. This will lead to prolonged latent and active phases of labour. If this condition is allowed to continue without treatment, the woman will become exhausted and will begin to show signs of distress, especially if she is unable to rest, sleep or eat. It is important to differentiate between primary hypotonic uterine action and false labour. If the membranes are ruptured, labour will be augmented, if not, the woman will receive medication to relieve pain and stress (*pethidine* and Aterax®). If the contractions disappear after the effect of the medication has worn off, she was in false labour. If not, it is accepted that she is in true labour. The woman must be assessed to exclude CPD, malpresentation and fetal distress, only then can labour be augmented.
- *Secondary hypotonic uterine action.* This condition is due to uterine exhaustion after a period of what we considered to be 'normal labour'. CPD should be excluded before this woman is augmented. In the presence of CPD, caesarean birth is the usual obstetrical management.

Hypertonic uterine dysfunction

- *Hypertonic lower segment.* This condition occurs mainly in primiparous women during labour and is relatively rare. The woman has much pain and this is due to a slightly elevated basal uterine tone and very strong, regular contraction (often four to five every 10 minutes). Sometimes the midsegment of the uterus contracts with more force that the fundus. There is little or no progress and no evidence of CPD. The management consists of psychological and physical support and encouragement. The woman may also need analgesia and intravenous fluids. *Oxytocin* is contraindicated as it may make the situation worse. If these measures are not successful birth is often by caesarean

section. This condition seldom recurs in a subsequent pregnancy.
- *Incoordinated uterine action.* With asymmetrical uterine action there is complete asynchronism of the impulses originating in each cornu of the uterus. Strong contractions may alternate with weak ones. The minor contractions are entirely ineffective. The major ones do bring about some cervical dilation but much less effectively than normal waves. Incoordinated uterine action can also occur with normotonic, hypotonic or hypertonic contractions. The lack of polarity leads to inability of the uterus to dilate the cervix. Progress is extremely slow under these circumstances. In the case of a colicky uterus, pacemakers appear all over the uterus. The contraction pattern is irregular with some contractions weak and others strong; sometimes coupling occurs where contractions are paired or even tripled. In addition there may be slow or no progress. Pain is present all the time and often out of proportion to the intensity of the contractions. Management consists of applying the rule of P's to ascertain any causes or precipitating factors, which must be corrected. Psychological support and good analgesia are important. *Oxytocin* is indicated when contractions are considered to be inadequate. With proper management, most of these women will deliver vaginally, though the incidence of forceps and vacuum deliveries are high.
- *Constriction ring and retraction ring.* A true constriction ring is very rare in modern obstetrics. It is a ring of the myometrium that goes into tetanic contraction around the fetus. It cannot be felt externally with abdominal palpation. The diagnosis is in most cases first made at caesarean birth. A constriction ring must be distinguished from a retraction ring. The latter is a ridge formed at the junction of the lower and upper segments. With CPD, where the lower segment expands, the ring moves upward in the direction of the umbilicus. When it reaches an abnormally high level it

is called a pathological retraction ring or Bandl's ring.

Cervical dystocia

Cervical dystocia means a rigid cervix, which, despite good uterine contractions, is unable to dilate. There may be underlying psychological reasons and/or physical causes. Cervical dystocia includes two main groups:

▶ *Primary cervical dystocia*. Primary cervical dystocia may mean a structurally normal cervix that does not open and relax. This cervix is associated with the tension and pain of a difficult labour. This is the rigid cervix of incoordinated uterine action causing prolonged labour. Epidural analgesia is the answer to this condition although a caesarean birth may be necessary. Primary cervical dystocia may also be due to a rigid cervix caused by an anatomical abnormality of the cervical tissue or nerve supply, making dilatation impossible. Occasionally the medical practitioner will do an incision of the rim of the cervix.

▶ *Secondary cervical dystocia*. The cervix may be scarred as a result of previous births, operations or cancer. Oedema of the cervix can be caused by an anterior or posterior lip of cervix becoming nipped between the hard fetal head and the pelvic girdle. The swollen cervix cannot dilate as easily. However, sometimes the woman cannot restrain herself from bearing down, it is an almost uncontrollable urge, and epidural analgesia would bring immense relief. Do not talk to her harshly or scold her as it will not help and make her feel even more out of control.

Should epidural analgesia not be available the woman may be advised to turn over on her elbows and knees, so that her shoulders are lower than her buttocks. By doing this, pressure is relieved from the swollen cervix. Supporting the vulva and perineum firmly during a contraction with one hand while talking to her gently and confidently during a contraction will help her to get through this difficult time while

the cervix slowly dilates. If cervical dystocia is not treated, the whole cervix may rupture or eventually slough off. This is called an annular detachment of the cervix.

Emergencies during childbirth

Presentation and prolapse of the umbilical cord

The umbilical cord is presenting when the cord is lying in front of the presenting part but the membranes are still intact. With umbilical cord prolapse the membranes are ruptured. The cord may either be at the pelvic inlet, in the vagina or prolapsed through the introitus. Cord prolapse has a reported incidence of approximately 1 in 200. The fetal mortality rate is high and there are increased maternal complications from the use of operative procedures. With emergency guidelines in place and practised by health care professionals these figures could come down dramatically.

With cord prolapse the blood supply to the fetus is cut off when the umbilical cord is compressed between the presenting part and the maternal pelvis. If not managed correctly this will lead to the death of the fetus.

Always exclude cord prolapse or presentation after rupture of the membranes (spontaneous or artificial) by performing a vaginal examination and auscultating the fetal heart rate. Prolonged fetal bradycardia or severe variable decelerations often accompany cord prolapse due to the resulting cord compression. It is of importance to note that nearly 50% of cord prolapses occur during the second stage of labour.

Management protocol

Management depends on several factors but mainly gestational age, fetal viability, underlying cause for the cord prolapse, cervical dilation and the need for transfer to a hospital with the facility to perform a caesarean section.

No interference is indicated under the following circumstances:

▶ When the fetus is dead.

- When there is a congenital abnormality incompatible with life.
- When extreme prematurity is present and the fetus is not viable.

Under these circumstances there are no indications for caesarean birth and vaginal delivery is awaited.

When the fetus is found to be alive and viable (estimated weight at or more than 1 kg) and the woman is not fully dilated:

- With the cord protruding through the introitus, gently replace it in the vagina or wrap it loosely in a warm, wet sterile towel saturated with warm saline solution.

Unnecessary handling will result in vessel spasm and fetal hypoxia.

- Digitally elevate the presenting part by vaginal manipulation, to prevent cord compression. With one finger on either side of the cord or both fingers to one side, exert upward pressure in an attempt to reduce the pressure of the presenting part on the cord. Maintain this continuously until the baby is delivered by caesarean birth.
- Confirm fetal wellbeing, should time allow, do continuous CTG or regular auscultation until birth of the baby.
- The woman is given oxygen (6 l/min) by facemask for a maximum of 10 minutes.

Table 26.5 Aetiology of cord prolapse

Fetal factors:	- Malpresentations (breech presentation, shoulder presentation, compound presentation and, rarely, face or brow presentation) often result in a high presenting part with poor application. This accounts for approximately 50% of cases. - Polyhydramnios: Excess amniotic fluid may cause the cord to be washed out when membranes rupture. Preferably membranes should be ruptured under controlled circumstances. - Prematurity accounts for 30 to 50% of cases and is mainly due to the small size of the presenting part and the high incidence of malpresentations in preterm labour. - Multiple pregnancy where prematurity, abnormal positions, abnormal presentations and polihydramnios are common. Ruptured membranes with a high presenting part, especially of the second twin, poses a high risk.
Maternal factors:	- CPD with poor application of presenting part. - High presenting part, especially in the multipara.
Cord and placental factors:	- Cord length: Especially when the length exceeds 80 cm. - Low implantation of the placenta.
Iatrogenic factors:	- Amniotomy without proper caution. Controlled, slow rupture of the membranes, with pressure on the presenting part from above, is preferable when performing rupture of the membranes in cases with a high presenting part. - While an extended head is flexed. - During internal version and breech extraction.

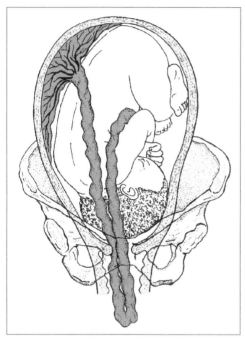

Figure 26.10 Prolapsed umbilical cord

Oxygen administration for longer than 10 minutes may be harmful to the fetus (Hofmeyer, 2003).

▶ Start intravenous Ringer's lactate or increase existing drip rate to increase placental perfusion.

▶ Stop *oxytocin* infusion if in progress to relax the contracting uterus.

▶ Tocolytic agents such as *hexoprenaline* (10 micrograms IV – as a single dose) may be administered slowly intravenously to stop contractions.

▶ The bladder may be distended with 500 ml of normal saline via an indwelling catheter which is then clamped until birth. If the full bladder relieves the pressure of the head on the cord sufficiently, digital elevation may be relieved.

▶ Continue to elevate the presenting part by positioning the woman in an exaggerated Sims' or knee-chest position, until birth can be accomplished.

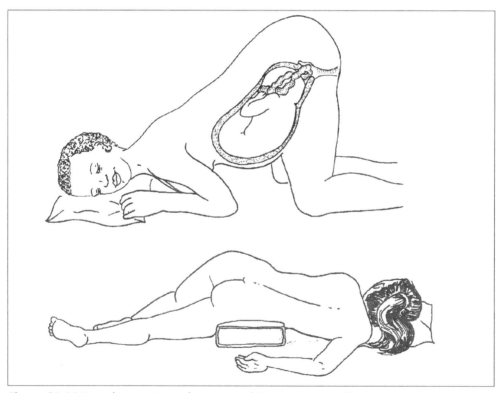

Figure 26.11 Knee-chest position and exaggerated Sims' position to relieve pressure on the umbilical cord

▶ All events should be recorded accurately.
▶ Transfer the woman to a hospital with facilities for caesarean section and neonatal care.

When the fetus is found to be alive and viable and the woman is fully dilated with the fetal head engaged in the pelvis, the baby must be delivered immediately. If progress is not fast enough the baby should be delivered by vacuum extraction. It is of great importance to exclude CPD under these circumstances.

Amniotic fluid embolism

An amniotic fluid embolism (AFE) is a complex disorder characterised by the abrupt onset of hypotension, hypoxia and consumptive coagulopathy but clinical manifestation varies greatly. Some women have only one of these symptoms while all three may be absent in other women.

Previously it was found that AFE occurs when amniotic fluid containing particles of human debris (e.g. vernix, hair, skin cells, meconium) enters the maternal circulation. Data now suggest a clinical picture similar to human anaphylaxis and unlike an embolic phenomenon as commonly understood.

During pregnancy, labour and birth there are ample opportunities for mixture of maternal blood and fetal tissue, yet in most cases these events are harmless. In certain women, however, such exposure initiates a complex series of physiological reactions mimicking those seen in human anaphylaxis and sepsis.

Clinical manifestation

In obvious cases the woman, in the late phases of labour or immediately postpartum, begins gasping for air and then rapidly suffers seizure or cardiorespiratory arrest which is complicated by disseminated intravascular coagulation (DIC), massive haemorrhage and death. Some women develop DIC without cardiorespiratory symptoms.

Management

A medical practitioner should be notified immediately and the midwife should start with the

> ### CRITICAL THINKING EXERCISES
> Ameena (G3 P2 term pregnancy) arrived at the hospital in strong labour. On entering the labour ward she said that she wanted to push. Her observations were done and the CTG was attached. The observations and fetal heart rate seemed to be normal. A midwife did a vaginal examination. She found her to be fully dilated, membranes bulging. The fetal head presented at station +1 and application was fair. The midwife proceeded to do an amniotomy. On rupturing the membranes the fetal heart rate decelerated to 80 bpm and recovered to 100 bpm after the contraction. An umbilical cord stretching closely over the fetal head could be felt on vaginal examination.
>
> 1. How could this situation have been prevented?
> 2. How should the attending care providers proceed from this point onward?

resuscitation efforts. Most women go through a transient period of systemic and pulmonary hypertension. Those women who survive long enough to receive any treatment other than cardiopulmonary resuscitation should receive therapy directed at oxygenation and support of the damaged myocardium. The management of maternal cardiac arrest is discussed in Chapter 22. Circulatory support with blood and component replacement is paramount.

In women who have not delivered and suffer from cardiac arrest, consideration should be given to emergency perimortem caesarean delivery (on the spot) in an effort to improve newborn outcome. However, when the woman is haemodynamically unstable, but has not suffered arrest, such decision-making becomes much more difficult.

Prognosis

The prognosis depends to an extent on how efficiently emergency measures were carried out.

In the United States the National Registry series indicate a 60% maternal mortality rate after an AFE. Neurological impairment is common in survivors. Neonatal survival rate is 70% but almost half suffer residual neurological impairment.

Shoulder dystocia

With shoulder dystocia the anterior shoulder gets impacted behind the symphysis pubis. Most midwives who have been present at a birth complicated by severe shoulder dystocia have vivid recollections of this stressful event and the minutes between delivery of the baby's head and the rest of the body can seem like hours. Shoulder dystocia usually occurs with large babies (more than 3.5 kg) when delivery of the head is not followed by delivery of the shoulders.

Definition and incidence

Due to variations in definitions and incomplete documentation, it is difficult to accurately report the true incidence of shoulder dystocia. Most authors reserve the definition of shoulder dystocia for births that required at least one manoeuvre to deliver the impacted shoulder. Using this definition the incidence of shoulder dystocia is approximately one in 300 vaginal births.

Diagnosis

You will recognise shoulder dystocia by the following signs:
▶ Commonly there is difficulty in completing the extension of the head and the hairy scalp slides out with reluctance.
▶ When the forehead appears it is often necessary to press the perineum back to deliver the face.
▶ There is definite recoil of the head back against the perineum.
▶ Due to friction with the vulva, the head is incapable of movement and therefore restitution rarely takes place.
▶ Traction from below and pressure from above fail to deliver the baby.

Risks for shoulder dystocia

Shoulder dystocia cannot be predicted, from either clinical characteristics or labour abnormalities, with any degree of accuracy. Therefore efforts to reduce the problem should be directed towards ensuring that birth attendants are aware of contributing factors, but above all are skilled in the management of this condition when it occurs. Effective implementation of emergency procedures can prevent fetal hypoxia and death.

The following associated risk factors have been evident:
▶ Fetal macrosomia (a larger than average fetus). Although shoulder dystocia is more common in larger babies (usually more than 3 500 g) almost half of the cases occur in infants weighing less than 4 000 g.
▶ Maternal obesity.
▶ Diabetes mellitus.
▶ A history of large siblings.
▶ When the birth attendant does not allow restitution to take place but forces the baby's head into a direction.
▶ Post-term pregnancy.
▶ *Oxytocin* induction or augmentation of labour.
▶ Prolonged second stage of labour.
▶ Mid-pelvic delivery – use of either forceps or vacuum extraction.

The effects of shoulder dystocia

Shoulder dystocia can cause significant fetal and neonatal morbidity and mortality and increased morbidity to the woman due to the problems associated with this emergency.

Management guidelines

The following guidelines may be helpful in the management of shoulder dystocia:
▶ The midwife should send urgently for at least two assistants to help with the delivery, one of which is a skilled medical practitioner or midwife.
▶ She should calmly explain to the woman what happened and ask for her full cooperation. There are only four or five minutes in which to deliver the baby before brain

Problems associated with shoulder dystocia	
Maternal complications	**Fetal complications**
▶ Haematomas and lacerations in the birth passage with possible bladder and rectum injuries. ▶ Manipulations and interventions lead to puerperal sepsis. ▶ Uterine rupture. ▶ Blood loss. ▶ Psychological trauma and stress.	▶ Brachial plexus injuries, resulting in an Erb-Duchenne's palsy (40% reported recovery at one year), and less commonly in a Klumpke's palsy (72–92 % recovery at one year). ▶ A higher incidence of fractured clavicle. ▶ Mental retardation, slow learning and speech defects. ▶ Severe asphyxia and death.

damage and possible death occurs, therefore she must work quickly and efficiently.

▶ Move the woman to the side of the bed with her buttocks hanging slightly over the edge and her legs supported by the assistants. This way there will be more space to apply downward pressure on the fetus.

▶ Place the woman in an exaggerated flexion position (McRobert's manoeuvre). The assistants can assist the woman on either side, by pushing and holding her legs so that her knees should almost touch her shoulders. This manoeuvre does result in flattening the sacrum relative to the maternal lumbar spine and thereby increasing the anteroposterior diameter of the pelvis (see figure 26.12).

▶ Cut a wide episiotomy to ensure a speedy delivery once the shoulder is dislodged.

▶ Firm suprapubic pressure, directed downwards and away from the pubic bone, is exerted on the side of the fetal back and toward the fetal chest, using the palm of the hand. This will usually dislodge the impacted shoulder, while gentle downward traction is applied on the fetal head by another midwife. Steady traction must be maintained until the shoulder appears under the symphysis (see figure 26.13).

▶ Do not use fundal pressure at any stage. This will only impact the shoulder further against the symphysis.

▶ If unsuccessful at this stage, deliver the posterior arm by locating the posterior shoulder in the birth passage and sweeping the arm in front of the fetal chest. Once the posterior arm is delivered, proceed to deliver the anterior shoulder by sweeping the arm in front of the fetal chest.

▶ If this fails, rotate the baby. This is done by putting two fingers on the anterior aspect of the anterior shoulder. Put pressure against the shoulder so that it moves through 180 degrees through the face-to-pubis position, to bring the posterior shoulder forward and make it anterior. Continue by placing two fingers on the anterior aspect of the newly posterior shoulder. Put pressure against the shoulder moving it towards the symphysis pubis. The arm and head must move together to facilitate rotation and reduce the risk of injury. This manoeuvre is called the screw principle of Woods.

▶ When you need to break the clavicle, do so in an outward movement. This may assist the delivery process by reducing the bisacromial diameter of the shoulders.

▶ The Gaskin manoeuvre is used where the woman is assisted to her hand and knees in order to relieve shoulder dystocia.

▶ The Zavanelli manoeuvre can also be used (see box on page 26-43).

Injuries to the genital tract and uterus

These injuries are usually incurred during the second stage of labour and involve the birth

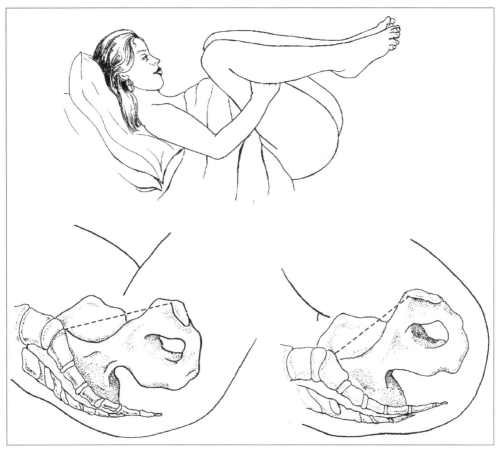

Figure 26.12 Technique to relieve shoulder dystocia. McRobert's manoeuvre during which the pelvic curve is straightened

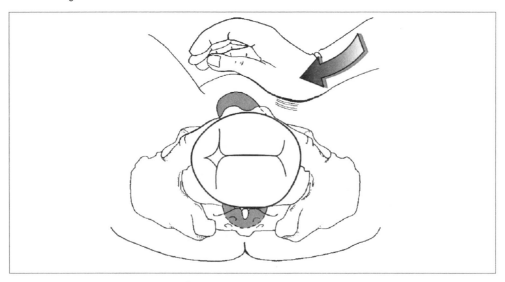

Figure 26.13 Correct application of suprapubic pressure

The Zavanelli manoeuvre

▶ The head of the fetus is returned to the occipitoposterior or occipitoanterior diameter.
▶ The head is flexed and slowly pushed back into the birth canal.
▶ The fetal status is assessed via electronic fetal monitoring or a hand-held ultrasound device while preparing for emergency caesarean birth.
▶ Personnel skilled in neonatal resuscitation should be in attendance at the caesarean birth.
▶ A review of 103 published cases of this manoeuvre from 1985 to 1997 revealed a 92% success rate with no reports of fetal injuries in those born by caesarean birth. This success rate is remarkable for a relatively new procedure for which almost all care providers noted no previous experience.

Source: Sandberg, 1999:312.

---

passage and surrounding structures. They may include injury to the urinary tract, haematomas, cervical tears and rupture of the uterus. The latter three are discussed in Chapter 21.

Injuries to the bladder and urethra, and occasionally the ureters, may occur with instrumental delivery and during caesarean section. Neglected obstructed labour may result in pressure necrosis of adjacent structures, especially the bladder, and result in fistula formation. These women usually show signs of incontinence or stress incontinence in the puerperium. Although the latter form of injury is less common in areas with good obstetric care, it still occurs in rural areas of South Africa.

In a nutshell

▶ Each labour ward should have a written protocol or drill for obstetric emergencies (for example cord prolapse or shoulder dystocia). Labour ward staff have a responsibility to learn, memorise and rehearse this protocol.
▶ All pregnant women should be considered to be at risk for preterm birth, as 50% of all preterm births occur in women with no identifiable risk factors.
▶ With preterm labour and pPROM and a estimated fetal weight of less than 1500 g, the woman should be transferred to a level 2 or 3 hospital with neonatal care facilities and experienced staff.
▶ When the problem of preterm labour or pPROM arrises, the woman should be prepared for the birth of a preterm child by introducing her to the neonatal intensive care staff and providing information about Kangaroo care and breastfeeding of the preterm infant.
▶ Injuries as a result of shoulder dystocia are likely to be followed by litigation. One way to decrease liability is to provide comprehensive objective documentation of the events in the woman's records.
▶ Abnormal labour occurs if there are differences in the normal relationships among any of the P's affecting labour.
▶ The best method for delivery of a term breech presentation is an elective caesarean section.
▶ The persistent posterior face presentation (mentum posterior) must be delivered by caesarean section.
▶ Always consider the woman's HIV status before doing any intervention.

References

Ball, J. H. S. 1996. Obstetric emergencies. In: Bassin, J. (Ed.) *Topics in obstetrics and gynaecology*. Johannesburg: Julmar Communications.

Bennett, V. R & Brown, L. K. (Eds.) 1999. *Myles textbook for midwives*. Thirteenth edition. Edinburgh: Churchill Livingstone.

Boulvain, M. & Irion, O. 2002. Stripping/-sweeping the membranes for inducing labour or preventing post-term pregnancy (Cochrane Review). *The Cochrane Library*, Issue 3, 2000. Oxford: Update Software.

Brocklehurst, P. & French, R. 1998. The association between maternal HIV infection and perinatal outcome: A systematic review of the literature and meta-analysis. *British Journal of Obstetrics and Gynaecology*, July-September (105):836–848.

Bruner, J. P., Drummond, S. B., Meenan, A. L. & Gaskin, I. M. 1998. All-fours manoeuvre for reducing shoulder dystocia during labour. *Journal of Reproductive Medicine*, 43(5):439–443.

Clark, S. L. 1990. New concepts of Amniotic fluid embolism. *Obstetrics and Gynecological Survey*, 45(6):360–368.

Creasy, R. K., Gummer, B. A., & Liggins, G. C. 1980. System for predicting spontaneous preterm birth. *Obstetrics and Gynecolog*, 55(9):692–695.

Cronje, H. S. 1996. Preterm labour and premature rupture of the membranes. In Bassin, J. (Ed.) *Topics in obstetrics and gynaecology*, Johannesburg: Julmar Communications.

Cunningham, F. G., Gant, N. F., Leveno, K. J. et al. 2001. *Williams Obstetrics*. Twenty-first edition. New York: McGraw-Hill Book Company.

DoH (Department of Health.) 2002. *Guidelines for maternity care in South Africa*. Second edition. Pretoria: Department of Health.

DoH (Department of Health.) 2002. *Saving Babies: Third Perinatal Care Survey of South Africa*. Pretoria: Department of Health.

Economy, K. E. & Abuhamad, A. Z. 2001. Calcium channel blockers as tocolytics. *Seminars in Perinatology*, October 25 (5):264–271.

Enkin, E., Keirse, M. J. N. C., Neilson, J., Crowther, C., Duley, L. & Hodnett, E. 2000. *A guide to effective care in pregnancy and childbirth*. Third edition. New York: Oxford University Press.

Gherman, R. B., Goodwin, T., Murphy et al. 1997. The McRoberts' maneuver for the alleviation of shoulder dystocia: How successful is it? *American Journal of Obstetrics and Gynecology*, 176(3):656–661.

Hannah, M. E., Hannah, W. J., Hewson, S. A. et al & the Canadian Multicenter Postterm Pregnancy Trial Group. 1992. Induction of labor as compared with serial antenatal monitoring in posterm pregnancy: A randomized controlled trial. *New England Journal of Medicine*, 326:1587–1592.

Hannah, M. E., Hannah, W. J., Hewson, S. A. et al for the term Breech Trial Collaborative Group. 2000. Planned caesarean section versus planned vaginal birth for breech presentation at term. *The Lancet*, October 356: 1375–1383.

Hannah, M. E., Hannah, W. J., Hodnett, E. D. et al. 2002. Outcomes at 3 months after planned caesarean vs planned vaginal delivery for breech presentation at term. *The Journal of the American Medical Association*, April 287(14):1822–1831.

Hofmeyer, G. J. 2003. Maternal oxygen administration for fetal distress (Cochrane Review). *The Cochrane Library*, Issue 2. Oxford: Update Software.

Hill, W. C. & Lambertz, E. L. 1990. Let's get rid of the term 'Braxton Hicks contractions'. *Obstetrics and Gynecology*, 75(4):709-710.

Johnstone, F. D. & Myerscough, P. R. 1998. Shoulder dystocia. *British Journal of Obstetrics and Gynaecology*, August (105):811–815.

Kenyon, S. & Boulvain, M. 2000. Antibiotics for preterm premature rupture of membranes (Cochrane Review). *The Cochrane Library*, Issue 2. Oxford: Update Software.

Khong, T. Y. 1998. Expression of endothelin-1 in amniotic fluid embolism and possible pathophysiological mechanism. *British Journal of Obstetrics and Gynaecology*, July 105:802–804.

Leigh, T. H. & James, C. E. 1998. Medicolegal commentary: Shoulder dystocia. *British Journal of Obstetrics and Gynaecology*, August 105:815–817.

Lowdermilk, D. L., Perry, S. E. & Bobak, I. M. 1999. *Maternity nursing*. Fifth edition. St Louis: Mosby.

Marivate, M. 1996. Maternal injuries. In: Bassin, J. (Ed.) *Topics in obstetrics and gynaecology*. Johannesburg: Julmar Communications.

Mclean, M., Walters, W. A. W. & Smith, R. 1993. Prediction and early diagnosis of preterm labor: A critical review. *Obstetrics and Gynecological Survey*, 48(4):209–225.

Newman, R. B., Gill, P. J., Wittreich, P. et al. 1986. Maternal perception of preterm uterine activity. *Obstetrics and Gynecology*, 68:765.

Nolte, A. G. W. (Ed.) 1998. *A textbook for midwives*. Pretoria: J. L. van Schaik.

Petro, G. A. 1998. Prolapse of the umbilical cord. *Principles and practice in the PMNS, Continuing Perinatal Education,* February 12(1):20–24. Observatory: Department of Obstetrics and Gynaecology.

Phillips, R. C. 1996. *Family-centered maternity and newborn care*. St. Louis: Mosby.

Rouse, D. J., Owen, J. & Hauth ,J. C. 1999. Active-phase labor arrest: Oxytocin augmentation for at least 4 hours. *Obstetrics and Gynecology*, 93(3):323–328.

Sandberg, E. C. 1999. The Zavanelli maneuver: 12 years of recorded experience. *Obstetrics and Gynecology*, 93(2): 312–317.

Simpson, R. S. 1999. Shoulder dystocia, nursing interventions and risk-management strategies. *Maternal and Child Nursing*, 24(6):305–310.

Tsatsaris, V., Papatsonis, D., Goffinet, F., Dekker, G. & Carbonne, B. 2001. Tocolysis with Nifedipine or beta-adrenergeic agonists: A meta-analysis. *Obstetrics and Gynecology*, Part 2, May 97(5):840–847.

Van Coeverden de Groot, A. A. 1997. Post-term or prolonged pregnancy. *Continuing Perinatal Education*, August 11(2):4–11.

Van Iddekinge, B. 1996. Preterm labour and premature rupture of the membranes. In: Bassin, J (Ed.) *Topics in obstetrics and gynaecology*. Johannesburg: Julmar Communications.

Wood, C. 1994. Postdate pregnancy update. *Journal of Nurse-Midwifery*, 39(2):110S.

Woods, D. L. (Ed.) *Perinatal education programme. Manual 1. Maternal care*. Cape Town: PEP.

Chapter 27

Operative obstetrics and the role of the midwife

Edith Zodwa Moosa

Introduction

Operative procedures are interventions usually performed by experienced medical practitioners in order to correct a problem or prevent fetal and maternal complications, which may result from an existing risk factor such as obstructed labour. However, an experienced and advanced midwife may perform some of these operative procedures in an emergency, where a medical practitioner is not immediately available, and the life of the fetus or the woman is at risk.

Basic midwifery considerations for operative obstetrics

The medical practitioner or advanced midwife explains the procedure to the woman and obtains her informed consent. The midwife acts as a witness to the consent and ensures that the woman fully understands the implications, the type and extent of the intervention procedure, as well as the associated risk factors. The woman must, after the explanation, be willing to give consent without coercion. If the midwife is in any doubt, the woman should be referred back to the medical practitioner. Any available significant other may be included in the discussion if the woman so wishes. In the case of an emergency, where the woman is not in a position to give consent, a legal guardian or surrogate must give consent. Should they not be available, a commissioner's consent must be obtained.

The midwife needs to stay with and monitor the woman and the fetus (where applicable) until the procedure is commenced and completed. Clear communication with and reassurance of the woman is of utmost importance at this stage, in order to prevent anxiety, which is very characteristic of any operative procedure. The midwife also plays a major role in patient advocacy to ensure that the woman's rights are not violated.

Preparation of the woman is done according to the type of procedure and the policy of the unit or institution, or as requested by the medical practitioner. Strict privacy and confidentiality must be maintained at all times and accurate recording of all the interventions must be done in order to ensure continuity of management and to prevent medico-legal risks.

Termination of pregnancy

Termination of pregnancy is deliberate ending of pregnancy in order to expel the non-viable fetus. Termination of pregnancy can be performed for many reasons such as a method of family planning, due to rape, etc. The focus in this chapter is the termination due to complicated pregnancy (e.g. maternal life-threatening disease or fetal abnormalities).

Grounds for termination of pregnancy

According to the Choice on Termination of Pregnancy Act of 1996 a pregnancy may be terminated:

(a) Upon request of a woman during the first 12 weeks of the gestation period of her pregnancy.

(b) From the 13th up to and including the 20th week of the gestation period if a medical practitioner, after consultation with the pregnant woman, is of the opinion that:
  (i)   the continued pregnancy would pose a risk of injury to the woman's physical or mental health; or
  (ii) there exists a substantial risk that the fetus would suffer from a severe physical or mental abnormality; or
  (iii) the pregnancy resulted from rape or incest; or
  (iv) the continued pregnancy would significantly affect the social or economic circumstances of the woman.

(c) After the 20th week of the gestation period if a medical practitioner, after consultation with another medical practitioner or a registered midwife, is of the opinion that the continued pregnancy:
  (i)   would endanger the woman's life; or
  (ii) would result in a severe malformation of the fetus; or
  (iii) would pose a risk of injury to the fetus.

Methods of termination

Considerations before the procedure

The South African Choice on Termination of Pregnancy Act (Act No. 1891, 22 November 1996) stipulates certain specific circumstances under which a termination can be done. The Act further stipulates specific prerequisites for termination. All midwives and medical practitioners must adhere to the Act before a termination of pregnancy can be performed.

The procedure must be performed in a private room with two people in attendance, which are the medical officer or midwife and another person to provide emotional support. Strict aseptic conditions and universal precautions against HIV infection must be maintained.

First trimester (gestational age of 12 weeks or less)

Ripening (priming) of the cervix is commenced by inserting *misoprostol* 600 mcg vaginally, usually two to four hours prior to the procedure. If the cervix fails to dilate after four hours, a repeat dose of *misoprostol* is given the next day.

Manual vacuum aspiration is then done, using a single or double valve syringe and canula (Kanaman canula). Alternatively, the suction curettage may be done under a paracervical block or general anaesthetic. An oxytocic agent may be given during or after the procedure in order to prevent haemorrhage (*oxytocin* 10 IU intravenously or intramuscularly).

After 12 weeks gestation

The procedure may only be performed by a medical practitioner in a secondary or tertiary centre, which is equipped to handle complications. Prostaglandins (*prostaglandin* E_2 preparations or *misoprostol* 600 mcg vaginally) are administered orally or vaginally for ripening of the cervix in order to initiate expulsion of products of conception. Laminaria tents or the cuff of an indwelling urinary catheter may also be used to dilate the cervix. *Oxytocin* 20 IU in one litre of intravenous fluid can be given to facilitate expulsion of products of conception and prevent excessive haemorrhage. Dilatation and curettage under general anaesthetic may be necessary if expulsion is not complete or severe haemorrhage is present.

Hysterotomy

Hysterotomy is the surgical removal of a non-viable fetus by means of an incision in the uterus and should only be considered under extreme circumstances where the life of a woman is threatened and other methods are contraindicated or have failed. The procedure is not recommended due to the associated high morbidity rate, such as uterine rupture with subsequent pregnancies and implant endometriosis.

Complications of termination of pregnancy

The immediate complications are haemorrhage due to trauma to the uterus, incomplete expulsion of products of conception or a hypotonic uterus. Infection is a major complication due to poor technique or pre-existing septic focci. The woman may later present with effects of psychological trauma due to guilt feelings. Furthermore, cervical incompetence can result in habitual abortions or preterm labour with subsequent pregnancies if cervical trauma occurred. Rhesus allo-immunisation may take place if an Rh-negative woman was pregnant with an Rh-positive fetus.

Specific midwifery management

Before the procedure the midwife must ensure that the woman is offered the opportunity of counselling and encouraged to express her concerns, so that they are attended to. She should also refer the woman for further counselling if the need arises to ensure psychological preparedness and/or aftercare. Strict confidentiality and privacy must be maintained. Observations of vital signs and psycho-emotional state of the woman are done in order to have a baseline for further observations during and after the procedure. The midwife must also ensure that the woman has given informed consent and that it is valid. Medications are given as prescribed by the medical practitioner, such as a tranquilliser prior to the surgical procedure to allay anxiety and relax the woman.

The midwife's participation during this procedure is voluntary and she has the responsibility to inform the employer and the medical practitioner timeously of her intention not to participate, giving enough time for a replacement.

The woman should be observed closely during the procedure, that is, her vital signs must be monitored for signs of shock and her psycho-emotional state checked. If the method of cervical ripening is used, the woman must be observed for onset of contractions, progress and amount of vaginal bleeding.

Specimens of the products of conception should be saved, preserved and/or sent for histology, according to the policy of the institution, or as requested by the medical practitioner. Accurate recording must be done and any abnormalities noted and reported immediately for prompt management.

After the fetus has been expelled, the woman should be cared for in a quiet environment to promote adequate rest. If the procedure is performed on an outpatient basis, the woman should be allowed to rest for a minimum of four hours. Every 30 minutes the vital signs must be assessed for signs of shock and pad checks must also be done to identify excessive haemorrhage. Check the mucous membranes for pallor, the psychological state of the woman and for any side effects of the drugs used.

Before discharge, the woman must be fully assessed for signs of shock and haemorrhage. She should be informed to report to the nearest health care facility if vaginal bleeding is excessive or persists beyond seven days. Regular personal and vulval hygiene must be emphasised to prevent infection. Advice on family planning should be given, so as to prevent an unwanted pregnancy or to allow her time for full recovery, both emotionally and physically. The type of recommended contraceptive will depend

---

Termination of pregnancy

Abortions are a major cause of early pregnancy deaths (less than 24 weeks gestation) in South Africa. In 1998, 26 out of 42 early pregnancy deaths were as a result of sepsis and haemorrhage following unsafe induced abortions. When the statistics of 1998 is compared with that of 1999–2001, there is a slight increase in the early pregnancy deaths to an average of 49 deaths per year.

---

mainly on the woman's individual needs and circumstances. *Anti-D immunoglobulin* is given if the woman is Rh-negative.

Arrangements should be made for her to access continued emotional support and counselling (Perinatal loss is discussed in Chapter 28). The partner or family may be included in the discussion if the woman so wishes. The woman is then discharged if stable, and is given a follow-up appointment for one week later.

Ectopic pregnancy

An ectopic pregnancy is the implantation of the fertilised ovum (or developing blastocyst) outside the uterine cavity, usually in the fallopian tubes and rarely in the ovary, abdominal cavity or on the cervix.

Anything that disturbs tubal function or structure and delays the passage of the fertilised ovum along the fallopian tube to the uterus, can lead to an ectopic pregnancy, including:
▶ Previous salpingitis
▶ Previous tubal surgery
▶ Abnormal tubal function
▶ Congenital narrowing of the fallopian tube
▶ Endometriosis

Current use of an intra-uterine contraceptive device can be another factor to consider, as can the fact that assisted fertilisation is also associated with a higher rate of ectopic pregnancy.

Tubal pregnancy

A tubal pregnancy is the most common and occurs in 95% of all ectopic pregnancies. Develop-ment of the pregnancy occurs between the mucosa and the muscular layer of the fallopian tube. A tubal pregnancy may progress to a tubal rupture, tubal abortion, spontaneous resolution or chronic ectopic pregnancy. A woman with a tubal pregnancy will present with a history of amenorrhoea, persistent lower abdominal pain, occasional sharp or stabbing pains, nausea and vomiting, vaginal bleeding or a slight or brownish continuous discharge and a persistent headache. On examination the uterus is enlarged due to vascular congestion and the abdomen is tender and muscle guarding is present. When tubal rupture occurs, the following will present: a sudden, excruciating lower abdominal pain, fainting, signs of shock, such as pallor, a weak rapid pulse, hypotension, collapse and epigastric or shoulder pain (referred pain).

The following investigations may be performed to diagnose the problem:
▶ Human chorionic gonadotrophin (HCG) estimation to diagnose pregnancy.
▶ Ultrasonography to identify and locate gestational sac.
▶ Laparoscopy (rarely) to visualise pelvic and abdominal structures.
▶ Culdoscopy to detect presence of blood in the pouch of Douglas.

Tubal pregnancy is an emergency, which requires immediate expert management. A medical practitioner must be called or the

---

Ectopic pregnancy and maternal mortality

Ectopic pregnancy is the second major cause of early pregnancy deaths in South Africa, primarily due to delay in diagnosis and intervention. Emergency management is of utmost importance to prevent maternal deaths. Problem recognition with subsequent incorrect management is an avoidable factor that must be addressed.

---

woman should be referred to a level 3 hospital after stabilisation (see Chapter 21 for the emergency management and resuscitation).

The woman should be put on complete bed-rest and an accurate history must be obtained to confirm diagnosis. The following are observed:
▶ Pulse and blood pressure for signs of shock.
▶ Skin colour for pallor.
▶ Mental state for listlessness, disorientation and level of consciousness.
▶ Vaginal bleeding for colour, amount, odour and consistency.
▶ Severity of abdominal pain.

Intravenous therapy (Ringer's lactate) should be commenced to maintain fluid and electrolyte balance and combat shock (see Chapter 21). Oxygen is then administered if necessary and an indwelling catheter is inserted to empty the bladder and monitor urinary output. The woman has to be prepared for the operation and the midwife needs to ensure that informed consent for the operation is obtained by the medical practitioner. The midwife must reassure and support the woman in order to allay anxiety. It is of paramount importance that an accurate record is kept of all midwifery assessments and interventions.

An emergency laparatomy must be done to control the haemorrhage and evacuate blood from the abdominal cavity in a ruptured tubal pregnancy, and to perform a total or partial salpingectomy. Conservative laparascopic surgery may be done for an unruptured tubal pregnancy.

The most common complications of an ectopic pregnancy are severe haemorrhage, shock and death if immediate diagnosis and appropriate intervention are not implemented timeously.

Abdominal pregnancy

This is an extremely rare type of pregnancy where the fertilised ovum is extruded into the abdominal cavity. The trophoblast attaches to the abdominal organs. Rarely, the pregnancy advances to term, resulting in compression deformities and growth restriction. The baby is delivered through a laparatomy and the placenta and membranes are left in situ to prevent haemorrhage. These are later re-absorbed into the general circulation. Alternatively, the fetus may die and calcify (a litopaedion).

Versions

A version may occur either spontaneously or by manipulation. The two types of versions which are performed in obstetrics are the external cephalic version and the internal podalic version.

The role of the midwife

According to the South African Nursing Council's directive for the Diploma in Midwifery: *An external version for a transverse lie should be taught in the case of a woman in early labour and in the transverse lie of the second twin after the first has been delivered. Version in these cases is attempted only where a medical practitioner is not available.*

Research highlight

A version is the manipulation of the fetal presentation or lie during pregnancy or labour. This procedure is rarely performed in modern obstetrics because of the fetal and maternal risks it carries, especially in the South African situation where a great percentage of women are HIV-positive. Most obstetricians prefer an elective caesarean section in order to avoid these risk factors.

However, according to research done in Italy, Thailand, Europe and the United States some obstetricians still consider an external cephalic version at or near term a better option to trial of labour or an elective caesarean section with their resultant increase in fetal and maternal morbidity and mortality rates as well as increased costs.

Source: Bergström, 1992; Gifford, Keeler & Kahn, 1995; Zhang, Bowes, & Fortney, 1993.

External cephalic version

This is the turning of the fetal head towards the mother's pelvis by manipulation through the mother's abdominal wall so that the fetal head lies above the pelvic brim. An external cephalic version is indicated in a transverse lie, breech or shoulder presentation (oblique lie) at the 37th week of pregnancy or at the onset of labour. It is also performed in malpresentation of the second twin after the first has been born.

An external version is absolutely contra-indicated in the following conditions:
▶ Multiple pregnancy before birth of the first twin.
▶ Placenta praevia.
▶ Ruptured membranes.
▶ Antepartum haemorrhage.
▶ Cephalopelvic disproportion.
▶ Gross fetal abnormalities.
▶ Severe pre-eclampsia.
▶ HIV seropositivity.

It is relatively contraindicated in preterm labour, intra-uterine growth restriction, a Rhesus-negative woman and previous caesarean section.

A version may result in the following:
▶ Prelabour rupture of membranes.
▶ Preterm labour.
▶ Placental separation and antepartum haemorrhage.
▶ Rupture or knotting of the umbilical cord or fetal distress.
▶ Birth asphyxia or intra-uterine death.
▶ At times, the position achieved may be worse than the original one, for example turning a breech presentation into a brow presentation.
▶ Rupture of the uterus may also occur, especially in a scarred uterus.

Preparation

An external cephalic version is best done at about the 37th week of pregnancy because:
▶ The liquor is adequate for manipulation.
▶ The fetus is less likely to revert back to the previous presentation.

Before attempting a version, informed consent must be obtained from the woman after the procedure has been clearly explained and discussed with her. Privacy must be maintained. The bladder must be emptied for comfort and easy manipulation. A tranquilliser, tocolytic drug or sedative may be given, as prescribed, before the procedure, in order to relax the woman and her uterine muscles. She may be placed in a Trendelenburg position one hour before the procedure, in order to dislodge the presenting part from the pelvis. The woman is placed on her back on a firm surface, with the hips and knees slightly flexed.

The following are monitored and recorded as a baseline to compare with further monitoring during and after the manipulation:
▶ Maternal pulse and blood pressure.
▶ Fetal heart rate and rhythm (preferably using a CTG).

Any abnormalities identified should be reported to the medical practitioner and will result in the procedure being cancelled. A sanitary pad is applied over the vulva in order to identify any drainage of liquor and haemorrhage.

The procedure
The clinician's hands must be warmed and the abdomen and hands should be dusted with talcum powder if either are moist.

The clinician stands on the woman's side. The presenting part is gently dislodged from the pelvis using one or both hands. One hand is placed on the head, the other on the breech. The fetal head is kept flexed and moved towards the pelvis (nose first) with one hand while the other hand brings the breech towards the fundus. The fetus is kept as flexed as possible. This position is kept while the fetal heart rate is being auscultated. If the fetal heart rate is normal, the version is continued until the head is over the pelvis and the breech is in the fundus. The end of the bed is then lowered. If the fetal heart rate slows down or becomes irregular, the fetus is turned back to its original presentation. If the first attempt is unsuccessful, an interval of at least three minutes must be allowed before the next attempt.

During the procedure the midwife should stay with the woman and reassure her. Maternal and fetal observations must be continued and recorded, and abnormalities, such as fetal heart rate abnormalities, haemorrhage or rupture of membranes must be reported promptly. The woman should also be observed for any pain and discomfort, as well as for possible side-effects to the medication administered.

Aftercare
After the procedure the woman should be positioned in the (left) lateral position and be

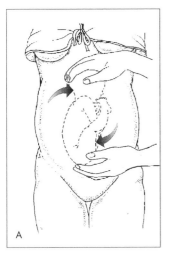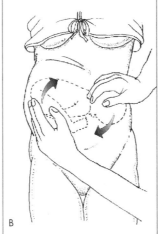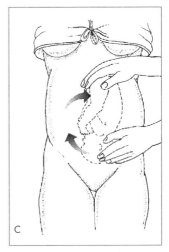

A   B   C

Figure 27.1 External version

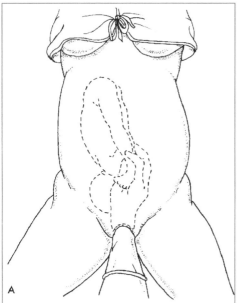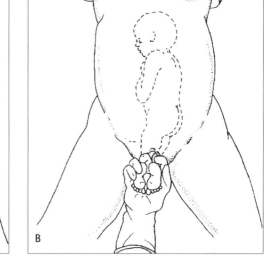

Figure 27.2 Internal podalic version

allowed to lie down for about four hours. The following should be observed every five minutes for 15 minutes, then every 15 minutes for one hour, and then hourly thereafter until no abnormalities are present:

▶ Maternal pulse and blood pressure for signs of shock due to internal haemorrhage.

▶ Fetal heart rate and rhythm for signs of fetal compromise.

▶ The uterus for contractions, which will indicate onset of labour.

▶ Excessive (or diminished) fetal movements due to early fetal compromise.

▶ Any other abnormalities, for example pallor, localised abdominal pain and vaginal bleeding.

A light meal or snack is given to the woman before she goes home and her partner, relative or friend should accompany her. A follow-up appointment should be made for a week later, or earlier if any of the above-mentioned abnormalities occur, after which she should be admitted or referred to a hospital or medical practitioner. This is necessary for further observation and management, or prompt emergency intervention if necessary, such as caesarean section.

The version may be repeated after a week if the first attempt failed. Further investigations must be done if the second attempt fails.

Causes of failed version

Causes for a failed version may include a large fetus and/or inadequate liquor, signs of fetal distress, maternal obesity causing difficult manipulation, tense woman who fails to relax her abdominal muscles and uterine abnormalities such as a bicornuate uterus.

Internal podalic version

This is an internal manipulation by which the medical practitioner inserts his/her hand through the fully dilated cervix and grasps the fetus by the feet, pulling him gently through the cervix and vagina. The fetus is then delivered in the same manner as a breech presentation. This procedure is performed only in extreme emergencies, where a caesarean section is not possible. Internal podalic version is indicated:

▶ In a transverse lie of a second twin.

▶ Where an external cephalic version has failed.

▶ Rarely in a transverse or oblique lie with a fully dilated cervix and intact membranes.

Internal podalic version should never be attempted in the presence of:

▶ Cephalopelvic disproportion.
▶ Rupture of membranes exceeding one-hour duration.
▶ Uterine scars.
▶ An incompletely dilated or rigid cervix.
▶ Any condition which predisposes to uterine rupture, such as prolonged labour or hypertonic uterine action.

Caesarean section

Caesarean section is the surgical procedure whereby the fetus is delivered through an incision in the uterus after 26 weeks gestation. It may be done under general anaesthetic, epidural or spinal anaesthesia. The incidence of caesarean sections is increasing. There seems to be an increased consumer demand for caesarean section on social grounds. As the caesarean section rate goes up, however, so does maternal mortality and morbidity.

Before attempting a caesarean section there needs to be a clear indication that it is well motivated.

Indications

Maternal indications include the following:

▶ Obstructed labour.
▶ Previous uterine surgery.
▶ Antepartum haemorrhage, such as placenta praevia and abruptio placentae.
▶ Severe maternal disease, such as eclampsia, renal disease or severe diabetes mellitus.
▶ Other various conditions, including failed induction, elderly primigravida, active genital herpes simplex, failed assisted delivery and poor obstetric history.

Fetal indications include fetal distress, cord prolapse, malpresentation and fetal abnormalities, such as hydrocephalus or siamese twins.

Types of caesarean section

Classical caesarean section. A vertical or longitudinal incision is made in the upper uterine segment. It is performed when a lower uterine segment incision would endanger the life of the woman or fetus, for example, in prematurity of less than 32 weeks, anterior placenta praevia or constriction ring dystocia. It is seldom performed because of the high risk of scar dehiscence during subsequent pregnancy and labour.

Lower segment caesarean section. A transverse incision is made in the lower uterine segment, usually after 32 weeks gestation. Of all caesarean sections 98% are of this type because the uterine scar heals faster than in an upper uterine segment incision and there is a slimmer chance for uterine rupture during subsequent pregnancies. This is mainly because the lower uterine segment has more fibrous tissue and less muscle. Compared to classical caesarean section there is usually less blood loss in the lower segment incision.

Elective and emergency caesarean section

Elective caesarean section is a planned caesarean section where the decision is made during pregnancy and the operation is performed before onset of labour. An emergency caesarean section is unplanned and performed urgently before or during labour because of adverse conditions affecting the woman and/or the fetus.

Advantages and disadvantages of a caesarean section

When complications exist, a caesarean section is the best and safest method of delivery. It can be combined with surgical sterilisation and is convenient for women requesting a caesarean section for social reasons.

There is, however, an increased rate of postpartum complications such as haemorrhage, sepsis and venous thrombosis. Post-operative pain and discomfort from the surgical incision causes delayed ambulation and inability to cope with the baby, and there is interference with the early maternal–child bonding.

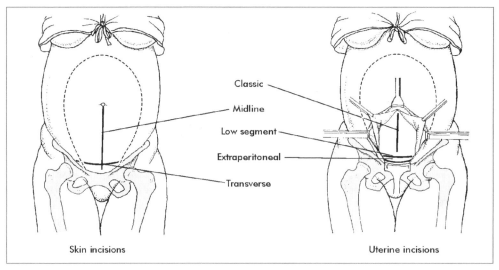

Figure 27.3 Skin and uterine incisions for caesarean section

Complications and dangers associated with caesarean section

Maternal complications	Neonatal complications
▶ Haemorrhage due to uterine atony. ▶ Poor haemostasis of uterine and abdominal wounds and sepsis, especially where infection pre-exists or where the woman's immune system is compromised, as in HIV-positive women. ▶ General anaesthetic complications. ▶ Failed endotracheal intubation and concomitant aspiration pneumonia. ▶ Amniotic fluid embolism. ▶ Venous thrombosis, resulting in thrombo-embolism. ▶ Injury to the bladder and/or ureters. ▶ General complications of abdominal surgery. Later maternal complications and/or dangers include: ▶ Uterine scar dehiscence. ▶ Endometriosis of the scar. ▶ Psychological and emotional problems due to a traumatic experience prior to the caesarean section and a feeling of failure and loss of self-esteem.	▶ Transient tachypnoea (wet lung syndrome) as a result of lung fluid not being squeezed out of the lungs as in a vaginal delivery. ▶ Birth asphyxia due to general anaesthesia, especially if there is a delay in extraction of the baby. ▶ Birth injuries resulting from instruments used. ▶ Prematurity due to incorrect calculation of gestational age.

Specific midwifery management of caesarean section

Elective caesarean section

The woman should be admitted before the day of operation. However, the period of admission depends on the indication for the caesarean section and the degree of stabilisation needed. Orientation to the ward environment and the nursery is necessary so that the woman is familiar with the surroundings. The pre-operative procedures and preparations should be explained to the woman and her support person so as to allay any anxiety. They should both be encouraged to express their concerns and ask questions, so that any misconceptions can be clarified. The partner or support person should also be encouraged to support and motivate the woman and to watch the birth of the baby if possible.

The midwife should ensure that the obstetrician obtains informed consent from the woman and checks that it is valid. The anaesthetist who discusses the anaesthetic with her then assesses the woman. If necessary any investigations and tests are done, such as full blood count and blood grouping. Skin preparation is then done according to the policy of the institution. A sedative may be prescribed by the obstetrician, to be given the night before the operation to ensure a good night's sleep.

For the six hours prior to the operation no food or drink must be given. *Sodium citrate* 0.3 mg or *magnesium trisilicate* is administered orally prior to going to the operating theatre, so as to prevent Mendelson's syndrome. *Metraclopramide* (Maxolon®) may be administered to facilitate emptying of the stomach as this is delayed in pregnant women and increases the risk of Mendelson's syndrome, even after starving.

Identification of the woman should be done before leaving the ward. An indwelling catheter is inserted to drain the bladder and prevent injury to the bladder during the operation. Intravenous therapy may be commenced in the ward or operating theatre prior to induction of general anaesthesia or spinal/epidural anaesthesia. The woman's support person must be allowed to be present during the operation after adequate discussion and preparation. Photos of the birth of the baby may also be taken if the woman so wishes and the hospital policy allows it.

Emergency caesarean section

This operation is not anticipated and as a result, all the above interventions are done in a great hurry. The staff may experience problems in obtaining informed consent, especially where a language barrier exists. The woman, partner and family members may become very anxious and need extra support and reassurance from the midwife before and after the caesarean section.

Post-operative management

Immediate care of the baby. The baby should be shown and given to the mother as soon as possible, preferably in theatre if spinal/epidural anaesthesia is used. One of the major causes of anxiety in a post-caesarean woman is if she is unable to see her baby. If necessary the baby is resuscitated, and transferred to the neonatal nursery for observation. Once stable, the baby is then 'roomed-in' with the mother under close observation for any further complications.

If the mother has chosen to breastfeed, she should be helped to put the baby onto the breast as soon as both mother and baby are ready. This will facilitate bonding and stimulate lactation. The woman should be assisted with each feed and handling of the baby until she is able to cope on her own.

Comfort needs of the woman. The woman is transferred to a firm comfortable bed and put in semi-Fowler's position once she is fully conscious, for easy respiration and to facilitate drainage of lochia. The medical practitioner may prescribe analgesia for pain and/or a sedative to promote rest and sleep. The midwife should ensure that the ward environment is relaxing and peaceful to ensure rest and sleep.

Safety needs of the woman. The following routine postpartum observations are done:

▶ After general anaesthesia the woman's level of consciousness must be assessed half-hourly until the woman is fully conscious, and thereafter four-hourly to identify any anaesthetic complications.

▶ Temperature, pulse, respiration and blood pressure half-hourly for the first two hours and four-hourly thereafter to identify any signs of shock, which may result from effects of anaesthetic, excessive bleeding from atonic uterus or suture line.

▶ Observe the abdominal wound frequently in the first 24 hours for bleeding.

▶ Wound drainage devices, such as portovac for amount, colour and consistency.

▶ Urinary output for amount and colour for the first 24 hours. Bloodstained urine must be reported, as it may be a sign of bladder injury. Diminished urinary output may be a sign of dehydration or injury to the ureters.

▶ The effectiveness of analgesia and sedatives given.

▶ Presence of pain and its location. For example, incision pain is a sign of tight sutures or infection, abdominal pain may be due to flatus or subinvolution, throat pain can occur from intubation, headache from pyrexia and breast pain may be due to engorgement.

▶ The legs and groin must be observed daily for redness, swelling and tenderness – signs of venous thrombosis and thrombo-phlebitis, which are all associated with post-caesarean bed-rest or reluctance to move.

▶ The colour of the skin and mucous membranes for pallor and cyanosis, which may be a sign of anaemia or pulmonary embolism.

▶ The wound must be kept as dry as possible to prevent infection. A light dressing may be applied. The sutures are removed (before or after discharge) only on the obstetrician's request, usually alternate sutures on day five and remaining sutures on day seven.

Nutritional needs of the woman. For the first 24 hours an intravenous therapy of one litre Ringer's lactate or a postsurgical electrolyte maintenance solution should be continued eight-hourly. The rate of flow and infusion site (for swelling and redness) must be observed regularly. After 12 to 24 hours, clear oral fluids may be commenced if bowel sounds are present or flatus has been passed. A regular diet should be resumed on about the third post-operative day after general anaesthesia and a bit sooner after spinal/epidural anaesthesia.

Elimination needs of the woman. The indwelling catheter drains into a urine bag, which must be emptied at least four-hourly or when full. The catheter is usually removed 24 hours postoperatively, if no complications (such as haematuria) exist. Thereafter, the woman should be encouraged to void urine every one to two hours. The bladder must be gently palpated for distension after voiding. The midwife should enquire daily whether there has been a bowel action. A mild aperient may be prescribed on the third or fourth day if there has been no bowel action. Early ambulation facilitates passage of flatus.

Hygienic needs of the woman. A vulval toilet is performed on the woman four-hourly for the first 24 hours. She is encouraged to clean herself under supervision until she feels competent to do so. A full wash is given on the first day and thereafter she is assisted when necessary. Mouthwashes are given frequently until she is able to brush her teeth unassisted. The woman is encouraged to shower as soon as she is able. The wound is then protected with a plastic dressing. Assistance must also be given with the grooming of hair.

Mobility needs of the woman. Early ambulation should be encouraged to prevent venous thrombosis and thromboembolism. Passive and active leg exercises should be performed from day one to prevent venous thrombosis. Deep breathing and coughing should start at the same time to prevent hypostatic pneumonia. If spinal/epidural anaesthesia was used, the woman is allowed out of bed only once sensation has completely returned to prevent risk of injury.

Discharge planning

The midwife should specifically inform the woman to avoid strain and pressure on the abdominal wound and lower back by lifting heavy objects, for example. She should also be informed about the indication for the caesarean section and the importance of giving birth in hospital with subsequent pregnancies. The danger signs, which need urgent medical attention, such as sudden vaginal bleeding, offensive lochia, severe abdominal pain and fever should all be explained. The woman should then be advised to come for a postnatal check-up whenever problems arise or after six weeks for family planning counselling.

Forceps delivery

Forceps delivery is an instrumental delivery used to extract a baby's head during the second stage of labour in a cephalic presentation, or an after-coming head in a breech presentation. Forceps are used mainly for the purposes of traction, that is to bring the head down in order to deliver the baby. The incidence varies between 5% and 15%, depending on the community being served. In modern obstetrics, the incidence of the use of low outlet forceps (Wrigley's) is associated with the increased popularity of epidural anaesthesia.

Indications and contraindications for the use of forceps

Maternal indications for the use of forceps
The following maternal conditions may indicate the use of forceps:
- Maternal distress or exhaustion where a woman is unable to bear down during the second stage of labour.
- Maternal disease, for example in cardiac disease, because bearing down will exert strain on the heart and may result in cardiac failure.
- In severe hypertension or pre-eclampsia, where the strain of bearing down will further increase the blood pressure and put the woman at risk for eclampsia.
- Following recent operations (for example eye, brain and abdominal operations so as to prevent rupture of the suture line).
- Following haemorrhage and other complications.
- In trial of scar after previous caesarean section or myomectomy.
- An accidental dural tap during administration of epidural analgesia, where bearing down would result in cerebral complications.
- A rigid pelvic floor and/or perineum.

The indications are relative and the use should be considered individually. Practices such as companionship, upright positions for birth, *oxytocin* augmentation for slow progress in the second stage, not using a time limitation for the second stage of labour and waiting for epidural anaesthesia to wear off will reduce the need for instrumental deliveries.

Fetal indications for the use of forceps
Fetal indications include:
- To shorten the second stage of labour in fetal distress.
- To shorten the second stage of labour in prolapse of the umbilical cord.
- To facilitate descent of the presenting part, for example in the occipitoposterior position, face presentation and failure of internal rotation of the head.

Contraindications for forceps delivery
A forceps delivery is contraindicated when:
- The woman does not give consent.
- The woman is uncooperative or confused.
- The cervix is not fully dilated.
- Cephalopelvic disproportion is present.
- The operator is incompetent or inexperienced.
- Inappropriate presentations such as brow presentation, compound presentation and transverse or oblique lie.

Possible complications of forceps delivery	
Maternal	**Fetal**
▶ Trauma, resulting in bladder and urethral injuries. ▶ Atony of the bladder. ▶ Nerve injuries. ▶ Fracture or dislocation of the coccyx. ▶ Soft tissue injuries. ▶ Haematoma of the birth canal. ▶ Uterine rupture. ▶ Cervical and vaginal tears. ▶ Perineal and rectal tears. ▶ Postpartum haemorrhage and shock. ▶ Infection may also occur as a result of manipulations and bruising of soft tissues.	▶ Asphyxia neonatorum if prolonged hypoxia occurs. ▶ Periventricular haemorrhage infarction. ▶ Soft tissue injuries and lacerations of face and scalp from application of forceps. ▶ Facial nerve injuries, such as facial and brachial nerves, due to pressure of the forceps. ▶ Cerebral nerve palsy. ▶ Umbilical cord compression. ▶ Fetal death.

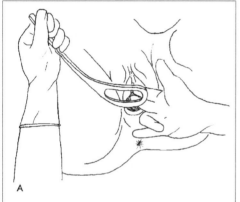
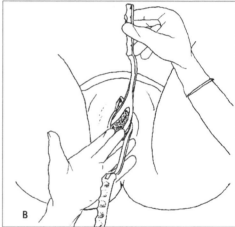
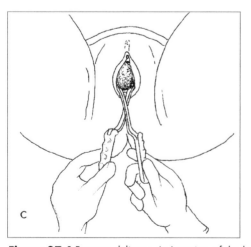
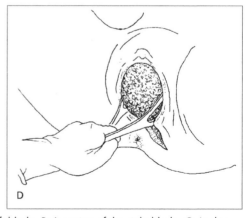

Figure 27.4 Forceps delivery. A: Insertion of the left blade, B: Insertion of the right blade, C: Locking of the blades, D: Gentle traction is applied to deliver the head. Episiotomy is cut when the perineum is bulging.

Causes of failure of forceps delivery

The possible causes of failure of forceps delivery may include:

▶ Inadequate assessment of the woman in order to identify or anticipate complications such as fetal abnormalities, cephalopelvic disproportion and pelvic tumours.

▶ Incorrect application of forceps by an inexperienced practitioner. The cervix may be caught between the blades, incorrect estimation of the station or position of the head and a uterine constriction ring holding the baby back.

Management

The procedure must only be performed by a skilled medical practitioner or, when not available, a skilled experienced midwife with a qualification in advanced midwifery. Prerequisites are that the head must be engaged and the cervix fully dilated with ruptured membranes. The bladder must be empty to prevent trauma to the bladder. The woman must receive adequate analgesia or anaesthesia.

The woman and her support person should be given a full explanation of the indications and how the procedure will be done and a written consent must be obtained. A midwife should remain with the woman throughout the procedure to give support and encouragement. The midwife also has a responsibility to ensure that all the prerequisites were met.

Equipment for resuscitation of the baby should be prepared, as well as a pre-warmed incubator. A sterile delivery pack and the relevant obstetric forceps are then prepared. The midwife should monitor the maternal and fetal heart rate pattern throughout the procedure. The time of application of forceps and the time of delivery must be noted and recorded.

Postpartum care of mother and baby

Routine care of the baby is given, unless resuscitation is necessary (see Chapter 16). The baby must be admitted to a high-care neonatal unit for early identification of any possible

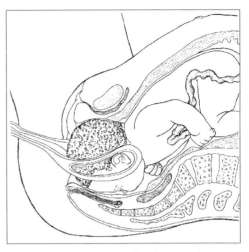

Figure 27.5 The relationship between the curve of the forceps and the pelvic curve

complications, such as signs of periventricular haemorrhage infarction.

The woman has a high risk of traumatic and atonic postpartum haemorrhage so she should be closely observed for early identification of complications so that these are attended to promptly. Vital signs and vaginal bleeding should be observed half-hourly for the first two hours and then four-hourly thereafter for the next 12 hours, or until stable.

Vacuum extraction

Vacuum extraction (ventouse) is the extraction of the baby by means of the suction of a vacuum cup on the fetal scalp. There are two types of cups available. One has a rubber tube, which extends from the metal cup to a pump and creates the suction as well as handle, chain and base plate that allows traction to be applied. A second type of cup is a one-piece reinforced silicone cup and handle combined. The vacuum cup and handle is connected to a hand pump or electrical pump with a gauge. This allows the strength of negative pressure to be controlled.

This procedure is performed only by a medical practitioner or midwife with advanced midwifery training in an emergency where a medical practitioner is not immediately available.

Indications and contraindications for the use of vacuum extraction

Vacuum extraction can be used where there is a delay in the second stage of labour due to maternal exhaustion or severe maternal disease. It may also be performed in cases of previous caesarean section to prevent strain on the scar.

A vacuum extraction delivery is performed to flex and/or rotate the head in malposition of the fetus or to facilitate delivery where fetal distress exists during the second stage of labour.

Vacuum extraction is absolutely contra-indicated in the following conditions:
‣ Moderate or severe cephalopelvic disproportion.
‣ Fetal head 3/5 above pelvis (preferably it should be not more than 1/5 head above the pelvis).
‣ Malpresentations (for example breech, face, brow and shoulder presentations).
‣ A macerated fetus.
‣ Preterm birth.
‣ When the woman is uncooperative.

Relative contraindications include a cervix that is not fully dilated, fetal congenital abnormalities such as hydrocephalus and anencephaly or intra-uterine death.

Management and the procedure

The woman is managed as in a forceps delivery. The vacuum extraction must be done under strict aseptic precautions and universal

---

Vacuum extraction delivery

In South Africa, this vacuum extraction delivery is not recommended as it results in abrasion and bruising of the fetal scalp. This exposes the baby to a high risk of HIV infection through the scalp injury. A forceps or caesarean section delivery is preferred.

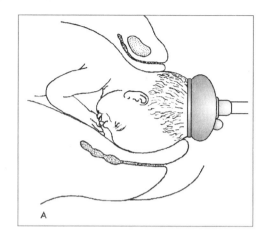

A

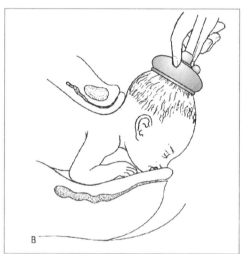

B

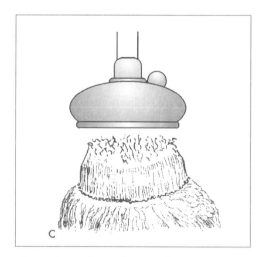

C

Figure 27.6 The application of the vacuum extraction and the resulting chignon

Advantages and disadvantages

Advantages of using the vacuum extractor:
- The vacuum extractor takes up less space in the pelvis than the forceps.
- There is less or no damage to maternal tissues.
- The fetal head is not fixed and as a result rotation will take place automatically.
- Flexion and rotation of the head are facilitated.
- The procedure is relatively easy to perform.
- Fetal intracranial pressure is significantly less than with forceps delivery.

The disadvantages are that the delivery is slower and the vacuum cup may slip off the head and cause trauma to the scalp.

Vacuum extraction

The maximum number of pulls during traction must not exceed *three*, that is, 'Dislodge the head, Descend the head and Deliver the baby'. With each pull noticeable descent should be present. The maximum cup detachments are *two*.

precautions against HIV transmission must be maintained throughout the procedure. The membranes should be ruptured. After determining the position of the head the medical practitioner positions the cup on the fetal head over the occiput, or as close to it as possible. It is then connected to sterile tubing and the pressure pump. Care should be taken that part of the cervix or vagina is not trapped between the fetal head and cup. The assisting midwife monitors the negative pressure of the vacuum closely, which must not exceed 0.7 to 0.8 kg per square centimetre at any time. An artificial caput succedaneum is allowed to form before the operator applies traction. Traction on the head must only be applied during uterine contractions.

The midwife should monitor and record the maternal vital signs and fetal heart rate during the procedure. The time of application of the vacuum cup, number of pulls and detachments and the time of birth must all be

Possible complications	
Maternal	**Fetal**
▶ Lacerations of the vagina and cervix resulting in traumatic postpartum haemorrhage, which is common, although less than with forceps delivery. ▶ Damage to the bladder, especially if the bladder was not emptied prior to the procedure. ▶ Infection to the genital tract. ▶ Psychological trauma due to failure to extract the fetus.	▶ Formation of a large circumscribed caput known as a 'vacuum chignon'. ▶ Abrasions, necrosis and ulceration of the scalp if the cup was left on too long, or improper traction was applied. ▶ Cephalohaematoma formation in 10 to 15% of babies with subsequent anaemia and hyperbilirubinaemia. ▶ Subaponeurotic bleeding due to rupture of capillaries in the scalp. ▶ Asphyxia neonatorum due to prolonged hypoxia or cerebral damage. ▶ Cerebral irritation. ▶ Periventricular haemorrhage infarction due to trauma or severe hypoxia. ▶ Infection due to scalp wounds.

recorded. Caesarean section is indicated if a vacuum extraction fails.

The baby should be resuscitated if indicated and the condition recorded. The baby is then transferred to a neonatal high-care unit for close observation and further management.

Symphysiotomy

Symphysiotomy is the separation of the symphysis pubis during delivery, which may occur spontaneously or be surgically induced. The surgical incision is made into the ligaments and fibro-cartilage of the symphysis pubis so as to enlarge the diameters of the pelvic cavity and thereby enhance delivery of the fetus. The procedure is performed mainly to overcome borderline cephalopelvic disproportion, in neglected cases of prolonged labour, where the caesarean section risk is too high, to facilitate delivery in prolonged labour and for women who are anaesthetic risks.

It is rarely performed in modern obstetrics, where good antenatal care, early detection of risk factors such as cephalopelvic disproportion, is available as well as efficient expert intrapartum care for management of the risk factors.

Destructive operations (embryotomy)

Destructive operations are performed to decrease the fetal size to enable easier delivery thereof, such as hydrocephalus. It can only be performed on a dead unborn fetus where the cervical dilatation is advanced in order to save the woman's life. In modern obstetrics, where adequate antenatal care and diagnosis exist, these procedures are very rarely necessary. These procedures are very traumatic for all concerned.

References

Beischer, N. A., Mackay, E. V. & Colditz, P. 1997. *Obstetrics and the newborn*. London: W. B. Saunders.

In a nutshell

- Although operative obstetrics have life-saving aspects, it also increases the risk of complications for mother and baby.
- During an operative intervention the midwife has a professional responsibility to provide a safe, therapeutic environment for the woman and her baby.
- The midwife should protect the mother's and baby's rights by effectively fulfilling her patient advocacy role, such as ensuring that all the prerequisites for each procedure are met.
- By effectively making use of the nursing process in the care of the mother and baby, the midwife will ensure that specific potential risk factors are identified early and managed promptly.
- The midwife should provide the woman with adequate information regarding the indication(s) for the procedure as well as specific health education to enable her to cope with self-care and subsequent childbirth.
- The midwife should involve the woman and her support person/s in all decisions made about her care, as well as that of her baby.
- The midwife should act within the parameters of the legal and ethical guidelines for midwifery practice.
- During an emergency, in the absence of a medical practitioner, an experienced midwife trained in advanced midwifery can perform an external cephalic version, a forceps delivery or a vacuum extraction.

Bennet, V. R. & Brown, L. K. 1999. *Myles textbook for midwives*. Edinburgh: Churchill Livingstone.

Bergström, S. 1992. External cephalic version and daily post-versional maternal self-assessment of fetal presentation. A prospective study. *Gynaecologic and Obstetric Investigation*, 33(1):15–18.

Bergström, S., Höjer, B., Litjestrand, J. & Tunell, R. 1994. *Perinatal health care with limited resources*. London: Macmillan Press Ltd.

Biswas, A., Chakraborty, P. S., Das, H. S., Bose, A. & Kalsar, P. K. 2001. Role of destructive operations in modern day obstetrics. *Journal of Indian Medical Association*, 99(5):248, 250–251.

Bjorklund, K. 2002. Minimally invasive surgery for obstructed labour: A review of symphysiotomy during the twentieth century. *BJOG: An International Journal of Obstetrics and Gynaecology*, 109(3):236–248.

Booyens, S. W. (Ed.) 2001. *Introduction to health services management*. Lansdowne: Juta.

Cronje, H. S., Grobler, C. J. F. & Visser, A. A. 1996. *Obstetrics in Southern Africa*. Pretoria: J.L. van Schaik.

DoH (Department of Health). 2002. *Guidelines for maternity care in South Africa*. Second edition. Pretoria: Department of Health.

DoH (Department of Health). 2002. *Saving Mothers: Second report on confidential enquiries into maternal deaths in South Africa 1999–2001*. Pretoria: Department of Health.

DoH (Department of Health). Maternal, Child and Women's Health. 1997. *Guidelines for termination of pregnancy (TOP) implementation*. Pretoria: Government Printers.

Enkin, M., Keirse, M. J. N. C., Neilson, J., Crowther, C., Duley, L. & Hofmeyr J. 2000. *A guide to effective care in pregnancy and childbirth*. Third edition. Oxford: Oxford University Press.

Gifford, D. S., Keeler, E. & Kahn, K. L. 1995. Reductions in cost and caesarean rate by routine use of external cephalic version: A decision analysis. *Obstetrics and Gynaecology*, 85(6):930–936.

Gupta, U. & Chitra, R. 1994. Destructive operations have a place in developing countries. *International Journal of Gynaecology and Obstetrics*, 44(1):15–19.

Larsen, J. 1996. *Obstetrics in peripheral hospitals*. Durban: DEPAM.

Llewellyn-Jones, D. 1999. *Fundamentals of obstetrics and gynaecology*. London: Mosby.

Maharaj, D. & Moodley, J. 2002. Symphysiotomy and fetal destructive operations. *Best Practice and Research in Clinical Obstetrics and Gynaecology*, 16(1):117–131.

Moore, M. L. 1983. *Realities in childbearing*. Philadelphia: W.B. Saunders.

Mothers choosing caesareans. 2002. *Caesarean sections: UK midwifery archives*. http://www.radmid.demon.co.uk/cs.htan

National Committee for the Confidential Enquiry into maternal deaths. 1998-2000. Changing patterns in Maternal Mortality in South Africa. Paper presented at the 20th Conference on Priorities in Perinatal Care in South Africa. 6–9 March 2001. Drakensberg Gardens: KwaZulu-Natal.

Nel, J. T. 1995. *Core obstetrics and gynaecology*. Durban: Butterworth.

Nolte, A. G. W. (Ed.) 1998. *A textbook for midwives*. Pretoria: J.L. van Schaik.

Odendaal, H. J., Schaetzing, A. E. & Kruger, T. F. 2001. *Clinical gynaecology*. Lansdowne: Juta.

Oxorn, H. 1986. *Human labor and birth*. New York: McGraw-Hill.

Pattinson, R. C. & Nyasulu, D. 1998. Maternal mortality related to early pregnancy loss in South Africa. Paper presented at the 7th World IAMANEH Conference 2000. 2–5 April 2000. Stellenbosch University, Cape Town.

SANC. 1987. *Diploma for registration as a midwife. One year course: Directive*. Pretoria: SANC.

Searle, C. & Pera, S. A. 1999. *Professional practice – a Southern African nursing perspective*. Sandton: Heinemann.

Sellers, P. M. 1997. *Midwifery*. Vol. 2. Kenwyn: Juta.

South Africa. 1996. *Choice on Termination of Pregnancy Act, 1996. No. 1891*,

22 November 1996. Pretoria: Government Printers.

Tarig, T. A. & Korejo, R. 1993. Evaluation of the role of craniotomy in developing countries. *Journal of the Pakistan Medical Association*, 43(2):30–32.

WHO (World Health Organisation). 1997. *Post-abortion family planning: A practical guide for programme managers*. Geneva: WHO.

WHO (World Health Organisation). 2000. *Managing complications in pregnancy and childbirth: A guide for midwives and doctors*. Geneva: WHO.

Zhang, J., Bowes, W.A. Jnr. & Fortney, J.A. 1993. Efficacy of external cephalic version: A review. *Obstetrics and Gynaecology*, 82(2):306–312.

Chapter *28*

Perinatal loss: Counselling and support

Joanita de Kock

Introduction

Experiencing loss is an inevitable part of our existence as human beings. This can be the loss of a function, job, friend, health or many other events. The most intense loss is that of the death of a long-awaited offspring – the newborn baby. When a fetus or baby dies, or is given for adoption, the parents and family grieve because they experience the shattering pain of losing a child.

Grief is not only experienced after a spontaneous or induced abortion, intra-uterine death (IUD) or neonatal death, but also in cases where congenital abnormalities are diagnosed, the decision is made to give the baby for adoption, a sick or preterm baby is born, or where infertility prevents couples from having their own child. When a baby is born with congenital abnormalities, the parents and family grieve because they have lost their image of a perfect child. When a baby is born preterm or with a severe illness, the parents grieve the loss of a healthy child.

Due to the impact of grief on the wellbeing of parents and families, more emphasis should be placed on bereavement counselling for families. We as midwives cannot replace the loss these parents experience, but we can recognise and acknowledge their grief, and guide and support them through their grieving process.

The experience of loss

The grieving process

The person who has undergone loss, no matter what the cause of that loss may be, will experience the various stages of the grieving process. People's reactions may differ within the grieving process. For example, the experience of a mother whose baby has died will differ from a mother whose child was born with a congenital abnormality.

Going through a grieving process takes time. Two people in the same situation, for example, husband and wife, will not have common experiences of that situation nor grieve for the same period of time. There are, however, indications that the most intense level of grief lasts three to six months after the incident but it may last for two to three years. There are some individuals that will never complete the grieving process because of unresolved grief.

Throughout the years authors have describe the grieving process differently. Murray-Parkes (in Jolly, 1987:7) divided the grieving process into the following stages:
) disbelief
) developing awareness
) acceptance

Elizabeth Kubler-Ross (1969) is well known for her classic work on bereavement. She identified the following stages (in Weston, Martin and Anderson, 1998:9):
) denial
) anger
) bargaining
) depression
) acceptance

There are many ways to classify and describe the process of grief that these parents experience. The following classification will be used in this chapter:
) shock and disbelief
) anger
) intense grief and guilt
) equilibrium and depression
) reorganisation and acceptance

Shock and disbelief

Initially when parents hear the bad news of their baby's death, sickness or impairment, they will be shocked and in disbelief. They are often calm but show some tears of sadness. They cannot believe what they have heard and that it is happening to them. There is the hope that the medical or nursing personnel have made a mistake in their diagnosis. They hope that the baby will be born alive and normal, or that the problem will disappear. The full implications of their loss are so enormous that the parents try to 'buy time' to absorb the reality of the situation. It is important to understand that shock and disbelief are ways that the mind protects itself from the onslaught of emotional pain that is about to be experienced. Therefore it is vital not to 'push' the reality of what has happened on the parents – even if they are in complete denial. This stage can last a couple of hours or even a few weeks.

The parents may experience physiological symptoms such as dizziness, tachycardia, palpitations, anxiety, restlessness, sweating, pallor, nausea and vomiting, as well as other gastrointestinal symptoms.

Anger

The parents revolt against the situation because the pregnancy did not progress the way they have anticipated. They feel angry and frustrated at not being able to prevent the loss. Unfortunately, they may need to put the blame of the loss on somebody, therefore they often blame the medical or nursing personnel. Their anger at this time is often unrealistic. They will blame, for example, the obstetrician for not diagnosing or treating a condition earlier even if it was impossible to do so. Some people will be angry with God. Some believe that they are being punished for something that they have done wrong. The parents may blame each other for being the cause of the loss. In this way a husband may blame his wife for giving birth preterm or not being able to conceive.

It is important to realise that the parents'

reactions are based on intense feelings of pain, failure, guilt and confusion. No matter what responses the parents express, the midwife must not become defensive or minimise and deny these feelings. Listen to the parents' feelings and continue to give them sensitive care, as these feelings are understandably very real to the parents.

Parents try to bargain with themselves as well as the medical and nursing personnel. In the case of Christians they may bargain with God to spare their child, others will make offerings and perform rituals to obtain the mercy of the gods or ancestors. The parents will do anything as long as their child's life can be saved. Some parents will say: 'I will be a good father/mother if my baby survives'.

Intense grief and guilt

This is the stage where the loss has become a reality. The parents are no longer in denial. They are intensely emotional and very sad. Their loss is constantly on their minds together with pronounced feeling of emptiness. They will experience feelings of meaninglessness, abandonment, injustice and vulnerability.

All parents experience feelings of guilt. Most of these feelings are unsubstantiated. They may feel that they caused the loss in one way or another. A mother may feel that she caused a fetal abnormality because she ignored the fact that she was tired early in her pregnancy. This belief may be aggravated if it is associated with taboos and folklore. Women who have been told not to lift their arms high during the pregnancy, because this may cause the baby's cord to wind around its neck, may be devastated by guilt if they have a stillborn child with cord strangulation as the possible cause. They will remember times they reached for objects on top shelves, or washed high cupboards and feel intensely guilty. The fact that there is no connection between the action and the fetal outcome should be carefully explained to the mother.

More feelings of guilt are usually involved when congenital abnormalities are present. If there are too many feelings running riot the

mother may not be able to move forward through the healing process of grief.

Equilibrium and depression

This is the stage where the intense grieving period has passed. The parents are still grieving but their emotions are less intense. They are no longer receiving the same level of support they had in the beginning. At this stage the parents may feel abandoned and alone in their grief. They are not only lonely, also yearn for their baby and for what could have been. Life continues around them, but not yet for them. This stage can continue for years.

Other feelings that may be experienced are isolation, feelings of failure, helplessness, despondency and some remaining feelings of guilt. By this time most of the parents are back at work although they may feel listless and unmotivated. They will probably perform only what is expected of them without any focus or creativity. These parents may experience chronic low moods, social withdrawal, impaired memory, less concentration and sleep or loss of appetite. The progress through this stage is much slower than the parents would have preferred it to be.

There is a substantial higher incidence of depression, somatisation and obsessive-compulsive behaviour in women six months after a pregnancy loss when compared to women who gave birth to live babies during the same time period. There is, however, a very fine line between normal grief and pathological depression that requires psychiatric counselling.

Reorganisation and acceptance

This is the stage where the parents gradually start to find an interest in life around them again. They become less and less preoccupied with their loss and start to work on their old relationships and possibly form new ones. Parents will never forget their loss, but they will gradually experience less intense pain.

Those who lost their baby will start to accept the death during this phase. Parents whose child was born sick or with congenital abnormalities, will accept their loss of a healthy or normal child and begin to adapt to the care routine that the situation requires of them.

Implications for the midwife

By understanding the different stages of the grieving process that the parents experience, the midwife will be better equipped to guide and support them. The midwife should be realistic in her expectations of the parents' reactions and her actions should be guided appropriately.

It is very difficult to determine the exact stage of the grieving process a person is experiencing at a given time. It can also be a combination of stages. A person does not end one stage completely before entering the next stage. It can be seen as a complete process through which a person has to go before there is acceptance of the loss. Grief is an individual experience that can differ tremendously from person to person and each situation is unique.

Although the word 'parents' is used when discussing the loss of a baby, it must be stressed that the mother and father will not experience the grieving process in exactly the same manner.

Certain events may cause temporary regression in the grieving process such as the expected date of birth, birthday of the baby, another baby born in the family or any similar event. These events may cause a resurgence of memory, emotion and pain.

The experience of the mother

A baby's death has a deep impact on all mothers, but each woman has an individual way of dealing with grief. Every mother's grief is strongly affected by her own personality, previous experiences, her culture, her religious beliefs and family relationships.

The mother often experiences the loss more intensely and therefore her grieving period is generally longer than that of the father. The pregnancy had formed a greater part of her day-to-day existence and by its effects on her mind and body it is therefore

more of a reality for the woman. This is intensified at the time of labour and birth. The father's relationship with the baby is more psychological from the start; therefore his experience of the loss is different to that of the mother who grieves the loss of a part of herself. Because the mother may still be grieving after the father has resolved his grief, this can lead to relationship discord and even serious marital problems. Effective communication and marital counselling can prevent these problems.

In general mothers talk more openly about their experiences than their partners do. Mothers tend to express their feelings whereas fathers tend to withdraw.

The experience of the father

Many healthcare workers concentrate on the mother and her grief. Therefore the father may easily feel left out. His first reaction is to protect his partner when he observes her pain. He has his own grief to work through however. The father often feels frustrated and helpless during the delivery and in his inability to protect her from pain. He fears that his spouse might encounter complications and experience pain. A Swedish study indicated that in the case of an intra-uterine death (IUD) the father prefers that the baby should be delivered as soon as possible, preferably by caesarean section. He does not feel comfortable with his wife carrying a dead fetus. The father may consider and accept a vaginal delivery after the advantages and disadvantages have been discussed with him and he realises that this is better for his partner (Samuelsson, Rådestad & Segesten, 2001).

The father is exposed to many more aspects of the baby's death than most people recognise. He is usually the one who has to do the painful task of informing friends and family about the loss. While the mother is still in the hospital, the father goes home alone to an environment where everything might have been prepared for the new baby. Traditionally men are expected not to show tears and to be the stronger partner.

The experience of the siblings

The siblings can feel insecure because they know something has happened but do not understand entirely. Their understanding of death will be determined by their developmental phase. Siblings may feel that they are to blame in some way because they were not excited about the arrival of the baby and scared about sharing their parents' attention with the newcomer. They may also show signs of behavioural changes such as naughtiness; problems at school or regression such as bedwetting again.

It is often the siblings that bring reality back to the home. They demand their physical entertainment and attention such as food, activities or promised outings while the parents may not be necessarily ready for it yet. The siblings often have their own unique ways of comforting their parents. Grief in children is not always obvious because some children hide their own grief so as not to upset their parents.

Family and friends

The grandparents will also experience a crisis. They have not only lost a grandchild but must witness the devastating pain and grief of their own children. The reaction of other family members and friends can differ, ranging from committed long-term support to complete avoidance of the parents. Sometimes they feel uncertain on how to approach the parents and are scared that they might upset them. Often the parents feel frustrated and isolated. Usually the amount of support that parents receive from family and friends will decline after a period of time after the loss, which will add to their sense of loneliness.

Social and cultural diversity

Loss and grief has no social and cultural boundaries and is experienced in each of the many different groups in South Africa. Except for the Western culture, very little information is available on how any of the other cultural groups in South Africa experience perinatal loss and what their expectations are. The midwife is advised to be sensitive to other cultural and social groups. She should never force her own beliefs and practices on anyone. Even if the midwife is not familiar with a specific group or culture, she should still be sensitive to their specific needs by following the verbal and nonverbal clues of the women. For example, if a woman comes from a conservative background, she may not appreciate touch, empathetic tears and many people expressing sorrow, whereas a woman from a large extended family will feel lost and abandoned if not surrounded by her family members, who are expressing their sorrow with her. By raising their awareness about their own culture, midwives will increase their understanding of other cultures.

Different forms of loss

There are different forms of loss that an individual may experience during and around the perinatal period. The unique features of each will now be discussed.

Early pregnancy loss

An early pregnancy loss can either be an unexpected, spontaneous abortion or a planned termination of pregnancy. A woman may have decided upon a termination of pregnancy as part of her family planning (fertility control) or because of unforeseen circumstances such as congenital abnormalities of the fetus. The fact that a woman decides on the termination of a pregnancy does not necessarily mean that she did not want the pregnancy. Every type of termination, even as part of family planning, will be experienced as an enormous loss. Previously these women were denied the right to mourn their loss. It is now recognised that no loss can be too small for women to mourn about. The only difference with these women is that they usually do not have the same amount of support because no one or only a few people knew about the pregnancy. Furthermore, society often does not allow them to grieve for a long period of time.

Intra-uterine death (IUD)

It has been described in several studies that the amount of grief experienced is directly related to the duration of the pregnancy. Therefore the parents with a full-term IUD may experience more intense grief than a loss at 28 weeks or even a first trimester pregnancy loss.

In many cases an IUD is diagnosed before birth. These parents face all the pain and grief even before 'meeting' their baby. About 30 years ago these parents were denied the right to grieve over their babies because it was believed that attachment did not take place before the birth of the baby. During the last few decades these parents' pain and grief have been acknowledged. The parents may experience intense grief and disappointment over the loss of their baby. They may experience the same emotions as after a neonatal death. Some parents describe it as being unfair because these babies did not even have a chance at life – they died even before being born.

Parents with an IUD also face the possibility of the fetus undergoing maceration. Maceration means to become soft by soaking. The skin of the fetus softens and peels off. The skull bones loosen and become movable while the abdomen becomes distended with blood-stained fluid. Showing the parents their macerated baby is a real challenge and this will be discussed later in the chapter.

Neonatal death

The parents of a baby that dies after birth usually have had the chance to see and possibly hold their baby while it was still alive. Sometimes difficult decisions have to be made around the care of the baby. In some instances the mother might still be too sick to visit her baby in the neonatal intensive care unit (NICU). These mothers have to rely on others to bring them information about their babies.

Congenital abnormalities

Many babies born with congenital abnormalities will die before, or soon after birth. This is not the case with all babies with congenital abnormalities. The parents are often very concerned about the risk of their baby dying. In many instances the full implications of the congenital abnormality will only be known days or weeks after the birth of the baby. Even when very small abnormalities are present the parents may be upset. Parents may feel that they are not good enough to produce a normal child. They may experience feelings of rejection, followed by guilt at having such thoughts. These parents go through a process of grief because they experience a loss, the loss of their perfect child (which every parent expects). When a baby with congenital abnormalities dies the parents experience a second loss, namely, the loss of their beloved baby. As such, the parents have to accept the death of the baby, as well as the baby's abnormalities. At one specific stage, for example, they may accept the abnormalities but not necessarily the loss of their child or visa versa.

Preterm or sick neonate

The parents of a sick or preterm neonate grieve the loss of the healthy baby they expected. Often the staff in the neonatal unit may disregard this grief and they believe that the parents should feel happy because the baby is alive. The parents often experience conflict in this regard. They would have preferred a healthy full-term baby, which they could cuddle and care for and may feel excluded at not being able to perform their main role as parents. These duties have been taken over by strangers. The mother may feel a failure for not carrying the baby to full term. In addition, the parents will be concerned about the possibility that the baby may die and the possible financial implications. Visiting a baby in the NICU is time consuming and costly. Transport difficulties to and from the hospital might add to their feelings of guilt.

Giving the baby up for adoption

Even though a mother who gives her baby up for adoption chooses to do so and may go through the legalities of the process, it does not necessarily mean that she wanted to do so. Due to her circumstances her decision may have been based on what will be best for the baby.

Bonding already took place in utero. All the mothers who give their babies up for adoption will grieve the loss of their babies. Their grief is often delayed and takes longer to resolve. It is unlikely that they anticipate the strong maternal feelings that are experienced after the birth. Society and family do not always recognise their grief. Sometimes the mother gives her baby up for adoption without any friends or family knowing about the pregnancy and therefore has no support.

Infertility

Infertile couples often have a less acute grieving process, but the problem remains indefinitely and tends to take longer to work through. They grieve the loss or absence of their fertility. This loss is often unrecognised and underestimated by family and friends. The infertile couple might withdraw from friends who started with a family out of jealousy and pain. Society and cultural beliefs expect people to produce children, which places a bigger burden on the couple.

Caring for the bereaved

The midwife's role is to care for these grieving parents from when they start realising the extent of their grief and it must be ensured that nothing interferes with the normal initiation of their grieving process. The following aspects act as guidelines in caring for people who have experienced a loss. They are based on research and on the vast experience of caregivers. Every individual and situation is unique, resulting in different bereavement behaviour. Adaptations should therefore be made to accommodate these differing needs.

Breaking the news

A woman will easily become suspicious that something might be wrong with her pregnancy.

The midwife should be honest even when death or abnormalities are suspected. This will promote a trusting relationship between the woman and the midwife, which the woman will need desperately later. On the other hand, if the woman feels she cannot trust the midwife in the beginning, why should she trust her later? Where possible, both parents should be present when breaking the news. In the case of a single parent, a relative or close friend may be present. Privacy should be maintained. Parents often prefer that the obstetrician, paediatrician or doctor inform them about the bad news. If the obstetrician, paediatrician or doctor is not available, the midwife should inform the parents as soon as possible rather than leaving them in uncertainty. Their questions should be answered as accurately as possible.

Supporting the bereaved family

Support for the bereaved family has many aspects and includes the full spectrum of care for the family. This ranges from being sensitive when the bad news is delivered to referring the family for counselling and support groups. The single most important aspect of support is to be able to listen to the parents (or family). Give them time to express their feelings freely. No words of advice will help them now; they just need someone to listen to them unconditionally. Using phrases like 'You still have your other children to be thankful for' or 'You can fall pregnant again' will frustrate the parents even when they are meant well. At this stage the parents are not interested in their other children or another pregnancy. They want the child they lost. Do not avoid them for they already feel extremely lonely. The midwife's physical presence will indicate her emotional availability and willingness to share their experience of loss. A caring midwife will help the parents understand that their emotions are natural and real. The midwife must show confidence in her ability to cope with the crisis.

Verbal and non-verbal communication methods such as quietness, therapeutic touch and positive body language can be used. There is no harm in shedding a few tears in the presence of the parents as long as the midwife stays in control and it does not impede the care given to the parents. The parents usually experience this as confirmation that the midwife really cares.

Care may be sought from other support people and organisations such as social workers, psychologists, the hospital pastoral team or the parents' own religious advisers. Refer these parents to perinatal support groups where available. Many parents will experience comfort and support by talking to other parents in the same situation.

The parents should be referred for genetic counselling and the opportunity of an autopsy should be offered to them if congenital abnormalities are present or the cause of death is unknown. This provides them with a concrete reason for the death and relieves their sense of guilt.

Parents might have a great number of questions. They might repeat the same questions because there is too much information to absorb while they are simultaneously trying to deal with their emotions. Answer their questions patiently in a factual yet sympathetic manner, or refer them to a more knowledgeable person.

Showing the baby to the parents

In the case of a sick or abnormal baby, encourage the parents to visit the baby regularly in the NICU. Most of them have never seen a preterm or very sick baby before. These parents are usually scared because they are trying not to bond with their baby because of their fear of death. Encourage them to touch their baby and participate in the care. Saying 'hello' to this baby is an essential requirement to helping them say 'goodbye' later.

Previously it was common practice that a woman was not allowed to see or hold her baby after the baby died. Currently parents are advised to see and hold their babies after death, even when a baby is macerated or congenital abnormalities are present. By seeing and holding their baby, they will move on through the grieving process. They can no

longer deny the death of the baby. Acceptance of death will come sooner. When parents see their baby with congenital abnormalities after death, firstly they begin to comprehend that the baby could not have lived with the severity of the abnormalities. They are given a cause of death, which is very important for them. Secondly, the parents realise that their baby has many normal and beautiful features, not only abnormalities.

When the death of the fetus is known before birth, the possible contact with the baby should be discussed with the parents prior to the delivery. Unless the parents ask to see the baby immediately after the birth or death, the baby should be washed before showing the parents. Dressing the baby and wrapping him in a clean blanket will make the baby more presentable. Before showing the baby to the parents, inform them about his colour, temperature and appearance so that it is not a shock to them. It is always better to show the baby as soon as possible after the death or birth while the body is still warm. The baby should be carried in the same way as a live or normal baby would have been carried. The normal features of an abnormal infant/fetus should be presented to the parents first. They need to realise that their baby was not only abnormal, but also had beautiful features. Thereafter the parents can decide whether they want to look at the abnormalities.

Encourage the parents to hold the baby but they will need support. Many parents will need some privacy with the baby to express their feelings freely. No limit should be placed on the time spent with the baby for these parents need enough time to say 'hello' and 'goodbye' to the baby at the same time. Offer the parents the opportunity to see their baby again later. This opportunity should also be offered to parents who did not want to see their baby initially. More encouragement is needed where congenital abnormalities are present. Parents always imagine the abnormality of their baby to be worse than it really is, and the longer the delay before seeing the baby the more such a delay will influence their perception in a negative manner. No parent should, however, be forced to see or hold their baby. Religion and culture may also play a role in their decision to view and hold the baby and this should be respected.

For some women the performance of religious rites at the birth of the baby is important and the midwife should be prepared for and sensitive to the parent's request for blessing, baptism or other ritual dedication of the deceased. Some religious groups insist that these be done at the moment of death or birth and any delay may result in more feelings of guilt for the parents.

Collecting memories

Saving as many memories as possible helps most parents in their grief. Memory items may include any of the following:
▶ Identification bands.
▶ A lock of hair.

▶ Foot and handprints.
▶ Cord clamp.
▶ Cardiotocograph printout.
▶ Sonar photo.
▶ Photographs of the baby.
▶ A card with the weight, length and head circumference of the baby.

These items may be presented to the parents in the form of a 'book of remembrance', which will help them in their bereavement.

The parents should be encouraged to name their baby and the midwife should use the name too.

Other aspects of care

Most women may prefer to be in a private room, although some may decline the offer. If possible place the woman in an area where she is protected from hearing other babies crying. Inform all staff members (including housekeeping personnel) and patients nearby

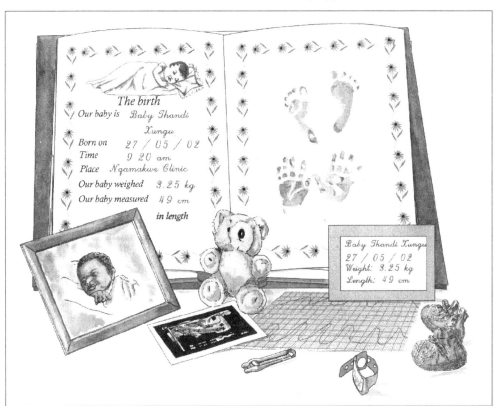

Figure 28.1 Memories of the baby

Guidelines on how to take a photo of a dead baby

Photographs provide not only proof of the baby's existence but are one of the most important memories of a baby that did not survive. A lot of effort should be put into it to make the baby as presentable as possible for the photograph. A dead baby or fetus should always be washed and dressed, or if not possible, wrapped in a blanket, before a photograph is taken. Green theatre cloths will look clinical, and so will the sluice room or medical apparatus in the background. One of the most effective ways to position the baby or fetus is to put it on or against two or three pillows. The baby should be positioned in the most natural way possible (see Figure 28.2 B). Through positioning bruises and abnormalities should be hidden. A parent may even hold the baby in his/her arm (especially in the case of a macerated baby where it is best to have some distance). The parents may want to have a family photograph taken.

Instant photographs seem like an easy option, but they fade over time and should rather be avoided. Black-and-white film disguises discolouration and bruising. Twins should be photographed together even if the one is alive and the other dead, to help the parents to come to terms with the reality.

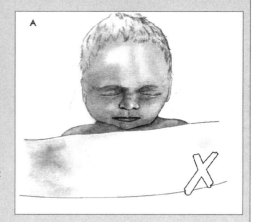

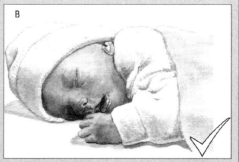

Figure 28.2
A: 'Clinical' picture of a dead baby that should be avoided.
B: More natural position of the baby with an exposed hand and a softly draped blanket.

about her loss. This will protect the woman from unnecessary remarks and questions. One of the biggest needs of these women is to be comforted by their family and friends and unrestricted visiting hours should therefore be allowed. A limited number of (preferably experienced) midwives should be allocated to this mother, which will facilitate the building of a trusting relationship.

Ensure that the woman's lactation is suppressed from the second trimester (e.g. by *bromocriptine*). Sedatives should not be prescribed routinely for they might delay the grieving process.

The parents most often do not realise that they have to register the birth as well as the death of the baby. The midwife should advise

them on this, as well as on funeral arrangements. When the woman is still hospitalised, the funeral should be postponed until she is able to attend. The midwife's decision on whether to attend the funeral of the baby will depend on her own preference. Some midwives feel that they want to support the family in this way and find it helpful for their own emotions during this difficult time.

To ensure comprehensive care of the parents a checklist should be compiled. Examples of items that can be included in such a list are:
▶ The name of the baby.
▶ Different professional people the woman has been referred to.
▶ Memories of the baby collected and given to the parents.

◗ Autopsy requested and specific information given to the parents.

Such a checklist will ensure that no aspect of care is left out and it will rule out the possibility of repetition.

> **CRITICAL THINKING EXERCISE**
> Compile a checklist that can be used by day and night staff in your unit to ensure continuity of care for bereaved parents.

Follow-up care

The woman is often discharged soon after the death of the baby. Many questions will only arise after her discharge from hospital in the weeks that follow. The midwife should provide the parents with the contact details of the midwives and physicians who were caring for her and her baby so that they can contact them if they wish to do so. Postnatal appointments should be made with great care for the parents may feel traumatised by coming back to the same institution. Ensure that the personnel who will be in contact with the woman during the appointment are informed about the loss. The midwife should contact the woman approximately a month after discharge to see how she is doing and to assess for possible pathological grief. Pathological grief is when the grief is prolonged, abnormally intense, delayed or the reaction is distorted or inhibited. Approximately one in five women will experience pathological grief, which should be referred appropriately.

The parents should be advised to delay the next pregnancy for at least six months to allow their grief to run its course. Having another baby before completing the grieving for the previous baby may result in the new baby unintentionally being connected to the hopes, emotions or feelings of the lost baby.

Midwives often do not recognise the parents' anxiety and concerns in the next pregnancy. These parents will need extra care and support, especially up to the comparative gestation or time period when they lost the previous baby.

Caring for the caregivers

It is unavoidable that the loss experienced by the parents will also greatly affect the midwives who are caring for them. Traumatic stress is caused not only by the death of a baby but a maternal death and even a traumatic delivery can be a profoundly negative experience for the caregivers. Prolonged exposure to such situations may make it more difficult for the caregivers to cope. Traumatic stress is associated with physiological and psychological symptoms such as tachycardia, raised blood pressure, recurrent images or nightmares, irritability, aggressive episodes, withdrawal and sleep disturbances, to name only a few. It is unavoidable that a person's professional performance will later be affected.

The emotional burden placed on the midwife is now being increasingly recognised. Often the South African midwife may have to

> **CRITICAL THINKING EXERCISES**
> Mary is a 23-year-old primigravida who was 37 weeks pregnant. She delivered a fresh stillborn after which a true knot in the umbilical cord was found. Her husband attended the delivery and has been supporting her throughout.
>
> 1. What are the normal feelings that the parents may experience over the next couple of months?
> 2. How will you best support this woman and her family?
> 3. Which preparations are necessary before showing the baby to the parents?
> 4. What memory items can you collect for the parents to take home?
> 5. How does this woman experiences loss in her particular culture?
> 6. What aftercare are you planning for this woman?
> 7. If you were fully involved in the care of this woman and family, what support would you like to receive from your colleagues?

move from the delivery of a stillbirth to the delivery of a live baby within 15 to 30 minutes and she runs an exhausting emotional gamut in doing so. In addition, these midwives work long shifts with heavy workloads. There are rarely any formal debriefing or counselling opportunities available to them.

Midwives should strive to support one another better under these difficult circumstances. Good team spirit and support from fellow team members are essential for the emotional health of midwives and other caregivers. The midwife manager should create a supportive environment for all staff members working under these stressful circumstances, including debriefing sessions where the midwives can express their feelings. The staff should be educated on bereavement counselling and how to cope with such stress. Midwives can also make use of other staff members such as the hospital minister or a counsellor for support. Without proper support the midwives would not be able to continue this very important service, which will lead to less support and care of the parents and families in the future.

References

Alexander, K. V. 2001. The one thing you can never take away: Perinatal bereavement photographs. *American Journal of Maternal/Child Nursing,* May/June 26(3):123–127.

Antonacci, M. 1990. Sudden death: Helping bereaved parents in the PICU. *Critical Care Nurse*, April 10(4):65–66, 68, 70.

Basson, T. A. 1995. The psychosocial implications of the loss of a fetus or baby. Doctoral thesis. University of Port Elizabeth, Port Elizabeth.

Bennett, V. R. & Brown, L. K. (Eds.) 1999. *Myles textbook for midwives.* Thirteenth edition. Edinburgh: Churchill Livingstone.

Caelli, K., Downie, J. & Letendre, A. 2002. Parents' experiences of midwife-managed care following the loss of a baby in a previous pregnancy. *Journal of Advanced Nursing*, July 39(2):127–136.

Casarett, D., Kutner, J. S. & Abrahm, J. 2001. Life after death: A practical approach to grief and bereavement. *Annals Internal Medicine*, February 134(3): 208–215.

Chambers, H. M. & Chan, F. Y. 2002. Support for women/families after perinatal death (Cohrane Review). In *The Cohrane Library*, Issue 1. Oxford: Update Software.

Cowles, K. 1996. Cultural perspectives of grief: An expanded concept analysis. *Journal of Advanced Nursing,* February 23(2): 287–294.

In a nutshell

▶ Grief is not only experienced after spontaneous or induced abortion, intra-uterine death (IUD) and neonatal death, but occurs also in cases where congenital abnormalities are diagnosed, the baby is given up for adoption, or the baby is sick or preterm. Grief is also experienced by couples who are unable to have children.

▶ The support and care given by the midwife should be individualised because every person experiences the grieving process in a unique way and at their own pace.

▶ The midwife should offer the parents the opportunity to see and hold their baby, even if the baby is macerated or has congenital abnormalities.

▶ Memories including photographs, footprints, hair and identification bands should be collected and offered to the parents.

▶ Midwives should encourage parents to express their grief freely.

▶ The best way to support the parents is to spend time listening to what they have to say.

▶ Staff members working with these parents are also entitled to a fair amount of support.

Cunningham, F. G., Gant, N. F., Leveno, K. J., Gilstrap III, L. C., Hauth, J. C. & Wenstrom, K. D. 2001. *Williams obstetrics*. Twenty-first edition. New York: McGraw-Hill Book Co.

De Kock, J. 1992. Ouers se belewenis van die dood van 'n baba met kongenitale afwykings. Ongepubliseerde M(Cur) skripsie. Randse Afrikaanse Universiteit, Johannesburg.

Ekblad, S., Marttila, A. & Emilsson, M. 2000. Cultural challenges in end-of-life care: Reflections from focal groups' interviews with hospice staff in Stockholm. *Journal of Advanced Nursing,* March 31(3):623–630.

Enkin, M., Keirse, M. J. N. C., Neilson, J., Crowther, C., Duley, L., Hodnett, E. & Hofmeyr, J. *A guide to effective care in pregnancy and childbirth.* Third edition. Oxford: Oxford University Press.

Geyer, N. 2001. Caring for the cared: Secondary traumatic stress. *Nursing Update,* November:20-22.

Hattingh S. 2001. Critical insident stress debriefing in health and emergency care workers. *Africa Journal of Nursing and Midwifery,* November 3(2):23–26.

Janssen, H. J. E. M., Cuisinier, M. C. J, de Graauw, K. P. H. M. & Hoogduin, K. A. L. 1997. A prospective study of risk factors predicting grief intensity following pregnancy loss. *Archives of General Psychiatry,* January 54(1):55–61.

Janssen, H. J. E. M., Cuisinier, M. C. J, Hoogduin, K. A. L & de Graauw, K. P. H. M. 1996. Controlled prospective study of the mental health of women following pregnancy loss. *Obstetrical & Gynecological Survey,* September 51(9):512–514.

Johnston, P. G. B. 1998. *The newborn child.* Eighth edition. New York: Churchill Livingstone.

Jolly, J. 1987. *Missed beginnings: Death before life has been established.* Berks: Austen Cornish Publishers Limited.

Klaus, M. H. & Kennell, J. H. 1976.

Maternal-infant bonding. Saint Louis: Mosby.

Klaus, PH. 1996. Commentary: Grieving a newborn loss calls for more than a rigid prescription by caregivers. *Birth,* December 24(4):216–217.

Laakso, H. & Paunonen-Ilmonen, M. 2001. Mothers' grief following the death of a child. *Journal of Advanced Nursing,* October 36(1):69–77.

Lundqvist, A., Nilstun, T. & Dykes, A. 2002. Both empowered and powerless: Mothers' experiences of professional care when their newborn dies. *Birth,* September 29(3):192–199.

Mabaso, M. S. & Uys, L. R. 1990. The experiences of black parents/caretakers with the births and care of a child with profound congenital defects. *Curationis,* June 13(1/2):33–36.

Modiba, L. M. 1997. The experience of mothers who gave birth to stillborn babies. Mini dissertation. Rand Afrikaans University, Johannesburg.

Nolte, A. G. W. (Ed.) 1998. *A Textbook for midwives.* Pretoria: J.L. van Schaik Publishers.

Primeau, M. R. & Recht, C. K. 1994. Professional bereavement photographs: One aspect of a perinatal bereavement program. *Journal of Obstetric, Gynecologic and Neonatal Nursing,* January 23(1):22–25.

Samuelsson, M., Rådestad, I. & Segesten, K. 2001. A waste of life: Fathers' experience of losing a child before birth. *Birth,* June 28(2):124–130.

Schott, J. & Henley, A. 1996. *Culture, religion and childbearing in a multiracial society.* Oxford: Butterworth-Heinemann.

Theut, S. K., Pederson, F. A., Zaslow, M. J., Cain, R. L., Rabinovich, B. A. & Morihisa, J. M. 1989. Perinatal loss and parental bereavement. *American Journal of Psychiatry,* May 146(5):635–639.

Weston, R., Martin, T. & Anderson, Y. (Eds.) 1998. *Loss and bereavement: Managing change.* Oxford: Blackwell Science Ltd.

Winchester, A. M. A. 1999. Sharing bad news. Nursing *Standard*, March 13(26):48–52.

Woods, J. R. & Esposito, J. L. 1987. *Pregnancy loss: Medical therapeutics and practical considerations.* Baltimore: Williams & Williams.

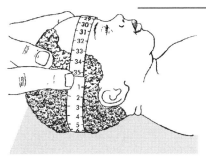

Section **7**

Newborn care

Chapter 29

Routine care of the healthy newborn

Angie Hennessy

Introduction

The aim of this chapter is to provide the midwife with the necessary skills and knowledge in order to attend to the normal infant's needs. Although the normal infant and the sick or preterm infant require a different focus of care, many of these basic principles remain the same. These principles will be discussed separately or as an integrated whole in this chapter. Routine care of the infant is extremely important as knowledge of the normal parameters and needs of an infant allow the midwife to care for her patient in the best possible manner.

Adaptation to extra-uterine life

The birth process of any infant results in a great amount of stress being placed on the infant regardless of the method of delivery, whether it be via normal vaginal delivery or caesarean section. The infant undergoes a number of physiological changes, which pre-

Terminology

Preterm: Infants born before the completion of the 37th gestational week.

Term: Infants born between 37 and 42 gestational weeks.

Post-term: Infants born after the 42 gestational week.

Small for gestational age (SGA): Infants born with a birth weight of less than the 10th percentile at any gestational age.

Large for gestational age (LGA): Infants born with a birth weight greater than the 90th percentile at any gestational age.

Low birth weight (LBW): Infants with a birth weight of less than 2 500 g.

Very low birth weight (VLBW): Infants with a birth weight of less than 1 500 g.

Extremely low birth weight (ELBW): Infants with a birth weight less than 1 000 grams.

pare the infant for the external environment. These adaptations occur simultaneously and are interdependent.

Circulatory adaptations

Once the umbilical cord is cut and clamped, the umbilical arteries and vein constrict. This causes the systemic blood pressure to rise. The ductus venosus closes due to lack of venous return from the clamped cord and forms the ligamentum venosum two to three days after birth. A decrease in pulmonary vascular pressure occurs due to respiratory adaptation, which causes pressures in the right atrium and right ventricle to decrease.

Pressures in the left atrium and left ventricle increase due to increased systemic vascular resistance. These pressure changes result in closure of the foramen ovale. Optimal lung functioning causes high levels of oxygenation. Fetal haemoglobin has a higher affinity for oxygen than adult haemoglobin, resulting in greater oxygen saturation of the blood. This higher oxygen level causes vasoconstriction of the ductus arteriosus. Another factor influencing the closure of the ductus arteriosus is the cessation of prostaglandins from the maternal blood supply.

Venous blood from the body now enters the right atrium from the inferior and superior vena cava. Deoxygenated blood flows to the right ventricle and then through the pulmonary arteries to the lungs. The blood is then oxygenated by the pulmonary circulation and returns to the left atrium via the pulmonary veins. It then passes trough to the left ventricle. Oxygenated blood is transported to the systemic circulation via the aorta (see Figure 29.1).

Pulmonary adaptations

The systemic vascular resistance is now greater than the pulmonary vascular resistance. The main stimuli that assist the initiation of breathing are hypoxia, hypercapnoea (increased PCO_2 levels) and acidosis. This occurs due to decreased or insufficient placental blood flow during maternal contractions. Acidosis, hypoxia and hypercapnoea

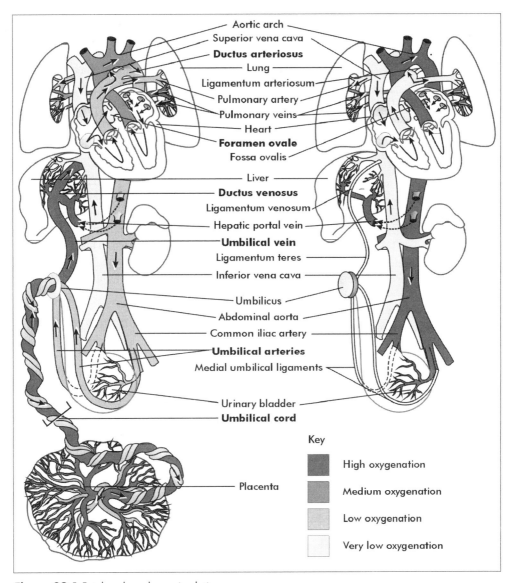

Figure 29.1 Fetal and newborn circulation

trigger chemoreceptors in the aorta and carotid arteries. These stimulate the respiratory centre in the brain to correct the disturbances by taking deep gasping breaths.

During a normal vaginal delivery, the infant's chest is compressed in the birth canal. Approximately one third of lung fluid is expelled from the lungs at this stage. Once the chest is delivered, the chest recoils and the lungs are filled with air. Inspiration and expansion of the lungs take place. Other stimuli that promote initiation of breathing are cold, light, touch and noise.

Air enters the lung with the first deep breaths causing lung fluid to move interstitially where it is drained by the lymphatic system. The pulmonary vessels dilate in response to the increased oxygen. Pulmonary vascular resistance decreases to adult values within the first few weeks of life.

Adaptation of other systems

The neurological system has matured in the optimal environment of the uterus where everything has been provided when needed: thermoregulation, protection, nutrition, gaseous exchange and waste product removal. After birth, the infant is now exposed to a loud, bright environment with much activity. The neurological system becomes highly stimulated in these new surroundings. The infant is alert and ready for interaction, which provides an excellent opportunity for bonding with the parents within the first hour.

The endocrine system also has to adapt after birth. In utero, fetal blood glucose was regulated by glucose concentrations in the maternal circulation. Glucose was exchanged with other nutrients via the placenta. After birth, the infant has to regulate his own blood glucose levels. It is therefore important to give the infant an initial feeding of colostrum or formula milk as soon as possible in order to provide him with a ready glucose supply. This in turn will prevent hypoglycaemia with all its negative effects.

The term neonate has glycogen stores greater than that of an adult, which provides him with adequate energy stores. Glycogen is broken down or metabolised into glucose that will then be used during the period of transition after birth. It is important to remember that glycogen metabolism is inhibited when the infant is stressed causing a reduction in energy availability (see Chapter 31).

The infant uses brown fat stores to provide and regulate an optimal core temperature. As the infant cannot shiver to create heat, it is important to keep him warm by covering the head and skin surface with blankets or clothing.

The special senses including eyes and ears are fully functional at birth. The infant's eyes take a few days before they can focus properly. This should be explained to the parents when seeing their infant for the first time.

During fetal development the amount of space in the uterus was reduced. This forced the infant into physiological flexion, which is crucial for proper progress in childhood development. The infant now has a chance to explore the concept of space but will always feel more secure in a flexed position (page 29-32).

During a stressful episode (such as birth or reduced oxygen supply), blood flow to the kidneys and gastrointestinal system are reduced owing to autoregulation of blood flow. This can justify a delay in optimal functioning of these systems until blood supply is optimised. The renal system was functional in utero by producing and excreting urine, which facilitates the readiness to function optimally at birth. The gastrointestinal system was producing meconium in utero but no excretion has yet occurred. This is, however, possible during an hypoxic incident, where the infant passes meconium into the amniotic fluid (see Chapter 31).

Characteristics of a normal infant

An infant is considered 'normal' when born at term with a one-minute Apgar score of seven or more out of ten. No resuscitation should be necessary after birth. The infant's birth weight should range between 2 500 and 4 000 g. No congenital abnormalities or abnormal clinical signs should be observed during the physical examination and the infant should not present with any problems before discharge.

Characteristics of a sick or preterm infant

A sick or preterm infant may have a one-minute Apgar score of less than seven and resuscitation may be necessary after delivery. Birth weight is not a reliable indicator of health as an infant of any weight can present with illness. During the physical examination, abnormalities are found. These can either relate to prematurity or congenital abnormalities. A congenital abnormality is considered as any anomaly that the infant is born with, including structural and functional defects. These infants generally need advanced medical attention with admission to high care baby units or neonatal intensive care units. Table 29.1 provides a number of warning signs which the midwife should be alert for.

Table 29.1 Warning signs of a sick newborn infant

Skin	▶ Cyanosis ▶ Pale skin colour ▶ Hypothermia ▶ Poor perfusion
Signs of respiratory distress	▶ Audible expiratory wheeze or grunting ▶ Nasal flaring ▶ Tachypnoea ▶ Sternal recession ▶ Rib retraction ▶ Oxygen needs above 21% (room air)
Cardiovascular system	▶ Low blood pressure ▶ Tachycardia ▶ Abnormal heart sounds ▶ Weak or abnormal pulses
Central nervous system	▶ Hypotonia ▶ Hypertonia ▶ Apathy or lethargy ▶ Tremors or jitteriness ▶ Bulging or sunken fontanelles ▶ Irritability and high-pitched crying
Gastrointestinal tract	▶ Frequent vomiting ▶ Abdominal distension

General care

Identification of the infant

Identification of the infant should be considered as a vital piece of information that needs to be confirmed. When receiving an infant, the identification bands should be checked with the attending midwife and/or parents. The infant should be identified on one wrist and one ankle with all the necessary details present. These details will depend on the hospital or clinic policy, but should include the infant's surname, date of birth, mother's details and attending obstetrician.

Vital observations

Vital data for the healthy newborn should be recorded four-hourly for the first 24 hours, and then twice daily if all observations are within normal limits. These act as baselines as some infants are discharged 6 to 24 hours after birth. Parameters for the healthy newborn infant are as follows:

▶ *Heart rate*: 110–160 bpm
▶ *Respiration rate*: 30-60 breaths per minute
▶ *Axillary temperature*: 36.5–37.2 °C
▶ *Oxygen saturation*: 90–100% in room air (21% O_2)
▶ *Mean blood pressure*: Greater than gestational age
▶ *Blood glucose*: 3 mmol/l–7.2 mmol/l

There is no need for the last three parameters to be done routinely unless indicated by abnormalities presenting in the newborn. For example, an infant presenting with signs of respiratory distress or cyanosis should have an oxygen saturation determined to establish the possible need for oxygen administration, or if an infant is very sleepy and fails to feed effectively, the blood glucose should be tested to ensure that it is not low. If the equipment is

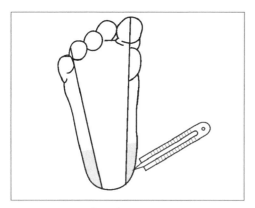

Figure 29.2 Heel prick areas

available, however, it is safer to obtain a baseline record of all parameters on admission of the infant for early detection of abnormalities.

Capillary samples to assess blood glucose are taken from the infant's heel. This sample should only be obtained from the outermost area on the lower quarter of the foot (see Figure 29.2). Blood glucose assessment can be done when indicated, such as for readings above or below the above-mentioned parameter.

Gestational age determination

Gestational age is an estimated age related to the maturity of the fetus. Gestational age gives the midwife a good indication of the condition to expect when receiving or delivering an infant. Although gestational age is needed for a correct level of preparedness in any delivery, it is not always available or reliable. Gestational age can be determined by the last menstrual period or first sonar, but it is often found that the specific date is not known or that no sonar was performed. Under these circumstances, the midwife can assess the gestational age of the infant by different methods where the physical and neurological features are observed and scored using a standardised scale.

There are two scales that can be used to assess gestational age:
▶ The Dubowitz maturity scale assessment of gestational age consists of two sections, assessing 11 physical and 10 neurological aspects. This scale looks at extensive criteria, which reduces its user-friendliness.

▶ The Ballard scale score is a simplified version based on the Dubowitz maturity scale. Neuromuscular (five items) and physical maturity (six items) are assessed. The infant can score from −1 to 5 for each of the items. Once assessed, the score is calculated from both sections and the maturity rating table is consulted. This table allows the midwife to correlate the score with the appropriate gestation in weeks. Gestational age can be determined from 20 weeks to 44 weeks gestational age (see Figure 29.3).

Growth assessment

Weighing, head circumference and length determination are methods of determining whether the infant's nutritional needs are being met in terms of growth and weight gain. These need to be measured accurately in the correct manner to prevent unreliable results. Weight is also used for the calculation of feeding, fluids, urine output and medication.

The length of the infant is measured from crown to heel, either by the use of a special measuring board, or by placing the infant on a flat surface with the measuring tape next to the infant. If possible, two people should perform the measurement, where one holds the infant and the other measures the infant. The infant should be held in a stretched-out position, with knees and ankles together against the surface. The measurement is then read from the tape measure. Normal length measurements range between 48 and 53 cm in term infants (see Figure 29.4).

To measure head circumference, measure the maximum occipitofrontal diameter of the infant's skull. The tape measure is positioned anteriorly above the eyebrows and to the most prominent posterior part of the occiput. This reading can be influenced by moulding and caput of the head. In these cases, the readings should be repeated at a later stage. Normal head circumference varies between 33 and 37 cm for the term infant (see Figure 29.5).

All measurements should be plotted on a growth chart in order to establish whether the

Neuromuscular Maturity

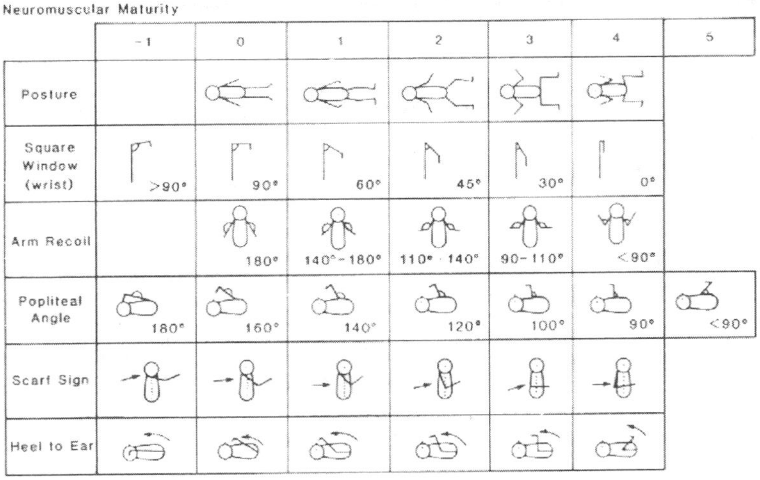

	-1	0	1	2	3	4	5
Posture							
Square Window (wrist)	>90°	90°	60°	45°	30°	0°	
Arm Recoil		180°	140°–180°	110°–140°	90–110°	<90°	
Popliteal Angle	180°	160°	140°	120°	100°	90°	<90°
Scarf Sign							
Heel to Ear							

Physical Maturity

	-1	0	1	2	3	4	5
Skin	sticky friable transparent	gelatinous red, translucent	smooth pink, visible veins	superficial peeling &/or rash, few veins	cracking pale areas rare veins	parchment deep cracking no vessels	leathery cracked wrinkled
Lanugo	none	sparse	abundant	thinning	bald areas	mostly bald	
Plantar Surface	heel-toe 40–50 mm: -1 <40 mm: -2	>50mm no crease	faint red marks	anterior transverse crease only	creases ant. 2/3	creases over entire sole	
Breast	imperceptible	barely perceptible	flat areola no bud	stippled areola 1–2mm bud	raised areola 3-4mm bud	full areola 5–10mm bud	
Eye/Ear	lids fused loosely:-1 tightly:-2	lids open pinna flat stays folded	sl. curved pinna, soft; slow recoil	well-curved pinna; soft but ready recoil	formed &firm instant recoil	thick cartilage ear stiff	
Genitals male	scrotum flat, smooth	scrotum empty faint rugae	testes in upper canal rare rugae	testes descending few rugae	testes down good rugae	testes pendulous deep rugae	
Genitals female	clitoris prominent labia flat	prominent clitoris small labia minora	prominent clitoris enlarging minora	majora & minora equally prominent	majora large minora small	majora cover clitoris & minora	

Maturity Rating

score	weeks
-10	20
-5	22
0	24
5	26
10	28
15	30
20	32
25	34
30	36
35	38
40	40
45	42
50	44

Figure 29.3 Ballard scale
Source: Reproduced from Ballard, J. et al. New Ballard Score, expanded to include preterm infants. Journal of Pediatrics. September, 119(3): 417–423, © 1991 Mosby, with permission from Elsevier.

growth curve is correct for gestational age. In this manner problems of growth impairment can be identified early, which then has to be investigated further to determine the underlying cause.

Weight is the most sensitive parameter that indicates growth. The midwife would therefore be able to identify impaired growth by observing deviations in weight gain. Growth charts are convenient and easy to use as weight changes can be recognised quickly. The growth chart has a series of lines that form a comparison basis for what is normal, and what is expected from the normal infant. These lines are called percentiles and indicate whether the weight gain is above, within or below the expected average.

The 50th percentile indicates the median of

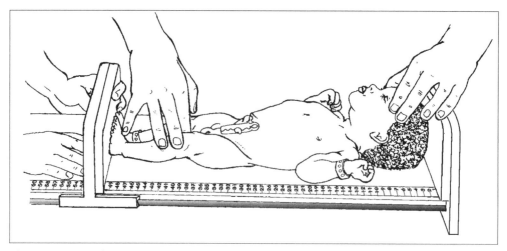

Figure 29.4 Length measurement

the growth chart with 50% of plotted weights above the line and 50% of plotted weights below the line. The 97th percentile indicates the normal upper limits of the chart with 97% of all plotted weights falling below the 97th percentile and only 3% of weights being plotted above this upper limit. These infants are considered to be very large. The normal lower limits or 3rd percentile indicates that only 3% of plotted weights should fall below this line. This shows that only 3% of infants should be plotted above or below the normal limits. These infants are then considered to be very large or very small (see Figure 29.6).

The healthy newborn infant loses up to 10% of its birth weight by days three to four after birth. Birth weight is usually regained by days

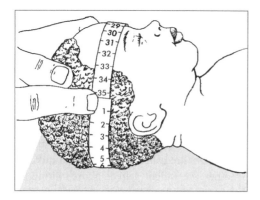

Figure 29.5 Head circumference

seven to ten. Weighing can be recorded every second day to monitor weight loss and gain. The infant should be weighed without clothes or diaper to obtain an accurate reading and on the same scale if possible. Swaddled weighing should be implemented to reduce an unnecessary stress response. The blanket used to wrap the infant in should be weighed before or after weighing the baby. The weight of the blanket is then deducted from the total weight.

Once the weights are measured monthly after discharge, the plotted dots can be joined to indicate the infant's growth curve. The growth curve must show movement in an upward direction. Rising growth curves show healthy infants, whereas flat curves should be warning signs of possible problems. A growth curve with a downward trend needs immediate action.

Physical examination

Each newborn has to be carefully assessed as soon as possible after birth for signs of problems, complications or genetic and congenital abnormalities. A short initial assessment is conducted directly after delivery, with a head-to-toe assessment once the infant leaves the labour ward. The physical examination is repeated prior to discharge. By doing a physical examination, the midwife assesses the infant's

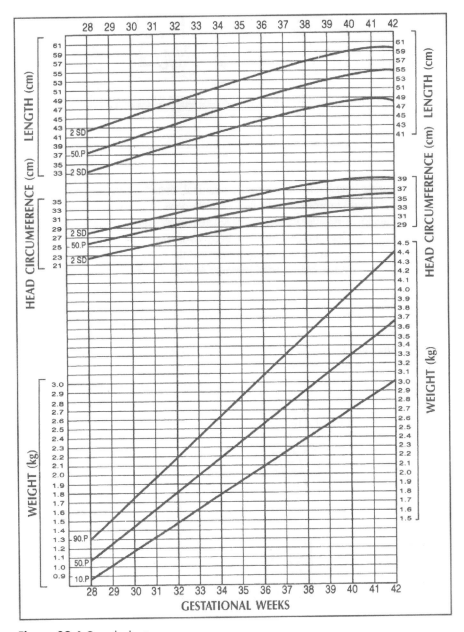

Figure 29.6 Growth chart
Source: Reproduced from Henning, P. A. An example of a perinatal percentile chart from
The examination of the newborn baby, 2002:16, with permission from Van Schaik Publishers.

health status, observes for signs of abnormalities or illness, and poor adaptation to extra-uterine life. This allows the midwife to diagnose actual and potential problems early.

The process of examination should be gentle, non-traumatic and conducted logically and systematically. It is important to inform the mother about the procedure and ask for her consent. If the mother wants to be present, she should be allowed to sit in during the examination. During the physical assessment all the normal expectations and appearances act as the baseline and findings are classified as either normal or a variation from the normal, and have to be recorded.

History

One of the most important aspects of assessment of the newborn is correctly obtaining a history. The history furnishes information on details and events prior to birth, the birth process itself, the infant's history and facts on social and family characteristics that are important for comprehensive care.

In order to assess the infant in a holistic manner, a complete maternal history is needed for accurate risk identification. The following aspects need consideration:

◗ Maternal age
◗ Obstetric history
◗ Antenatal history, including high-risk maternal conditions
◗ Psychological and social history
◗ Complete history of the labour and delivery of the infant

Apgar scores, possible resuscitation, administration of eye prophylaxis and vitamin K_1, identification, initial physical examination, and blood collected from umbilical cord (thyroid functions or Coombs tests) are all vital information when examining the newborn infant.

General principles

There are general principles applicable while examining the newborn. The parents should be involved, which alleviates parental anxiety and confirms normality in the infant. All equipment and supplies to be used should be cleaned and prepared before starting the assessment to ensure working order and accessibility. An examination area with adequate natural light decreases the risk of misinterpretation or wrongly made conclusions. Ensure that the infant will not be harmed or exposed to infection by removing all jewellery. Apply infection control principles with effective hand-washing. Take precaution to prevent hypothermia during the examination. Do not undress and expose the whole infant. Expose only the body area examined to minimise heat loss.

Special precautions may be needed with preterm and sick infants. If the baby is in an incubator, do not remove him but examine him inside. The oxygen head box or any oxygen administration devices should not be removed during the examination. Avoid traction on intravenous lines as they may become displaced. Switch off the phototherapy light to allow for correct assessment of skin colour and the infant's eyes. Comfort the baby during and after the examination by soft talking, touching, slow movements and cuddling (see DSC page 29-31).

Examination routine

The physical examination should be done systematically and thoroughly without missing any abnormalities or excluding systems, that is, from head-to-toe or according to the systems. The infant should be examined when awake and while peaceful and calm.

Perform all investigations that require a hushed environment and a non-crying infant first, including auscultation of the lungs, heart and abdomen. Disturbing procedures should be performed last, such as testing neurological reflexes. Make certain that once the physical examination is complete, all structural and functional components of the body have been assessed.

General examination

During the general examination the infant's identification, weight, length, head circumference, nutritional status, general appearance, colour, skin, hydration and lymph nodes need to be assessed. The general appearance indicates the infant's health status and whether the infant has any immediate problems, such as signs of respiratory distress. Gross congenital abnormalities are looked for, as well as a normal flexed posture and coordinated symmetrical movement of all limbs.

Colour. The normal colour of the skin is pink. This pink colour is caused by oxygenated blood in the capillaries under the skin. Abnormal skin colour includes the following:

▶ *Jaundice* is seen when the infant's skin has a yellow discolouration when pressed with the finger and then released. In deeply pigmented infants, jaundice may be identified more easily in the oral mucosa and the conjunctiva of the eye.

▶ *Cyanosis* can be peripheral or central. Peripheral cyanosis is blue discoloration of the hands and feet due to cold and vasoconstriction. Central cyanosis is serious and is evident when the tongue is blue. These infants generally have respiratory and/or cardiac problems (requiring immediate attention).

▶ *Pallor* is very pale skin that may indicate shock or anaemia. The capillary filling time is more than three seconds and the mucous membranes are pale.

▶ *Redness* can be caused by overheating, cold stress and polycythaemia. Episodes of crying can cause transient redness but this is normal.

▶ *Polycythaemia* occurs when the infant's haematocrit or haemoglobin is elevated giving the skin a red colour.

▶ *Mottled* skin refers to a blueish-pale colour and can be due to stress or infection. The cause should be isolated as it may be indicative of a serious problem.

Skin. The infant's skin has a pink colour and is soft, flexible and supple. In dark-skinned infants, this pink colour can be seen in the nail beds and oral mucosa. In preterm infants the skin is often very thin and transparent and capillary veins can easily be seen. Findings of the skin are as follows:

▶ *Vernix caseosa* is a white greasy substance covering the skin that is visible from the second trimester during pregnancy. No vernix caseosa is seen on a post-term infant. Green discoloration of the vernix may be due to meconium in the amniotic fluid.

▶ *Lanugo* are small, fine hairs found over the face, shoulders and back of the preterm infant as well as dark-haired infants.

Lanugo falls out spontaneously within a few months.

▶ *Skin peeling* off the hands and feet is normal, especially towards the end of the first week of life. Post-term, meconium-stained infants and intra-uterine growth-restricted infants can also present with skin peeling. Severe peeling of the palms and foot soles may indicate congenital syphilis.

▶ *Erythema toxicum* is a benign rash that disappears spontaneously. Multiple small erythematous areas with a central white-yellow papule cover the skin. Staphy-lococcal and candidiase skin infections have similar appearances and should not be confused with erythema toxicum.

▶ *Mongolian spots* are blue-grey skin dis-colourations found over the buttocks, shoulders and back of the infant. These marks are benign and become less prominent with time. They appear blue in colour due to delayed pigmentation of the skin area and are common in infants of Mediterranean and African descent.

▶ *Milia* are small white papules found on the nose and chin. They disappear spon-taneously and are formed by keratin plugs in the sebaceous glands of the skin.

Hydration. Hydration is assessed by looking at the following:

▶ Reduction or increase in weight
▶ Skin elasticity (skin turgor test)
▶ Moistness or dryness of mucous membranes
▶ Sunken or bulging fontanelles
▶ Normal sunken or swollen eyes

A dehydrated infant will be lethargic with reduced elasticity of the skin. The mucous membranes will be dry, the fontanelles and the eyes will be sunken, and there will be evident weight loss. Oedema in the newborn is not a normal occurrence and can be seen around the eyes, lower extremities, and on the dorsum of the hands and feet. It may indicate overhydration or more severe problems relat-ed to the heart or kidneys.

Lymph nodes. Palpable lymph nodes in the healthy newborn should be absent. If present at birth, it may indicate intra-uterine infection or congenital lymphoedema (Turner's syndrome).

Head-to-toe examination

Head. The head should be inspected for size and shape. The size of the head should be relative to the weight and length of the baby. The shape of the normal head of an infant is round and symmetrical and the head can be turned with ease from side to side. The cranial sutures can be felt. If you press slightly on the bone next to the sutures, separate movements of the bone can be felt, as they are not yet fused. Assess specifically for the following:

▶ *Moulding* occurs when the flexible skull has pressure on it in the birth canal causing re-shaping of the head. Moulding results from overriding of sutures, which are palpable, as ridges. The skull returns to its normal shape within the first week after birth.

▶ *Craniostenosis* results from early permanent closure of the cranial sutures and causes an abnormal head shape.

▶ *Meningocoele* and *encephalocoele* are midline defects where the skull bones did not close properly. The meningocoele contains meninges, whereas the encephalocoele contains meninges, cerebrospinal fluid and brain tissue.

▶ The infant's *hair* varies from sparse to thick and bushy. Hair is generally soft and fine. Hair strands can be separated easily and they do not stick to one another. A normal posterior hairline should be above the nape of the neck. A low hairline may indicate chromosomal abnormalities.

▶ The scalp must be observed for any injuries especially after caesarean section and assisted deliveries (forceps and vacuum). *Petechiae* on the scalp, face and neck may be a result of increased pressure on the head, impacted shoulders or from the umbilical cord tightly constricting the neck.

Four types of swellings can be found on the scalp:

▶ *Caput succedaneum* is diffuse oedema of the scalp caused by local injury of soft tissue on the presenting part, which may cross the fontanelles and suture lines. The swelling usually subsides in a few days.

▶ *Vacuum haematoma* is bleeding of soft tissue in the area of attachment to the vacuum extractor. The scalp has a raised purple area that is very painful with possible breakdown of skin. The lesion usually heals within a few days.

▶ *Cephalhaematoma* is bleeding between the skull and the periosteum that presents as swelling located to a specific cranial bone and does not cross the skull sutures. It is a result of a traumatic delivery. Possible complications for this infant include jaundice, anaemia, infection and possible linear skull fracture. The cephalhaematoma may persist for six to eight weeks.

▶ *Subaponeurotic haemorrhage* is extensive bleeding below the epicranial aponeurosis. This crosses suture lines and is generally caused by failed vacuum and forceps deliveries. The infant presents with swelling and bruising of the eyelids and behind the ears, and is at risk of anaemia and severe shock. Prompt treatment of the complications is crucial.

The anterior fontanelle is a diamond-shaped opening, approximately 2.5 cm x 2.5 cm, between the cranial bones found in the midline on the top of the head. This closes at approximately 18 months of age. The posterior fontanelle is a smaller triangular opening, approximately 0.5 cm, between the cranial bones a few centimetres backwards, but still in the midline. Both fontanelles should be soft and firm but level with the skull and not bulging or sunken. A third fontanelle can be palpated about three centimetres above the posterior fontanelle. This can present in infants with chromosomal abnormalities, but has also been found in normal infants.

Abnormalities that are reason for concern are:

▶ A very small or large head in proportion to the body.
▶ A flattened head (top, back and sides).
▶ Small forehead.
▶ Bulging or sunken fontanelles.
▶ Absence of fontanelles.
▶ Spreading of fontanelles.
▶ Rigid sutures.
▶ Visible or palpable indentation, laceration, bruising and protruding soft tissue from the scalp.

Face. The face is relatively small in relation to the head with the appearance of chubby cheeks that facilitate sucking. Observe for symmetry of the face, as well as location of the facial features. If the face is divided in three parts, the upper third is the forehead, the middle third the eyes, nose and ears, and the lower third the mouth and jaw. Take into consideration the parents' appearance and ethnic group when examining the face. The following skin lesions may be observed:

▶ *Capillary haemangiomas* are found on the forehead, eyelids, nose bridge or nape of the neck. They are commonly named 'stork's bite' or 'angel's kiss'. These tend to fade within two years but capillary haemangi-omas on the neck may take longer to fade.
▶ *Naevus flammeus* (port-wine stain) is a red-purple mark that does not reduce in size. It can be isolated to the face or spread to the meninges (Sturge-Weber syndrome).
▶ *Cavernous haemangiomas* (strawberry naevi) have a bright red colour and are normally positioned over the face, scalp, back and chest. These haemangiomas tend to grow before they reduce in size.

The size, shape and amount of cartilage of the ears may differ from infant to infant. The position for ears would be normal if an imaginary horizontal line from the top of the ears could be drawn to the corner of the eyes. Low set or rotated ears (not upright but leaning back-wards) often indicate anomalies in development, such as chromosomal or renal abnormalities. The infant's response (startle reaction or blinking) to sound or noise should be tested to assess the hearing ability.

A *pre-auricular sinus* is a blind-ended hole in front of the ear. It may be familiar and is normally benign. If recurrent infections occur removal of the sinus is possible. *Pre-auricular skin tags* can be present and are not necessarily abnormal although they are associated with certain syndromes and renal problems.

The infant will open his eyes if held in an upright or prone position, with some shielding from excessive light. Observe the eyes for correct positioning. The eyes should be horizontal with equal spacing between them. Squinting is common and improves with increased optic muscle strength. Assess for bilateral presence and size of eyeballs, as well as pupil reaction to light. The midwife should compare both eyes and note any *cataracts* (white or opaqueness over the cornea), *sub-conjunctival haemorrhage*, or severe squinting (*strabismus*). Observe for any swelling or dis-colouration of the eyelids due to a traumatic delivery. Epicanthic folds may be familiar, but are often found in chromosomal abnormalities such as Down's syndrome.

The newborn is an obligatory nose breather and patency of the nostrils is essential for effective breathing. Any obstruction or nar-rowing of the nose will result in breathing and feeding problems. The width of the nose is normally less than 2.5 cm. The nose bridge is generally flat at birth due to soft cartilage. A flat nose bridge can be attributed to Down's syndrome if other related dysmorphic features are found. Nasal flaring is associated with res-piratory distress and is not normal. Nasal flar-ing should be absent during breathing. The nasal septum must be straight and in the mid-line. The philtrum is the central groove run-ning from the nose to the top lip. If this is flat-tened or absent, the infant may present with *fetal alcohol syndrome*.

The mouth and oral cavity is difficult to examine and should be done with care:

▶ *Sucking blisters* are normal and may be seen in the middle of the upper lip.

▶ *Cleft lip* is seen easily and may involve both the soft and hard cleft palate. This is referred to as a *cleft palate*.

▶ *One* or *more teeth* may be present. No intervention is necessary until they cause problems for example, tongue laceration.

▶ *Retention cysts* (water cysts) on the gums are harmless and disappear spontaneously.

▶ *Ebstein's pearls* appear as white-grey marks on the palate and are of no significance. Ensure not to confuse these with oral thrush.

▶ The tongue should be pink and fit into the oral cavity proportionately. *Macroglossia* is an abnormally large tongue that protrudes from the mouth. It is associated with hypothyroidism, Beckwith syndrome and tongue tumours.

▶ *Milk crusts* found in the mouth are normally only present after a feed and are found on the tongue. The mouth is clean before the feed and the crusts can be removed relatively easily.

▶ *Oral thrush* (moniliasis) is a fungal infection that presents with white spots in the oral cavity. It is seen before and after feeding. The white spots are difficult to remove and generally cause bleeding on removal. The oral cavity is inflamed and red. This infection needs treatment to prevent it from spreading to other systems. Remember to treat the mother as well as her nipples/breasts, which may be the source of the infection.

The infant's jaw should be symmetrical and proportional to the face. A small lower jaw, (*micrognathia*) may indicate chromosomal abnormalities such as Trisomy 18. A skew jaw could be due to intra-uterine compression and may take a few months to correct.

Neck. The neck of an infant is relatively short, but recognisable without skin folds or webbing. A webbed neck can indicate congenital syndromes like Turner's syndrome. A skew neck may be attributed to intra-uterine compression. The presence of swelling, sinuses and fistulas of the neck must be assessed, for example, thyroid enlargement. The trachea should be straight and in the midline. The neck should move easily, indicating mobility and function of cervical vertebrae and attached muscles. The clavicles should be felt to ensure their presence and position, and fractures should be excluded.

Chest. The size of the term infant's chest is approximately the same as the head circumference. The shape of the chest is cylindrical with similar anterior-posterior diameter and lateral diameters. There are 12 pairs of ribs, which are more horizontal than adult ribs. During breathing the infant uses the diaphragm, which is seen with abdominal movement. The nipples are situated in line with the middle of the clavicles. The nipples are clearly evident and have a raised bud. Breast tissue can be felt when palpated but it should not be squeezed if enlargement is noticed as this could cause mastitis. This enlargement can be due to maternal oestrogen, and nipple discharge may also be present.

Respiratory system. The skin colour should be pink with no signs of peripheral or central cyanosis. The nostrils and nasal passages should be free of obstruction with no nasal flaring.

▶ *Periodic breathing* is normal where the infant had periods of faster and slower breathing rates. The infant can have episodes of normal breathing alternating with no breathing attempts lasting between five to ten seconds. This usually occurs during REM sleep.

▶ *Apnoea* is no breathing for more than 20 seconds or shorter but associated with bradycardia (less than 100 bmp) and colour changes such as cyanosis or pallor may accompany it. Normal respiration is between 30 to 60 breaths per minute.

The infant must be assessed for any signs of respiratory distress as mentioned below:

▶ *Tachypnoea* is a breathing rate greater than 60 breaths per minute.
▶ *Sternal recession* and *intercostal retraction* assists in strenuous breathing by using auxiliary muscles and bones to increase lung spaces and internal pressures in the lung.
▶ *Expiratory grunting* is a compensatory mechanism where the infant tries to maintain a pressure in the lungs to prevent the alveoli from collapsing.
▶ *Central cyanosis* (see under Colour on page 29-13).

Normal chest sounds are bilateral and symmetrical when auscultating the anterior, lateral and posterior aspects of the chest at the level of the apex, mid-lobes and lower lobes. No stridor, rales, wheezing or crepitations should be heard.

Cardiovascular system. Although skin colour has already been assessed, abnormalities may indicate cardiac defects. Normal perfusion or peripheral circulation can be observed on the fingertips and toes as a capillary refill of less than three seconds. To measure capillary refill press the fingertips or toes gently between two fingers, release and measure the time lapse before it returns to the original colour. Delayed time of more than three seconds shows fair or poor perfusion. Blood pressure should be assessed to obtain baseline data.

The following pulses are to be palpated to ensure adequate circulation of blood to all extremities:
▶ Carotid
▶ Brachial
▶ Radial
▶ Femoral
▶ Popliteal
▶ Foot pulses (dorsalis pedis).

A bouncing pulse accompanied by a heart murmur can indicate a *patent ductus arteriosus* (PDA). Reduced pulses and blood pressure differences between limbs may indicate *coarctation of the aorta* (see Chapter 31).

A normal heart rate varies from 110 to 160 bpm. The apex beat of the heart is normally at the fourth intercostal space on the nipple line. If heard at a different rib space, enlargement may be present. This can be confirmed with X-rays if available. Listen to the presence, intensity, rate and rhythm of the heart sounds and the presence of any murmurs. Observe how the heart rate is influenced by the baby's activity. *Tachycardia* presents when the heart rate is greater than 160 bpm.

Abdomen. The normal appearance of the abdomen is slightly prominent due to diaphragmatic respiration. The sides protrude laterally and upwards. A distended abdomen can be caused by excess air in the stomach, enlarged abdominal organs and ascites (fluid-filled abdominal cavity). A sunken-in (scaphoid) abdomen may indicate a *diaphragmatic hernia* or *oesophageal atresia*. Presence of abdominal muscles must be established. Absence of abdominal muscles is called *Prune belly syndrome* due to the prune-like appearance of the abdomen. Bowel sounds can be auscultated to ensure peristalsis of the intestines and colon.

Skin covers the abdominal surface, with the umbilical cord protruding more or less centrally. Two umbilical arteries and one umbilical vein should be visible on inspection of the umbilical cord stump. Only one artery can indicate renal anomalies. No bleeding should be seen. An infected umbilical stump is called *omphalitis*. Abdominal wall abnormalities include *umbilical hernia*, *exomphalos* and *gastroschisis*.

The abdomen is soft on palpation and the infant should not appear to be stressed (no crying) or in pain during palpation. Palpate the abdomen gently to examine the liver. The normal liver border is palpable just below the right costal margin. The bladder, spleen and kidneys can be palpated although this needs extra skill. Abdominal masses should be reported.

Excessive vomiting (possible oesophageal stenosis) and drooling (possible oesophageal atresia) must be reported swiftly.

Diaper area. The inguinal area must be examined for femoral pulses, lymph nodes, and possible inguinal hernias. *Inguinal herniation* normally occurs in the preterm male infant where intestines pass through the hernia into the scrotum. This is extremely painful and may require surgical correction. The anal sphincter is visible below the genitalia of the infant. Patency of the anus can be tested by gentle insertion of a rectal thermometer, but there is a lot of controversy about this method. Meconium is the first stools passed and can confirm rectal patency unless the meconium has escaped through a vaginal fistula in the female infant. *Anus imperforatum* occurs when the colon and anus fail to connect. Surgical correction is necessary. Constipation and diarrhoea are abnormal findings and should not be left unattended.

The hips must be examined to exclude *congenital hip dislocation*. Hip dislocation is the dislocation of the femur head out of the acetabulum, most often caused by developmental dysplasia of the hip. It is characterised by asymmetrical lengths of the legs with one knee higher than the other one and the skin fold of the buttocks on the one side higher than the other one.

When examining the genitals the midwife should address the following:
◗ Gender
◗ Ambiguous genitalia
◗ Gestational characteristics
◗ Abnormalities
◗ Discharge
◗ Micturition

The term female infant has a prominent labia majora which covers the labia minora and most of the clitoris. In preterm females, the labia majora is less visible with a prominent labia minora and clitoris. Enlargement and increased pigmentation of the clitoris may occur in dark-skinned infants. The genitals may be bruised and oedematous after a breech delivery. *Vaginal tags* (hymeneal mucosal tags) are common and they will resolve spontaneously during the first few weeks of life. A white, mucoid vaginal discharge may be present and results from secretion of antenatal oestrogen. This usually disappears after a few weeks. Vaginal haemorrhage also occurs occasionally due to the presence of maternal hormones. The urethra is positioned between the clitoris and the vagina. The vaginal opening is larger than the urethral opening and is situated between the urethral opening and anus.

The sizes and shapes of the male penis vary. The glans of the penis is covered with loose skin that cannot be retracted to expose the glans. The scrotum is inferior to the penis and has horizontal folds on it when mature. The testes of a term infant can be observed with gentle palpation of the scrotum. The scrotum of a preterm infant can be empty on palpation (undescended testes) with less horizontal skin folds. Scrotal swelling may present due to breech delivery or a hydrocoele. A *hydrocoele* is an accumulation of fluid in the tunica vaginalis. It is painless and resolves voluntarily.

The normal position of the urethral meatus is at the front tip of the penis. *Hypospadia* refers to a urethral opening lower than the normal position. It can be under the glans, on the shaft or on the perineum. *Epispadia* refers to a urethral opening above the normal position. This therefore opens on the dorsal surface of the penis. These infants should not be circumcised as the extra foreskin can be used for reconstruction purposes.

Limbs. With a normal infant's musculo-skeletal system, you can expect symmetrical left and right sides of the body and symmetrical limbs. Movements of the limbs are coordinated, mainly flexed and towards the midline. Asymmetrical movement is observed as an obvious difference in the use of one limb compared to the limb on the other side. It is most often caused by injury of the one that is used less, such as fractures or paralysis.

The limbs are proportionate to the body and they are similar in size. Posture, muscle tone and movement of the baby should be assessed. Normal posture consists of flexion and limb movements. These are symmetrical when observing the degree of physical activity of the baby.

Swelling of a limb may be caused by infusion infiltration, oedema, fractures or possible infection. *Fractures* are associated with a lack of movement of the involved area, swelling and intense pain response when manipulated or touched.

Amniotic bands can cause indentations or even amputations of fingers, toes, arms and legs. A range of incomplete limbs occurs due to genetic factors and environmental factors, including teratogenic drugs and radiation. Injury to the brachial plexus during birth can result in nerve injury with upper arm, lower arm or total arm paralysis.

The hands are open or flexed. Each hand has five fingers next to each other, but not attached to each other, and without overriding or crossing. Each finger has three joints, except for the thumb that has two joints. Nails are present on all fingers. The palms each have two clear transverse folds. Single transverse creases can be indicative of chromosomal disorders such as Down's syndrome.

The legs are symmetrical and most often kept flexed to the abdomen with the knees together. They are used in synchrony to kick or extend and return to flexion. The legs are the same length with the knees at the same height, as well as the skin folds of the buttocks symmetrical in line. The feet can be turned from side to side and return spontaneously to midline. Each foot has five toes that are next to each other, but not attached to each other, without overriding, crossing or large spaces inbetween. Movement of the limbs through the normal ranges is without any discomfort or pain.

 ▶ *Polydactyly* is the presence of additional fingers or toes, more than five per hand or foot.
 ▶ *Syndactyly* or *webbing* of the fingers or toes occurs when parts or full areas of the fingers or toes are fused, either by skin, or bone and skin.
 ▶ *Short limbs* refer to abnormally short arms

and/or legs in proportion to the rest of the body, usually associated with dwarfism.
 ▶ *Talipes equinovarus* (clubfoot) is the inward turning of the foot.

Back. The spinal cord is in a straight line with the head, if observed from a posterior angle, and slightly curved if observed from the side. There should not be any indentations, openings or masses on the surface of the back. *Spina bifida* is incomplete joining of the vertebral arches resulting in exposure of the spinal cord and/or meninges. Tufts of hair situated on the spine may indicate an occult spina bifida.

Central nervous system. The head, brain and spinal cord are crucial requirements for proper neurological functioning, and abnormalities thereof will always result in abnormalities of their related functions. Monitoring of the baby's ability to maintain his body temperature, blood glucose, normal breathing and heart rate assesses the autonomic system.

Motor functions are observed as the baby's ability to maintain his posture: a full-term infant is able to maintain mainly flexion or fetal position without assistance. A preterm infant tends to extension or an inability to maintain fetal position without assistance, but he will attempt to flex. A full-term infant also has strong enough muscle tone so that resistance can be easily observed if you try to straighten an arm or leg. Movements of the limbs are symmetrical, smooth and often deliberate. Important motor functions are latching and sucking. Grasping of your finger if you put it in the palm of the hand is an indication of the motor functioning of the upper limbs, while kicking with the legs indicates lower limb functioning.

 ▶ *Extension* is the straightening of parts of the body or the whole body, usually associated with prematurity or stress.
 ▶ *Hyperextension* is extension accompanied by rigidity that makes it difficult to flex the limbs or the body, often associated with increased intracranial pressure, neurological

damage or stress. *Hyperflexion* is flexion of a part of the body or the whole body accompanied by rigidity that makes it difficult to extent the limbs or the body, often associated with neurological damage.

Higher brain functions (see Table 29.2) are assessed by the observation of appropriate responses and behaviour, such as lusty crying when uncomfortable or if pain is experienced, but also to be able to be soothed when the cause of the discomfort is removed and the baby is cuddled or breastfed. The level of consciousness and behaviour must be evaluated. The normal newborn is alert and interested in the immediate environment. It is also possible to make eye contact with the baby. Signs of reduced levels of consciousness include excessive irritability, drowsiness or lack of response during examination, apathy and coma.

▶ *Paresthesia* is sensory loss or the inability to feel stimuli, usually as a result of nerve damage.

▶ *Paralysis* is the inability to use motor muscles, usually as a result of nerve damage.

▶ *Lethargy* is a general poor response to demands associated with a lack of energy and interest in the surroundings.

▶ *Floppiness* is a very poor response to the surroundings accompanied by weakness and limited conscious movement.

The sensory functions are observed as a response to sensory input, such as movement of a limb on physical touch or an attempt to withdraw from painful stimuli such as a heel prick. An infant should also respond to noise, bright lights and taste, either by deliberate behavioural responses or changes in heart rate and breathing. Very important sensory responses are the seeking and rooting reflexes, where the baby will open his mouth and turn the head to root for a nipple with touch of the cheek or sensation around the mouth.

Table 29.2 Newborn refexes

Newborn reflex	Description of reflex
Sucking reflex	When the lips of the infant are stimulated, the mouth will open to start sucking.
Rooting reflex	When the cheek of the infant is stimulated, the head will turn in the direction of the stimulus, and he will open his mouth.
Palmer grasp	This should be a bilateral response where the infant will close his hand in response to pressure in the palm of his hand, for example by a finger.
Moro reflex (startle reflex)	This reflex is seen when the infant gets a fright or during testing, where the infant's head and neck are lifted off the mattress slightly with a hand under him. He is then allowed to fall a few centimeters into this supporting hand. The infant responds to this rapid movement by extending his arms with open hands. The arms are then flexed back to his midline and the hands are closed.
Stepping reflex	When the infant is held upright with his feet touching a flat surface, alternative stepping motions will be made by the lower limbs.
Babinski reflex	When pressure is applied to the soles of the infant's feet, he will extend or flex his toes.

▶ *Unresponsiveness* is a total lack of response, even to pain, and it is a very worrying sign.
▶ *Inappropriate response* is either a stronger response or overreaction to the stimuli, or a much poorer response than normal to the stimuli, and is often associated with prematurity.

Additional information that contributes to the assessment of neurological maturity include:
▶ The levels of consciousness.
▶ The infant's sleep-wake pattern.
▶ Crying.
▶ Response to stimuli such as bright light, noise and position changes.
▶ Response to comforting such as swaddling, developmentally supportive positioning or holding.

Abnormalities that need to be reported are:
▶ Prolonged periods of sleep (for example passed feeding time) or no deep sleep at all.
▶ Inability to cope with stimuli with explicit stress cues (see DSC on page 29-29).
▶ Inability to be comforted.

Thermoregulation

Temperature control is essential for the newborn and should be observed four-hourly for the first 24 hours and then eight-hourly if it is normal and stable. An axillary temperature range of 36.5–37.2 °C is acceptable and should be measured for at least three minutes. Temperature taken rectally would indicate the core temperature, but this practice has a high risk of injury to the infant, including perforation of the colon. If the infant is cold, he can be warmed under a radiant warmer, in a warm blanket with added clothing or preferably by skin-to-skin contact with the mother or father.

A neutral thermal environment with a temperature between 24–28 °C should be provided especially during assessment and nursing of the infant. Such an environment reduces the energy expenditure of infants in order to maintain their temperature, without increas-ing oxygen consumption, reducing energy stores or brown fat supplies. Infants battling to maintain their temperature may need assistance via an incubator. This can also be a warning sign of possible infection.

The control of the external environment includes the reduction of convection by preventing a draft, especially if the infant is nursed on a radiant warmer, in order to maintain a stable room temperature. It also implies the control of radiation by prevention of direct sunlight on the infant and to make sure that the temperature probe of the radiant warmer is efficiently attached and in working condition. The infant should be bathed in water of approximately 37 °C. Conduction should be controlled by preventing skin contact with cold surfaces, such as a scale or stethoscope, and by using warmed linen, hands and instruments. Evaporation can be minimised by reducing the exposed surface area of the infant through developmentally supportive positioning, increasing the humidification of air surrounding the infant (use cling wrap, perspex or clothing) and by preventing wet skin areas from being exposed to air (keep covered when bathed).

Vitamin K$_1$ (Konakion®)

Administration of vitamin K$_1$ (Konakion®) has become routine practice in most of the institutes in South Africa as one dose of Konakion® prevents the occurrence of haemorrhagic disease in the newborn. Konakion® is administered soon after birth in the postnatal ward. It may be administered in the labour ward but this is not recommended due to the possible risk of confusion between Konakion® and *oxytocin*. A Konakion® dosage of 1 mg is administered by intramuscular injection in the anteriolateral aspect of the mid-thigh.

Eye prophylaxis

In order to prevent opthalmia neonatorium or gonococcal conjunctivitis in the newborn infant, administration of a single application of *chloramphenicol* ointment is recommended as prophylaxis. Although gonorrhoea is less prevalent, many mothers are asymptomatic. The newborn is infected when exposed to the mucous membranes of the birth canal. Administration of this ointment may be delayed by an hour so as not to interfere with the initial bonding between mother and infant. The ointment is oil based and reduces the infant's spontaneous eye contact and visual response to parental interaction.

Initial feeding and fluid requirements

The mother should make an informed decision regarding the type of nutrition that the infant is to receive before the infant is delivered. If the mother has chosen breastfeeding, it should be initiated within the first hour after delivery if her condition allows. If formula feeding is chosen, a cup feed, spoon feed or bottle feed should be available within the first hour of delivery for the initial feed of the infant if his condition allows it. This improves bonding and the mother's confidence.

Routine management of the infant

Normal infants with no health problems do not need to be woken up routinely for vital observations. The infant should wake up spontaneously every three to four hours for feeds. During these awake periods the midwife may conduct the necessary observation of the infant. A sleeping baby is a growing baby and should not be disturbed unnecessarily. The newborn infant should not, however, sleep for periods longer than five to six hours to prevent development of hypoglycaemia.

The infant's body can become tender from frequent handling which will be uncomfortable and painful. Interaction with infants should occur when they are naturally awake and they should be allowed to rest undisturbed when sleeping. Infants cry for a reason and cannot be 'spoiled', so they should be attended to when they cry.

Umbilical cord care

The umbilical cord stump should be checked for effective clamping during the initial obser-

vations. If bleeding is present, the cord must be double secured by adding an additional clamp. To reduce the risk of further bleeding, the original clamp should not be removed.

At approximately seven to ten days post-delivery the stump becomes necrotic and separates from the umbilicus. Cleaning of the cord should be carried out during diaper changing and it should be left exposed (out of diaper) if possible to prevent excessive contact with urine. Plain water can be used if no signs of inflammation and infection are present. Surgical spirits and alcohol swabs are bacteriocidal agents and reduce the risk of omphalitis. Antibiotic solutions should only be used when signs of omphalitis are confirmed. Cord care should be performed three- to six-hourly or as prescribed. The selected solution is used to clean the stump and umbilicus by applying firm strokes from the tip to the base of the stump/cord. Be careful not to pull at the umbilicus while cleaning.

Research highlight

Recent research has linked the cessation of bacteriocidal care of the umbilicus to an increased prevalence of omphalitis.

Source: Janssen et al 2003. To dye or not to dye: A randomised, clinical trial of a triple dye/alcohol regime versus dry cord care. Pediatrics. 3(1):15–20.

Diaper changing

Urine and stools are generally passed soon after birth, although it is still normal for urine output to start from 24 hours of age and stools from 48 hours of age. Once the micturation is commenced, a normal urine output is a minimum of six to eight times every 24 hours. The first stools passed are called meconium. Meconium is thick, sticky and dark green in colour. Meconium stools are passed for the first few days until the consistency of the stools gradually changes. Transition stools are those changing from meconium to normal stools and they occur between three to five days after birth. These are green-yellow in colour and have a grain-like appearance. Looser yellow stools with a scrambled egg appearance are normal and occur from day five onwards.

The frequency of stools passed varies depending on the type of feeding received. Infants can pass two to five stools in 24 hours. Frequency of stools is not significant unless the particular infant's pattern changes, or the infant demonstrates other indications of constipation as well, such as abdominal distension and discomfort. The buttocks and genitalia are cleaned with water and a clean cloth or cotton wool in a top to bottom manner. This reduces the transference of stools and related organisms (such as *Escherichia Coli*) into the vagina. A barrier substance can be applied to the area to prevent unnecessary exposure to excrement, such as colour and fragrance-free petroleum jelly. If the buttocks appear red and skin integrity is reduced, a zinc and castor oil cream may be beneficial.

Eye, nose, mouth and ear care

The eyes, nose and mouth should be cleaned during routine care of the infant before feeding time. The eyes and nose may be cleaned with damp cotton wool to remove any crusted secretions. If the secretions become purulent with signs of infection, they should be observed and reported. A new piece of cotton wool should be used for each eye to limit cross-infection from one eye to another. The mouth should be cleaned as well. The buccal cavity and mucous membranes should be inspected regularly for signs of oral thrush. If neonatal teeth are observed in the oral cavity, they should be left to fall out spontaneously. No ear buds or other objects should be inserted into the newborn infant's ears as these can cause extreme damage. The external pinnae may be cleaned with a damp face cloth.

Skin care

Skin care can be done at any time or after bathing when a moisturiser (aqueous cream) should be applied to the infant's skin. It is also important to observe skin integrity during handling to identify any possible problems.

After bathing the infant it is important for the skin to be dried well, but the skin should not be rubbed causing friction – rather press gently with a soft towel. If the skin develops an infection, early diagnosis, referral and appropriate intervention are essential, especially due to the high risk of a superficial infection spreading and becoming a systemic infection as a result of permeable skin.

Bathing

The newborn infant may generally be bathed on the second or third day after birth once temperature regulation is stable. However, due to our current situation with the HIV/AIDS epidemic, infants are being bathed much earlier. Possible indications for early bathing include severe meconium staining, offensive odour possibly due to chorio-amnionitis/amniotic fluid infection syndrome, and contamination of maternal blood or stools. In rural settings where mother and infant are discharged shortly after birth, it is unacceptable to take home a 'dirty' infant. Bathing has to be delayed if the infant is preterm or if any pathology is suspected. The midwife should make a decision on the timing of bathing after considering the specific circumstances.

Vernix protects skin and kills bacteria. It does not need to be removed as it is absorbed and disappears after a few days. Cold stress can occur due to a rapid decrease in temperature of the newborn and it should be prevented at all costs. The infant's temperature should be measured before and 30 minutes after bathing to ensure optimal heating. If the temperature is less than 36.7 °C before bathing, bathing should be delayed until the temperature has improved. Parental involvement should be encouraged as far as possible and all mothers, especially primigravidae, should know how to bath the infant before discharge. It is generally recommended to limit bathing to two to three times a week and even less if the infant is unstable. It is recommended to bath a preterm infant in cooled-off boiled water at approximately 37 °C. The infant should not be immersed in the water for longer than five minutes at a time.

Commercial products can be used but a product that is scent- and colour-free may be more baby-friendly, such as aqueous cream. These products should not be shared between infants, as this will increase the risk of cross-infection. Individual soap bars should not be left in damp or wet areas that could promote the colonisation of organisms. Cross-infection can be reduced with adequate hand-washing and the disinfection of communally used items, such as the baby bath. Bathing can be an extremely stressful experience for the newborn and swaddled bathing should be considererd. The infant should be identifiable on one hand and one foot and ensure that the identification bands are still legible after the bath. The infant should then be dressed in a suitable manner with two layers of clothing in order to maintain optimal body temperature. Depending on the infant's thermoregulatory ability, and the environmental temperature, one or two blankets may be used.

Sleeping position

The recommendation is that all healthy term infants or unmonitored infants should be put to sleep on their backs (supine position) to reduce the risk of possible suffocation with the infant's feet positioned at the bottom of the cot. The infant's head is to be turned to the left or right side to prevent possible aspiration of vomitus in the case of emesis. If the infant is placed in a side-lying position, the infant's arm closest to the mattress must be stretched out forwards to prevent rolling into a prone position (see Figure 29.7).

Preterm or high-risk infants can sleep in the prone position when continuously monitored. If not monitored, these infants should also be placed in the recommended supine positions as explained above. It is important that these infants be positioned in flexion (according to developmentally supportive care principles) in this recommended position.

Sleep-wake cycle

All infants should develop a normal sleep-wake cycle where the infant awakes for demand feeding and interaction. A period of sleep should then follow which allows the infant time to rest and grow. Infants experience different phases of sleep and progress from deep sleep, light sleep, and drowsiness to eventual waking. During the first few months, the infant will spend most of his life sleeping.

Infection control

Infections can be transferred to the newborn by vertical or horizontal transmission. Vertical transmission occurs when the infection is passed from the mother to the infant. The infection may be transferred in three possible ways:

▶ *Transplacental contamination* occurs when pathogens cross the placenta to the fetus, for example, rubella.
▶ *Ascending infection* occurs when the pathogen passes through the cervical mucous plug, chorion and amnion. This normally happens before delivery when their barrier function is less optimal (such as chorio-amnionitis/amniotic fluid infection syndrome or after rupture of membranes).
▶ *Intrapartum infection* occurs during the delivery when the infant is exposed to

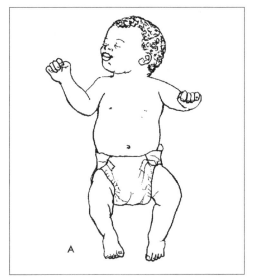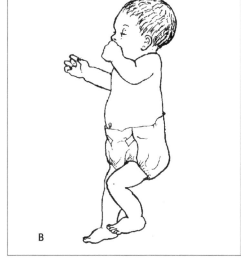

Figure 29.7 Correct sleeping positions

various pathogens while passing through the birth canal, such as gonococcal conjunctivitis and HIV.

Horizontal transmission takes places when pathogens are transferred to hospital equipment via hospital staff and then transferred to the infant. These infections are termed *nosocomial infections*. The pathogens causing nosocomial infections tend to be more resistant and difficult to treat with the available antibiotics. This fact contributed to the ongoing problem of pathogens becoming 'super bugs', such as *Klebsiella*, with an increased resistance to antibiotics.

As a midwife, your number one defence against infection is a correct and effective hand-washing technique. Hands and body surfaces should be washed immediately after direct or indirect contact with the infant, regardless of whether gloves were worn or not. This practice is to reduce exposure to body fluids as far as possible. Hand jewellery provides a mode of transport for organisms and should not be worn during patient care.

Gloves, masks, eye protection and non-sterile aprons or gowns should be used as barrier methods when the risk of exposure to body fluids is high. Barrier precautions reduce exposure to blood, body fluid, secretions, excretions and other contaminated fluids during routine or invasive procedures. If resuscitation is necessary, prevent mouth-to-mouth ventilation as far as possible by using a one-way breathing valve or mask-bag ventilation.

Patient-care equipment should be cleaned regularly to prevent the spread of pathogens to skin, mucous membranes and clothing. Soiled linen should be separated from other linen and stored in plastic bags, to be rinsed and washed separately from unsoiled linen. These procedures should be done in designated areas with adequate sharps disposal and sufficient working space to reduce the risk of accidental needle-stick injuries.

All visitors and children should be screened for contagious infections before entering the nursery to reduce the amount of pathogens that the newborn may be exposed to. Furthermore, all staff should be educated and trained with regard to correct infection control principles in order to reduce the risk of infection as far as possible. Unit and hospital policies should be in place for quick reference and detailed procedures.

Signs of infection in the newborn infant may include:

- Unstable thermoregulation (hypothermia or pyrexia)
- Signs of respiratory distress (tachycardia, tachypnoea, apnoea and cyanosis)
- Hypoperfusion with cold extremities
- Hypotension
- Abnormal skin colour (pale, mottled or grey)
- Hyperglycaemia or hypoglycaemia
- Emesis
- Poor feeding
- Abdominal distension
- Lethargy
- Hypotonia
- Bleeding tendencies

If these signs are observed, the midwife should document all abnormalities clearly and report them to the attending physician. Once the infant starts to present with signs of infection, early diagnosis will prevent unnecessary complications.

Antiretroviral treatment

HIV/AIDS is rapidly becoming a leading cause of immunodeficiency in the South African neonatal population with vertical mother-to-child transmission increasing morbidity and mortality for these infants. The following medications are used in different combinations and must be administered according to the latest available regime as recommended by the clinic or hospital.

Zidovudine (ZDU), also known as *azidothymidine* (AZT), functions by inhibiting reverse transcriptase and/or termination of the DNA chain intracellularly. However, this has toxic effects on the newborn, including macrocytosis, anaemia and neutropenia. AZT may be administered orally or intravenously.

Nevirapine and *lamivudine* (3TC) also interfere with viral reverse transcriptase. Little information on neonatal side-effects is however available, but no symptoms have been reported as yet. This medication is given orally. It should be protected from light and stored at room temperature.

Jaundice

Physiological jaundice (*hyperbilirubinaemia*) is common during the first week of life and presents in 45 to 60% of newborn infants of which some resolve spontaneously. (Physiological jaundice that does not resolve spontaneously is then classified as pathological jaundice.) Jaundice appearing within the first 24 to 36 hours after birth is considered to be abnormal with serum bilirubin levels elevated above normal ranges. It is caused by a number of factors (see Chapter 31). Conjugated bilirubin is excreted by the newborn but unconjugated (free) bilirubin crosses the blood–brain barrier. Unconjugated bilirubin has an affinity for fatty tissue and is best observed in the sclera, skin and mucous membranes. Once situated in the brain, neuronal tissue is stained and the basal ganglia are injured resulting in kernicterus, with severe consequences (see Chapter 31).

Bilirubin is excreted in two ways. Phototherapy causes the bilirubin to oxidise into water-soluble products, which are then excreted in the urine and stools. The stools will be brown-green in colour. If phototherapy is to be done at home, carefully monitoring of temperature and fluid intake is essential. Bilirubin is converted into water-soluble isomers, which can be excreted in the liver without being conjugated. Blue, green and violet fluorescent lights can be used for phototherapy. It is critical that the infant's eyes are closed during phototherapy as this bright light will cause damage to the retina. Eyepads should be removed during feeding. Coloured lights can make the working environment unpleasant and distort the skin colour of the infant. Fibre-optic 'bili-blankets' are more effective as there is no need to shield the infant's eyes. Another advantage of this method is that the infant can be held during phototherapy.

Hyperbilirubinaemia is diagnosed by drawing blood for serum bilirubin levels. These levels are then compared to the infant's weight and age to give an indicator of the seriousness of the elevated levels. Phototherapy is used to reduce these elevated bilirubin levels in the newborn.

Infants usually need between two and three days of phototherapy although this varies from infant to infant, and may be even less in a healthy full-term infant. Assessment of improved skin colour is not a reliable indicator of reduced bilirubin levels and therefore serum tests should be redone to confirm results.

The midwife should inform the parents about the physiology of jaundice and phototherapy so that bonding and breastfeeding continue as normal as possible. This will also reduce their fears of possible complications. The infant may be taken out from under the phototherapy light for short periods of time for breastfeeding, but it must be remembered that frequent interruptions will extend the time period of phototherapy. The infant may initially be lethargic with reduced enthusiasm to feed. Nasogastric feeds can be given until energy levels return to normal if necessary.

Fluorescent lights used for phototherapy should be positioned 45 to 50 cm away from the infant for maximum irradiance. A large skin surface area should be exposed to the light and therefore all clothes should be removed. The diaper should be left on as skin rashes caused by phototherapy can reduce skin integrity and predispose the infant to skin breakdown. Position changes should be frequent to facilitate maximum exposure of skin. Thermoregulation should be monitored as these infants may develop hyperthermia due to the added heat source. Intake and output must be monitored carefully as much body water is lost via radiation and evaporation (*insensible water loss*). If bottlefed, an additional 25% milk can be added to the total fluid volume, especially if diarrhoea occurs. Breastfeeding mothers should increase the frequency of feeds to meet the increased fluid requirements. No additional water is needed for breastfed infants as long as frequent breastfeeding takes place.

Side-effects of phototherapy include:
- Hyperthermia
- Dehydration
- Skin rashes
- Lethargy
- Abdominal distension
- Hypocalcaemia
- Sensory-visual deprivation
- Lactose intolerance
- Loose stools

Circumcision

At birth, the foreskin is attached to the glans of the penis. This skin only separates between the age of three and six years. It is therefore advised not to force the foreskin backwards for any reason including cleaning purposes, as this will cause scaring of tissue and possible phimosis at a later stage. *Phimosis* may occur when the front of the foreskin constricts, preventing it from being pulled back over the glans.

The decision to circumcise a male infant remains the responsibility of the parents and informed consent must be obtained before the procedure is performed. Circumcision can be performed within the first week of life, but a decrease in complications is seen when surgery is delayed until one year of age. No medical benefits or indications are evident to motivate circumcision during this stage of life. Phimosis occuring in early childhood years is an indication for this procedure. Circumcision is contraindicated with hypospadia, infection, bleeding disorders and jaundice. Possible complications may include infection, haemorrhage, and ulceration of the glans.

Preparation of baby's records

The Road to Health chart must be completed for every infant delivered. This card holds vital information about the delivery and neonatal history. Weight and growth progress are monitored on the chart, as well as recording of all immunisations received. Mothers should be made aware of the importance of this card and that it should be looked after. This card should also accompany the child when seeking any medical attention.

The birth of the infant must be registered by the parents with the Department of Home Affairs. They should complete all the necessary documentation for submission as soon as

Table 29.3 South African Immunisation Schedule

Age	Immunisation required
Birth	BCG (Bacille Calmette-Guérin) polio drops
6 weeks	Polio drops Hib (Haemophillus influenza type B) DTP (diphtheria, tetanus and pertussis) Hep B (hepatitis B)
10 weeks	Polio drops Hib DTP Hep B
14 weeks	Polio drops Hib DTP Hep B
9 months	Measles
18 months	DTP Polio drops Measles
5 years	DT (diphtheria and tetanus) Polio drops

possible. It is also the parent's responsibility to register the child with the medical aid, if they are members of a medical aid.

Immunisation

BCG and polio drops are usually administered within five days of birth. The infants of an HIV-positive mother must also receive immunisation unless the baby shows clinical signs of progressive AIDS. Each baby must receive his first immunisation before discharge and the importance of these immunisations should be explained to the parents. If the baby did not receive his first immunisation during hospitalisation, the mother should be advised to visit her nearest clinic as soon as possible. A com-

pleted Road to Health immunisation chart must be given to the parents for future use and the next immunisation must be discussed with the parents.

Baby Friendly Hospital Initiative

The World Health Organisation (WHO) and the United Nations Children's Fund (UNICEF) introduced the Baby Friendly Hospital Initiative in 1991. Its main aim was to encourage and support practices of breast-feeding. Although this becomes controversial in terms of HIV/AIDS, the midwife should apply baby-friendly principles where applicable. This initiative is centred on the following ten steps:

1. A written policy of breastfeeding should be communicated to all healthcare staff.
2. All healthcare staff should be trained with the necessary skills and knowledge for the implementation of the written policy on breastfeeding.
3. All pregnant women should be informed about the management and benefits of breastfeeding before delivery.
4. Mothers who choose to breastfeed should be assisted in allowing the infant to suckle within the first hour of life.
5. Mothers should be shown how to breastfeed and how to express their milk if they are separated from their infants for a particular reason.
6. No artificial feeds, including water, should be given to the infant except breast milk unless otherwise prescribed due to medical reasons (such as maternal medication secreted in breast milk that may affect the infant).
7. Rooming-in should be implemented. Rooming-in refers to the newborn infant staying in the mother's room during the period of hospitalisation. This technique has advantages for the mother and infant. Bonding is facilitated as the mother gets to know and interpret her infant's needs. The mother gains confidence and

competence when handling the infant and she will be more comfortable at the time of discharge. Demand breastfeeding is facilitated if that were the choice of feeding. Rooming-in reduces the infection risk of the newborn infant. The infant has a tendency to grow the bacteria present on the mother's skin as opposed to the antibiotic-resistant organisms responsible for nosocomial infections. Staff demands are also reduced, as the mother becomes the infant's primary caregiver.

8. Feeding the infant on demand should be encouraged.
9. According to the WHO, artificial teats and pacifiers should not be provided to breastfed infants to reduce the possible risk of nipple confusion. Although this is true for healthy term infants, sick or preterm infants benefit greatly from a pacifier and will lose their sucking reflex if it is not stimulated.
10. Breastfeeding support groups should be established and mothers should be referred to them following discharge.

Infant stress and Developmentally Supportive Care (DSC)

When dealing with the vulnerable population of neonates, which includes term and preterm infants, it is necessary to protect them as far as possible from the detrimental effects of the unfamiliar extra-uterine environment. Although there are differences between term and preterm infants, it is important to apply the DSC principles to all newborns in order to improve developmental outcomes.

As medical technology improves, the neonatal mortality rate decreases. Although this is seen as a positive advancement, the preterm infant experiences short- and long-term effects that are not as positive as we would like. In spite of the improved technology, sick and preterm infants tend to present with more stress than they can cope with. They experience morbidity related to immatu-

rity of their organ systems and to their concurrent disease states.

Stressors experienced by a neonate

Sleep interruptions, supine positioning, routine and excessive handling, loud sounds, unattended crying, reduced sucking opportunities, and social and medical interactions have unfavourable developmental effects. Other stressors include painful procedures and noxious oral medication. Strong smells, noise and bright lights are some of the other negative stimuli the infant experiences while in the hospital, clinic or neonatal intensive care unit (NICU). These stimuli are direct causes of stress that result in disorganised stimulation of the developing sensory systems. These sensory systems are therefore stimulated at the wrong time or out of sequence, which may influence morbidity.

Internal disturbances related to the infant's illness and/or any disturbance of internal homeostasis that demands compensation in one or other way, are also stressors. These stressors include hypoglycaemia, hypothermia, acid-base disturbances, fluid and electrolyte disturbances, hypoxia, hyperoxia, side or adverse effects of medication, pain or discomfort and several more. The compromised infant does not have the ability to tolerate such stressors.

Indicators of stress in the neonate

The *Miller-Keane Encyclopaedia and Dictionary of Medicine, Nursing and Allied Health* (1997) defines stress as the sum of biological reactions to any adverse stimulus including physical, mental, or emotional, internal or external, that tends to disturb the homeostasis of any organism. A stressor is further defined as any factor that disturbs homeostasis resulting in stress.

The neonate shows signs of stress by using three main systems, namely the autonomic system, the motor system and state organisation.

The above responses demonstrate communication abilities of the infant to express positive and negative responses besides the physiologically observable autonomic and visceral

Table 29.4 Neonatal stress cues

Autonomic system	Motor system	State organisation
▶ Colour changes ▶ Hiccupping and sneezing ▶ Gagging and spitting up ▶ Increased or decreased heart rate ▶ Blood pressure fluctuations ▶ Changes in respiration patterns or rate ▶ Temperature instability ▶ Apnoea ▶ Vasoconstriction and pallor ▶ Decreased gastric motility ▶ Increased secretion of cortisol, adrenaline and catecholamines (inhibit optimal repair of damaged tissue and normal growth)	▶ Generalised hypotonia ▶ Flaccidity or floppiness ▶ Hyperextension of extremities or body ▶ Splaying of fingers and toes ▶ Facial expressions, including grimaces and frowns	▶ Irritable behaviour ▶ Sleep disturbances ▶ Inappropriate behaviour

responses. From these methods of communication, one can assess the infant's behaviour as well as the physiological parameters to determine whether medical, nursing or social interventions are beyond the infant's coping mechanisms. An infant's communication to show stress is divided into physiological cues and behavioural cues.

These behavioural cues and physiological cues supply the midwife with the best information base in order to make the necessary alterations to caregiving techniques and the environment, that would facilitate the reduction of infant stress. However, it requires caregivers who are sensitive to these cues.

Short- and long-term outcomes

The short-term outcomes, such as increased heart rate, increased respiration rate, skin colour changes, blood pressure fluctuations, fluctuating saturation levels or desaturation and temperature instability, are specifically related to physiological instability or increased stress levels.

Preterm and sick infants who survive the NICU experience have a higher prevalence of long-term outcomes such as cognitive, sensory, motor and developmental problems. The preterm infant with fewer complications is also faced with developmental problems, which may manifest during school-going years. These infants are prone to the following developmental problems:

▶ Learning disabilities
▶ Lower intelligence proportion
▶ Attention deficit disorders
▶ Impulsiveness
▶ Visual motor impairments
▶ Space orientation disturbances
▶ Language comprehension and speech difficulties
▶ Affective vulnerability and altered self-esteem

Birth weight, gestational age, clinical course and related complications play a large role in the determination of outcomes for preterm and ill infants.

Infants admitted to the NICU are predominantly nursed in the supine position during the initial weeks of life, which consequently facilitates the development of extensor muscle groups over flexor muscle groups and results in postural pathology. Incorrect body positioning results in postural deformities, including hip abduction and external rotation, ankle eversion, retracted and abducted shoulders, neck hyperextension and shoulder elevation, and cranial moulding, which in turn impedes developmental milestones of head control, rolling, sitting, crawling and walking.

Other long-term problems and complications related to prematurity and illness include:

▶ Cerebral palsy
▶ Visual impairment
▶ Hearing impairment
▶ Growth restriction
▶ Epilepsy
▶ Chronic lung disease
▶ Hydrocephalus
▶ Bronchopulmonary dysplasia
▶ Periventricular haemorrhage infarction
▶ Retinopathy of prematurity
▶ Necrotising enterocolitis

These infants are also susceptible to disease and have poor resistance to infection. They often require long-term developmental and functional rehabilitation, including treatment by speech therapists and audiologists, occupational therapists and physiotherapists.

Developmentally Supportive Care (DSC)

The above-mentioned negative outcomes can be reduced through Developmentally Supportive Care (DSC), which is a simple and effective method of reducing these complications by modifying the environment that the infant is exposed to and consequently minimising the impact of the NICU environment.

DSC is an approach introduced during the 1980s that has been defined by the National Association of Neonatal Nurses as 'care of an infant to support positive growth and development'. It allows for the stabilisation of physiological and behavioural functioning, which may ultimately improve the developmental outcomes. Infant behaviour is observed to determine what modifications to the environment and infant care is needed in order to improve the developmental outcomes.

These interventions may include control of one or more elements of the external environment influencing the tactile, vestibular, gustatory, olfactory, auditory and visual systems in such a manner that it facilitates and supports the neurodevelopmental and physiological stability of the newborn infant.

The principles of DSC

The principles of DSC include individualised, family-centred care with minimal and appropriate handling and positive touch of the preterm infant, initiation of cluster care for nursing activities, specific positioning, non-nutritive sucking, and manipulation of the external environment to reduce negative stimuli (noise and light reduction, positive smell stimuli). These interventions result in decreased stimuli and increased rest periods to the benefit of the infant. The principles are applicable to term and preterm infants although the focus will be different when dealing with the latter.

The family is seen as a crucial contributor to the infant's care and should therefore be involved in decision-making, as well as the physical implementation of DSC. By having a family-centred approach, the preterm infant's potential development is enhanced and interpersonal relationships (bonding) are improved between the family and their infant.

To provide individualised care, the infant's unique behaviour and physiological cues are used as a foundation for interactions and interventions. In other words, the infant himself determines to a large extent the care provided by a midwife who is sensitive to the infant's stress cues and needs. Structure is given to a 24-hour period by clustering care, where the infant's behavioural cues are taken into consideration to establish whether he is ready for the intervention/s. Interventions are grouped together to allow minimal handling and to provide for longer periods of rest with fewer interruptions.

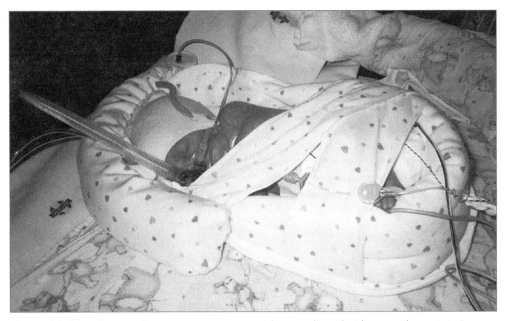

Figure 29.8 Developmentally supportive positioning (photograph used with parental permission)

The principle of appropriate handling and touch refers to slow, gentle movements while maintaining boundaries (see positioning principles) throughout care. Touch should only be done using flat palmar surfaces of the hands or fingers and not the fingertips to ensure equal distribution of pressure. Tickling touch, friction and hard touching are prohibited to prevent uncomfortable or painful touch. If painful procedures have to be executed, such as a heel prick, pain management has to be provided with it (the administration of sucrose, for example) to minimise pain and to prevent any negative associations with touch. Placement of hands on the infant during and after care allows the infant to self-regulate and become calm. Skin-to-skin contact is facilitated whenever possible, and if convenient through the application of kangaroo care. Swaddled bathing is promoted as far as possible to allow easier adjustment to the water and to prevent bathing from becoming a traumatic experience. This holds true for swaddled weighing of the infant as the containment gives the infant an added sense of security. The infant is wrapped in a blanket during the procedure to maintain a flexed position. This also reduces a hypersensitive startle reflex to fright.

Developmentally supportive positioning includes midline orientation, hand-to-mouth activity, fetal flexor position and containment (fetal position) to promote self-soothing and self-regulation behaviours (see Figure 29.8).

Positioning is characterised by rounded shoulders, curved back, hands in midline near the face (midline orientation), knees together flexed towards the stomach and the neck in neutral position. The infant can be positioned supine or in a lateral (left or right) position. Prone positioning can be used if the infant is being monitored. Positioning and three-dimensional containment are obtained by using linen or specifically designed soft equipment, gel mattresses, sheep skin, soft toys or other suitable material.

These positions all contribute to neurobehavioural development of the preterm infant. The positioning principles aim at simulating the uterine environment. This is particularly important for the preterm infant who is born lacking physiological flexion, has low muscle tone and is exposed to static positioning in the incubator, which is further complicated by gravitational forces.

Non-nutritive sucking allows the infant to suck on his own thumb or a pacifier. This not only has a calming effect on the infant, but also maintains the sucking reflex to ensure optimal functioning when transition to oral feeds occur, as the preterm infant is at risk to lose the sucking ability if it is not stimulated. Non-nutritive sucking provides positive tactile stimulation to the oral area in comparison to all the negative stimuli such as intubation and suction, and in that sense may contribute to an easier transition to oral feeds in comparison to an infant who only experienced negative stimuli.

Another aspect of DSC is the manipulation of the infant's external environment. The physical environment is altered by minimising excessive noise, reducing bright lighting and the prevention of strong odours or inhalation of chemicals. Noise levels may be reduced by turning down the volume or silencing the continuous sounds of the monitors (not the alarms), nursing the infant in an incubator instead of an open radiant warmer, using ear muffs and not switching on any radios or televisions in the infant's environment.

Lighting may be reduced through the use of a screen between the infant's face and the lights, for instance a pillowcase on the top of

Outcomes of DSC
▶ Improved respiratory status.
▶ Earlier transition from nasogastric tube feeds to oral feeds.
▶ Increased self-regulatory abilities.
▶ Physiological stability.
▶ Reduced morbidity.
▶ Improved neurological organisation (seen by appropriate behaviour).
▶ Improved growth and weight gain.
▶ Diminished length of hospitalisation.
▶ Reduction in cost of hospitalisation.
▶ Improvement in neurodevelopmental outcomes at 24 months corrected age.
▶ Bonding and acceptance by the family is better with enhanced feelings of security.

the incubator or over the crib, or an eye mask or any other protective measures.

Strong odours can be reduced by selective use of cleaning solutions for cleaning of the incubators. Nursing staff and parents should be educated not to wear perfume or cologne when handling the infant and to wait until hands are dry when sprayed with a chemical solution before approaching the infant.

The role of the newborn caregiver is to develop an individualised plan in conjunction with the parents and family, and to adapt the environment and caregiving methods to the infant's behavioural competencies, which will result in the facilitation of the infant's ability to optimal self-regulation.

All these aspects are difficult to control as they require cooperation from all the role players. Adequate education is needed to ensure that all staff and families are aware of the infants' needs and that the principles of developmentally supportive care are adhered to.

Kangaroo care

The principles of kangaroo care, better known as Kangaroo mother care, are congruent with DSC principles. Kangaroo care is a method of skin-to-skin contact where the parents or family members place the infant, dressed only in a

Principles of DSC
1. Individualised infant care
2. Family-centred approach
3. External environmental manipulation (light, noise and smell)
4. Handling, positive touch and vestibular care
5. Non-nutritive sucking
6. Developmental supportive positioning (flexion, three-dimensional containment and midline orientation)
7. Cluster care (clustering care activities)

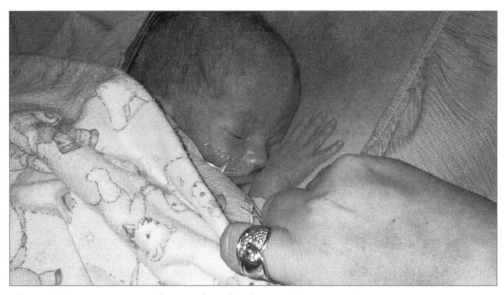

Figure 29.9 Kangaroo care (photograph used with parental permission)

diaper on the chest between the breasts in a flexed position (see Figure 29.9). Exclusive breastfeeding is promoted with kangaroo care but this is not always possible taking the reality of personal preference and HIV/AIDS into consideration. Mothers who choose formula feeding can also care for their infants in this way.

Kangaroo care has many advantages for the neonate and the parent. Skin-to-skin contact causes the release of growth hormone (somatotropin) resulting in rapid weight gain in the infant and possibly an earlier discharge of the low birth-weight infant. The upright position improves pulmonary function and oxygen saturation, as well as promoting physiological stability. The infant tends to sleep better with toleration of longer interaction periods as well as improved self-regulatory behaviours. Body temperature of the infant is maintained by the mother's ability to regulate her own body temperature according to her infant's temperature. This is called thermal synchrony. Fathers tend to overheat their infants, as they do not have this ability of temperature control.

Parents become more confident in handling their infants, which helps with bonding. Mothers tend to be more relaxed which promotes breastmilk production and longer breastfeeding time periods after discharge. Parents with an infant in the NICU visit more frequently and a sense of calmness enables more effective coping mechanisms.

It is necessary to emphasise again the importance of DSC for the preterm and ill newborn for the reasons mentioned above. It is also important though to be flexible enough to accommodate the healthy and/or full-term infant who develops a need for and has the ability to cope with more stimulation. It is crucial to be sensitive to the infant's own behavioural cues and respond accordingly to provide the best individualised care at the infant's specific developmental phase.

Going home
Discharge planning

Discharging an infant that is normal or was sick previously is often an unnerving and anxious experience for parents as they realise that they are now the sole caregivers of their child. Transition from the clinic or hospital to home can be stressful for families. A well-informed parent, however, is better equipped when going home and would feel more confident during the discharge process, even for a normal full-term infant. Effective discharge information must be offered to parents to assure that they are informed enough to take the best possible care of their child.

Before the infant and mother can be discharged, the midwife needs to be certain of the mother's coping abilities with her new infant. The midwife should assess the mother's skills of routine care which include feeding and hygiene.

Feeding

Offer information applicable to the type of feeding the mother has decided on. If it is breastfeeding, inform the mother about the principles of feeding on demand, how to determine if the infant is drinking enough, variations in stools that the infant may have, the breastfeeding diet that the mother should follow and any potential problems she may encounter, as well as what to do about them.

If the mother has decided on formula feeding, inform her about the type and amount of formula feed the infant should drink, how to mix the formula feeds, how to sterilise the cup, spoon, bottles and teats and store them, the potential problems she may expect and what to do. Growth should also be monitored and recorded on the Road to Health chart. In both cases the mother should also be informed about whom to contact if she needs advice, such as a support group or helpline.

Hygiene needs

The parents should receive at least one bath demonstration before discharge but ideally, they should have bathed their baby themselves. Proper hygiene care must be demonstrated to parents, including buttock and cord care, eye care and mouth care. They must also be informed about the use of cleaning agents, ointments, and oils. Plain aqueous cream remains the best and safest product.

General information

A complete physical examination should be repeated before discharge to ensure that a healthy infant is sent home. Routine handling should be explained with emphasis on the infant's needs of comfort, rest and sleep. A stable room temperature without any draughts should be maintained in the infant's room. The mother has to be informed about normal body temperature of an infant, that infants often cannot maintain the stability of their own temperature and that special precaution should be taken with a warm or cold environment, as well as how to take these precautions. Lightweight bedding and blankets should be used. No pillows are preferable to reduce the risk of SIDS and suffocation, and the infant should be placed on his back to sleep. Ensure immunisation is given before or as soon as possible after discharge. This is to be recorded in the Road to Health chart.

Identification of abnormalities or healthcare problems

Parents should be told about the signs and symptoms their child could have which require medical help. These include lethargy, poor feeding, vomiting, fever (pyrexia), diarrhoea, abdominal distension, bleeding, jaundice and unsettledness. Medical help should be sought by visiting a clinic, doctor or emergency facility after hours.

Parents should also be taught about emergency care, including the principles of basic cardiopulmonary resuscitation. The telephone numbers of whom to contact when there is a problem should also be provided. If the high-risk infant needs to go home with any special equipment or monitors, the parents need to be informed about the use and the care of this equipment, as well as whom to contact if there is a problem.

Medication

Any medication that the infant needs after discharge should be explained to the parents, preferably in a written form. Write down all of the medications, the dosages, the route and the time that it should be given for the parents. Also explain the side-effects to them. Assure that enough of the medication is given to the parents or that they have received a prescription to last them until their next follow-up visit or end of course (e.g. antibiotics or antiretroviral medication).

Follow-up and referral

A healthy infant should have a follow-up examination six weeks after delivery. A physical examination should be done including assessment of growth. This will also include assessment of developmental milestones. These details must be filled in on the infant's Road to Health chart. Immunisation needed at six weeks can also be given and recorded. The mother should be assessed regarding her coping skills at home.

Preterm and sick infants need to be followed up more frequently by a paediatrician. Inform the parents about the importance of developmental milestones and that they will be checked with their follow-up visits. Infants born preterm or with complications could experience certain delays in their developmental progress and the parents should be made aware of this. It is therefore important for them to know what the normal developmental milestones are.

Parents have to be informed about the need for any special follow-up arrangements or referrals if any problems are identified during follow-up visits. This includes all facets of the multidisciplinary team.

Community resources

Primary health care clinics in the vicinity can meet the normal needs or minor ailments of the infant. Community nurses are trained in the care of general ailments. If further care is needed, the community nurse can refer the mother to another source of help. Private practising midwives may also be consulted on areas of concern. Family and community involvement provides the mother with a support system in order to help her in caring for her infant.

The role of the family

Being a new parent, whether for the first time or not, is a frightening, intimidating but at the same time wonderful experience. The importance of the midwife's role in supporting the family through this new territory will now be discussed.

It is each infant's right to have an empowered parent and an involved family. According to the Standards for Nursing Practice by the South African Nursing Council, it is the right of the high-risk and normal newborn infant to receive not only basic nursing but also warmth and 'cuddling'. These standards also acknowledge the infant as an unusually vulnerable human being that has the right to confidentiality, privacy, protection and informed consent with refusal of procedures where applicable. The standards should be interpreted as the rights of their parents to be their advocates. It is here where it becomes the responsibility of the midwife to empower parents so that they can fulfil their role as the primary care providers for their child. Empowerment is defined as the process of increasing personal, interpersonal and political power, which enables individuals or collectives to improve their life situation.

When working with new parents the midwife may find that they experience feelings of frustration, lack of involvement and not being in control of their infant's care and condition while he is still in the hospital. All of these emotional stressors influence the parenting experience. The infant's parents are ultimately responsible for all medical care their infants receive. Mothers and fathers often want to participate in the many decisions that are necessary in caring for their infant. Healthcare providers should therefore support and encourage their participation. Parents need to be empowered in order to take the best possible care of their children, which begins in the hospital and continues for life. It can therefore be concluded that it is the right of an infant to have his parents involved and empowered. In this way, it is ensured that the infant's best interests are upheld and that their rights are not ignored.

Pregnancy and the transition to parenthood

is recognised as a period of stress and change during which mothers and fathers master parenthood. Few new parents are prepared for the impact a baby will have on their lives and even under the best of circumstances, this change will be very stressful for them.

It is therefore unimaginable what parents must go through when a preterm baby, a sick infant or an infant with abnormalities is born, or when a baby dies. The parents and families of these special babies are never prepared for these events. It is therefore important to keep in mind that the newborn infant's parents are very vulnerable and need guidance regardless of the infant's medical condition. Parents of preterm or sick infants need even more care and guidance during this period of grief and adaptation (see Chapter 28).

Parents regard the midwife as an expert in the day-to-day care of babies. Therefore they expect authoritative advice regarding various aspects, such as how to bath a baby or identify the developmental milestones. The role of the midwife, however, is much more than just giving information and demonstrations. The midwife is crucial to ensure that family-centred care is effective with the best possible outcomes, helping these parents to cope and to resume their normal, functional role in which they can make the best decisions for their child.

The support of parents will differ in each situation and the midwife should acknowledge each parent as an individual. There are no rigid rules to follow, therefore by assessing each parent's understanding of the situation, how they cope with stressful situations and what their needs are, the midwife can offer the best advice and guidance for each different circumstance.

Information

Talking to the parents often helps to determine their ongoing needs and provide the necessary information. It also establishes communication and builds a trusting relationship. Keep the parents informed as soon as something new has developed. Be careful not to give too much information – keep it factual and short, but give consistent information. If different information is given to parents, they will no longer trust the healthcare providers. When they ask a question which the midwife does not know the answer to, she should admit it and try to find out the answer from someone who might know. Never provide an answer that is not evidence-based.

Assess their understanding of the situation. When stressed or concerned, people do not absorb everything they are being told. Also make sure that the information given to them corresponds with their particular situation. For instance, if they have just been informed about the need for phototherapy they may be disappointed about a delayed discharge. Assess their knowledge and skills before providing them with information, for example, ask them if they have ever changed a baby's diaper or if they know anything about jaundice before you start explaining and demonstrating.

If possible, use the same caregivers for consistency. This builds trusting relationships in which both the parents and the caregivers feel comfortable and it contributes to a much more positive experience of hospitalisation.

Feelings

Allow the parents the opportunity to express the different emotions they are experiencing and acknowledge the different phases of their adaptation to the situation with their associated emotions. Never judge parents on the emotions they may show, even if it is anger that is directed at you. Assure them that it is normal to experience those conflicting feelings. The midwife should be a good listener and encourage them to express their feelings.

Participation

For parents to be empowered, it is crucial to let them participate in their child's care and the decision-making around the planned care. The principle of informed consent throughout hospitalisation is critical. Always ask them, if possible, for permission before handling their child or performing a procedure on the child.

Fulfil any promises that you have made to the parents. If you promised to phone them when the doctor arrives, do so. If you cannot or if it is not possible, tell them so. Trust in the relationship between parents and the midwife is of extreme importance.

Parents must be able to visit the child as often as they like and should never be treated as visitors but always as part of the multidisciplinary team. Encourage activities like taking photographs and ask them to bring personalised items such as soft toys or a blanket.

Involve them in the actual physical caretaking of their infant as much as possible. If the infant is very ill and unstable, at least involve them with positive touch methods. If their infant is stable they can become involved with routine care such as diaper changing or cord care, building up to taking full responsibility for basic care if the infant's condition allows it.

Environment

Allow parents some time alone with their child. Privacy tends to be the last priority in a busy unit, but parents need these private moments for bonding. If there are no separate cubicles or rooms available, a mobile screen could be used. Make the bonding experience a personal one – give the family as much time with their baby as they need without compromising the infant's health. The midwife sometimes forgets how uncomfortable a special care unit is for parents. If possible, ensure that comfortable chairs are available and offer to dim the lights.

Diversity of families

Be sensitive to what parenting means in the specific culture of the parents. Consider the different family structures that may exist, especially in the South African context. Currently nuclear families are not the norm any more, but single-parent families are on the increase. Extended families are still common especially in the rural areas. Parents of different socio-economic status also have different needs. Try to accommodate these different beliefs and needs wherever possible (see Chapter 2).

Involvement of the rest of the family members and friends

Involve siblings and grandparents as much as possible because the newborn infant has entered an existing family unit and needs to be introduced to each family member. They will be playing important roles during the rest of the baby's life and the sooner they are introduced, the better the opportunity for bonding with the rest of the family. Siblings may easily feel left out. Include them in the care of the infant by giving them certain tasks, such as holding the nasogastric tube during feeds, or to by bringing the baby something special like a soft toy or a drawn picture.

The newborn as an individual

The newborn is a stranger to the family. Introduce him by calling the baby by his name. Identify special characteristics, for example, point out his dimples or his beautiful hair. Share personalised information about the infant with the family, such as 'he likes to suck his finger'.

In a nutshell

▶ Normal adaptation to extra-uterine life is imperative for external survival.
▶ Growth assessment and the physical examination are skills that the midwife needs to master for early identification of problems and abnormalities.
▶ DSC and kangaroo care are beneficial to the infant and should be implemented as far as possible.
▶ Discharge planning should be complete to equip the parents with coping tools.
▶ The importance of family-centred care and the parents' involvement is emphasised.

References

Als, H. 1986. A synactive model of neonatal behavioral organization: Framework for the assessment of neurobehavioral development in the premature infant and for support of infants and parents in the neonatal intensive care environment. In: Sweeney, J. K. (Ed.) The high-risk neonate: Developmental therapy perspectives. *Physical and Occupational Therapy in Pediatrics*, 6:3–55.

Als, H. 1999. Reading the preterm infant. In: Goldson, E. (Ed.) *Nurturing the premature infant: Developmental interventions in the neonatal intensive care nursery*. New York: Oxford University Press.

Ballard, J. L., Khoury, J. C., Wedig, K., Wang, L., Eilers-Walsman, B. L. & Lipp, R. 1991. New Ballard Score, expanded to include extremely preterm infants. *The Journal of Pediatrics*, September 119(3):417–423.

Becker, P.T., Grunwald, P.C., Moorman, J & Stuhr, S. 1991. Outcomes of developmentally supportive nursing care for very low birth weight infants. *Nursing Research*, May/June 40(3):150–155.

Beischer, N.A., Mackay, E.V., and Colditz, P.B. 1997. *Obstetrics and the newborn: An illustrated textbook*. Third Edition. W. B. Saunders Company Ltd.

Bellefeuille-Reid, D. & Jakubek, S. 1989. Adaptive positioning intervention for premature infants: Issues for paediatric occupational therapy practice. *British Journal of Occupational Therapy,* March 52(3):93–96.

Bohin, S., Draper, E.S. & Field, D.J. 1999. Health status of a population of infants born before 26 weeks gestation derived from routine data collected between 21 and 27 months post-delivery. *Early Human Development*, 55:9–18.

Bennett, V.R. and Brown, L.K. (Eds.) 1999. *Myles textbook for midwives*. Thirteenth edition. London: Churchill Livingstone.

Deacon, J & O'Neill, P. (Eds.) 1999. *Core curriculum for neonatal intensive care nursing*. Second edition. Pennsylvania: W. B. Saunders Company.

De Groot, L., v. d. Hoek, A,. Hopkins, B. & Touwen, B. 1993. Development of muscle power in preterm infants: Individual trajectories after term age. *Neuropediatrics*, 24:68–73.

De Vos, A.S. (Ed.). 1998. *Research at grass roots: A primer for the caring professions*. Pretoria: Van Schaik.

Enkin, M., Keirse, M. J. N. C., Neilson, J., Crowther, C., Duley, L., Hodnett, E. & Hofmeyr, J. 2000. *A guide to effective care in pregnancy and childbirth*. Third edition. Oxford: Oxford University Press.

Fowles, E.R. 1999. The Brazelton neonatal behavioural assessment scale and maternal identity. *MCN*, November/December 24(6).

Glass, P. 1999. The vulnerable neonate and the neonatal intensive care environment. In: Avery, G.B., Fletcher, M.A. & MacDonald, M.G. (Eds.) *Neonatology: Pathophysiology and management of the newborn*. Fifth edition. Philadelphia: Williams & Wilkins.

Guntheroth, W. G. 1995. Crib death: *The sudden infant death syndrome*. New York: Futura Publishing.

Harrison, V. C., Keet, M. P. and Shore, S. C. L. 1996. *The newborn baby*. Third edition. Cape Town: Juta & Co Ltd.

Henning, P. A. 2002. *The examination of the newborn baby*. Pretoria: Van Schaik Publishers.

Janssen, P. A., Selwood, B. L., Dobson, S. R., Peacock, D. & Thiessen, P. N. 2003. To dye or not to dye: A randomised, clinical trial of a triple dye/alcohol regime versus dry cord care. *Pediatrics*, January 111(1).

Jorgensen, K. M. 2000. *Developmental care of the preterm infant: A concise overview*. Second edition. In conjunction with Children's Medical Ventures: p.1–4.

Kristensson-Hallström, M. I. 1999. Strategies for feeling secure influence parents' participation in care. *Journal of Clinical Nursing*, 8(5):586-592.

Merenstein G. B. & Gardner, S. L. 1998. *Handbook of neonatal intensive care*. Fourth edition. New York: Mosby.

Miller-Keane Encyclopedia and Dictionary of Medicine, Nursing, and Allied Health. 1997. Sixth edition. New York: W.B. Saunders Company.

National Association of Neonatal Nurses (NANN) 2000. Infant and Family-Centered Developmental Care: Guideline for Practice. Unpublished.

Pollack, H. A. & Frohna, J. G. 2002. Infant sleep placement after the Back to Sleep Campaign. *Pediatrics*, April 109(4).

Seidel, H. M. et al. 1995. *Mosby's guide to physical examination.* Third edition. St Louis: Mosby.

South African Nursing Council (SANC). 1992. *Standards of nursing practice.* Pretoria: SANC.

Sudia-Robinson, T. M. & Freeman, S. B. 2000. Communication patterns and decision making among parents and health care providers in the neonatal intensive care unit: A case study. *Heart & Lung: The Journal of Acute and Critical Care,* 29(2):143–148.

Symingtom, A. & Pinelli, J. 2002. Developmental care for promoting development and preventing morbidity in preterm infants (Cochrane Review). In: *The Cochrane Library*, 1:1–37. Oxford: Update Software.

Taquino, L. T. & Lockridge, T. 1999. Caring for critically ill infants: Strategies to promote physiological stability and improve developmental outcomes. *Critical Care Nurse*, 19(9) December 64–79.

Vento, T. & Feinberg, E. 1998. Developmentally supportive care. In: Cloherty, J. & Stark, A. (Eds.) *Manual of neonatal care.* Fourth edition. Philadelphia: Lippincott–Raven Publishers.

WHO (World Health Organisation). 1986. The growth chart: A tool for use in infant and child health care. Geneva: WHO.

Woods, D.L. (Ed). 2001. *Perinatal education programme. Manual 4. Primary newborn care.* Cape Town: Perinatal Education Trust.

Yeo, H. 1998. *Nursing the neonate.* London: Blackwell Science Ltd.

Young, T. E. & Mangum, B. 2000. *Neofax: A manual of drugs used in neonatal care.* Thirteenth edition. New York: Acorn Publishing.

Interesting web pages:
http://kangaroo.javeriana.edu.co
www.neonatology.org
www.neonatalnetwork.com
www.kangaroomothercare.com

Chapter **30**

Nutrition

Carin Maree and Seugnette Rossouw

Introduction

The baby's nutritional needs form an integral part of parenthood. Parents are faced with the decision on how and what to feed from early in the pregnancy. They expect the midwife to guide them to make the correct decision and to support them in carrying it out. Midwives have to know about the different types of infant feeding, particularly regarding the nutritional, economic and social advantages and differences among the methods and types available. Parents need to be assisted to make this decision early in the pregnancy and should then be provided with well-designed, well-written and well-illustrated information. We must remember that previous experiences and the attitudes of the mother and those of friends, family members and caregivers all play an important role in the mother's final decision.

Optimum nutrition during the first year of life is crucial in the current and future growth and development of a child. Positive feeding experiences can enhance fine motor skills and provide opportunities for important social interaction during infancy.

Infancy is characterised by a very rapid growth rate. The provision of adequate proteins, calories, vitamins and minerals to support optimal growth is essential in both breastfeeding and infant formula feeding.

Normal physiology of the newborn's gastrointestinal system

The newborn has an adequate ability to digest, absorb and metabolise milk feeds, although some of these functions are limited. Enzymes are available to denaturalise proteins and catalyse monosaccharides and disaccharides (simple carbohydrates). There is a deficiency in production of pancreatic amylase in the newborn baby, resulting in impaired utilisation of polysaccharides (complex carbohydrates). Fat absorption is also limited because of deficient levels of pancreatic lipase, which limits the absorption of fat, especially with the intake of baby feeds that are high in saturated fatty acids, such as cow's milk. If the woman is not breastfeeding, the above-mentioned should be taken into consideration when choosing a formula for bottle feeding.

Of the gastrointestinal organs the liver is the most immature. This results in reduced levels and activity of the enzyme glucuronyl transferase and deficiency in forming plasma proteins. Infant nutrition should therefore be appropriate and not add additional strain on the immature liver. The newborn liver stores less glycogen at birth than in later infancy, which consequently may result in hypoglycaemia. However, it can be prevented with early and effective breastfeeding.

The capacity of the newborn's stomach is about 60 to 90 ml, which gradually increases as the baby gets older. Therefore the newborn requires small and frequent feeds.

Rapid peristaltic waves with simultaneous non-peristaltic waves are present in the oesophagus. Together with the immature, more relaxed cardiac sphincter, it means that regurgitation can commonly occur. All these elements should be taken into consideration when feeding the newborn baby.

Fluid and energy requirements

Normal fluid requirements for a full-term, healthy baby with a birth weight of more than 2.5 kg can be calculated as follows:

Day 1	60 ml/kg/24 hours
Day 2	90 ml/kg/24 hours
Day 3	120 ml/kg/24 hours; if tolerated well
Day 4	150 ml/kg/24 hours

Variations of this fluid requirement schedule occur as well, but all the approaches are geared towards a formula of 150 ml per kg per 24 hours around day 5.

The food requirements of a healthy baby include:
- *Energy*: ± 462 kJ/kg/day (110 kcal/kg/day)
- *Protein*: 2–3 g/kg/day

Expected body weight of the infant

Parents are normally very concerned that their baby is not thriving and not 'getting enough' milk, especially when the baby is being breastfed. The major concern is that they are unsure of the amount of milk the baby takes with every feed.

The following advice, which indicates a well-fed baby, may be offered to parents:
- The normal newborn should sleep 3 to 4 hours between feeds.
- After feeding, the baby should be satisfied and relaxed or sleeping.
- Voiding urine in normal light-yellow colour: 6 to 10 wet diapers per day.
- Stools are soft, pasty and with the typical characteristics of the type of feeding the baby is receiving.

Another way to identify adequate weight gain is to calculate the expected body weight of the baby. In estimating body weight, it is firstly

---

Calculation of expected body weight

Formula: expected weight of the baby at the end of three months = birth weight + 30 g/day x 90 days minus the first 10 days.

Example: In a baby with a birth weight of 3.2 kg, the expected weight at three months can be calculated as follows: =   3.2 kg + (80 days x 30 g per day)
=   3.2 kg + 2.4 kg
=   ± 5.6 kg at the end of the third month

Variations from this calculation may occur, because babies grow in their own, unique way and may show a more rapid weight gain.

---

important to allow for some weight loss immediately after birth till around the tenth day after birth. Normally a subsequent weight gain of around 30 g per day until the end of the third month is then assumed.

Choices of infant feeding

Parents need to choose between exclusive breastfeeding, pasteurisation of breast milk and formula feeding. This decision should be an informed one and the midwife plays an important part in guiding the parents to choose a method of feeding. Commercially prepared infant formulas include a variety of options with different characteristics, depending on the baby's needs.

General principles in choosing an infant feeding are as follows:

▶ The most important principle is that the method has to provide adequately for the infant's nutritional needs.
▶ The parents should be informed that breastfeeding is the best choice.
▶ They should also be informed about the implications of their choice in terms of cost and the availability thereof, as well as the impact on the woman's lifestyle.
▶ The feeding method must be acceptable to the parents and they must make the final choice, as they have to live with it.
▶ Once they have made the choice, the midwife has to accept it without displaying any prejudice or negativity.
▶ Maintain a supportive environment where the woman feels safe to express her feelings and concerns without fear of

Table 31.1 Comparison of the composition of human and cow's milk

Types of milk	Protein (g)	Fat (g)	Carbohydrate (g)	Calories per 100 ml	mg per 100 ml				
					Iron	Sodium	Potassium	Calcium	Phosphorus
Breast milk	1.2 g: 60% lactalbumin 40% casein	3.8 g	7.0	293 kJ (70 kcal)	0.076	15	60	35	15
Cow's milk	3.4 g	3.7 g High in saturated fat	4.8	276 kJ (66 kcal)	0.05	50	15	120	95

rejection. The midwife should also be sensitive to the individual, the family and the economic and cultural factors that may influence their decision.

It is unethical to advertise formula feeding as breastfeeding is internationally regarded as the optimum feeding method for newborn babies. Accurate information is therefore essential in assisting parents to make this important decision.

Cow's milk does not supply all the essential nutrients the growing infant needs. It can lead to malnutrition, anaemia and gastrointestinal disturbances such as possible diarrhoea. Cow's milk is high in saturated fat. Absorption is limited due to the deficient levels of pancreatic lipase in the neonate.

Breastfeeding

Characteristics

Human milk has the ideal composition for the infant's needs. It is also safe, free of contamination and is at the correct temperature. In addition there is the psychological benefit to the maternal–child relationship due to the close nesting of the baby to the woman's skin during breastfeeding. The rhythm of the woman's heartbeat and the warmth of her skin enhance the sense of peaceful security for the baby. The woman also develops a feeling of union with her baby and will experience a deep sense of accomplishment and satisfaction. Breastfeeding promotes involution of the uterus and weight loss.

Breastfeeding is a very economical form of feeding and is always available. The protection against infection can be viewed as an additional saving in terms of fewer visits to the doctor and the time saved for the working woman. Breast-feeding appears to offer protection against diabetes, obesity, allergies and arteriosclerosis, although the evidence is inconclusive and studies were only recently initiated. The anti-infective factors of breastfeeding are numerous. There are immunoglobulins, maternal antibodies, lymphocytes and macrophages in breast milk. These anti-infective factors limit the multiplication of bacterial and viral pathogens in the gastrointestinal tract. The enzyme lysozyme and the iron-binding protein lactoferrin, have to be taken into consideration for their non-specific inhibitory action on bacterial growth. Lactoferrin also aids with iron absorption. The gut pH is decreased by the production of lactic acid and acetic acid in the gut and bacterial growth is inhibited. *Lactobacillus bifidis* colonises the gut of a breastfed baby and assists in maintaining a low pH. Human milk therefore contains a growth factor, which facilitates the bacterial growth and colonisation of *Lactobacillus bifidis* in the gastrointestinal tract. The immature gastrointestinal tract of the newborn easily digests human breast milk. Furthermore, breastfed infants grow at a satisfactory although slower rate beyond three months.

Physiology

The birth of the placenta causes a decrease in the maternal levels of oestrogen and progesterone, followed by an increase in the level of the hormone prolactin. Nipple stimulation during feeds increases the prolactin level, which is raised further by the patterns of pressure and release of the baby's mouth on the areola. Prolactin is secreted from the anterior pituitary gland and stimulates the production of milk in the alveolar cells of the breasts. The production of prolactin and therefore milk is hampered by the use of nipple shields, poor positioning of the baby and a weak sucking effort.

The hormone oxytocin is responsible for the contracting of the smooth muscle surrounding the alveoli. Contraction of these muscle bands is responsible for squeezing the produced milk into the ductal system.

The 'let-down reflex' takes place when the baby latches on the breast and begins to suckle. Stimulation of the nerve endings in the areola results in the posterior pituitary gland secreting oxytocin. Oxytocin causes the myoepithelial cells surrounding the alveoli and the lactiferous sinuses to contract and eject the milk.

The hypothalamus controls the pituitary gland and therefore the let-down reflex is influenced by the environment, maternal fear, anxiety, pain and stress. Signs of the let-down reflex include:

▶ Uterine cramps accompanied with increased lochia (especially during the first few days).
▶ A feeling of 'pins and needles' in the breasts.
▶ Milk leaking from the other breast.
▶ A change in the baby's swallowing pattern from quick sucks to clear swallowing.
▶ Gulping and milk in the corner of the baby's mouth.
▶ A feeling of relaxation in the woman.

Source: Mohrbacher & Stock, 1997:32.

The first milk to be ejected is known as *foremilk*, which is more watery and has less nutritional value. It is very important to lessen the baby's thirst first.

Hindmilk is ejected after the let-down of foremilk and it is rich in fats and nutrients. *Colostrum*, which is the yellow milk the baby will receive in the first few days, is high in nutrients and immunities. At the same time it is of smaller volume, which means that the baby should be fed more often.

Antenatal preparation

The establishment of breastfeeding should start during the antenatal period. Any breastfeeding problems and queries should be

Table 30.2 Composition of human breast milk

	Colostrum (during the first few days of lactation)	Mature human milk
Protein	▶ Consists of five times more proteins than mature milk. ▶ 20% of proteins are casein. ▶ The majority of the other 80% protein is IgA (secretory immunoglobulins). ▶ The rest is whey proteins of which lactoferrin and lysozyme are the most important.	▶ Consists of less protein than colostrum. ▶ Predominantly whey proteins. ▶ Contains IgA, IgG, IgM, lactoferrin and lysozymes.
Fat	▶ Less than in mature milk.	▶ Low content in foremilk. ▶ Higher concentration in hindmilk, therefore there is a greater energy content with a higher satiety value. ▶ 50% of the energy is provided by fat.
Carbohydrates	▶ Less than in mature milk.	▶ Lactose to be converted to glucose and galactose.
Vitamins and minerals	▶ Higher in sodium than mature milk. ▶ Trace elements bound to proteins to form part of enzyme.	▶ Dependent on maternal nutritional status. ▶ Contains iron, copper, zinc, manganese, chromium, molybdenum, cobalt, selenium, iodine and fluorine.

managed with skill and consideration in order to empower the woman to make an informed decision about the best method to feed her baby.

Giving information and sharing facts during the antenatal period is important as women are very open and responsive during pregnancy and eager to make the best decisions that will positively influence the health of their babies. Literature on breastfeeding should be available and health talks during antenatal visits should encourage good breastfeeding practices.

Breastfeeding skills

Breastfeeding is a learned social behaviour and no one is born with the skill. It requires confidence and consistent information and support. The Ten Steps for Successful Breastfeeding should be practised.

Positioning the baby

Positioning the baby is important to ensure proper latching on and comfort during feeding. The woman needs to sit or lie in a well-supported and comfortable position so that no extra strain is placed on her breasts or muscles, while she relaxes and enjoys the experience. The principle is to bring the baby to the breast and not the breast to the baby. The baby's body should face the mother.

Breastfeeding while sitting up

Ensure that the woman is comfortable with her back supported and straight – leaning over the baby will cause strain in the neck and back as well as poor latching on. The woman may use pillows under the arms to support and relax her. If the woman is comfortable with this position, she has to ensure that the baby is also properly supported by using pillows to take his weight. Therefore she does not need to hold the baby – even the tiniest baby can become very heavy within a short period of time. A woman with high breasts will need a few pillows to support the baby at breast height. A large-breasted woman, however, may only need a diaper-roll to lift and support the breast high enough for correct

---

The Ten Steps for Successful Breastfeeding

Every facility which provides maternal services and care for newborn infants should implement the following practices:
- Routinely communicate a written breastfeeding policy to all healthcare staff.
- Train all healthcare staff in the skills necessary to implement this policy.
- Inform pregnant women about the benefits and management of breastfeeding.
- Help women to initiate breastfeeding within half an hour of birth.
- Show women how to breastfeed, and how to maintain lactation even if they should be separated from their infants.
- Do not give newborn infants any food or drink other than breast milk, unless medically indicated.
- Practise rooming-in and allow women and infants to remain together through 24 hours a day.
- Encourage breastfeeding on demand.
- Do not give artificial teats or pacifiers (also called dummies or soothers) to breastfeeding infants.
- Foster the establishment of breastfeeding support groups and refer women to them on discharge from hospital or clinic.

---

latching on, while keeping the baby's nose uncovered. Some large-breasted women prefer this position with a football hold position of the baby's head, because it gives them more control over their baby's head.

Breastfeeding while lying down

Encourage the woman to try different positions lying down until she and her baby are comfortable. Again she may need pillows to support herself and the baby. Depending on the size of the breasts the woman may want to roll over when the baby has finished feeding on the one breast – the process is easier when she holds the baby close to the chest as she rolls

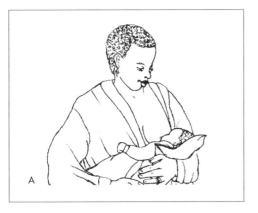
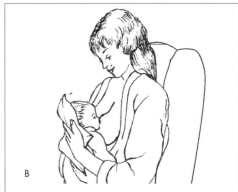
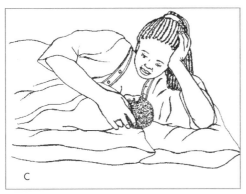
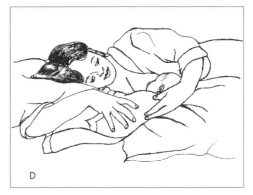

Figure 30.1 Examples of breastfeeding positions: A: Cradle hold; B: Modified football hold; C: Lying down to breast feed; D: Football hold lying down

over. The baby should be supported at the level of the breast with his ear, shoulder and hip in a straight line and his head very slightly tilted back, so that he can swallow easily and not pull back at the breast. The baby's body should be well supported so that he feels secure. Lying down is also comfortable after having a caesarean birth.

Latching on to the breast

Babies have to learn how to latch on properly in order to suckle correctly, get enough milk and become satisfied. Women, on the other hand, have to learn how to breastfeed their babies correctly. Latching on may be started through stimulating the rooting reflex by brushing the baby's lips with the nipple. As response the baby will open his mouth wide and the tongue will move down to prepare the mouth for latching on and suckling.

The purpose of supporting the breast is to make the breast firmer for latching on and to keep the breast away from the baby's chin during feeding so that he remains on the breast correctly. The following techniques may be used to support the breast while latching on is attempted:

▶ *C-hold*: Thumb on top and four fingers underneath the breast allows gentle support without distortion of the nipple. Correct placement of the fingers is well behind the areola.
▶ *Cigarette or scissor-hold*: The woman holds her breast between the index and middle fingers. Because the woman's fingers are unable to stretch as far apart as the thumb and fingers in the C-hold, they may get in the baby's way as he tries to latch on and prevent him from taking the breast far enough into his mouth, which can result in sore nipples.

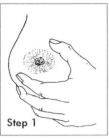
Step 1

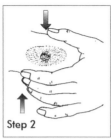
Step 2

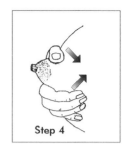
Step 3

Step 4

Figure 30.2 The nipple sandwich hold

Signs of good latching on

▶ Baby has taken most of the areola, and in case of small areolas, some of the surrounding breast tissue.
▶ The baby's chin is pressed into the breast.
▶ The baby's nose is resting on the breast.
▶ The baby's lips are flanged out and relaxed.
▶ The tongue is cupped beneath the breast.
▶ The nipple is on the back of the tongue.

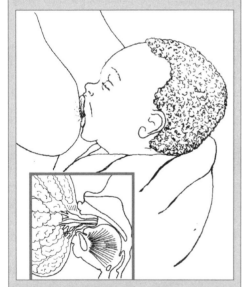

Figure 30.3 Position of the infant's mouth over the areola

▶ *Nipple sandwich hold*: The woman first uses the C-hold technique correctly and squeezes her thumb and fingers gently together. This makes the round-shaped areola area more oblong and supplies the baby with a narrower part to latch on to. The woman then pushes in towards her chest wall to help the nipple protrude, which makes grasping for the baby easier. Finally the woman pushes in more with her thumb than with her fingers to make the nipple point slightly upward towards the roof of the baby's mouth. Only then should the woman encourage her baby to open his mouth wide and pull him in close.

Using neonatal reflexes

The rooting and sucking reflexes occur spontaneously when the baby's lips or cheek are brushed with the nipple – the head turns towards the stimuli and the baby opens his mouth. Sometimes the baby will start with suckling movements before latching on. Initial swallowing occurs till weeks 9 to 12 following birth, from the posterior part of the tongue. This is one of the reasons why the baby should take more than just the nipple and surrounding tissue into the mouth when latching on, in order to place the nipple as far posterior on the tongue as possible for swallowing. The extrusion reflex is prominent for the first nine weeks of life and this reflex results in 'pushing' or moving food or milk out of the mouth when placed anterior on the tongue. Poor latching on with nipple placement on the tongue will result in the nipple been pushed out of the mouth by the baby. When the woman excludes these possibilities during latching on, she will quickly notice a suck-swallow rhythm. The baby will make two to three deep suckling movements, followed by a slight pause and then only the swallowing will occur.

The first feed

The baby should be breastfed as soon as possible after birth. It is common practice to put the baby to the breast as soon as possible after delivery. The outcomes of this are:

▶ Establishment of mother–child bonding.
▶ Encouragement of suckling response in the baby.
▶ Hormonal response to suckling stimulates lactation.

Breastfeeding should occur every two to three hours or on demand, whichever comes first, during the day and night. No supplementation with formula or glucose water should be given. Until breast milk is established, both breasts should be used at each feeding, starting on the breast that was used to end the previous feeding. Be careful not to give the woman a list of steps on do's and don'ts because this may cause anxiousness if she does not follow it to the letter.

Explain to the new mother that the let-down reflex may take up to five to seven minutes to occur. To ensure conditioning and effective let-down she should allow enough time for feeding on one breast as long as it is comfortable.

Frequency of feeding

The traditional practice of three- or four-hourly feeds is not appropriate to establish breast milk or feeding the newborn. The newborn needs to be fed as frequently as possible – and by breastfeeding alone. Frequent breastfeeding may result in:

▶ an increase in maternal milk stimulation.
▶ an improvement in the woman's confidence about her ability to feed her baby.
▶ less breast discomfort associated with engorgement.
▶ a reduction in the development of sore nipples.

Taking the baby off the breast

Encourage the woman to keep the baby on a breast long enough to ensure he receives the right balance of foremilk and high calorie hindmilk. When the baby is satisfied, he will come off the breast spontaneously or fall asleep. If the woman decides to take the baby off the breast before he has finished, she first has to break the suction to avoid damage to the sensitive breast tissue. Suction can be broken in the following ways:

▶ Press down on the breast near the baby's mouth.
▶ Pull down on the baby's chin.
▶ Insert a finger into the corner of the baby's mouth.

Common breastfeeding problems or anxieties

Anxiety about the baby 'not getting enough milk'

Encourage the woman to keep track of the baby's wet diapers and bowel movements. A normal urine output of a minimum of six to eight times per 24 hours and two to five bowel movements a day for a baby less than six weeks of age are indicators of adequate milk intake. If the baby is thriving and gaining weight after the first ten days of life, he is getting enough milk.

Breast fussiness during the early weeks of breastfeeding

Possible reasons for breast fussiness:

▶ *Fussiness since birth to one week*: Have the baby checked for any medical problem and consider poor latching on, hypertonia, delayed or inhibited let-down reflex.
▶ *Fussiness between the second and fourth day*: Possible reasons may include engorgement of the breasts and forceful or inhibited let-down reflexes.
▶ *Fussiness between one and four weeks in a baby who previously breastfed well*: Nipple confusion may be a reason if the baby received artificial nipples as well. Also consider thrush, ear infection, a change in the taste of the mother's milk or the development of an own temperament.

Forceful let-down reflex

If the baby is choking and pulls away from the breast, the cause may be a forceful let-down reflex or overabundant milk supply. The best positions for breastfeeding are those in which the baby's head and throat are higher than the breast.

Foremilk–hindmilk imbalance

This sometimes happens when a baby is switched from breasts too soon and he receives too much of the watery lactose-rich foremilk and not enough of the fatty high-calorie hindmilk. Lactose stimulates gut peristalsis and results in green, watery stools with poor weight gain. The baby will experience poor satiety and take some time before he settles down.

Colicky baby

A fretful baby who refuses to settle down at the breast may contribute to early weaning off the breast or severe engorgement leading to mastitis. A good idea is to assist the woman by demonstrating a few ways to settle the fretful baby. Be careful not to discourage the woman by giving her too much information or making her feel guilty.

The woman can be advised to nurse the baby before he is fully awake. If he is crying and fussing, she can rock and cuddle him enough to settle him down – then she can latch him on properly for feeding. Swaddling may make the baby feel safe and relaxed. The diaper should be changed before feeding. During breastfeeding the woman should remove competing stimuli from the environment, or try another breastfeeding position. It is important that she is reassured.

Flat or inverted nipples

Assist the woman to ensure good latching on by the baby. A flat or inverted nipple will normally not cause a problem as the baby does not suckle to the nipple but takes in a good amount of areola and breast tissue during correct latching on.

Sore and cracked nipples

Sore nipples are a sign of poor latching on. The baby does not take the breast deeply enough into his mouth and will not be able to milk the breast well. Encourage the woman to try another position or to relax and stimulate the baby for proper opening of the mouth before latching on. It is important that she continues to breastfeed the baby. Discontinuing breastfeeding or applying ointments does not help: on the contrary, these preparations have been shown to have a negative effect on breastfeeding.

> **Note**
>
> The only factor that has been shown to both prevent and treat nipple trauma is good positioning of the baby at the breast.
>
> *Source:* Enkin et al, 2000.

Cracked nipples may be caused by poor latching on technique, improper breast pumping, candidial infection, irritating substances like soap and alcohol or creams and ointment applied to the nipples which can result in eczema or dermatitis.

The woman should be helped with the baby's positioning and latching on. The woman should express a small amount of milk before feeding to stimulate let-down and ensure proper latching on. The use of analgesics is advised, when necessary, and emotional support is essential.

Breast engorgement

Engorgement may develop from the third to fifth day, especially if the baby was not fed often or long enough. Engorgement causes the nipples to become flat and the skin on the breast taut, making latching on and feeding difficult and resulting in refusal of the breast. Encourage the woman to express enough milk to soften the areola so that latching on will be possible. Frequent breastfeeding will also lessen the occurrence of engorgement and it will subside. The application of warm, moist compresses immediately prior to breastfeeding may be beneficial as it stimulates the let-down reflex and helps the milk to flow. Gentle massage from the chest wall towards the nipple in circular motion will also help let-down. The use of cold compresses between feeds can reduce swelling and relieve pain. Remind the woman to switch back to warm, moist compresses 10 to 15 minutes prior to the next feeding. Do not restrict maternal fluid intake, because restriction does not reduce breast engorgement. Make sure the woman wears a comfortable, well-fitting bra to support her breasts properly.

Mastitis

Mastitis is the term generally used to refer to any inflammation of the breast as it is difficult to determine the cause of breast inflammation (infection or a plugged duct). It is possible for the woman to run a low-grade fever without a bacterial infection. A tender, red or sore lump in a lactating breast in the absence of fever is probably a plugged milk duct. Mastitis is not usually a contraindication to continue breastfeeding.

Mastitis is treated with heat, gentle massage and frequent breastfeeding. The woman should also contact her doctor for treatment while she continues to breastfeed.

Soaking the breasts in a warm bathtub or applying hot wet packs between feeds may be of help. To stimulate milk flow the woman should massage the affected area in gentle circular motion. Breastfeeding the baby frequently on the affected side will keep the milk flowing freely and prevent engorgement. The woman may benefit from wearing a bra which is a size larger or one that has a different cut to relieve any pressure on the milk ducts. Encourage her, if possible, to go to bed with her baby and remain there until she feels better. This will also promote frequent breastfeeding.

Postnatal support

It is a natural occurrence that after the birth of the baby and the excitement of having a new baby, the woman may frequently find taking care of her baby is both physically and emotionally exhausting. At such times she may be particularly liable to abandon breastfeeding, especially in a hospital with an early discharge policy. The provision of formula milk in the puerperium ward may also contribute to the cessation of breastfeeding. During this period when lactation is becoming established maternal milk supply may be affected by anxiety, tiredness and improper breastfeeding practices. By keeping the baby with the woman and assisting her with breastfeeding techniques continuous breastfeeding can be encouraged.

Contraindications to breastfeeding

Known contraindications to breastfeeding are mostly relative in nature. The midwife needs to sit down with parents and discuss the options before a final decision is taken. Important variables such as maternal, infant and personal circumstances, the home environment and the availability of equipment, and the level of support at home and at work all need to be taken into account. Individualising the final decision is therefore essential for successful breastfeeding.

Contraindications will include the following:

▶ Maternal infection with the Hepatitis C virus (HCV).
▶ Serious, debilitating maternal disease, such as any debilitating cardiac disorder or advanced cancer.*
▶ Active, untreated maternal tuberculosis.*
▶ Positive history of previous maternal puerperal depression, psychosis or bonding difficulties.
▶ HIV/AIDS infection although it is a relative contraindication (see Chapter 19 for choice of feed).
▶ Galactosaemia.*
▶ Maternal substance abuse: cocaine, nicotine and alcohol.*

Absolute contraindication

Maternal lifestyle requirements

Diet

During pregnancy, deposits of fat are laid down. These deposits will later be used as energy stores for breastfeeding. Most women, however, need an extra 400 to 600 kcal (1 680–2 520 kJ) per day. Most women experience an increase in hunger and thirst while they breastfeed the baby. Food should be rich in iron, proteins and vitamins A, C and D. The extra energy requirements can be made up from a variety of sources. High salt or sugary snacks should, however, be discouraged because although they are quick to prepare and contain high calories, they generally contain few nutrients (vitamins or minerals). Good examples of high-caloric food, which also take little time to prepare, are wholewheat sandwiches, wholewheat toast, fruit, biscuits and cheese.

Fluid requirements

Between 8 to 10 glasses of water or fluid should be drunk daily. Breastfeeding women should be encouraged to establish a routine of having a drink before, while they are feeding and after breastfeeding the baby. It is also a good idea to prepare a drink to take during the night while breastfeeding. This extra fluid should come from a variety of sources, but excessive amounts of fruit juices and caffeine-containing beverages should be limited. Continuing to drink 500 ml of milk per day will provide extra calcium, riboflavin, protein and energy. Alcohol in excess will inhibit the let-down reflex.

Rest and sleep

Enough rest and sleep are essential requirements for successful breastfeeding. The woman should be assisted to identify adequate sources of support so that she is able to have sufficient time to relax and rest. During the postpartum period this is important for the physiological recovery of the woman, as well as for the establishment of breastfeeding and lactation. It is a good general practice for the woman to sleep when her baby is asleep.

Medications

Most medications taken by the woman will be secreted in her breast milk, although it will be a rare indication to stop breastfeeding.

▶ *Anti-infective agents.* Most anti-infective agents are present only in small amounts in the woman's breast milk. This makes toxicity unlikely, but there is the potential for non-dose-related adverse effects. Drugs to avoid during breastfeeding are *ciprofloxacin, chloramphenicol*, Ethambutol®, Plaquenil®, *metronidazole*, Oxacillin®, *sulfamethoxazole, tetracyclines* and *metronidazole*. Some drugs are not systemically available when taken by the woman; others have the potential to alter the newborn baby's bowel flora resulting in diarrhoea. Allergic reactions such as rash or fever are also potential side-effects.
▶ *Anticonvulsants.* The use of anticonvulsants during breastfeeding is not associated with adverse effects, but their safety in long-term follow up remains unstudied.

Expressing breast milk

Sometimes it happens that a period of separation occurs between mother and baby. The baby was either preterm, required intensive care or was transferred to another hospital for advanced medical management. If the woman wants to breastfeed the baby, consistent information and support should be provided. The goals are firstly to maintain milk production and secondly to preserve and store the expressed milk safely and to keep it as clean as possible for later use.

The method and technique used to express breast milk will differ from woman to woman. The simplest method to use is hand-expressing. This method is workable and provides a way to relieve fullness of breasts and ensure

---

Guidelines for expressing milk

▶ Always wash the hands thoroughly before expressing.
▶ Express milk in familiar and comfortable settings without distractions.
▶ Apply heat to the breast first and then follow with a gentle massage.
▶ Use a gently rhythmic motion, which mimics the suckling of a baby.

proper latching on during the early days of breastfeeding. The needs for expressing milk differ when you compare the needs of the above example with those of a woman who has been separated from her newborn. It is very important to assist the woman in adapting to a method by encouraging realistic expectations. A number of factors can influence the amount of milk the woman may express:

▶ Ability to stimulate the let-down reflex.
▶ Time lapsed between previous expressing or feed and current attempt to express.
▶ The skill and technique she uses to express.
▶ The woman's level of comfort while she is expressing.
▶ The woman's stress level.
▶ Time of day.

Marmet technique

This method combines gentle expressing with breast massage, stroking and shaking to stimulate the milk-ejection reflex. The entire procedure should take aproximately 30 minutes.

Traditional technique

With this method the woman positions her index finger and thumb above and below the areola, away from the nipple. She then presses towards the chest wall with the fingers and then presses the fingers behind the nipple to stimulate milk flow. This technique also takes about 30 minutes to empty the breasts. Hand techniques of expressing should not hurt. If it does, the woman is probably squeezing the breast or pulling on the nipple.

Breast pumps

Available breast pumps can be either motor-operated, resulting in a regular suction and release method, or hand pumps that use a draw-and-hold-method. The following guidelines are important:

▶ The woman should always ensure and maintain clean and hygienic conditions before, during and after expressing.
▶ She should follow the guidelines for pumping instructions closely.

▶ Pumping should not be painful – if it is, the woman should stop and check that the nipple is centred and the alignment is correct.

Storing expressed milk

Collect the milk in a clean container, preferably plastic, as immunological factors tend to adhere to glass. Special milk storage bags are available in different ranges. The milk storage bags are designed for storing expressed milk, while the freezer milk bags are used for freezing expressed milk. Ensure that the stored milk is labelled and dated.

Recommended storage norms:
▶ Term colostrum expressed within 6 days of delivery:
  ✦ at 27 °C–32 °C: 12 hours.
▶ Mature milk:
  ✦ at 15 °C: 24 hours.
  ✦ at 19 °C–22°C: 10 hours.
  ✦ 25 °C: 4–6 hours.

Storage in a freezer:
▶ In a freezer compartment located inside a refrigerator: 2 weeks.
▶ In a self-contained freezer unit of a refrigerator: 3 – 4 months because of variation in temperatures associated with frequent opening and closing of freezer door.
▶ In a separate deep freezer at a constant –19 °C: 6 months.

Handling and thawing expressed milk

Frozen human milk should be thawed under cool running water with the gradual addition of warmer water until it is thawed and heated to room temperature. A sealed container with frozen milk can also be submerged into heated water. Inform the woman never to heat the milk directly on the stove. A microwave oven should not be used to thaw human milk, as high temperatures will destroy valuable components in the milk. Additionally microwave ovens heat liquids unevenly, resulting in 'hot spots' that may burn the baby. Thawed milk can be refrigerated for up to 24 hours but should not be refrozen.

Cup feeding

When a baby cannot be put to the woman's breast, he can be fed with the expressed mother's milk or formula milk, using a small cup. This may help the baby to take the breast easier and prevent the so-called nipple confusion. When compared to drinking from a bottle, drinking from a small cup results in the baby using less oxygen and his breathing effort also decreases. A cup is easier to clean than a bottle and it reduces the prevalence of gastroenteritis.

Breastfeeding in the neonatal intensive care unit

Preterm babies will develop the ability to be breastfed as their age increases and their reflexes become more mature. The mothers, however, need constant support and encouragement to express milk and maintain milk production. A few women are unable to make the transition from expressing milk to breastfeeding.

Guidelines to follow

When the baby is stable and can be held, the woman should be encouraged to hold the baby close to her naked breast, even during gavage or cup feeding. This will promote rooting reflexes and stimulate the hormonal let-down reflex.

Readiness to breastfeed the preterm baby

Indications of readiness to breastfeed the preterm baby include:
▶ The baby's general progress and condition.
▶ The ability to maintain body temperature outside the incubator.
▶ Coordination between suckling, swallowing and breathing.
▶ General tolerance of gavage feeds.

An effective position for breastfeeding the small preterm baby is the cross-cradle hold, where extra head support is provided. At first the preterm baby will make little suckling movements or lick the nipple, but the feeding skill will develop rapidly in most cases.

Breastfeeding in special situations

Caesarean birth

The woman is still able to breastfeed her baby but she may require additional support and guidance to establish successful breastfeeding. The basic guidelines to promote breastfeeding are all applicable:
▶ Breastfeeding should be started as soon as the woman and baby are comfortable.
▶ Suggest that the woman use relaxation-breathing techniques to manage discomfort and pain. Administer analgesics as prescribed to relieve acute pain before breastfeeding.
▶ Assist and encourage the woman to feed her baby frequently every two to three hours.
▶ Advise the woman to sleep and rest when the baby is sleeping.
▶ Provide information on the different breastfeeding positions available and assist and encourage the woman to try them out until she is comfortable with one position in particular. Start with the football hold position – this will prevent the baby from accidentally kicking the incision.

Neonatal jaundice

Breastfeeding can continue in the healthy full-term newborn with physiologic hyperbilirubinaemia. If the jaundiced baby is lethargic and suckling poorly, the woman can express breast milk, which will be administered to the baby. This will also ensure adequate milk production.

Breastfeeding twins

Breastfeeding is possible with twin births. If the babies are full term and healthy, breastfeeding can start immediately after birth. Simultaneous feeding promotes the rapid production of the milk needed for both babies. The milk that would be lost in the let-down reflex is also made available to one of the twins. When only one baby is awake and hungry, the woman

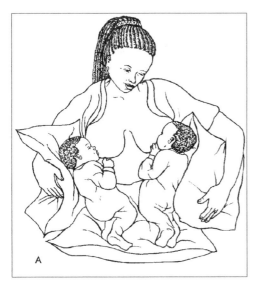

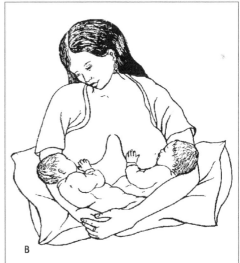

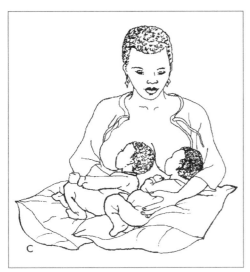

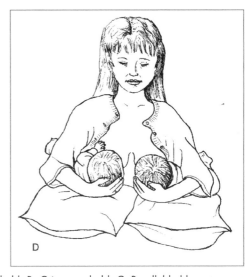

Figure 30.4 Breastfeeding postions for twins: A: V-hold; B: Crisscross hold; C: Parallel hold; D: Double footbal hold

should feed singly. The woman should alternate breasts when feeding each baby, to avoid favouring one breast for one infant. The suckling patterns of babies vary and therefore the breasts should be alternated.

Possible simultaneous breastfeeding positions include:

▶ *Combination cradle and football hold*: The woman sits with one baby in the cradle hold and the other in football hold.

▶ *Crisscross hold*: The woman sits with both babies in the cradle hold crisscrossed in her lap, with their heads in the crooks of her arms. One baby will be pressed against the woman, while the other baby's body will be pressed against its sibling.

▶ *Parallel*: The woman sits with the babies' bodies extended in the same direction. One baby is in the cradle hold with his head in the crook of the woman's arm and his body across her lap. The other baby's body extends in the same direction as his sibling's off the woman's lap, with his head supported by his mother's hand and arm.

▶ *Double football hold*: The woman sits with both the babies in the football hold, lying on pillows at the woman's side.

Interventions to promote breastfeeding

The following practices will promote breast-feeding:

▶ Assist the woman to help her baby to establish a correct suckling technique.

▶ Follow nursing practices with the absence of rigid feeding time schedules.

▶ Demonstrate and assist in suitable positioning of the infant at the breast to achieve correct latching on. Correct suckling for breastfeeding is defined as a wide-open mouth, with the tongue under the areola and expressing milk through slow, deep suckling.

▶ Prompt early breastfeeding during the first hour of life with close skin-to-skin contact, between the woman and her baby.

▶ Frequent breastfeeding or feeding on demand practices and rooming-in facilities.

▶ Careful control of drugs administered to the woman and baby to prevent the use of drugs that suppress milk production or sedate the baby.

▶ Midwives have to directly model the importance of breastfeeding by encouraging demand feeding with no formula supplementation and discouraging the emphasis on infant formula products.

▶ Increased information and support to breastfeeding women following discharge. If the newborn is unable to nurse immediately, introduce early breast pumping two-to three-hourly for 20 minutes per session bilaterally – this increases oxytocin production and subsequent milk production.

Alternative infant feeding

Basic choices

If the mother is for some reason unable or unwilling to breastfeed the baby and a substitute is needed, a choice is available from two groups:

▶ *Whey dominant breast milk substitutes* are specially formulated for the normal baby in the weight group 2.5 kg to 3.5 kg. Examples in this group are Nan 1, S26, S25 Gold, Infa Care 1, Similac PM60/40, and Cow's Gate Premium.

▶ *Casein dominant breast milk substitutes* are normally given to the hungry, big baby with a weight greater than 3.5 kg. This group includes formulas such as Lactogen 1, SMA, New SMA, Pelargon, Similac and Cow and Gate Plus.

It is important to note that special formulas are available for specific indications such as allergies and lactose intolerance. The South African Ethical Code for the Marketing of Breast Milk Substitutes (SA Code) controls the marketing, labelling and quality of breast milk substitutes. The midwife should keep up to date on the best formulas available for a particular baby.

Feeding schedules

The baby's hunger should determine the feeding schedule. Demand feedings involve feeding when the baby indicates readiness, while scheduled feedings are arranged according to predetermined intervals, usually every three or four hours. Four-hourly feeds will require six bottles and three-hourly feeds will require eight bottles of feed for a 24-hour period.

Feeding positions

Eye and skin contact still remain important strategies to promote parent–infant bonding, for example holding the baby in the cradle position (see Figure 30.5).

Preparation of bottles

Wash the hands properly with soap and water. All utensils, bottles and nipples must be cleaned by washing them with soap and water and they should be thoroughly rinsed afterwards. Before re-use, boil all equipment for at least 20 to 25

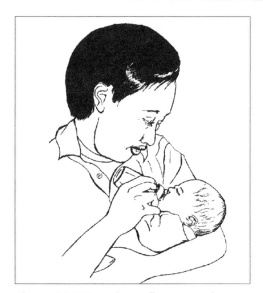

Figure 30.5 Using the cradle position when bottlefeeding an infant

minutes in water. Ensure that the insides of bottles and nipples are not touched with the hands.

Follow the directions provided by the manufacturer on the tin to prepare the formula with regard to the amount of water needed per scoop of powder. For example: one scoop (provided in the tin of milk powder) per 25 ml of boiled, cooled-down water.

Calculate the volume of fluid required for the feeds by using the baby's current weight (after day 3):
4 kg x 150 ml fluid for 24 hours
    4 x 150 ml/24 hours
       = 600 ml fluid/24 hours
Calculate the number of bottles needed if the baby feeds every four hours:
24 hours ÷ 4 hourly feeds = 6 bottles
    600 ml per 24 hours ÷ 6 bottles
       = 100 ml in each bottle

Calculate the amount of milk formula needed:
1 scoop per 25 ml water (or other directions from the manufacturer)
    100 ml = 4 scoops
    600 ml = 24 scoops

Therefore, six bottles can be prepared in advance, and refridgerated, to cover the baby's feeding needs over 24 hours, or 100 ml can be made up when needed.

Preparation of bottles:
Pour exactly 100 ml of boiled, cooled-down water into each bottle. Only then add the four scoops of milk powder. It is important to level the scoops before adding the milk powder to the water. Boiled, cooled-down water is used because the boiling process destroys all microbacteria. Cooled-down water will not destroy the heat-sensitive vitamins.

Another method is to pour 600 ml of boiled, cooled-down water to a clear jug and then to add the 24 scoops of milk powder. Six bottles can then each be filled up to the 100 ml mark.

Warming the formula is optional but room temperature is the acceptable norm for infant feeds. Any milk remaining in the bottle after feeding should be discarded, since leftover milk is an excellent medium for bacterial growth.

How to burp the infant

All babies will swallow air while feeding. This does not always cause discomfort. If a baby gulps loudly during the feed or becomes fussier as the feeding progresses, the baby needs to burp. The baby can be held upright against the shoulder, allowing air to escape naturally, or he can be laid down on the left side. He can also sit on the woman's lap with his chin supported between her thumb and index finger. Patting the baby's back gently while bending him slightly forward will bring up a burp. This will prevent regurgitation of milk accompanying the 'wind' and distension of the stomach.

Conclusion

Breastfeeding is the best way to feed a newborn baby but it always remains the final decision of the woman. Midwives should support the woman in her decision and promote breastfeeding practices as far as possible. When breastfeeding is chosen, the baby is usually put to the breast shortly after birth, if possible. During the period of hospitalisation and thereafter assistance should be given to the woman to choose a comfortable position. She should be advised on support techniques to stimulate milk flow and correct latching. Accurate and consistent information for the management of problems is essential.

If the mother chooses not to breastfeed her baby, the midwife should still assist her and give correct information on the selection and preparation of the feeding. In the case of a formula-fed baby, the importance of a comfortable position and eye contact between woman and baby should also be discussed.

References

Baker, H. M. 2002. *Nutrition and dietetics for health care*. Tenth edition. Edinburgh: Churchill Livingstone.

DoH (Department of Health), UNICEF. 2000. *South African breastfeeding guidelines for health workers and health facilities*. Pretoria: DoH.

Dungy, C. L. et al. 1992. Effect of discharge samples on duration of breastfeeding. *Pediatrics*, (90):223–237.

Ladewig, P. W. 1998. *Maternal-newborn nursing care: The nurse, the family and the community*. Fourth edition. California: Addison-Wesley.

Lawrence, R. 1994. *Breastfeeding: A guide for the medical profession*. Fourth edition. St Louis: Mosby.

Lawrence, R. 1995. The clinician's role in teaching proper infant feeding techniques. *Journal of Pediatrics*, 125(6):S112–S117.

Louw, J. 2001. Protection, promotion and support of breastfeeding. A historical perspective. *Geneeskunde*, January/February 43(1):38–43.

Mohrbacher, N. & Stock, J. 1997. *La Leche League International: The breastfeeding answer book*. Revised edition. Illinois: Schaumburg.

Neifert, M. R. 1998. The optimization of breastfeeding in the perinatal period. *Clinics in Perinatology*, 25(2):227–253.

Nolte, A. G. W. 1997. *A textbook for midwives*. Pretoria: J.L. van Schaik.

Wong, D. L. (Ed.) 1999. *Whaley & Wong's Nursing care of infants and children*. Sixth edition. St. Louis: Mosby.

Chapter 31

The baby with special needs

Carin Maree

Introduction

In order to effectively care for the baby with a health problem or disorder, it is crucial to understand the normal physiology of every topic of discussion first and then to relate it to the underlying pathophysiology of the specific disorder.

For this reason a system-related approach was used in this part of the book, with the following principles in mind:

▶ The relevance and attainment of the history and assessment of each system is fully understood/mastered as discussed in Chapter 29.

▶ The normal related physiology and anatomy are mastered as well as the adaptation of the newborn from intra-uterine to extra-uterine life (see Chapter 29).

▶ Stress cues are recognised and acted upon as outlined in Chapter 29, as well as the application of Developmentally Supportive Care (DSC).

The management of the newborn is based on the following principles:

▶ As far as possible preventing problems from occurring.

▶ Identifying and accurately diagnosing problems.

▶ Ensuring early intervention and/or appropriate referral for prompt management. The interventions are based on the following principles:

◆ Replace what is missing.

◆ Support what is necessary.

◆ Take over a physiological function.

◆ Minimise the workload on the organs or energy demand.

◆ Minimise the risk of complications by using the gentlest treatment with the best results.

◆ Use appropriate medication.

Holistic care is of critical importance with an emphasis on maintenance of internal homeostasis, stress reduction, DSC and a family-centred approach.

The concepts of holistic care are used recurrently during the discussions regarding the infant with a health problem or disorder. Stress reduction, DSC and the family-centred approach are discussed in more detail in other chapters of the book. The maintenance of internal homeostasis has not yet been addressed. As it forms a very important part of the approach in the care of the sick baby, it will be briefly discussed in the following section.

Maintenance of internal homeostasis

Internal homeostasis is the optimal internal environment of the baby that accommodates the optimal functioning of the body's cells with minimal stressors adding to the cells' demands. Optimal functioning of the body cells implies the ability of the cells to do what they are supposed to do efficiently: for example, impulse conduction of the nerve cells, or muscle contraction of the cardiac cells; to make the necessary adjustments if there is a higher demand, in the presence of an infection, as well as to grow at the expected pace.

Groups of cells form organs and groups of organs become systems to work together as an individual infant. They are all finely tuned and coordinated to execute all the normal duties expected of a living being, as well as to increase in order to grow. These normal duties require energy and involve various activities. Any problem that occurs will require an additional amount of energy and activities in order to be overcome.

Preterm and ill infants already have to cope with some disturbance of internal homeostasis due to their prematurity or illness, for which they often lack the ability or reserves. By the maintenance of internal homeostasis, they are given the best possible opportunity for recovery and healing, and to continue with normal functions and growth.

The following crucial aspects of internal homeostasis have a general impact on cell functioning and therefore on functioning of the systems, healing and growth:
▶ Temperature
▶ Oxygenation
▶ Blood pressure or tissue perfusion
▶ Acid-base balanc.
▶ Fluid and electrolyte balance
▶ Nutrition with special reference to blood glucose
▶ Removal of waste products
▶ Hormones with specific reference to stress hormones versus growth hormones

Internal homeostasis implies that the infant is infection free, pain free and not experiencing the side-effects of medication.

It is not possible to achieve perfect internal homeostasis for all infants but it is very important to restore any disturbance as soon as possible without waiting for the situation to become critical. In this sense it is the midwife's responsibility to identify the disturbance of internal homeostasis and to respond appropriately by either restoring homeostasis or referring the baby for the necessary interventions. Referral may even imply transfer to another institution for specialised care.

The different aspects of internal homeostasis will be addressed as part of the relevant systems responsible for their maintenance, but first pain management will be briefly dealt with in the following section.

Pain management

Previously it had been the belief that infants do not feel pain. Evidence though proves that infants, both full term and preterm, are very sensitive to pain and remember it. Unfortunately they are unable to tell where and how they feel pain, but they respond to pain with signs of physiological and behavioural stress (see Chapter 29).

Causes of pain can be touch, pressure, vibration, sudden movement, heat, cold, acidosis, alkalosis, hypoxia, strong taste, strong smell, noise, light on the retina, tissue damage due to invasive procedures or trauma.

Pain management is given firstly to prevent the pain by eliminating the causes, such as exposure to cold surfaces, or maintaining the internal homeostasis. It can also be prevented by the administration of a painkiller before the exposure to pain from invasive procedures. If the baby is exposed to pain over a period of time, after surgery for example, it can be prevented by administration of a painkiller before the effects of the previous administration wears off.

The first non-pharmacological choice of pain management is a single drop of sucrose (white sugar and not dextrose or fructose) on the baby's tongue. The taste stimulates the release of endorphines that function as a painkiller. Take note that a drop on the tongue is not enough to influence the blood glucose or the gastrointestinal function. It has no side effects or contraindications, but the effect is weaker or slower in preterm infants of less than 32 weeks gestation. It is strongly recommended to administer a drop of sucrose before any invasive procedure or if signs of stress are present that may be related to pain.

Other non-pharmacological methods for reducing pain are appropriate positioning and skin-to-skin contact, preferably using Kangaroo care, but hand cupping will also do (see Chapter 29) as well as breastfeeding, if it is feasible for the infant's condition.

Pharmacological pain management has to be introduced in selected cases where the baby can be closely monitored, like in a neonatal intensive care unit. It has to be prescribed by the attending physician and all the medication requirements have to be met. The choices of pharmacological management are Tylenol®, *morphine* and *fentanyl*. Be careful not to administer a sedative only, such as *phenobarbitone* or *diasepam*, without the accompaniment of a painkiller, as the sedative suppresses the infant's response to pain, but not his experience thereof (that is: he feels it, but we don't see it).

The rest of the chapter should be read with these principles in mind. It should also be emphasised that in order to reach a conclusion on what would be the best care for the baby, further research should be done if there appears to be a disparity between the theory described in this chapter and the reality of the practice.

Shock and resuscitation

Shock

Stress occurs when there is an increase in demand for oxygen and nutrition at cellular level. *Shock* occurs when there is a cellular, metabolic and haemodynamic disturbance as a result of an inability to meet the cellular demand for oxygen and nutrition. It is a widespread process affecting all the organs and eventually results in cellular dysfunction and death. There are different ways to classify shock:

Shock in terms of *aetiology* refers to:
▶ Hypovolaemic shock due to dehydration or haemorrhage.
▶ Cardiogenic shock as a result of reduced cardiac output and hypoperfusion with consequential hypoxia or other severe disturbances of internal homeostasis.
▶ Neurogenic shock resulting from failure of peripheral vasoconstriction due to brain damage or local factors such as hypoxia or acidosis.
▶ Distributive shock when fluid moves into the third space or the interstitial space, as is the case with sepsis and anaphylaxis.

Shock in terms of *effects* or outcomes refers to:
▶ Compensative shock where perfusion is poor but the blood pressure is still within normal limits.
▶ Decompensative shock where all systems are failing, including the blood pressure.

Shock can also be classified in terms of the *different stages or phases* thereof, namely:
▶ Compensatory shock which is when autoregulation takes place to ensure perfusion to vital organs.
▶ Progressive shock occurs when compensation is failing.

▶ Refractory shock is characterised by multi-organ failure and death.

It is a life-threatening situation if an infant is in shock and it requires emergency interventions or resuscitation, irrespective of the causes or classification thereof. All systems are involved and the sooner appropriate interventions are initiated, the better the outcomes will be.

The first warning signs of shock are signs of stress (see Chapter 29 on stress and DSC). Shock is present if the signs of stress persist, the infant does not respond to the normal stress reduction measures taken, and there are clinical signs of hypoperfusion of the different systems with compensation. These clinical signs include lethargy, tachycardia, tachypnoea, reduced bowel sounds and feeding intolerance, oliguria, cool and moist skin with peripheral cyanosis, temperature fluctuations and acid-base disturbances.

If the infant's condition deteriorates, there are signs of the different systems failing such as unresponsiveness, bradycardia, hypotension, bradypnoea or apnoea, feeding intolerance and abdominal distension, oliguria or anuria, central cyanosis, hypothermia, severe acid-base disturbances and clotting disturbances. It is important to respond quickly as the infant's condition can become irreversible and result in death.

Prevention is crucial, but if not possible, the outcomes depend on early diagnosis and appropriate management. Appropriate management includes the principles of resuscitation, to identify and eliminate the cause as soon as possible and to eliminate or reduce all other stressors (see Chapter 29).

Resuscitation

Resuscitation refers to emergency interventions to re-establish lung and heart function to ensure oxygen perfusion to all areas of the infant's body, but especially to the neurological system so as to prevent tissue damage due to hypoxia.

Prerequisites for successful resuscitation are knowledge, skills, preparedness, the ability to make competent decisions and to prioritise the sequence of interventions with smooth co-ordination. Basic resuscitation refers to the interventions necessary to keep an infant alive if there is only one person available to intervene. Advanced resuscitation refers to further skilful interventions to stabilise an infant with the use of medical technology.

Preparation for resuscitation: Hazards
Preparation refers to being prepared in terms of prevention or early identification of hazardous risk factors. These risk factors include the identification of factors from the history of which the DOOM-factors are important at birth:
▶ **D** = drugs given to the mother or infant
▶ **O** = old/age of infant, especially gestational age
▶ **O** = other previous or current problems
▶ **M** = meconium in the amniotic fluid

Preparation also involves being prepared in terms of a safe environment, such as preventing obvious hazards like sharp edges, exposed electrical wires and an open incubator. It also includes the prevention of hidden hazards of which the most important are hypothermia, infection and insensible water loss. Other hidden hazards include hyperoxia, faulty or inadequate equipment, expired drugs, noise, bright lights or the lack of positive identification of the infant.

Another important hazard is the use of unskilled, incompetent, inadequate and/or negligent staff. This can be avoided through education of staff for emergency interventions. It is also essential to ensure that adequate emergency equipment is available and that it is functional, such as oxygen and accessories, suction unit and accessories, lighting, monitors, infusion pumps and a mechanical ventilator or an oscillator. An emergency trolley should be available that is adequately equipped for basic and advanced resuscitation and there should be a warm, flat surface with efficient lighting on which to handle the infant.

An important part of preventing hazards is to follow the available protocols regarding all aspects of care of an infant.

Preparation for resuscitation: Hello

'Hello' refers to assessment of the infant's response to tactile stimulation, which is an indication of his neurological functioning or responsiveness. Tactile stimulation is experienced immediately after birth, when the infant is exposed to room air, which is cooler than the familiar intra-uterine environment. Thereafter the baby is dried and warmed and an appropriate response would be crying.

In other circumstances tactile stimulation would be given with physical touch. An appropriate response to soft touch may be a change in the breathing pattern or other vital signs, or a deliberate attempt to respond to the touch or movement. The appropriate response to painful touch, such as a heel prick, is crying with a deliberate attempt to pull away from the painful stimulus.

Warning signs of deterioration or inappropriate responses to tactile stimulation can vary from slow or sudden behavioural changes to irritability, agitation, seizures, poor reflexes, lethargy or unresponsiveness, usually associated with clinical signs of shock.

Preparation for resuscitation: Help

'Help' refers to the interpretation of the warning signs or inappropriate responses to tactile stimulation and the immediate decisions that have to be made regarding emergency interventions.

These decisions include whom to contact or consult to assist, what interventions to take, where to do it, what emergency equipment to use and how to do it. The implication of these decisions is that a specific person/s take responsibility for leading the resuscitation process.

Basic resuscitation

Airway. An open airway is obtained through clearing the airway of obstructive secretions by positioning the infant's head in 'sniffing

---

Basic resuscitation and advanced resuscitation

The sequence of basic resuscitation can be summarised as H H H A B C:
▶ Hazards
▶ Hello
▶ Help
▶ Airway
▶ Breathing
▶ Circulation

Advanced resuscitation includes the above plus D D D E E F F F F G:
▶ Drip
▶ Drugs
▶ Defibrillation (in exceptional cases)
▶ Endotracheal intubation
▶ Electrolytes
▶ Fluid
▶ Feeding
▶ Formal assessment
▶ Final diagnosis
▶ General aspects

The focus of advanced resuscitation is to stabilise the infant and initiate advanced care to prevent illness, facilitate recovery and improve health.

---

position'. This is a slight extension of the head with the face in midline (not hyperextension and not flexion). It may be necessary to use a suction device to clear the airways. This is the first step of resuscitation and is a prerequisite for the following steps.

Breathing. The next step will be to facilitate breathing. Assess for the presence of breathing, as well as the quality thereof. If there is spontaneous comfortable breathing, emergency interventions are not required and assessment can be continued to determine the possible cause for what the concern was, or if it is a newborn, the infant can be given to the mother.

Oxygen should be administered with a funnel, mask, nasal cannula, head box or CPAP-driver if there are spontaneous breathing attempts but with signs of respiratory distress such as nasal flaring, accessory muscle use, tachypnoea, rib and/or sternal recession and grunting or stridor. The first choice is a CPAP-driver and second choice is nasal cannula, while a head box should only be used if nothing else is available.

If breathing attempts are absent or poor, oxygen should be administered with a mask and ambubag or mechanical ventilation. It is critical to obtain a proper seal with the mask over the nose and mouth, to maintain an open airway by holding the head in sniffing position with the chin lifted, and to maintain a rhythmic tempo of approximately 30 to 40 breaths per minute. Use chest movement as an indicator of successful bagging in terms of the volume administered. Chest movement can only be obtained if there is a proper seal, an open airway and an efficient volume of air ventilated. However, it is important to only obtain chest movement and not to force more air into the lungs in order to prevent pneumothorax or other pressure-related complications.

Mechanical ventilation with a mask and ambubag can be maintained for as long as necessary together with cardiac compressions if required, until a suitably skilled professional can continue with advanced resuscitation and insert an endotracheal tube for continuous mechanical ventilation or oscillation.

Circulation. Circulation or the presence of a pulse has to be determined as soon as breathing is established, after two breaths. It can be assessed by connecting the infant to a cardiac monitor, listening to the heart rate with a stethoscope or feeling for a carotid or brachial pulse. Continue with assisting the breathing if the heart rate is more than 80 beats per minute.

Circulatory assistance by means of cardiac compression is necessary if the heart rate is less than 80 beats per minute. The important considerations for successful cardiac compressions include:
▶ The *correct placement* of two fingertips at approximately 1 cm lower than the nipple line on the lower third of the sternum.
▶ The correct *depth of compressions* at

approximately a third to half of the chest from the front to the back.
▶ Maintaining a *tempo* of approximately 100 compressions per minute.
▶ Maintaining a *ratio* of one breath followed by three compressions.

The basic resuscitation to maintain breathing and circulation should be continued until a skilled professional person can continue with advanced resuscitation.

Advanced resuscitation
Although advanced resuscitation must be done by a skilled and competent professional, it is important for all nursing staff to know the steps so that they can assist and prepare for it.

Drip. As soon as possible a drip should be put up for intravenous fluid, either via umbilical catheterisation or peripheral infusion. The safest solution is to use a volume expander (normal saline 0,9% or Ringer's lactate). All infusions must be administered through an infusion pump and there should be no free-running infusions on an infant. It should be calculated according to the infant's weight. If it is a newborn, it can be calculated at 60 ml/kg/24h, with boluses calculated as 10 ml/kg/bolus (administered over 20 to 30 minutes) if the blood pressure is low. If the infant is older than one day, the fluids should be calculated as discussed on page 30-2. Haemacel®, plasma or other colloid solutions are not routinely used during resuscitation, but in selected cases they may be prescribed by the attending physician.

Drugs. Emergency drugs can be used if indicated, of which the most common are *epinephrine* (adrenaline) if the heart rate is lower than 80 bpm and *naloxone* to reverse the effects of anaesthetics and other drugs given to the mother. It is crucial to administer the *correct drug* at the *correct dose* through the *correct route* at the *correct frequency*. Protocols should be available on the use of drugs, and staff should be informed about it.

Endotracheal intubation. Endotracheal intubation can also be done before an infusion is inserted, as it provides an opportunity for long-term artificial ventilation, as well as a route for administration of some of the drugs, such as *epinephrine* (adrenaline) and *surfactant*. Ventilation with an ambubag can continue after intubation but it is recommended to attach the infant as soon as possible to a mechanical ventilator or oscillator, as ventilation is more stable and the person would be free to assist with other tasks. Important aspects for successful intubation include:

▶ A functional laryngoscope with the correct straight blade.
▶ Correct size ET-tube.
▶ Correct procedure.
▶ Efficient stabilisation of the tube.
▶ Confirmation of the placement of the tube with air entry bilateral and X-rays.

The midwife should have knowledge of endotracheal intubation as it is a specialised skill, but she may be expected to prepare and assist during the procedure. More information can be found in advanced neonatal care literature. It should preferably be included in the policies.

Electrolytes. Breathing and circulation remain the first priorities throughout resuscitation. If these are successfully maintained, it is important then to assess the blood glucose levels, the acid-base balance with an arterial blood gas analysis and other electrolyte disturbances by blood sampling for laboratory investigations. Any disturbances need to be corrected appropriately as prescribed by the attending physician.

Fluids and feeding. Fluids and feeding refer to the necessity to replace the volume expander with the prescribed infusion, such as potassium-free Neonatalyte® for the newborn, and calculated according to the infant's weight (see Chapter 30).

It is recommended that the infant is kept nil per mouth until bowel sounds are present. A nasogastric tube should be inserted to obtain free drainage of the gastric contents if the infant has been artificially ventilated and abdominal distension has subsequently been observed.

Formal assessment. Once all the above criteria are met a full physical examination of the infant should be conducted. Special investigations may be necessary, either to make a diagnosis, to confirm a diagnosis, or to assess the infant's response to treatment such as a blood gas, X-rays or bloods for laboratory investigations.

Final diagnosis. A final medical and nursing diagnosis is then made and planning is done regarding the treatment, management and nursing care, depending on the diagnosis.

General aspects. Important information should be communicated to all the relevant role players. For example, the paediatrician or attending physician must be informed about the results obtained. The parents need to be counselled and their informed consent obtained for further management. Record keeping should be completed, the area must be cleaned, the emergency trolley and equipment cleaned and restocked and all other uncompleted tasks should be taken care of.

Resuscitation

Resuscitation refers to the emergency interventions to provide perfusion to all systems (especially the brain) in order to maintain life. It requires skilled staff who will make competent decisions and execute the resuscitation procedure according to the sequence of priorities. The quicker and more competently it is executed, the better the outcome will be for the infant, irrespective of the initial cause. The midwife has an important role in resuscitation because she is often the first person to identify a high-risk infant, and may be the only one present for a period of time. Her skills can therefore make the difference between life and death.

Respiratory conditions

Introduction

Respiratory disorders are the most common health problems in the neonatal period. They may be related to anatomical, functional or physiological problems. The anatomical disorders are related to the physical or anatomical component of the respiratory system, which include the bony structures, the airway responsible for conduction of air, the functional airway or alveoli, the nerve supply and the systemic blood supply, as well as the pulmonary blood supply. The functional or physiological disorders refer mainly to problems with ventilation (inhalation and/or exhalation) and gas exchange.

Respiratory anatomical structures are essential for proper ventilation, which is an important requirement for gas exchange. Proper gas exchange is in turn required for all bodily functions and for the provision of oxygen for aerobic metabolism. It therefore plays an important role in energy production, as well as acid-base homeostasis.

Respiratory distress can be described as an additional respiratory effort of the infant to provide in the oxygen demand, irrespective of the cause. If the infant fails, it becomes life-threatening or fatal as all the organs will be affected. Please note that respiratory distress is not the same as respiratory distress syndrome, which is hyalin membrane disease.

Abnormalities of the respiratory system may be due to congenital abnormalities or they may be acquired. It usually results in deviations in ventilation and/or gas exchange.

Ventilation problems result in poor air entry and are indicated when any of the following conditions are present:

▶ The use of accessory muscles, such as nasal flaring.
▶ Abnormal breathing sounds such as stridor, grunting or wheezing.
▶ Abnormal chest movement, such as asymmetrical movement, rib retractions or sternal recession.

Abnormalities in gas exchange are indicated by skin colour changes that are usually central cyanosis or mottledness, desaturation or saturation fluctuations. The systemic impact of abnormalities in gas exchange may be observed as stress cues, acid-base disturbances, hypoxia, hyperoxia, hypocapnoea, hypercapnoea or other disturbances of internal homeostasis.

Respiratory functions may change for a number of reasons and they may not always be due to a respiratory abnormality or disorder. Tachypnoea (respiratory rate of more than 60 per minute) is often a compensatory mechanism for an additional demand for oxygen as is the case with stress, metabolic acidosis, anaemia, cardiac disorders or other disturbances of internal homeostasis. Bradypnoea (a respiratory rate of less than 40 per minute) may be a compensation for metabolic alkalosis or decreased levels of carbon dioxide. However, tachypnoea or bradypnoea can also be a result of a respiratory disorder or problem. It is therefore important to assess the patient as a whole and not to focus on a single system in making a diagnosis.

The special investigations used to assist in the assessment of the respiratory system include saturation monitoring, chest X-rays, arterial blood gas analysis and bronchoscopy. Ultrasonography can also be used, as well as laboratory tests such as culturing of a sputum specimen. See Chapter 29 regarding assessment of the respiratory system.

The most commonly used methods for respiratory assistance from least invasive to most invasive are as follows:

▶ Nasal prongs.
▶ CPAP-driver.
▶ Mechanical ventilation.
▶ High-frequency ventilation or oscillation.

'Gentle ventilation' is ventilation that is as close as possible to the physiological parameters (see Chapter 29). This includes lower pressures and a respiratory rate of less than

The management of respiratory conditions

In the management of respiratory conditions the main focus should be the maintenance of internal homeostasis and stress management through the implementation of Developmentally Supportive Care in order to reduce the oxygen demand and to facilitate optimal respiratory functioning (see Chapter 29). Other measures to prevent or limit respiratory problems include 'gentle ventilation' or using the least invasive respiratory assistance, which is suitable for the individual infant, and to wean as soon as possible from respiratory assistance.

60 per minute. Oxygen toxicity is prevented by close monitoring and maintaining partial oxygen pressures (PaO$_2$ 50 to 80 mmHg) or oxygen saturation of preferably less than 95%. It is important to humidify and warm the oxygen and to use sterile circuits for mechanical ventilation, as well as to apply the infection control protocols. Pharmacological treatment also plays a major role in the management of respiratory problems, as well as surgical interventions or other invasive procedures such as inserting an intercostal drain for a pneumothorax.

The conditions that will now be discussed occur commonly in the neonatal phase and their outcomes are dependant on timely identification, fast decision-making and appropriate management in the delivery room.

The conducting airways (nose, trachea, bronchi and bronchioli) are relatively small in diameter in comparison to those of an adult but they allow symmetrical and bilateral air entry with ease according to the infant's needs.

An *airway obstruction* refers to a partial or full blockage of the conducting airway. It may be the result of a congenital defect or an acquired stenosis (see the discussions on structural defects). It may also be caused by obstructive secretions, such as a mucous plug, inflammation of the airway as with an infec-

tion, the presence of meconium or an obstructed endotracheal tube.

As the diameter of the conducting airway is small, anything entering or occupying space in the airway can potentially cause an obstruction big enough to decrease the conduction of air and cause respiratory distress. The clinical picture and outcomes are influenced by the severity, the cause and other factors such as gestational age:

▶ The *severity* thereof is determined by the size of the obstruction, if it is a partial or full obstruction and the location that determines the number of alveoli that are not ventilated. A tracheal obstruction is, for example, much worse than an obstruction of a bronchus to a part of a lobe.

▶ If the *cause* thereof is a congenital defect, respiratory distress will be present from birth, but if it is an acquired obstruction, it might occur any time. An outstanding sign is that *audible air entry is absent lower than the obstruction* and sudden deterioration is a common feature.

▶ *Other factors* that play a role include
  ◆*gestational age*: the lower the gestational age, the worse the outcomes
  ◆*birth weight*: the lower the birth weight, the worse the outcomes.

The diagnosis can be confirmed with X-rays if there is time and the baby's condition allows it. The outcomes for an obstruction can vary from being undetected to life threatening.

The first and most important step in the treatment of the airway obstruction is to obtain an open airway by preventing an obstruction and if it could not be prevented, to remove it as soon as possible. Mucous plugs can be prevented by administering warmed and humidified air, even if it is administered through nasal prongs or in a head box, as well as by suctioning thick secretions and following with appropriate physiotherapy. It may be very helpful to rinse with lukewarm normal saline to loosen the mucous plug before suction. Respiratory infections have to be prevented in order to avoid the production of thick secretions and inflammation of the conducting airway. They have to be treated as early as possible if they could not be prevented. Mechanical obstruction by the endotracheal tube can be prevented through placing it correctly, securing it properly and suctioning according to the baby's needs. Careful positioning and handling of the infant are crucial to prevent the endotracheal tube from kinking or becoming displaced. The endotracheal tube has to be removed if it is kinked or displaced, and replaced with a new one. If the cause is congenital or acquired stenosis, referral for surgical correction is essential. It is possible for a baby on a mechanical ventilator to present with the same symptoms if the ventilatory circuit is disconnected, so check the whole ventilatory circuit.

Management of an obstructed airway

The management of obstruction of airway cases focuses on establishment of an open airway as soon as possible and support with the necessary respiratory assistance. It is also important to maintain internal homeostasis, reduce stress and to provide support and advice for the parents.

Structural deformities of the conducting airways

The nose develops as part of the mid-face and already has bilateral open nostrils in the first trimester. The trachea and oesophagus originate from the endoderm, as they elongate and separate during the fourth week of gestation and then mature. The bronchi develop from the trachea and in turn give origin to the bronchioli and later to the alveoli.

Congenital structural deformities of the conducting airways originate in the early phases of embryology due to inherited, environmental or multifactoral conditions, such as *choanal atresia*. *Acquired structural deformities* are usually related to injury followed by scar formation, for example, tracheal stenosis caused by endotracheal intubation.

Choanal atresia

Choanal atresia is a unilateral or bilateral membranous or bony obstruction of the nasal passage. This is a congenital abnormality often associated with other congenital abnormalities such as CHARGE syndrome (**c**oloboma, **h**eart disease, **a**tresia choanal, **r**estricted growth and development, **g**enital hypoplasia and **e**ar anomalies).

Newborns are compulsory nose breathers. Choanal atresia causes a full airway obstruction with severe respiratory distress after birth, as newborns with this condition are unable to breathe through the mouth except when they are crying. The infant is therefore pink when crying, but turns cyanotic when not crying, with gasping attempts and severe respiratory distress.

The diagnosis is confirmed with failure to insert a nasal endotracheal tube or nasogastric tube, or if the tube coils back. An oral airway has to be inserted as soon as possible as the immediate prognosis is very poor and the mortality rate high without an artificial open airway. An oral airway may be efficient to relieve the respiratory distress but it may also be necessary for oral intubation, with or without mechanical ventilation. The tube must be well secured to prevent the risk of accidental extubation. Early referral for surgical repair is essential, as well as providing the parents with the necessary support and information. The outcomes after surgical correction can be very good without long-term complications.

Cleft lip and/or palate

A *cleft lip and/or palate* can be classified as an abnormality of the upper conducting airways, as well as an abnormality of the gastrointestinal tract. As the gastrointestinal outcomes are more severe, the condition will be discussed further on pages 31-67 to 31-68.

Tracheal stenosis

Tracheal stenosis refers to a narrowing of the trachea, either due to a congenital defect associated with syndromes, or acquired after injury. The stenosis causes a partial airway obstruction. The signs and symptoms depend on the severity of the obstruction. Stridor is present if it is severe, as well as other signs of respiratory distress. If respiratory compensation is needed, as in stressful circumstances, the slight obstruction of a small tracheal stenosis can result in respiratory distress.

The treatment of a tracheal stenosis depends on its severity. If it is severe enough to cause respiratory distress, a tracheostomy and/or referral for surgical correction is necessary. If the stenosis is not severe it might be sufficient to prevent crying and any other activities that may require respiratory compensation or an increase in oxygen demand. It is critical to prevent inflammation of the airway as the swelling worsens the obstruction. Respiratory assistance with oxygen has to be provided if signs of respiratory distress are present. The expected outcome may vary from a very good prognosis to very poor, or even death, depending on the severity of the obstruction and the efficiency of treatment.

Tracheo-oesophageal fistula and tracheo-oesophageal atresia

A *tracheo-oesophageal fistula* is an abnormal anatomical communication between the trachea and the oesophagus. *Tracheo-oesophageal atresia* refers to an interruption of the trachea or oesophagus (see Figure 31.1A). These are congenital defects occurring as separate defects, together or commonly in association with other defects, such as cardiac defects or gastrointestinal anomalies. It forms part of the VATER syndrome (vertebral anomalies, anal atresia, tracheo-oesophageal fistula and radial or renal dysplasia) or VACTERL syndrome (vertebral anomalies, anal atresia, cardiac defects, tracheo-oesophageal fistula, renal agenesis and limb defects). The outcome for the babies with a combination of defects is worse than those with single defects.

A tracheo-oesophageal fistula (commonly referred to as TOF) and/or atresia originate as abnormal early embryonic developments. Several variations are possible (see Figure 31.1), with various signs and symptoms.

Common signs and symptoms include polyhydramnios during pregnancy, after birth respiratory problems and/or gastrointestinal problems.

A *proximal oesophageal atresia* and *upper tracheal fistula* (Figure 31.1B) are associated with a flattened abdomen, no air in the stomach and intestines on X-ray, severe choking while feeding, continuous drooling, aspiration pneumonia and difficulty or choking on attempts to pass a nasogastric tube.

A *proximal oesophageal atresia* and *tracheo-oesophogeal fistula to the distal pouch* (Figure 31.1C) are associated with an air-filled abdomen and intestines, continuous drooling and overflow during feeding with no feeds in the abdomen and no meconium, as well as difficulty to pass a nasogastric tube.

A *tracheo-oesophageal fistula without atresia,* is associated with coughing when being fed and aspiration pneumonia (see Figure 31.1D and 31.1E). The baby may develop abdominal, air-filled distension with mask-bag ventilation. The diagnosis will be confirmed with X-rays or ultrasonography. Barium swallow should be considered carefully before using it if a fistula is suspected to prevent aspiration and the resulting chemical pneumonia.

Early diagnosis and referral for surgical correction is crucial, especially if there is a history of polyhydramnios. The infant should be admitted to a neonatal intensive care unit for specialised care. In the event of respiratory distress, respiratory assistance should be considered. The baby has to be kept nil per mouth and the fluid must be replaced intravenously. Transparenteral nutrition (hyperalimentation) has to be initiated in approximately 24 hours to replace oral nutrition (see Chapter 30). Consider continuous low vacuum suction for saliva if there is unremitting drooling. Parental support is crucial, especially as the expected outcomes may vary from fatal (especially without surgical repair), to good with complications (such as chronic respiratory infections or feeding difficulty), to very good without any complications.

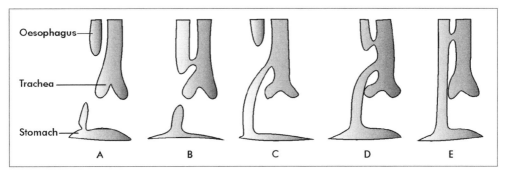

Figure 31.1 Different types of Tracheo-oesophageal fistula and Tracheo-oesophageal atresia.
A: Oesophageal atresia, B: Oesophageal artresia and upper tracheo-oesophageal fistula,
C: Proximal oesophageal artresia and tracheo-oesophageal fistula to the distal pouch, D and E:
Examples of tracheo-oesophageal fistula without artresia.

Diaphragmatic hernia

The diaphragm has developed by 24 weeks gestation in order to separate the abdominal and thoracic organs and to maintain normal breathing. A *diaphragmatic hernia* is a congenital defect where the abdominal organs herniate into the thoracic cavity through a defect in the diaphragm. It is caused by the diaphragm failing to close during embryonic development. The protruding abdominal organs invade the space and displace the normal thoracic organs. These organs may be small intestines with or without the stomach, and in severe cases the liver can protrude. The most severe complication is an underdevelopment of the lung on the side where the protrusion is found due to lack of space. The resulting complications are pulmonary hypertension and severe respiratory distress, as well as patent ductus arteriosus (see page 31-21).

A diaphragmatic hernia after birth is characterised by a very flat abdomen and a barrel chest, as well as severe respiratory distress with ventilation on the one side only. The diagnosis is confirmed with a chest X-ray where the abdominal organs will be visible in the chest cavity. Immediate interventions after birth should focus on resuscitation to provide adequate ventilation, including immediate endotracheal intubation, administration of surfactant and respiratory assistance. The respiratory assistance is usually mechanical ventilation, high frequency ventilation or oscil-

lation, as well as the administration of inhaled nitric oxide. If resuscitation was successful the infant must be admitted to a neonatal intensive care unit for specialised care. Early diagnosis and early referral for surgical correction is therefore very important as the outcomes may vary but the condition is usually associated with a very high mortality rate.

Acquired lung problems

Pulmonary air leaks

During normal breathing symmetrical, bilateral air entry and even distribution of air is expected in both lungs. The areas around the alveoli should be free of any air.

Pulmonary air leaks occur when the alveoli rupture and air leaks into the thoracic cavity and visceral pleura (*pneumothorax*), the mediastinum (*pneumomediastinum*), interstitial spaces around blood vessels or along lymphatics (*pulmonary interstitial emphysema* or *PIE-syndrome*), or into the pericardium (*pneumopericardium*). The alveoli can rupture spontaneously or it may be due to barotrauma, such as high pressure assisted ventilation or overdistension of alveoli with an ambubag. The removal of intercostal drains without proper closure of the site of insertion can result in an air leakage.

As soon as alveoli rupture, surface areas for gas exchange are lost, and the more alveoli rupture, the worse the gas exchange will be.

The leaked air occupies space in the closed chest cavity and prevents expansion of the alveoli during inhalation, with worsening respiratory attempts and deterioration of the infant. The associated signs and symptoms are respiratory distress, tachycardia and desaturation, as well as asymmetrical respiratory attempts, chest movement and audible air entry. Deterioration is sudden and can occur any time but is commonly found after resuscitation interventions or during assisted ventilation. It is possible, however, that the leakage is small enough to go undetected until the oxygen demand increases, during invasive procedures for instance. The diagnosis is usually confirmed with X-rays.

The specific management for the condition will be determined by the severity of the air leakage, the aim being to maintain efficient ventilation. In some cases it might imply respiratory assistance such as mechanical ventilation. If it is more severe, with poor response to such assistance, the insertion of an intercostal drain/s with an underwater drainage system may be necessary. This would require admission to a neonatal intensive care unit. It is vital to reduce the baby's stress to the absolute minimum so as to decrease the oxygen demand. The outcome is usually very good with early diagnosis and immediate appropriate intervention. However, there is the possibility of complications or even death.

Meconium aspiration syndrome

In term and post-term fetuses asphyxia in utero may stimulate peristalsis and relaxing of the anal sphincter, which results in the passing of meconium into the amniotic fluid. The presence of meconium in the amniotic fluid is recognised as a significant risk factor and aspiration may occur with the first breath at birth. It can be prevented by suctioning the nose and mouth at birth if meconium is present before the first breath is inhaled and before the body is delivered. Aspiration of meconium can occur in utero with repeated episodes of asphyxia leading to respiratory gasping. It is not possible to predict at birth if the baby has already inhaled meconium or not, and the principle is therefore that all newborns have to be suctioned if meconium is present in the amniotic fluid.

Aspiration of meconium that results in partial or full airway obstruction and respiratory distress, is known as *meconium aspiration syndrome*. It causes air-trapping in the alveoli resulting in poor gas exchange with poor oxygenation and an accumulation of carbon dioxide. Other outcomes include chemical pneumonitis, acid-base disturbances, suppression of surfactant production, inactivation of surfactant, development of pulmonary air leaks and bronchopulmonary dysplasia.

The focus for preventing meconium aspiration syndrome is the prevention of episodes of fetal asphyxia and suctioning before the first breath.

Management of meconium aspiration syndrome, if it could not be prevented, should include suctioning before first breath, endotracheal intubation with endotracheal suctioning as soon as possible after birth, respiratory assistance, repeated administration of surfactant and the establishment of internal homeostasis as soon as possible with reduction of stress. These babies require admission to a neonatal intensive care unit.

The expected outcome depends on the severity of the fetal asphyxia, the promptness and efficiency of resuscitation, and the presence of any complications. The prognosis may be very good but it could result in long-term neurological or other complications, or even death. It is therefore essential that the midwife prevents meconium aspiration at all costs, or refers the infant for specialised treatment as soon as possible.

Transient tachypnoea of the newborn (wet lung syndrome)

The lungs of the fetus are filled with lung fluid before birth. During movement through the birth channel, a third to a half of the lung fluid is compressed out of the lungs. The lung fluid left in the lungs is then displaced to the interstitial space during the first deep gasping breaths for slow absorption into the bloodstream. The alveoli can then fill with air, normal breathing continues and gas exchange takes place.

Transient tachypnoea of the newborn, also known as *wet lung syndrome*, is a condition where the normal absorption of lung fluid is delayed after birth, mainly as the result of a caesarean section. The birth process during caesarean section does not have the same mechanical pressure on the chest as normal delivery does to compress the lung fluid out. Newborn babies delivered via caesarean section show less deep gasping attempts after birth, resulting in less displacement of lung fluid to the interstitial space. More lung fluid may be found in the alveoli, resulting in a decreased gas exchange with a compensatory increase in the respiratory rate and the characteristic audible 'wet lungs' or crepitations. Other signs of respiratory distress may accompany it and the diagnosis can be confirmed with X-rays. There is no specific treatment other than to allow time for the absorption of the fluid. Respiratory support has to be considered, if necessary. Recovery is usually spontaneous within 24 to 48 hours and without any complications.

Hyaline membrane disease or respiratory distress syndrome

The production of surfactant in the alveoli takes place from about 24 to 28 weeks gestation, with the most production occurring from 34 to 36 weeks. The role of surfactant ('surface-active phospholipids') is to reduce the surface tension in the alveoli, which prevents them from collapsing after expiration and allows easy inspiration to follow. Surfactant activates alveolar macrophages and plays a role in the prevention of infection in the lungs. Surfactant production is increased by fetal stress hormones in cases such as maternal hypertension, retroplacental bleeding, maternal drug use and smoking. The production can be accelerated by the artificial administration of corticosteroids, namely, betamethasone or dexamethasone (Decadron®), which are given to women who

are in preterm labour or at risk of preterm labour. Surfactant production may be suppressed by maternal diabetes and hypocalcaemia and it is inactivated by meconium as found in meconium aspiration syndrome.

Hyaline membrane disease, also known as *respiratory distress syndrome*, is due to a surfactant deficiency in the lungs, which leads to respiratory distress. The surfactant deficiency is usually caused by preterm birth, at usually less than 34 weeks gestation. It can be aggravated by the presence of asphyxia and meconium if it is aspirated. A lack of surfactant results in a collapse of the alveoli after expiration and a large inspiratory effort is then required for the next breath. The characteristic signs and symptoms are grunting, which is an attempt to retain a certain amount of pressure in the alveoli to keep them open and prevent collapse, as well as other signs of respiratory distress such as intercostal and sternal recession. This clinical picture develops within the first few hours after birth and becomes progressively worse as the newborn tires because he has to work very hard to breathe.

The diagnosis of hyaline membrane disease is confirmed with the equal matt appearance of the lungs on an X-ray to various degrees of severity. Immediate management after birth requires endotracheal intubation with the endotracheal administration of surfactant and respiratory assistance, such as CPAP-drive mechanical ventilation or oscillation. If surfactant is not available for endotracheal administration, the infant will at least require respiratory assistance. It is important to maintain internal homeostasis and reduce stress levels to minimise the baby's oxygen demand and so his effort of breathing. The outcome with treatment is usually very good with quick recovery.

Bronchopulmonary dysplasia

The lungs begin to develop at about four weeks after conception. Most of the alveoli are developed by 24 weeks gestation, but they will continue to develop after birth till approximately ten years of age. Vascularisation of the alveoli takes place from 24 to 28 weeks gestational age and is more or less completed at 37 weeks, with further slow development thereafter. Repair of damaged alveoli and bronchi depends on their vascularisation to provide healing factors such as nutrients, oxygen, temperature and acid-base balance.

Bronchopulmonary dysplasia is a condition of alveolar and bronchial damage with permanent changes of the tissue and consequent oxygen dependency. It is acquired after birth. The alveoli and other lung tissue are very vulnerable during development. There is a high risk that growth may stop or changes occur in the lung tissue if an infant is exposed to any damaging factor during the development phase and there is a deficiency in healing factors. Damaging factors include high oxygen concentration, high pressure used for ventilation, atelectrauma or trauma due to collapse of alveoli with air-trapping, and prematurity, especially in association with disturbances of internal homeostasis such as acidosis and hypoxia. The longer the duration of exposure and/or the more intense the damaging factor, the worse the damage. The areas of bronchi and alveoli that are damaged decrease the surface area available for gas exchange, which results in a need for additional oxygen administration. It is characterised by tachypnoea, a tendency to tachycardia, hypoxia, hypercapnoea and respiratory acidosis. Signs and symptoms of respiratory distress will be present, such as sternal retraction, rales, increased secretions and an inability to be *weaned off oxygen*. The diagnosis will be confirmed with X-rays.

Bronchopulmonary dysplasia can be prevented by proper oxygen administration, by following the principles of 'gentle ventilation', maintaining internal homeostasis and reducing stress. Due to a baby not having the respiratory resources available to cope with loss of gas exchange surfaces, key treatment should be to prevent respiratory infection. Pharmacological assistance plays an important role, especially bronchodilators, steroids and diuretics. Again parental counselling is neces-

sary, as the respiratory damage is usually permanent, with very slow improvement, if any, in oxygen dependency. The mortality rate increases sharply if any additional respiratory complications occur or if the baby falls ill.

Respiratory infections

An infant's respiratory system is very vulnerable and is highly affected by the adaptation from intra-uterine to extra-uterine life. The baby may be even more susceptible if he is born preterm with an immature respiratory system and a compromised immune system in addition.

Respiratory infections refer to the invasion and growth of microbes in the upper or lower airways. It occurs most commonly after exposure to microbes in the external environment, such as chorio-amnionitis in utero, breathing contaminated air, mechanical ventilation, endotracheal intubation or suctioning with contaminated tubes. The infection may be localised or spread to all areas of the respiratory system as pneumonia, or it can spread further resulting in sepsis. These microbes may either be bacteria, fungi or viruses. The clinical picture will be very similar, but the specific cause will determine the management of the infection. Common signs and symptoms of a respiratory infection include general signs of stress and respiratory distress. The diagnosis is confirmed with X-rays, as well as a sputum specimen for culturing, CRP and FBC.

Prevention of respiratory infections is achieved mainly by adhering to general infection control protocol, as well by maintaining internal homeostasis and reducing stress. The main focus of treatment is antibiotic treatment for a bacterial infection. Antibiotic treatment can be prescribed for prophylaxis of a secondary infection if it is not a bacterial infection, i.e. fungal or viral infection, but it is controversial. Treatment of respiratory infections often includes respiratory assistance, such as oxygen administation or ventilatory support, bronchodilators and, although controversial, steroids. The outcome depends on the size of the surface area affected, the site or location and the infant's immunity. The cause may influence the outcome, in that viral, fungal and resistant bacterial infections are worse than bacterial infections which are sensitive to antibiotics. The outcome can vary from complete recovery to mortality.

Pulmonary hypoplasia/hypoplastic lungs and avascularisation of lungs

The conducting airways are formed more or less by 17 weeks gestation, followed by the development and vascularisation of the alveoli. The alveoli are usually sufficient in numbers to provide life-sustaining gas exchange from 26 to 28 weeks, in the absence of hyaline membrane disease, meconium aspiration and pneumonia.

Hypoplastic lungs or *pulmonary hypoplasia* refers to the condition when the lobe/s or lung/s do not develop and may be a result of any of the following factors:

 ▶ Multifactoral congenital defects, such as Potter syndrome.
 ▶ Mechanical constraint that prevents the development of alveoli (such as diaphragmatic hernia or severe oligohydramnios).

Hypoplastic lungs are not related to gestational age. There is a limited or absent surface area for gas exchange resulting in severe respiratory distress and poor response to any respiratory assistance. It is fatal if both lungs are hypoplastic. The infant does have an opportunity for survival if one lung only is affected, as in the case of a diaphragmatic hernia, but he will require respiratory assistance and admission to a neonatal intensive care unit. Poor ventilation and small lobe/s or lung/s are visible on X-ray.

Avascularisation of the lungs is associated with preterm birth and affects babies usually born at less than 26 weeks gestational age, as the vascularisation of the lungs is not yet sufficient to facilitate proper gas exchange. It

results in severe respiratory distress with poor response to respiratory assistance. The diagnosis is confirmed with chest X-ray.

The main focus for treating these conditions are as follows:

 ▶ Maximise ventilation, which includes the administration of surfactant.
 ▶ Respiratory assistance with oscillation or high frequency ventilation if possible, or at least with mechanical ventilation.
 ▶ Reduce stress and handling to limit the oxygen demand to the absolute minimum.
 ▶ Maintain internal homeostasis as far as possible.

Providing the parents with support and information is essential as these conditions are associated with a very high mortality rate or with long-term complications. Therefore, if the baby is born at an institution that cannot provide specialised care, he should be referred for admission to a neonatal intensive care unit.

Other causes of respiratory distress

Other causes of respiratory distress that were not discussed include injury of the respiratory centre in the brain, cot death (sudden infant death syndrome), drug-induced respiratory suppression, pulmonary hypertension, pulmonary haemorrhage and chronic lung disease in preterm babies or Wilson-Mikity syndrome. More information on these conditions can be found in advanced textbooks on neonatal and paediatric care.

The emphasis for respiratory conditions should be on prevention, early diagnosis, early appropriate intervention and symptomatic, supportive or corrective management. In some institutions it may mean the early identification of warning signs, resuscitation and referral to a tertiary institution. The main reason for this is that the survival of all the other organs relies heavily on the proper functioning of the respiratory system.

Cardiovascular conditions

Introduction

The cardiovascular system refers to the structures and functions necessary for perfusion of all the systems of the body. These systems all rely on the cardiovascular system to provide the blood supply with oxygen and nutrients. It is therefore critical for survival. In addition this system plays a major role in the removal of waste products, such as carbon dioxide, ureum, creatinine, excess hydrogen and toxins.

The assessment of the infant's cardiovascular system needs to be understood by taking the following into consideration:
▶ The interrelated effect of all the different systems.
▶ The normal anatomical development of the different systems.
▶ The adaptation from fetal circulation to normal circulation.
▶ The compensation of the cardiovascular system for an increased demand of oxygen and nutrition, as well as any other disturbance of internal homeostasis.
▶ The normal mechanisms of blood pressure maintenance.
▶ The difference between the pulmonary and systemic blood supply.
▶ Conduction of the heart.

The special investigations used to confirm or reject a diagnosis or to monitor the progress or response to treatment include chest X-rays, electrocardiography (ECG), ultrasonography (cardiac sonar) and radiological studies with contrast medium (cardiac catheterisation).

Management

The management of cardiovascular problems is mainly aimed at perfusion of the systems. Methods to enhance perfusion are stress reduction, minimising the oxygen and nutrient demands and maintaining the blood pressure, by implementing Developmentally Supportive Care and maintaining internal homeostasis.

Cardiovascular assistance is the replacement of volume in order to increase blood pressure, pharmacological support of blood pressure, interventions to adjust cardiac conduction, such as administration of drugs or cardioversion, and surgical correction of deformities.

The common cardiovascular conditions will now be discussed, as well as those that need immediate recognition and intervention in order to ensure the survival of the baby.

Blood pressure deviations

Infant blood pressure determines the amount of perfusion taking place in all the organs and tissue, and therefore the supply of oxygen and nutrients to the tissue. Normal blood pressure is the result of cooperation between several organs and internal homeostasis, which is maintained by a very complicated system of feedback and compensation. This regulatory process involves the following organs:
▶ the hypothalamus-pituitary-axis
▶ medulla oblongata
▶ thyroid gland
▶ adrenal cortex
▶ kidneys
▶ heart
▶ vascular system.

An accurate measurement of blood pressure can be obtained with an electronic blood pressure monitor. The ordinary baumonometer may be used for efficient measurement if care is taken to ensure the blood pressure cuff covers at least two thirds of the upper arm or the upper leg being used to measure the blood pressure.

Blood pressure deviations are referred to as decreased blood pressure or hypotension, and increased blood pressure or hypertension based on the calculations on page 31-19. Various factors can influence the blood pressure. A normal newborn, however, should be able to compensate and correct blood pressure deviations to ensure perfusion to all systems.

Determining infant blood pressure

Mean blood pressure (BP) is calculated as follows:

$$\text{Mean BP} = \frac{(\text{Systolic BP} + 2\ (\text{Diastolic BP}))}{3}$$

A practical quick reference to determine the baby's blood pressure status is as follows:

▶ The minimum mean blood pressure should be equal or more than the baby's corrected gestational age.

▶ The maximum mean blood pressure should be less than the corrected gestational age plus 30 mmHg.

▶ For example: The baby was born at 27 weeks gestational age and is now one week old. His corrected gestational age is therefore 28 weeks. The mean blood pressure then has to be between 28 mmHg and (28 weeks + 30 mmHg) = 58 mmHg.

Hypertension

Hypertension is most often caused by the following conditions:

▶ Renovascular anomalies.
▶ Intrinsic renal disease.
▶ Endocrine disorders.
▶ Medications
▶ Fluid overload.
▶ Cardiac defects with decreased pulmonary blood flow.
▶ Cardiac failure.

Hypertension is usually asymptomatic, until the signs and symptoms of haemorrhage or other complications appear. These signs and symptoms will depend on the particular area of haemorrhage or the particular organ that is affected. The outcomes related to hypertension may include intracranial haemorrhage, cerebrovascular incidents, cardiac failure and retinopathy of prematurity. Hypertension can easily be diagnosed though if the infant's blood pressure is monitored.

Treatment of hypertension as such includes fluid and/or sodium restriction, usually 150 ml/kg every 24 hours; diuretics such as *hydrochlorothiazide, spironolactone* or *furosemide,* and antihypertensive drugs, such as *hydralazine* or *propranolol,* prescribed by the attending physician.

Hypotension

Hypotension is also uncommon but it may be caused by the following conditions:

▶ Neurological damage, especially where the hypothalamus and medulla oblongata are involved.
▶ Dehydration or hypovolaemia.
▶ Medication.
▶ Sometimes due to cardiac conditions with pulmonary hypertension.
▶ Cardiac failure in a late/severe stage.
▶ The most common cause though is if the baby is in shock and may be beyond the compensatory phase of progressive shock (with failure of the compensatory mechanisms), or in refractory shock which is characterised by multi-organ failure and death (see pages 31-4 and 31-5).

A preterm newborn with immature vasoconstriction ability will have a tendency to develop hypotension. This has to be kept under control by preventing it from dropping lower than the lower limit for normal mean blood pressure as previously mentioned. Note that a preterm or very ill baby's blood pressure will be more easily influenced by factors such as stress or any cause that increases the demand for oxygen. If a cardiac defect is present with pulmonary hypertension, the probability is high for presentation with a relatively low systemic blood pressure.

Hypotension is characterised by general lack of energy and activities, poor capillary refill and often pallor or cyanosis. Hypotension can contribute to the failure of any organ or even multi-organ failure.

Treatment of hypotension may include:

▶ Fluid boluses with volume expanders, such as Ringer's lactate or normal saline 10 to 20 ml/kg over 20 to 30 minutes.
▶ Increased fluid administration of usually

180 to 200 ml/kg every 24 hours, depending on the infant's other clinical features.

▶ Administering inotropic agents such as *dopamine*, *dobutamine* or *isoproterenol*.

▶ The monitoring of the baby's vital signs is essential, as well as his intake and output.

With the above in mind, the critical healthcare issue with blood pressure maintenance will be to prevent any deviations, as it may be too late to wait until the deviation is obvious. Management would include:

▶ proper monitoring
▶ stress reduction
▶ maintenance of internal homeostasis
▶ accurate calculation and administration of fluid and nutrition
▶ proper medication management.

It is especially significant to diagnose and treat the underlying problem, as in the case of a cardiac defect with pulmonary hypertension, where more damage may be done through treating the systemic hypotension and thus aggravating the pulmonary hypertension. The blood pressure deviations have to return to normal limits, but it should be done gradually and in a stable manner over a few hours and not too sudden, as sudden changes or fluctuations put the baby at risk for intracranial haemorrhage.

Cardiac failure

The heart is one of the first functional organs in embryonic life. It is a hollow organ that fills with blood and pumps the blood out to the lungs and the systemic circulation. The function of the SA-node, conductive tissue and cardiac muscles is dependent on proper internal homeostasis in order to maintain effective conduction and contraction, as well as the ability to compensate for increased oxygen demands.

Cardiac failure without enlargement of the heart

Cardiac failure refers to an inability of the cardiac muscle to adjust to maintain normal blood pressure in order to meet the body's demand for oxygen and nutrients. Cardiac failure without enlargement of the heart can be caused by the following conditions:

▶ arrhythmias
▶ severe anaemia
▶ hypoxia
▶ acidosis
▶ electrolyte disturbances
▶ severe dehydration
▶ hypotension
▶ sepsis
▶ toxins
▶ medication, such as digitalis toxicity
▶ hypoglycaemia.

In the presence of these disturbances the cardiac muscle cannot continue to function effectively and indefinitely. Perfusion to all the organs decreases if the cardiac muscle loses its ability for effective contractions and consequently all of the organs deteriorate. Cardiac failure usually develops over a period of time, varying from a few hours to a few weeks, depending on the specific cause. If the cause is hypoxia, it may even be within minutes. The reduced perfusion is characterised by neurological deterioration resulting in a lethargic infant, initial tachycardia, tachypnoea, cool skin, poor peripheral perfusion, metabolic acidosis, and signs of stress and later unresponsiveness, hypotension, bradycardia and shock. It can result in death.

Congestive cardiac failure

Congestive cardiac failure is a dysfunctional cardiac muscle associated with enlargement of the heart. The causes are most commonly structural cardiac defects that affect the volumes and/or pressures involved during cardiac contractions. Other causes include fluid overload, renal dysfunction, hypertension and persistent fetal circulation. It is characterised by the signs and symptoms of cardiac failure, as well as cardiomegaly, hepatomegaly and failure-to-thrive. The progress is usually gradual.

Problems related to adjustment from fetal to adult circulation

The foramen ovale and ductus arteriosus are part of the normal fetal circulation (see Chapter 29). The foramen ovale is an opening in the atrial septum that allows blood flow from the right atrium to the left atrium, ventricle, aorta and ultimately to the placenta for oxygenation, while 'bypassing' the pulmonary circulation. The ductus arteriosus is a vessel between the pulmonary arterial system and the descending aorta which facilitates blood flow so that it 'bypasses' the lungs and flows to the placenta for oxygenation. Both the foramen ovale and the ductus arteriosus close and no longer function after birth due to the following combination of factors present as the newborn adapts to extra-uterine life:

▶ The decrease in pulmonary resistance if the lung fluid is expressed and the lungs are filled with air facilitates blood flow through the pulmonary circulation.

▶ A decreased pressure in the right atrium and an increased pressure in the left atrium result in the functional closure of the foramen ovale.

▶ The ductus arteriosus closes functionally if the resistance and the blood pressure in the lungs decrease after birth. Increased levels of oxygen are also a potent stimulant for constriction and closure of the ductus arteriosus.

The closure of the foramen ovale and the ductus arteriosus play a key role in the facilitation of distinct pulmonary and systemic circulations, with the pulmonary circulation's blood pressure approximately five times lower than that of the systemic circulation.

Patent ductus arteriosus

A *patent ductus arteriosus* occurs when the ductus arteriosus remains functional after birth. It is commonly due to increased

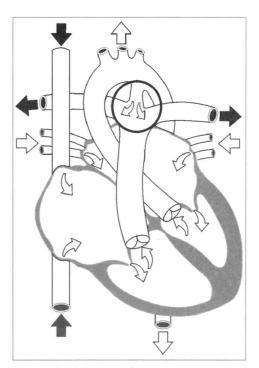

Figure 31.2 A: Patent ductus arteriosus

pulmonary blood pressure associated with structural cardiac defects or some respiratory conditions, which force blood flow through the ductus arteriosus from the lungs into the aorta and the systemic circulation. It may also be possible that the ductus arteriosus remains open if the systemic blood pressure is much higher (more than five times), than the pulmonary blood pressure. This may be the case with structural cardiac defects with pulmonary hypotension, which force blood flow through the ductus arteriosus from the aorta into the lungs. Other factors responsible for a patent ductus arteriosus are systemic hypertension, as in for example, with a fluid overload, and hypoxia which prevents constriction of the smooth muscles of the ductus, especially if the smooth muscles are immature as is the case with a preterm infant.

Patent foramen ovale

A *patent foramen ovale* refers to the foramen ovale that remains functional after birth. It is commonly found if the blood pressure in the right atrium remains high. It is most often caused by pulmonary hypertension either due to structural cardiac defects or respiratory conditions such as persistent pulmonary hypertension of the newborn. The result will be right-to-left shunt of blood via the foramen ovale.

Persistent fetal circulation

Persistent fetal circulation refers to the combination of both a patent ductus arteriosus and foramen ovale after birth. The most common causes appear to be prematurity and hypoxia, but it is also associated with several cardiac defects and syndromes such as:

▶ Pulmonary atresia.
▶ Congenital rubella syndrome.
▶ The effect of certain medications such as *indomethacin*, prostaglandins and *aminophylline*.
▶ Fluid overload where there is a wrong calculation or regulation of the baby's total fluid.

Persistant fetal circulation, or only a patent ductus arteriosus or foramen ovale, may however be life saving when it occurs simultaneously with some of the structural cardiac defects. Pulmonary atresia, for example, is where a patent foramen ovale is the only exit for blood from the right atrium and the only blood flow to the lungs is facilitated through the patent ductus arteriosus. These patients will not have any chance for survival without a persistant fetal circulation.

The clinical features and outcomes may vary and depend on the direction of blood flow and the associated pressures, as well as their specific causes. Most often it is initially asymptomatic, but gradually deteriorates with the clinical features of respiratory failure due to pulmonary hypertension, or cardiac failure due to cardiac overload. Initially there would be no murmur present. The common signs and symptoms later on include:

▶ An audible 'waterfall-like' murmur.
▶ Bouncing peripheral pulses.
▶ Relatively big differences in upper-limb and lower-limb blood pressures (more than 20 mmHg).
▶ Failure-to-thrive.
▶ Bronchopulmonary dysplasia.
▶ Chronic pulmonary infections.

The diagnosis is usually based on the clinical features and the observation of increased vasculature of the lungs on X-rays and cardiac ultrasonography.

The focus of treatment for persistent fetal circulation, patent ductus arteriosus and patent foramen ovale is the prevention of risk factors such as preterm birth, hypoxic incidents and fluid overload. Proper assessment, early diagnosis and early appropriate intervention will be the next step if it could not be prevented, or at least referral to a centre where advanced care can be provided. Cardiac ultrasonography within 24 hours after birth is recommended for a preterm infant to facilitate early diagnosis if the facilities are available. Appropriate interventions include stress reduction, fluid restriction (usually 150 ml/kg/24), prevention and/or management of disturbances of internal homeostasis and respiratory support. The decision to use pharmacological or surgical interventions to close the ductus arteriosus and/or foramen ovale or to keep it patent, is based on the associated problems, e.g. it will be kept open if the baby's survival depends on it. The ductus arteriosus can be kept patent with the administration of prostaglandins. The ductus arteriosus can usually be closed by administering oxygen, *ibuprofen* or *indomethacin*, but in some cases it has to be closed surgically.

The outcomes are mainly determined by the specific causes, associated problems and/or results of surgery. Spontaneous closure of the foramen ovale and/or ductus arteriosus is possible if the opening is not very big. The outcomes may be worse if there has been a delay in the diagnosis and treatment, and respiratory and/or cardiac failure are present. However, with early and appropriate intervention the outcomes are usually good.

Cardiac and great vessel structural defects

At three weeks after conception the heart has already begun forming and it is pumping at four weeks post-conception. From five to eight weeks the left and right sides of the heart divide, followed by the division between the atria and ventricles (or the upper and lower parts of the heart), division between the aorta and pulmonary artery, the development of the pulmonary veins and the different cardiac valves. The vascular system then subsequently develops rapidly and the fetal circulation is formed and functional at approximately eight weeks after conception. The placenta plays a very important role in fetal circulation but the infant has to adjust from fetal circulation to normal circulation at birth (see Chapter 29).

The *cardiac structural defects* are abnormal development of the cardiac structures, which may be because of chromosomal abnormalities,

such as Trisomy 13, 18 and 21, or some genetic abnormalities, like DiGeorge syndrome. Other causes include several multifactoral or environmental congenital conditions such as congenital TORCH-infections, fetal alcohol syndrome, maternal use of thalidomide, anticonvulsants, anticoagulants and antineoplastic medications. A high risk factor may be the mother's lifestyle as these abnormalities develop at the time when the mother is usually unaware of her pregnant status.

Respiratory distress appears in circumstances where there is an increased demand for oxygen, such as during stress, feeding and crying. These conditions are often undetected until it is too late. It has to be identified early and referred for follow-up treatment.

Based on the clinical appearance of the newborn after birth (after adaptation from fetal circulation to adult circulation), the defects can be classified into two main groups:

◗ *Acyanotic defects* are cardiac defects that may initially be asymptomatic, but gradually result in cardiac failure. If it is associated with pulmonary hypertension, the infant gradually develops respiratory oedema and respiratory failure.

♦ *Acyanotic cardiac defects with pulmonary hypertension* include hypoplastic left-heart syndrome, atrial septal defects, ventricular septal defects, atrioventricular canal or endocardial cushion defect, and coarctation of the aorta.

♦ *Acyanotic cardiac defects with pulmonary hypotension* includes a small stenosis of the pulmonary artery or one of the branches, and structural defects of the pulmonary vascular system affecting only a part of the lung, for example one lobe.

◗ *Cyanotic defects* result in mixing of oxygen-enriched blood with oxygen-depleted blood and thus there is decreased saturation and central cyanosis. As the infant is continuously in a relative state of hypoxia and has increased levels of carbon dioxide, he will compensate for the oxygen demand with increased heart rate and respiratory rate. A distinctive characteristic is that the baby's condition does not really improve with administration of additional oxygen. It worsens if there is any additional demand for oxygen, during oral feeding for example, or hypothermia, stress and pain. The baby tends to be lethargic with failure-to-thrive and there is slow recovery after incidents or interventions. Eventually respiratory and cardiac failure with disturbances of internal homeostasis, such as hypothermia, and acidosis, occur.

The cyanotic cardiac conditions can be further classified in terms of increased or decreased pulmonary blood flow. The implications of increased blood flow to the pulmonary system or pulmonary hypertension are decreased gas exchange and respiratory distress. The combination of a cyanotic cardiac condition and respiratory distress worsens the infant's condition, lessens his ability to compensate and adds to disturbances of internal homeostasis.

✦ Common examples of *cyanotic cardiac defects with pulmonary hypertension* include transposition of the great vessels, total anomalous pulmonary venous connection and truncus arteriosus. They are usually associated with low systemic blood pressure in addition to the above signs and symptoms.

✦ Examples of the *cyanotic cardiac defects with pulmonary hypotension* include tetralogy of Fallot, tricuspid atresia, pulmonary stenosis and pulmonary atresia. These are characterised by the above-mentioned signs and symptoms with normal or increased blood pressure.

The diagnosis for these conditions is based on the clinical picture, cardiac sounds, chest X-rays, cardiac ultrasonography and/or cardiac catheterisation.

The main nursing issues are stress reduction to lessen the demand for compensation and appropriate support to provide in the demand for oxygen and nutrition. Mainte-

nance of internal homeostasis is therefore crucial, as well as provision of additional oxygen supply as needed and pharmacological support. Counselling and support would be a key in preparing the parents for the long-term outcomes, which may vary from limited to life-threatening complications or even mortality.

Acyanotic cardiac defects

Hypoplastic left ventricle syndrome occurs with failure of the mitral valve to develop between the left atrium and left ventricle and consequently there is a lack of blood flow through the aorta to the systemic circulation and an underdeveloped left ventricle. The foramen ovale remains patent with shunting from the left atrium to the right atrium and right ventricle, resulting in hypertrophy of the right ventricle. An increase in the volume of blood pumped to the lungs leads to pulmonary hypertension. Oxygen-enriched blood flows back to the left atrium to repeat the route. The baby's survival depends on the patent ductus

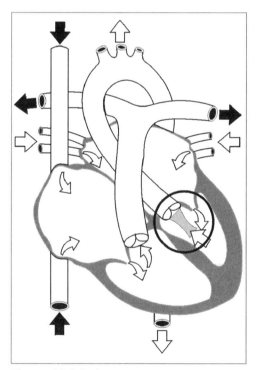

Figure 31.2 B: Aortic stenosis

arteriosus which shunts oxygen-enriched blood into the aorta and the systemic circulation. The infant will therefore initially be acyanotic but will gradually present with systemic hypotension, respiratory distress and right cardiac failure.

Aortic atresia is the complete obstruction of the aortic valve and aortic stenosis refers to a partial obstruction. The outcome of both these conditions is a lack of blood being pumped into the systemic circulation, resulting in hypotension. The accumulating blood in the left ventricle leads to increased pressure in the left ventricle and later hypertrophy, as well as in the left atrium. The foramen ovale remains patent with blood shunting from the left atrium to the right atrium due to the high pressure in the left atrium. The increased volume in the right chambers will lead to increased blood flow to the lungs and cause pulmonary hypertension and a patent ductus arteriosus that allows some oxygen-enriched blood to flow into the aorta and the systemic circulation. The infant is initially acyanotic with systemic

hypotension but his condition will deteriorate to respiratory and cardiac failure.

Atrial septal defect is the failure of the atria to divide completely, resulting in communication or shunting between the atria. The pressures in both atria are initially very similar, but the pressure in the right atria gradually decreases after birth, resulting in blood shunting from the left atrium to the right atrium. The increased volume in the right chambers leads to pulmonary hypertension and right cardiac hypertrophy that deteriorates to respiratory and cardiac failure. It is often confused with a patent foramen ovale, which is a temporary opening with the ability to close if the pressures are suitable.

A *ventricular septal defect* occurs when defective division of the ventricles leaves an opening between the ventricles of various sizes. The bigger the opening, the worse the shunting is from the one ventricle to the other. The direction of flow is determined by blood flowing from the

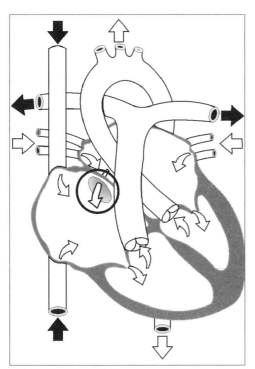

Figure 31.2 C: Artrial septal defect

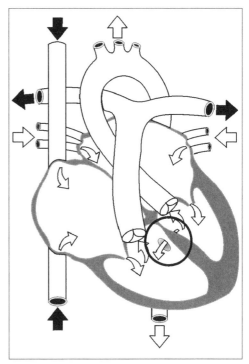

Figure 31.2 D: Ventricular septal defect

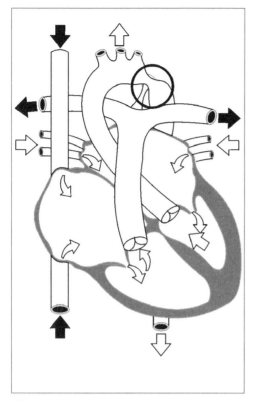

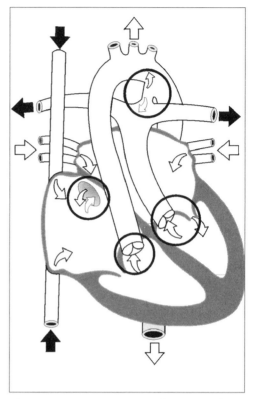

Figure 31.2 E: Coarctation of aorta

Figure 31.2 F: Transposition of great vessels

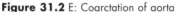

highest pressure to the lowest pressure that is usually from the left ventricle to the right ventricle, resulting in increased flow to the lungs and pulmonary hypertension, and gradual respiratory and cardiac failure. Ventricular septal defect is commonly associated with other cardiac defects.

Coarctation of the aorta refers to the constriction of the aorta. It is most commonly found in the aortic arch before the ductus arteriosus. The blood pressure in the aortic arch, the left atrium and left ventricle is high with high blood pressure in the right arm or both arms, while the blood pressure in the lower limbs, or the left arm and lower limbs is significantly lower, depending on the location of the coarctation. The blood pressure in both arms is relatively high and significantly lower in the lower limbs if the coarctation is found after

the ductus arteriosus. The pulmonary pressures depend on the patency of the ductus arteriosus, which is commonly patent resulting in pulmonary hypertension, especially if the coarctation is located after the ductus arteriosus.

Cyanotic cardiac defects

Transposition of the great vessels is a defect where the aorta arises from the right ventricle and the pulmonary artery from the left ventricle. If the transposition is the only abnormality, the baby will have two parallel blood circulations that are not connected. Blood will flow from the lungs to the left atrium, the left ventricle and via the displaced pulmonary artery back to the lungs with oxygen-enriched blood and at increased pressure. Concurrently the systemic circulation's blood will flow to the right atrium, the right

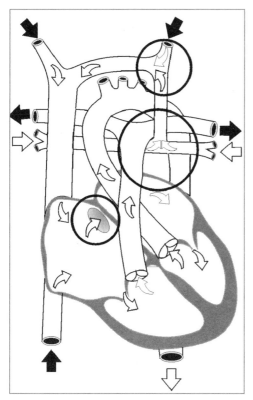

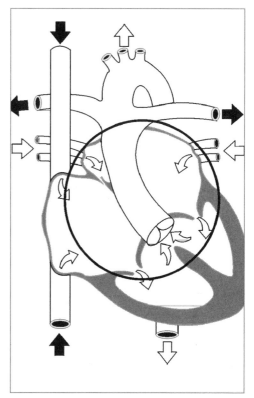

Figure 31.2 G: Total anomalous pulmonary venous return

Figure 31.2 H: Truncus arteriosus

ventricle and via the displaced aorta back into the systemic flow with oxygen-depleted blood. Babies with this condition, however, usually have other associated abnormalities, such as a ventricular and/or atrial septal defect, that aid survival because they allow mixing of oxygen-enriched and oxygen-depleted blood in the ventricle or atrium, as well as a patent ductus arteriosus that accommodates flow from the lungs to the systemic circulation. The increased pulmonary blood pressure remains a problem though.

Total anomalous pulmonary venous connection occurs when the pulmonary veins drain oxygenated blood directly or indirectly into the right atrium instead of the left atrium. It means that the oxygen-enriched blood from the lungs and the oxygen-depleted blood from the system are mixed in the right

atrium, and all return to the lungs, resulting in severe pulmonary hypertension and systemic hypotension. The infant's survival depends on the presence of a patent foramen ovale or atrial septal defect to allow some of the mixed blood to enter the left atrium, or via a patent ductus arteriosus to the systemic circulation.

Truncus arteriosus is the result of incomplete or abnormal division of the pulmonary artery and the aorta during organogenesis. As it is impossible for division of the ventricles if the pulmonary artery and aorta are not separated, a ventricular septal defect will also be present. The truncus or common artery usually overrides the ventricular septal defect, resulting in mixing of oxygen-enriched blood from the lungs and the oxygen-depleted blood from the system. The mixed blood is pumped through

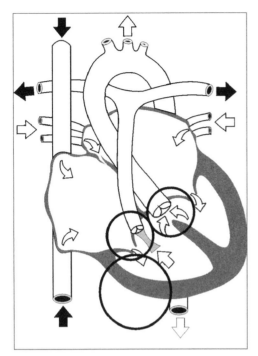

Figure 31.2 I: Tetralogy of Fallot

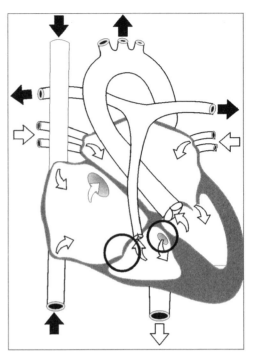

Figure 31.2 J: Tricuspid artresia

the common trunk supplying both the lungs and the systemic circulation. The biggest problem is related to the blood pressure that is the same in both circulations, which leads to severe pulmonary hypertension with systemic hypotension and results in respiratory and cardiac failure.

Tetralogy of Fallot is characterised by the combination of four cardiac defects:

- A ventricular septal defect.
- Stenosis of the pulmonary artery.
- The aorta overriding the ventricular septal defect.
- Hypertrophy of the right ventride.

Blood flow to the pulmonary circulation is very limited with consequent pulmonary hypotension and reduced oxygen-enriched blood, with mixing of oxygen-enriched blood from the lungs and the oxygen-depleted blood from the system through the ventricular septal defect. This results in cyanosis and hypoxia, with the systemic blood pressure normal to high.

Tricuspid atresia is the failure of the tricuspid valve to develop between the right atrium and right ventricle. This results in the inability of blood flow to the right ventricle with a consequent hypoplastic right ventricle, persistence of a patent foramen ovale and pulmonary blood flow only accommodated by a patent ductus arteriosus. The baby's condition is better if a ventricular septal defect is present in order to allow some blood shunting from the left to the right ventricle to flow through the pulmonary artery to the lungs.

Pulmonary stenosis is a partial structural obstruction of the pulmonary artery's valve and *pulmonary atresia* is a complete structural obstruction of the valve. In the case of a stenosis, there will be limited blood flow to the lungs, while there will be no blood flow through the pulmonary artery in the case of atresia. In both cases the infant's survival depends on the patency of the ductus arteriosus to contribute to pulmonary blood flow to provide oxygen-enriched blood. The foramen ovale often remains patent with shunting from

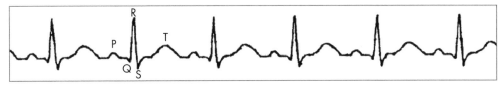

Figure 31.3 A normal electrocardiography

the right to the left atrium. Pulmonary hypotension with decreased oxygenation is present in spite of a patent ductus arteriosus, resulting in hypoxia and cyanosis with a normal to high systemic blood pressure.

Cardiac conduction abnormalities

Conduction of the heart develops from approximately three to four weeks and the conduction system's functionality increases in order to have normal sinus rhythm by 16 weeks in utero. A normal sinus rhythm at birth varies between 120 to 160 bpm, with a very quick response in rate to compensate for any changes in homeostasis, sleep, position or stress.

In normal cardiac conduction there is a spontaneous rhythmic discharge of electrical impulses from the sinu-atrial node (SA-node). The electrical impulses follow a specified conduction route to depolarise the cardiac muscle cells from the SA-node via the atria, atrioventricular node, bundle of His through the Purkinje fibres to the ventricular muscle, causing contraction of the cardiac muscle. Blood is pumped into the systemic circulation from the left ventricle, and into the pulmonary circulation from the right ventricle. Depolarisation is followed by repolarisation and relaxation of the cardiac muscle. This results in blood flowing from the systemic circulation into the right atrium and from the pulmonary circulation into the left atrium. The sequence is repeated to create and maintain blood pressure.

The normal conduction is reflected on an electrocardiography (ECG) as a P-wave that represents atrial depolarisation, followed by a QRS-complex that represents ventricular depolarisation, and then a T-wave that repre-

sents repolarisation of the ventricles. Other features of importance are the rate and regularity, the intervals, the sizes of the different waves and their deviations (positive or negative) from the baseline.

Abnormalities of cardiac conduction are disturbances related to electrical conduction of the cardiac nerve supply, which result in decreased cardiac function. They may either take the form of *abnormal rates*, such as bradycardia and tachycardia, or *disturbed rhythms* as in arrhythmias and heart blocks. Probable causes may include:

- Congenital inheritance, such as a congenital heart block.
- The effects of drugs, for example digitalis toxicity and epinephrine.
- Electrolyte disturbances, especially potassium and calcium.
- Other disturbances of internal homeostasis such as hypoxia, hypoglycemia and acidosis.

Abnormalities in the electrical cardiac conduction decrease the efficacy of the heart, decrease the blood pressure and therefore decrease perfusion to all the systems with a decrease in their effective function. The diagnosis is based mainly on the history, the clinical picture of the infant and a 3-lead and/or 12-lead electrocardiography.

Deviations include *tachycardia* or a heart rate of more than 160 bpm; *bradycardia* or a heart rate less than 100 bpm; *atrial flutter*; *atrial fibrillation*; *nodal rhythm*; *ventricular rhythm*; *ventricular flutter*; *ventricular fibrillation* and *ventricular tachycardia*. Other abnormalities include *atrial* and *ventricular extrasystoles*; the various heart blocks, i.e. first-, second- and third-degree heart block, and *bundle branch blocks*; the abnormalities

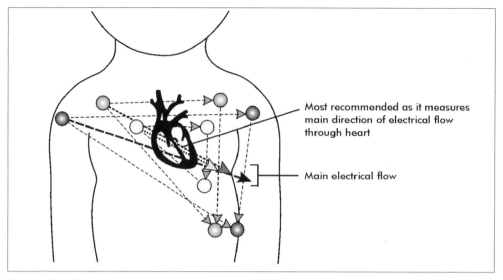

Most recommended as it measures main direction of electrical flow through heart

Main electrical flow

Figure 31.4 The position of ECG stickers

related to electrolyte disturbances, especially hypokalaemia, hyperkalaemia, hypocalcaemia and hypercalcaemia, and digitalis-toxicity.

The baby's clinical features are worsened in correlation with the severity of the deviation and the impact of this on contractility and blood pressure, varying from insignificant to mortality. Common initial signs and symptoms include lethargy, inability to feed, slow recovery after interventions or incidents and signs of stress. The longer the deviation persists, the worse the outcome will be, which includes a failure-to-thrive, respiratory failure, cardiac failure and finally multi-organ failure. The infant's condition becomes life-threatening if the heart rate exceeds 200 bpm, if it is less than 80 bpm or if there is *pulseless electrical activity*, i.e. electrical impulses are present, but the heart is unable to contract in order to create a blood pressure. *Asystole* is the failure or absence of electrical activity and is usually the result of a prolonged cardiac problem, hypoglycaemia, hypoxia, acidosis, pulmonary hypertension, hypothermia or any other cause of shock.

Important aspects of care for cardiac con-duction abnormalities, are early referral and diagnosis and to minimise the need for compensation by reducing stress. Early diagnosis can be done by interpreting at least one 3-lead ECG as part of the assessment of any newborn with special needs, irrespective of the risk factors. The 3-lead ECG can be done with a cardiac monitor, but it is vital to stick the ECG-stickers correctly so as to obtain a proper ECG pattern (see Figure 31.4). Referral is very important if any abnormalities are observed. The care of the baby thereafter depends on the particular abnormality.

In the functioning of the body the cardio-vascular system has a principal role and any defect or abnormality may therefore impact on all the other systems. The clinical pictures of these defects are not always that easy to recognise. They require careful observations, including the infant's ability to feed without deterioration, to obtain the blood pressure of all four limbs at least once, and to observe the ECG-pattern if any of the clinical pictures discussed are present. Early detection with early referral or intervention can thus help to prevent major complications.

Neurological conditions

Neurological disorders are common in the neonatal period, but they are often missed because of the difficulty in assessing the neurological system and its complexity. They are related to anatomical disorders and/or functional or physiological problems. The anatomy of the neurological system refers to the skull and vertebrae, the cerebral cortex, the midbrain and brainstem, the peripheral nervous system and the cerebral fluid system. In the neurological system the functions involve the sensory, motor, autonomic and the higher brain functions such as thoughts and emotions, which are all closely linked to the different body functions.

The neurological system is one of the first systems to develop but it is one of the last to mature (refer to Chapter 29 on the physical assessment of the neurological system). It is a very vulnerable system, which can be severely affected by injury and has limited ability to recover. The neurological system is sensitive to hypoxia, hyperoxia, increased levels of carbon dioxide, hypoglycaemia, hypothermia, hypotension or hypoperfusion, acidosis or alkalosis, fluid and electrolyte disturbances, as well as any accumulation of waste products such as ureum and creatinine, and therefore disturbances of internal homeostasis. In addition, it is sensitive to mechanical injury caused by pressure, sharp objects, prolonged vibration, friction and heat.

Increased intracranial pressure

Increased intracranial pressure can be the result of a number of cranial or neurological conditions including haemorrhage, injury, hydrocephalus, craniosynostosis and spina bifida. It usually presents with vague or general signs and symptoms including irritability, restlessness, bulging fontanelle, vomiting and lethargy. Systemic signs and symptoms include tachycardia and tachypnoea, and later on shock with bradypnoea and bradycardia. The important principles of management are to reduce stress and activity, to encourage slow handling and position changes (see DSC), as well as to position the infant in semi-Fowler's and to sedate him if restlessness is observed.

Several congenital abnormalities of the neurological system can be prevented by quality preconceptional care, especially by supplementing nutrition with folic acid and iron, maintaining a well-balanced diet, eliminating harmful substances such as alcohol, nicotine, drugs, radiation and preventing viral infections, especially the TORCH-infections (see Chapter 19 for preconception care).

The principles of management for the neurological system

▸ Protect the vulnerable areas or functions by applying Developmentally Supportive Care principles, such as reducing stressors, minimal and appropriate handling, appropriate positioning and pain management.

▸ Prevent problems or complications by maintaining internal homeostasis, especially the oxygenation, acid-base homeostasis, fluid and electrolyte homeostasis, blood pressure, nutritional status and thermoregulation.

▸ Stimulate functions appropriately to maintain them, with non-nutritive sucking for feeding, for example.

▸ Refer for surgical corrections in order to obtain maximum function, for example the insertion of a ventrico-peritoneal shunt for hydrocephaly.

▸ Use pharmacology to improve the condition, such as anticonvulsants for epilepsy.

▸ Initiate rehabilitation as soon as possible, such as occupational therapy, physiotherapy or speech-language therapy.

▸ Involve and educate the parents.

A principle that needs to be kept in mind for long-term outcomes of the neurological system is 'if you do not use it, you will lose it, but if you abuse it, you will also lose it'. It implies that specific neurological functions need appropriate stimulation or positive stimulation such as non-nutritive sucking to maintain the sucking reflex for feeding and to create positive oral associations (refer to Chapter 29 on DSC). 'Abuse', overstimulation or negative stimulation of the mouth and surrounding area may often occur, for example, by suctioning, intubation, routine cleaning of the mouth and nose and foul-tasting medication. A lack of stimulation of the sucking reflex, together with negative oral associations, result in an inability and reluctance of the infant to suck and feed after a period of illness. It can, however, be prevented with appropriate stimulation. The same applies for various other neurological functions.

Special investigations used for the neurological system include X-rays, cranial ultrasonography or brain sonar, electroechography (EEG), computed tomography (CT-scan), magnetic resonance imaging (MRI) and lumbar puncture (LP).

The most common conditions will be briefly discussed in the following sections, but bear in mind that the neurological system is a very complex system and there are many more conditions which can be studied in advanced neonatal nursing textbooks.

Intracranial bleeding

The growth of blood vessels or vascularisation into the membranes of the brain takes place with brain development from the embryonic phase, but it is vulnerable even at full term. Between 28 and 32 weeks when there is a 'growth spurt' of vascularisation the blood vessels are most vulnerable. A temporary capillary network, known as the germinal matrix, develops during this peak growth period and then disintegrates later to become part of the connective tissue. They are situated next to the ventricles in the brain. The vessel walls of the germinal matrix are thin and fragile, and are highly dependant on oxygen metabolism.

Subdural and subarachnoid bleeding

Mechanical pressure or injury from a Wrigley's forceps delivery, for example (one of the top ten causes of death of babies in South Africa), can easily cause rupture to the vulnerable blood vessels in the membranes of the brain. A *subdural bleeding* results if the bleeding is between the cerebral hemispheres and the skull, underneath the dura mater or outermost brain membrane. *Subarachnoid bleeding* refers to bleeding into the grooves of the cerebral hemispheres, known as the subarachnoid space.

The bleeding is aggravated by asphyxia or other internal disturbances. Cephalohaematoma or caput succedaneum may be present. Other signs and symptoms include:
- Bulging fontanelles.
- Neurological deterioration characterised by irritability or floppiness.
- Signs and symptoms of stress, such as tachycardia, tachypnoea and behavioural cues.
- Anaemia may also develop.

The outcome, however, depends on the location and degree of bleeding, as well as the duration and it can result in irreversible neurological damage. A brain sonar or CT scan is used to confirm the diagnosis and the main focus of treatment is the prevention of injuries during delivery, as well as prevention of disturbances of internal homeostasis as discussed on page 31-3.

Periventricular, intraventricular and intracerebellar bleeding/periventricular haemorrhage infarction

Periventricular, intraventricular and/or *intra-cerebellar bleeding* are associated with preterm birth, especially with the period between 28 to 32 weeks gestation age, as well as disturbances of internal homeostasis and cerebral blood flow changes. The vessel walls of the germinal matrix are easily damaged by hypoxia and other internal disturbances such as acidosis. The damaged vessels rupture easily when there are cerebral blood flow changes, which may be the result of hypoxia, hypercapnoea, hypoglycaemia, changes in blood pressure, hyperthermia, hyperthermia or sudden positional changes. A *periventricular* is when the bleeding remains in the area of the germinal matrix. *Intraventricular bleeding* occurs if the vessels are ruptured into the ventricle, while *intracerebellar bleeding* is when the bleeding extends into the cerebellum. They are all referred to as *periventricular haemorrhage infarction.*

The infant's clinical picture may vary from vague signs of stress (see Chapter 29) to severe shock (see pages 31-4 to 31-5) with signs of neurological deterioration and bulging of the fontanelles. Diagnosis will be confirmed with brain sonar or CT scan. Depending on the degree of bleeding, the outcome can vary from no complications at all to hypoxic-ischaemic encephalopathy or leucomalacia with permanent neurological damage.

Prevention is crucial, especially by maintaining internal homeostasis and preventing sudden changes in cerebral blood flow. Sedation has to be considered in some cases to reduce the risk of bleeding.

Hypoxic-ischaemic encephalopathy (periventricular leucomalacia)

A part of the development of the neurological system is an increase in the number of neurons, which peaks from 12 to 16 weeks. The neurons thereafter mainly grow and mature from the brain towards their end location, but do not increase further in number. From then the neural tissue has a very limited ability to regenerate, if damaged. The neurological system is highly dependent on aerobic metabolism of glucose, with a high sensitivity for disturbances of internal homeostasis, which may cause permanent damage. The following are considered to be damaging causes:

- Hypoglycaemia
- Hypoxia

- Increased carbon dioxide levels
- Acidosis
- Alkalosis
- Hypothermia
- Hypotension
- Fluctuating blood pressure
- Mechanical pressure causing bleeding or injury
- Other disturbances of internal homeostasis.

Hypoxic-ischaemic encephalopathy refers to irreversible general brain damage as a result of the previously listed causes. The infant presents initially with standard risk factors, irritability and stress cues and the condition then changes to lethargy, poor sucking, hypotonia and fluctuating breathing. It may worsen to seizures, unresponsiveness, apnoea and bradycardia and often results in mortality or survival with severe neurological disabilities.

Periventricular leucomalacia refers to irreversible damage of the white matter located next to the ventricles, where the germinal matrix develops during 28 to 32 weeks. It is often preceded by periventricular bleeding. The condition may initially be asymptomatic but is later characterised by weakness of lower limbs and motor spasticity. The long-term outcomes are often associated with motor disabilities, lower limb weakness, intellectual deficits and visual impairment.

The diagnosis is confirmed with brain sonar, CT scan or MRI. The main aim of the treatment for this condition is to prevent it by the maintenance of internal homeostasis (see page 31-3). If it could not be prevented, the focus will be on symptomatic treatment and referral for specialised rehabilitation.

Hydrocephalus

Cerebrospinal fluid (CSF) fills the intracranial ventricles and spinal cord, providing protection against mechanical pressure. It provides chemical protection as part of the blood–brain barrier and it is a transport medium for glucose, oxygen, carbon dioxide and the removal of waste products. CSF is produced by brain parenchyma, cerebral ventricles, areas along the spinal cord and the choroid plexus. The fluid circulates from the lateral ventricles to the third ventricle, the fourth ventricle, the spinal cord and the subarachnoid space where it is absorbed again. There is a fine balance between production and absorption. (Refer to an anatomy/physiology textbook for revision.)

Hydrocephalus is an excess of cerebrospinal fluid in the ventricles of the brain. It can be a result of any of the following:

▶ A decrease in absorption caused by congenital defects such as aquedactal stenosis or a Dandy-Walker cyst.
▶ Abnormalities due to TORCH infections or meningitis.
▶ An obstruction resulting from intraventricular bleeding.
▶ Excessive production which is usually inherited and very rare.

The signs and symptoms may be chronic or acute, with neurological signs of increased intracranial pressure (see page 31-31), an increase in the size of the head and signs of stress or shock. Sunset eyes may indicate neurological damage. Brain sonar, CT scan or MRI will confirm the diagnosis. The outcomes are determined by the severity and duration of the increased intracranial pressure, with a high mortality rate if not treated. With appropriate surgical intervention, such as ventriculo-peritoneal shunt, the outcomes are usually very good but have to be monitored in the long term.

The crucial principles in the management of hydrocephalus are the prevention of increased intracranial pressure, reducing stress (see Chapter 29) and early referral to a neurosurgeon for specialist treatment. Parental counselling and education are very important for long-term management.

Kernicterus

Unconjugated bilirubin is a result of red blood cell haemolysis and is fat-soluble so it can cross the blood–brain barrier. It is transported by albumin intravascularly and converted to conjugated bilirubin in the liver. Conjugated bilirubin is water-soluble, excreted by the bile and kidneys and it cannot cross the blood–brain barrier.

Kernicterus per definition means yellow staining and neuronal injury of the basal ganglia of the brain as a result of increased levels of unconjugated bilirubin that has crossed the blood–brain barrier. The high levels of unconjugated bilirubin can be caused by:

▶ Prematurity.
▶ Inefficient liver function due to liver immaturity.
▶ Illness of the liver.
▶ Haemolytic conditions, such as ABO/Rh incompatibilities.
▶ Congenital metabolic disorders, such as galactosaemia.
▶ Hypoalbuminaemia.
▶ Bacterial or viral infections.
▶ Disturbances of internal homeostasis, such as asphyxia, hypoxia and acidosis.

Signs and symptoms of kernicterus include jaundice, lethargy, high-pitched crying, weak sucking and hypotonia. Later on there is fever, hypertonia, opistotonus and upward gaze. The outcome of kernicterus is irreversible and usually includes hearing loss, cerebral palsy and mental retardation. Diagnosis is based on the clinical picture and confirmed when biochemical laboratory tests find high levels of unconjugated bilirubin.

Refer to page 31-66 regarding the treatment of hyperbilirubinemia in order to prevent kernicterus. If this is unsuccessful or it is too late, it may be necessary for a blood exchange transfusion to reduce the serum levels of unconjugated bilirubin.

Nerve injuries (cranial or peripheral)

Neuronal maturation occurs from the last trimester to several years postnatal. Nerves have a limited ability to regenerate once they are damaged. Injuries of the nerves can be caused by difficult labour and delivery, instrument-assisted delivery, abnormal presentation and pressure, such as infiltrated infusion, or by ischaemic injuries due to hypoxia or hypoperfusion. The injuries may involve cranial or peripheral nerves. Injuries may result in oedema and bleeding with temporary loss of function if the nerve is still intact. Permanent loss of function will result if the nerve is not intact or the soma of the nerve is injured.

The signs and symptoms will depend on the specific functions of the particular nerve which was lost, for example, paralysis or inability to move a muscle or group of muscles if it is a motor nerve; or paresthesia or lack of sense if it is a sensory nerve. It may be accompanied by intense pain, observed as restlessness, tachycardia, tachypnoea and other stress cues.

The main focus of management would be on prevention. If the condition could not be prevented, the emphasis is on early diagnosis and appropriate referral, to consult a neurologist for example. Further treatment may include protection of the affected area, such as:

▶ Pain management, stress reduction and appropriate positioning.
▶ Minimal stimulation if the cranial nerves are injured.
▶ To prevent complications due to lack of function, for example, to keep the eye closed and moist if it is a facial paralysis.
▶ To position a limb in anatomical position if it is a peripheral injury and by consulting a physiotherapist for specialist care.
▶ Follow-up treatment by a specialist, such as a neurologist, physiotherapist and occupational therapist for rehabilitation.

Seizures or convulsions

Neurological activity depends on the conduction of electrical impulses in the neurons. The conduction of impulses in turn relies on a suitable neuronal environment, including oxygenation, acid-base balance, nutrition, fluid and electrolyte balance and thermoregu-lation. If there are abnormalities in the neuronal conduction it can result in seizures or convulsions which are a symptom of an illness and not the disease itself.

Seizures or convulsions are involuntary and inappropriate motor responses due to excessive simultaneous electrical discharges in the neural tissue. The signs and symptoms may vary widely from unrecognisable or very slight, nearly unobservable twitches to clearly evident fits. There may be variations such as eye blinking or fluttering, rowing movements, smacking of lips, drooling, tonic extension or flexion of limbs, and jerking. The movements do not change, stop or respond to external stimuli, such as touch. Diagnosis is usually based on the history and an EEG. Other special investigations will be related to the possible causes such as genetic inheritance (epilepsy), acid-base disturbance, hypoxia, metabolic disturbances (such as hyperammonaemia), increased intracranial pressure, infections or withdrawal from maternal drugs.

The treatment and the outcomes are determined by the underlying cause. Keep in mind that the symptom and not the cause would be treated with the administration of anticonvulsant medication. It is therefore critical to arrange a referral for diagnosis and specialist treatment, to a paediatrician or neurologist.

Infections: Meningitis and encephalitis

The normal brain is protected against infection by a mature blood–brain barrier, as well as a mature immune system and internal homeostasis. The cellular lining of the blood–brain barrier or the meninges, develops from early in the first trimester but at full term it is still not fully matured and more permeable than that of an adult. During the peak growth of the germinal matrix at 28 to 32 weeks the blood supply to the brain increases. Any systemic infection, or microbes (bacterial, viral or fungal) that are then in contact with the vascular system have the potential to enter the brain and cause infection.

Meningitis is an infection of the meninges or the membranes that surround the brain. *Encephalitis* is an infection of the encephalon or brain tissue. The infection results in an inflammatory response with or without cell damage. It can contribute to increased intracranial pressure, seizures and other signs and symptoms of neurological deterioration, such as poor feeding, irritability or floppiness, inappropriate response to stimuli or unresponsiveness, as well as respiratory distress or apnoea, tachycardia and other disturbances of internal homeostasis, such as acidosis, hypothermia and hypotension. The infant demonstrates pain, flexion of the limbs and extension of the neck and the outcomes would be determined by the specific microbe/s involved and the effectiveness of treatment. Prognosis for viral and fungal infections is, however, usually very poor, often resulting in irreversible brain damage or death. Bacterial infections are easier to treat successfully with antibiotics and the baby may recover without complications, but they can also result in brain damage or mortality.

The diagnosis would be confirmed with brain sonar, CT scan or MRI, and blood tests such as blood cultures and CRP. An early diagnosis and treatment with broad-spectrum antibiotics would be very beneficial. Treatment should be reconsidered once the results of the cultures are available and further management of the condition should focus on preventing an increase in intracranial pressure, stress reduction (DSC), minimal handling and slow positional changes, semi-Fowler's position and maintaining internal homeostasis.

Neural tube defects

At three weeks the neural tube is formed and it is properly closed at four weeks gestational age, becoming the brain and spinal cord. Neural tube defects occur when the brain or spinal cord fail to close during this early developmental phase. The most common causes are:
▶ Chromosomal, such as Trisomy 18.
▶ Genetic, as in Meckel-Gruber syndrome.

▶ Multifactoral when there is a combination of genetically predisposed characteristics and folic acid and iron deficiency of the pregnant mother.

Encephalocele is an open area in the cranium or head which is usually covered with skin or mucous membranes but not with bone. *Spina bifida* is an opening in the spinal cord that bulges and is covered with skin or mucous membranes, containing cerebrospinal fluid only or neural tissue too. The skin and mucous membranes can rupture, resulting in a leakage of fluid. If there is a naevus in the midline of the spinal cord with hair on it, spina bifida is usually suspected, despite it being covered with skin and no bulging being present.

The prognosis depends on the location and amount of neural tissue involved, as well as whether there has been any damage. Encephalocele often results in brain damage or mortality and spina bifida often results in paralysis and/or hydrocephalus.

Prevention is paramount and all pregnant women should be instructed to follow a balanced diet with a supplement of folic acid and iron before and during pregnancy. Early diagnosis is otherwise of critical importance, as well as protection of the affected area against mechanical injury. Follow-up treatment would include referral to a neurosurgeon and genetic counselling.

Anencephaly and microcephaly

The peak development of the cerebral hemispheres is between 8 to 12 weeks. Abnormal development may be caused by genetic inheritance and multifactoral congenital disorders, especially associated with TORCH and HIV infections, maternal alcoholism and maternal cocaine abuse.

Anencephaly is the failure of development of the cerebral hemispheres during the embryonic phase. The upper third of the head is flattened with partial absence of skull. The infant can be a stillbirth or demonstrates only basic bodily functions without appropriate responses to external stimuli.

Microcephaly is partial development of the cerebral hemispheres resulting in a small upper third of the head with a high possibility of developmental delays.

Prevention is again crucial, especially the elimination of risk factors such as TORCH infections, alcohol and cocaine abuse. Once born, early diagnosis is critical, as well as genetic counselling and parental support. The main focus of management of the infant is on basic nursing care which supports the basic needs.

Craniosynostosis

The skull develops from early in the first trimester. At full term birth the different skull bones are joined, but not fixed, with the anterior and posterior fontanelles observable as gaps between the skull bones. The skull bones would still be mobile on assessment.

Craniosynostosis or preterm closure of the skull sutures may occur. The cause is not clear, but it results in the limitation of optimal brain growth. On assessment of the skull, the suture line/s may be prominent with an abnormal shape of the head. The fontanelles are most often closed as well. Later symptoms include signs of increased intracranial pres-

sure such as irritability, vomiting and lethargy, seizures and developmental delays in the long term. The diagnosis may be confirmed with a CT scan.

The main focus of management is the prevention of increased intracranial pressure with appropriate positioning, limited activities and handling, stress reduction through Developmentally Supportive Care and maintaining internal homeostasis, especially the blood pressure. The infant needs to be referred to a neurosurgeon as soon as possible for specialist treatment, which generally involves surgery to separate the sutures. The outcome is usually good, depending on the success of the surgical intervention.

The discussions in this section are a basic introduction to the neurological system. A key aspect to remember is the involvement and integration of this system with all the other body systems. A change in one system will thus have an impact on another and this emphasises the importance of maintaining internal homeostasis and stress reduction. Once again the midwife can make a critical difference in the outcomes of these patients by prevention, early identification of warning signs and early referral for specialist treatment.

Skin and thermoregulation

The importance of the skin is often underestimated in midwifery care, most probably because the problems relating to the skin are often not easily observable and require indirect methods of assessment. The main functions of the skin include the following:
- It provides a barrier to micro-organisms and toxins for protection against infection.
- It plays a major role in fluid and electrolyte homeostasis, particularly for fluid and electrolyte retainment, selective secretion and insensible water loss.
- It assists in thermoregulation.
- The elasticity of the skin accommodates movement of the limbs and body.

- The subcutaneous fatty layers serve as an energy store.
- The skin allows the synthesis of vitamin D which is in turn essential in calcium homeostasis.
- It is a principal organ for the sensory observation of heat, touch, pain and pressure.
- It is important for the facilitation of communication through touch.

Normal anatomy of the skin would include the epidermis or outer layer of skin, the dermis and the subcutaneous fatty layer. The *epidermis* consists of layers of non-living cells

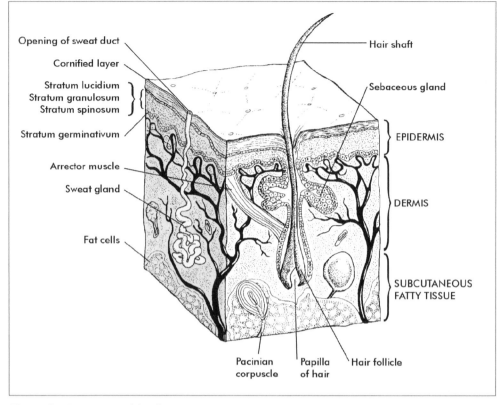

Opening of sweat duct

Cornified layer

Stratum lucidium
Stratum granulosum
Stratum spinosum

Stratum germinativum

Arrector muscle

Sweat gland

Fat cells

Hair shaft

Sebaceous gland

EPIDERMIS

DERMIS

SUBCUTANEOUS
FATTY TISSUE

Pacinian   Papilla   Hair follicle
corpuscle   of hair

Figure 31.5 Diagram of the skin

made of proteins and lipids which are closely packed together so that they form the 'bricks and mortar', known as the horny layer or stratum corneum. It is supported by the granular layer that is responsible for the production of new epidermic cells or keratinisation as the old ones are scaled off.

The epidermis is responsible for protection against the external environment, such as water, mechanical injury, bacteria, toxins and chemicals, and it prevents the loss of water and chemical substances from the internal environment. It contains melanin, which creates skin pigmentation and protects against ultraviolet light.

The dermis is a deeper layer of skin and develops from three to four months in utero. It consists mainly of collagen and elastin which gives the skin elasticity and the ability to stretch and return to normal. This layer is rich in nerve and blood supply and contains sweat glands, sebaceous glands and hair shafts.

Underneath the dermis is the *subcutaneous fatty layer* which is responsible for insulation, protection of internal organs and energy storage. The fatty tissue is deposited in the last trimester.

Critical aspects of the assessment of the skin are the history (gestational age, age after birth, and injuries to the skin), as well as the physical assessment for colour, temperature, dryness/moistness, oedema, elasticity/turgor, thickness and the presence of any other abnormalities such as rash, growths, injuries or discolouration. It is also important to observe the infant's behaviour to touch or other tactile stimulation. Additional special investigations for skin assessment are skin biopsy or skin specimen.

The assessment of the skin's function includes the ability of the infant to thermoregulate and the maintenance of the fluid and electrolyte balance (especially regarding

---

The neonatal skin and preterm skin

The *neonatal skin* has several unique characteristics which contribute to the severity of several skin conditions:

▶ The surface area of the skin is relatively large in comparison to the size of the body.
▶ The epidermis is thinner and more fragile than adult skin.
▶ Although the sweat glands are present, they are non-functional.
▶ The skin is covered with vernix caseosa at birth which has protective properties.
▶ It is more alkaline than normal skin and therefore has fewer antibacterial properties.
▶ Neonatal skin allows much more absorption than adult skin.
▶ Increased loss of water, known as insensible water loss, occurs through the skin.
▶ Neonatal skin can be easily irritated by chemicals such as soaps or perfumes, and has a higher risk for developing an allergic reaction.

The *preterm skin* differs from neonatal skin regarding the following:

▶ It is even thinner than mature neonatal skin, more fragile and provides less protection.
▶ It has less subcutaneous fat and more superficial capillary supply which contributes to the red appearance and less protection.
▶ The more preterm the infant is, the more the skin is covered with lanugo or fine hair and less with vernix caseosa.
▶ Preterm skin has less cohesion between the epidermis and dermis which makes it extremely vulnerable, easy to blister and therefore a weakened barrier.
▶ It has less collagen in the dermis and is therefore less elastic with increased risk for injury.
▶ Preterm skin is highly sensitive to touch due to a superficial and poorly protected nerve supply.
▶ Preterm skin heals and repairs slower than mature neonatal skin.
▶ Preterm skin, however, has the remarkable ability to mature within two to three weeks after birth so as to have the same characteristics as term skin, irrespective of gestational age.

---

insensible water loss). In special cases the assessment would include laboratory blood results for infection or allergies and the absorption of chemicals, such as testing the serum levels of the applicable chemical.

Skin injuries or trauma

The epidermis is responsible for protection against the external environment (temperature, chemicals, mechanical injury) and for preventing water loss and electrolytes from the internal environment. High-risk infants, however, are exposed to additional risk factors that may cause trauma or injury to the skin, such as:

▶ Invasive procedures.
▶ ECG-stickers.
▶ Use of adhesives to stabilise an infusion line or ET-tube.

▶ Temperature probe and saturation probes.
▶ The administration of tissue toxic intravenous drugs that can cause severe damage with infiltration in the tissue.

Because of the characteristics of neonatal or preterm skin, it is much more vulnerable and susceptible to injury or trauma. An additional contributory factor is the inability of the infant to change position or to complain about discomfort so there is complete dependency on the caretaker to observe discomfort and to respond appropriately to it. The trauma or injury would be worsened with the presence of internal disturbances such as hypoxia, acid-base disturbances, hypoglycaemia, hypothermia and hypotension.

Bruising of the skin is a result of rupture of capillaries due to pressure. It is often caused by difficult delivery with the use of forceps or vacuum delivery, or invasive procedures. The bruise remains localised and usually heals spontaneously within a few days.

Skin necrosis is initially observed as a white and later a purple or black discolouration or yellowish sloughing of a skin area due to cell death which is caused by severe hypoperfusion. It is irreversible with loss of function of the affected area, and can even result in the loss of a part of the body such as a limb or part of a limb. A common cause is irritation of an artery that has gone into spasm when an arterial line was inserted or blood was drawn for investigations. Another common cause is an infiltrated infusion that has been undetected for a prolonged period of time or when the contents of the infiltration is tissue toxic, for example, hyperalimentation or certain tissue toxic drugs. Prolonged pressure to an area can also cause necrosis, such as hard surfaces, drip lines or any other hard objects underneath the infant. The cause has to be removed as soon as possible and the attending physician should be informed immediately to decide on further treatment.

Blisters may be caused by heat, for example if the placement of the saturation probe is not changed often, or with the removal of adhesives. *Cuts* are commonly caused by caesarean section or invasive procedures.

The outcomes of skin injuries may vary from insignificant to severe complications depending on the size of the area affected, the amount of tissue involved, the cause of the injury and its treatment or management.

Prevention of skin trauma is of the utmost importance in the care of newborns. Injuries can be prevented by adhering to the following guidelines:

▶ Take care to eliminate any sharp or hard objects or edges.
▶ Heat sources, such as the saturation probe, need to be changed often. If it is preterm skin at least hourly and with full-term skin at least three-hourly.
▶ The use of adhesives should be kept to the absolute minimal and if necessary, hypoallergenic adhesives should be used. It

is recommended to use a protective barrier with the adhesives, such as pectin-based barriers like Granuflex®, especially on areas where adhesives have to be used often, such as the cheeks, to maintain an endotracheal tube in position. The frequency of removal has to be limited and it has to be done cautiously.

▶ Any infusion site, whether arterial line, transparenteral nutrition (hyperalimentation) or intravenous infusion, should be visible. The use of semi-permeable transparent adhesives, such as Tegaderm® or Opsite®, is recommended. The site has to be checked at least hourly for swelling or colour changes of the skin and must be reported immediately if observed.
▶ The skin can be strengthened to provide better protection against injury by the use of appropriate emollients to moisten the skin and maintain its pH.
▶ The skin has to be exposed for less than five minutes at a time to water during bathing in order to prevent the hydration of superficial layers as it reduces cohesion.
▶ Postpone the first bath after birth if there are any risk factors or reasons for concern present, so as to reduce stress.
▶ Unperfumed aqueous cream should be used as the first choice soap as well as emollient.
▶ If the skin is injured, clean the area properly with *saline* or *chlorhexidine in water*. Cover it preferably with a pectin-based barrier or semi-permeable transparent dressing.
▶ Antibiotic ointment should only be applied in cases of confirmed infection because it can be absorbed intravascularly.
▶ Any skin area affected deeper than the epidermis, or bigger than the palm of the infant's hand, must be referred for the specialist opinion of a surgeon or a dermatologist.
▶ In addition, bear in mind that the internal homeostasis is an important variable of the skin's condition and it should therefore be maintained at all costs.

If the infant is preterm or ill, bathing should be postponed to limit stress. Only 'top and tail' cleaning is done at times when the infant can cope with the stress. 'Top and tail' refers to cleaning the infant with cotton wool dampened with warm water on selected areas. Swaddled bathing may be introduced but should be limited to two or three times a week if the infant can cope with bathing (see Chapter 29 on DSC and bathing).

Skin infections

A normal adult skin has an acidity or a pH of 5.5 that has antibacterial properties. Neonatal skin is more alkaline with a pH of 6.34 and it has several other characteristics that contribute to a higher risk of infection (see Box on page 31-39). The vernix caseosa that is present at birth has antibacterial properties, however, preterm infants have limited amounts of vernix caseosa. The risk of infection and related complications increase with a compromised immune system that is associated with prematurity or illness. Common symptoms of a *localised skin infection* include redness, swelling, blistering, localised rash or puss formation. *Systemic infections* due to the skin's permeability and absorption ability are characterised by hypothermia, tachycardia and tachypnoea, as well as other signs of stress or shock. Hyperthermia, however, is uncommon in neonates with infections.

The midwife has the responsibility to maintain an optimal hygienic environment in order to prevent infection, which includes herself. Infection control principles (see Chapter 29), with special reference to hand-washing before touching the infant and minimal handling, is essential in order to prevent nosocomial infections. It is also important to maintain general hygiene for the infant through proper care of the eyes, ears, scalp, nails, umbilicus and buttocks, as well as by changing position at least three-hourly (see chapters on DSC and general care). It is recommended to delay the infant's first bath for two to three days in order to benefit from the antibacterial properties of the vernix caseosa, and also because of the amount of stress it generates. This is especially necessary if there are any risk factors or stress signs present. The exception will be if there is an intra-uterine infection present at birth or a strong suspicion of HIV.

The role of skin in disturbances of internal homeostasis

The characteristics of neonatal or preterm skin often contribute to disturbances of internal homeostasis, especially in the presence of illness. Neonatal skin is more permeable for transdermal or insensible water loss leading to dehydration. Preterm skin which is thinner than neonatal skin, with less subcutaneous fat, is even more susceptible. The water lost through the skin is not sweat, but only water while the sodium is retained. Contributing factors that increase insensible water loss are extended posture, lack of clothing, use of a radiant warmer, poor humidification of the immediate environment, drafts and overhandling.

Insensible water loss can result in hypernatraemia and general deterioration. The fluid loss contributes to hypovolaemia resulting in hypotension, poor perfusion to the systems, decreased functioning of the systems and an increased demand for oxygen and glucose to provide energy.

The infant responds with tachycardia and tachypnoea to compensate for the increased demand for oxygen and glucose, which in turn increases the demand even more. The energy stores of subcutaneous fat and brown fat are limited, especially in the preterm infant and consequently they are easily depleted. This is followed by hypoglycaemia, muscle breakdown (as an alternative energy source) and weight loss. Additional symptoms include poor feeding, hypothermia and an inability to cope with stress due to the lack of energy. The specific outcomes are very difficult to determine, as these characteristics of the skin are extra contributing factors to internal homeostasis. However, the predicted outcome is that the more preterm or compromised the infant's condition is, the worse the effect will be.

The main focus of management for this condition should be prevention. The general principles of prevention of insensible water loss for both term and preterm infants include:

▶ To maintain the flexed position (see Chapter 29 on DSC).

▶ To postpone the first bath.

▶ To cover the skin. If clothes or linen cannot be used, for example as with a critically ill neonate that needs to be observed on a radiant warmer, humid air can be 'trapped' around the infant by using a perspex shield or cling wrap a few centimetres from the skin.

▶ To use an oil-based barrier skin ointment such as unperfumed petroleum jelly to cover the skin and prevent water loss.

▶ To preserve as much of the glucose stores as possible through reducing the demand for oxygen and glucose by decreasing stress levels, providing appropriate nutrition and maintaining internal homeostasis.

Absorption of chemicals and other substances

Protection against the external environment, for example chemicals, is mainly done by the thick impermeable epidermis that acts as a barrier between the external environment and the capillaries in the dermis. The epidermis of neonatal skin is much thinner than normal skin, and the preterm skin is even worse. The dermis is rich in capillary supply, which lies very superficially in neonates. Vernix caseosa is present at birth, especially in term infants, and it contributes by forming a protective fatty layer on the skin to make it less permeable for dangerous substances.

Having a much thinner epidermis with a superficial capillary supply, an infant's skin becomes highly permeable for substances applied on the skin, which can be absorbed

into the bloodstream. The substances therefore may have systemic effects. Examples include absorption of iodine, used for cleaning wounds, or as an antiseptic ointment, resulting in *hypothyroidism*; alcohol resulting in *metabolic acidosis*; hexachlorophane resulting in *brain damage*; and perfumes or chemicals used in soap or cream resulting in allergic reactions. The blood levels of these chemicals increase in relation to the size of the surface area where applied, as well as the duration of contact.

The emphasis therefore is to withhold anything that contains perfume or colourants, e.g. baby soap, cream, washing powder, or any harmful chemicals like iodine found in disinfectant dressings or solutions, hexachlorophane that is used as a disinfectant, alcohol to clean the skin for invasive procedures, and salicilate used as an umbilical cord powder. It is recommended rather to use unperfumed aqueous cream as a replacement for soaps and creams, unperfumed petroleum jelly (Vaseline®) as a protective barrier and to use saline or chlorhexidine and water as a disinfectant solution for general purposes. Other disinfectant solutions and dressings have to be used only in justified cases, such as surgical procedures or in case of a confirmed bacterial infection, and then still with caution.

Touch sensitivity and touch aversion

The neonate's skin is rich in nerve and blood supply without the protection of a thick epidermis. It is therefore very sensitive to tactile stimulation or touch. *Touch sensitivity* is the increased intensity of the following negative experiences:

▶ *Sensory pain*, such as a heel prick.

▶ *Pressure*, due to a tightly strapped intravenous cannula for example.

▶ *Friction*, such as when the mother is rubbing the infant.

▶ *Heat*, for example the saturation probe.

▶ *Cold*, as experienced with cold hands or a stethoscope.

▶ *Continuous stimulation*, such as continuous feather-like touch with cotton wool.

Keeping in mind that the infant has the ability to memorise, it is clear why they demonstrate stress signs when touched, especially with repetitive procedures such as heel prick, but even with procedures such as bathing or massage. This stress response to touch is due to *touch aversion* or the negative association with touch, especially if the infant has been ill or preterm.

The outcomes are not life threatening, but contribute to morbidity, such as refusal to feed as a result of excessive negative stimulation of the oral area, or negative behaviour on attempts of the parents to cuddle the infant. The specific outcomes are related to the area/s affected, but they may be a general stress response to touch.

Treatment involves preventing the negative associations by using appropriate or positive touch, as discussed in Chapter 29.

Congenital skin disorders

Congenital skin disorders can be classified as disorders affecting large or all surface areas of the skin, or as affecting a local skin area. They are most commonly caused by chromosomal or genetic factors, and less commonly due to environmental or multifactoral causes. These abnormalities are obvious, visible and easy to recognise. The layers of skin affected and/or the specific area would determine the associated outcomes. An unfortunate outcome is that children with skin disorders are often excluded socially.

Congenital skin disorders affecting all or large surface areas

Albinism is a hereditary genetic condition associated with hypopigmentation or extreme lightness of the skin, hair and eyes, which results in severe sensitivity to ultraviolet light. *Ichthyosis* is a hereditary condition with excessive scaling of the skin. *Epidermolysis bullosa* is a genetic defect resulting in the formation of blisters over various parts of the body, from simple non-scarring blisters to numerous and large erosive lesions.

The *collodian baby* is born with a tight, unelastic, shiny, transparent skin membrane that cracks and peels off after a few days. The *harlequin fetus* on the other hand has hard and thick, grey or yellow scales that crack to form fissures between thickened plaques. It differs from *harlequin colour change* which is a temporary colour change of the baby to red on the one side and pale on the other side.

Pain, infections (especially with *Staphylococcus aureus*) and injuries such as tears or cracks are common complications of these skin conditions. The focus of the treatment is usually symptomatic in nature, such as moistening of dry or scaling skin, pain management and limiting activities that can aggravate the skin condition. It can be preventive as in using sun block for hypopigmented skin and limiting exposure to the sun. Maintaining optimal internal homeostasis for maximum skin functioning is very important, as well as diligent infection control. The outcomes are always permanent but the severity will be determined by the specific condition: the bigger the area or the deeper the affected area, the worse the outcomes, especially if there is a risk of infection. Albinism is often associated with skin cancer, especially if the skin is exposed to sunlight. Parental involvement and education are therefore of critical importance, as well as genetic counselling.

Congenital defects affecting localised surface areas

Pigmented naevi are dark brown or black flat spots that may or may not be hairy and can be found anywhere on the body. They are generally benign, but can be malignant or associated with other congenital abnormalities such as neurofibromatosis or tuberous sclerosis. A hairy nevus over the spine may indicate spina bifida or meningocele. Because of these associations it is important to do further investigations if they are observed.

Hemangioma refer to vascular skin lesions

which are usually raised, with involvement of subcutaneous tissue and they are red, brown or dark in colour. They can be found anywhere on the body in varying sizes and they often increase in number. The severity and associated signs and symptoms depend on the location and the size of the lesions. For example, if found on the neck, the hemangioma may displace the trachea causing obstruction of the airway, but they may be insignificant if found on an area such as the buttocks. The importance of hemangioma is their common association with other congenital disorders such as Kasabasch-Merritt syndrome and Klippel-Trenaunay-Weber syndrome, or their disturbing appearance.

Port-wine stain is a flat vascular pink, red or purple lesion as a result of mature dilated and congested capillaries underneath the skin. The lesion itself is not of much significance, but it is worrying because of the association with other congenital abnormalities, such as Sturge-Weber syndrome, which presents with a port-wine stain on the face, atrophic changes of the cerebral cortex, glaucoma, seizures, hemiparesis and mental retardation.

Early diagnosis is crucial to distinguish between benign and malignant naevi, as well as to determine any possible relationship with a congenital abnormality. Immediate consultation and referral for specialist care is therefore needed. The diagnosis will determine the appropriate treatment. If it is not associated with a congenital problem, the outcomes depend on the location and the amount of tissue involved. It there is an associated congenital abnormality such as neurofibromatosis, the outcome is usually not related to the naevi but to the associated problems of the particular congenital abnormality.

Temperature disturbances

Body temperature plays an important role in normal cell metabolism, with the recommended skin temperature being between 36.5 to 37 °C and the core or internal temperature at 37 to 37.5 °C for optimal cell function. Body temperature is a balance between the *gaining of heat* through metabolism and from the external environment versus the *loss of heat* to the external environment through exposure or drafts, for example.

The infant's body temperature is controlled internally by the hypothalamus mainly through adjustments of the metabolic rate, vasoconstriction to retain heat and vasodilation for heat loss. The insulation effect of the subcutaneous fat layer assists in retaining heat. Other factors of relevance in thermoregulation of infants include:

▶ Their large surface area in relation to body mass.
▶ Their posture where flexion prevents heat loss and extension increases heat loss.
▶ Their inability to shiver with limited or no ability to sweat.
▶ Internal homeostasis which is a requirement for metabolism to generate energy and heat. Internal homeostasis factors that are of significant importance for thermoregulation are oxygenation, acid-base homeostasis, fluid and electrolyte homeostasis and nutritional status.
▶ The heat generated through metabolism of energy stores is mainly through brown fat metabolism, with subcutaneous fat metabolism once the brown fat stores are depleted.
▶ Preterm infants have difficulty in increasing metabolism or making use of vasoconstriction and vasodilation.
▶ Influencing factors in the external environment, such as radiation, cold surfaces, drafts and water temperature.

Brown fat is vascularised fatty layers deposited around the great vessels, kidneys, adrenal glands, axillas, nape of the neck and between the scapulas. Brown fat will be deposited from 28 weeks and until three to five weeks postnatally. It is metabolised in the neonatal period for generation of energy and heat and cannot be replenished once used. The subcutaneous fatty layer underneath the dermis is responsible for insulation, protection of the

Management of temperature disturbances

Prevention of temperature disturbances is critical and should firstly be done by monitoring the infant's temperature (see Chapter 29), and treating the cause. In maintaining thermoregulation of an infant the main aims are, on the one hand, to *assist the infant with his own attempts* to thermoregulation by the maintenance of internal homeostasis and stress reduction. On the other hand thermoregulation is maintained with the provision of a *thermoneutral environment*, according to the infant's specific needs. This is done by, for example, adjusting the incubator's temperature to maintain the infant's temperature within normal limits, to prevent drafts and to clothe the infant if his condition allows it.

If a temperature deviation is present, it is essential to prevent sudden temperature changes, as the infant may go into a state of shock. Rather obtain normal core temperature slowly but efficiently through environmental manipulation. Limit the use of medication such as paracetamol for hyperthermia unless absolutely necessary.

internal organs and energy storage. The subcutaneous fatty tissue is deposited in the last trimester with the implication that preterm infants have very limited or no energy stores at all, and they therefore do not benefit from the insulation effect of subcutaneous fat either. Furthermore they tend to lie in an extended position, exposing greater areas to the external environment. Their body surface area is relatively larger in proportion to their body size, which increases the risk of loss of heat. Added to that they have a superficial and rich capillary supply to the surface area that is a transport medium for heat. Preterm infants are therefore at risk of losing much more heat than they are able to generate or retain.

Hypothermia occurs when the core temperature is less than 36.5 °C. If the body temperature decreases, the normal response is vasoconstriction to prevent further heat loss and increased metabolism to generate more heat. Vasoconstriction may be observed as pale and cool skin. The increased metabolism increases the oxygen and glucose demands. The oxygen demand is met by increased respiratory rate, increased heart rate and lack of energy for feeding and growth. The glucose demand is met through the use of glycogen stores, brown fat, subcutaneous fat and even muscle breakdown if the other stores are depleted, resulting in an inability to gain weight or failure-to-thrive. If the oxygen consumption is higher than the oxygen supply, the infant will experience hypoxia, anaerobic metabolism and metabolic acidosis, as well as weight loss. These in turn increase the oxygen and glucose demand and it becomes a vicious cycle, accompanied by signs of stress and decrease in functioning of all the systems.

The infant is at risk of *cold injury* if the core temperature decreases to less than 34 °C, which implies permanent damage of the thermoregulatory centre in the hypothalamus and an inability to regulate the body's temperature. Symptoms will include unresponsiveness and severe disturbances of internal homeostasis, especially acidosis and hypoxia. The skin often has an unusual reddish-pink colour or sclerema that may be very misleading, as it is due to oxygenated red blood cells that are trapped in the superficial capillaries as a result of poor perfusion. The low temperature, however, prevents the red blood cells from releasing the oxygen for metabolism to generate heat.

Cold injury is associated with a very high risk of death. The inability to thermoregulate is irreversible, which puts the emphasis of management on external control of the infant's temperature through the use of clothing and manipulating the environmental temperature.

Thermal instability usually occurs when the infant is too immature for appropriate thermoregulation and the body temperature is easily influenced by the external environment.

The body temperature fluctuates between hypothermia, normal temperature and hyper-thermia. This calls for close monitoring of the baby's temperature and making the necessary environmental adjustments. It is most often associated with gestational age, but improve-ment takes place as the baby gets older until he is able to maintain his own temperature within a few days to weeks.

Hyperthermia or *pyrexia* is a core tempera-ture of more than 38 °C. It is uncommon in the neonatal period as infants more often tend to suffer from hypothermia, even in cases of infection. Mature full-term infants can present with hyperthermia in association with infec-tion. Other causes of hyperthermia, especially in very ill and preterm infants, however, are external environmental factors, such as the radiant warmer or sunlight. Infants with hyperthyroidism tend to develop hyperther-mia due to the increased metabolism (see Chapter 29). An infant with hyperthermia is usually pink, warm and very restless. The

infant's temperature should be normalised by making the environmental adjustments.

The outcomes of temperature disturbances, which can be devastating and even result in death, include:
▶ Stress or shock
▶ Metabolic acidosis
▶ Hypoxia
▶ Hyperglycaemia or hypoglycaemia
▶ Lack of weight gain or weight loss
▶ Slow recovery or general deterioration with worsening disturbances of internal homeostasis.

This section dealt with the skin and ther-moregulation of the infant, as well as a num-ber of the associated problems. There are, however, many more related conditions which can be researched in advanced textbooks on neonatal care. Please keep in mind that all the information provided in this section should be examined as part of a holistic picture of the infant's care.

Renal and genitourinary conditions

The renal and genitourinary system refers to the kidneys, ureters, urinary bladder, urethra, internal and external sex organs. The main functions are fluid homeostasis, electrolyte homeostasis, acid-base homeostasis, calcium homeostasis, blood pressure control, produc-tion and activation of several hormones, and the removal of waste products, as well as the removal of drugs, metabolites and toxins. The renal system therefore plays a very important role in the maintenance of internal homeosta-sis. Another important function is the identi-fication of gender.

The nephrons are the basic functional units of the kidney. Each nephron consists of:
▶ A glomerulus which is a specialised capillary network.
▶ The Bowman's capsule, which is a membrane that surrounds the glomerulus and is in direct contact with it.

▶ The tubules that consist of proximal and distal tubules with the loop of Henle connecting them.

Each component plays a crucial role in kid-ney function. The glomerulus is responsible for the perfusion of the Bowman's capsule with blood that needs cleansing of waste products or to restore the balance of fluid, electrolytes or acid-base homeostasis. It is crucial for the survival of the nephron to maintain relatively stable blood pressure in the glomerulus as it consists of specialised single-layered capillary vessels that can easily collapse or rupture. This pressure is maintained through autoregulation of the kidney by the nephron itself.

The activities that take place in the nephron are responsible for excreting water, various electrolytes, metabolites, waste products, toxins and certain drugs. Reabsorption of water and electrolytes takes place, however, to maintain the infant's fluid and electrolyte homeostasis. The excretion or reabsorption of hydrogen and bicarbonate is crucial for acid-base homeostasis. Different electrolytes controlled by the kidneys are important for different bodily functions. The kidneys play a very important role in blood pressure maintenance through the excretion or reabsorption of water and sodium, as well as the production or activation of blood pressure hormones such as antidiuretic hormone and angiotensin.

The normal urine output of an infant is less than 1 ml/kg per hour for the first 24 hours, which is known as the prediuretic phase. A diuretic phase takes place approximately 24 to 48 hours after birth where the normal urine output increases to 4 to 7 ml/kg per hour. The post-diuretic phase occurs after 48 hours to maintain a normal urine output of 1 to 4 ml/kg per hour. Insensible water loss (IWL) can play a significant role in fluid loss and should be considered in the calculation of intake and output.

All the above contribute to the maintenance of internal homeostasis but any abnormalities of these phases may result in decreased urine output, oedema, hypertension or hypotension, irritability or floppiness, stress, tachycardia, tachypnoea, cardiac arrhythmias, metabolic acidosis and drug toxicity. A prolonged presence of these abnormalities will result in irreversible cell damage and can even lead to mortality.

An antenatal history of *oligohydramnios* is often an indication of congenital renal conditions. The assessment of the renal and genitourinary system should include:

▶ The physical assessment, especially of the skin, mucous membranes and fontanelles.
▶ The blood pressure.
▶ The relationship between intake and output.
▶ The genitals (see Chapter 29).

Special investigations include urine analysis such as dipsticks or laboratory tests, laboratory blood tests, ultrasonography or kidney sonar, renal scan or CT scan, magnetic resonance imaging (MRI) and cysto-urethrography. Genetic or chromosome studies may also be indicated due to the frequency of involvement of the renal system in inherited conditions.

Management of renal and genitourinary conditions

The main emphasis for management of problems relating to the renal and genitourinary system, is the prevention or early correction of disturbances of internal homeostasis. It implies oxygenation, acid-base maintenance, electrolyte maintenance, monitoring and maintaining blood pressure, thermoregulation, nutrition, reduction of stressors, accurate calculation of fluid intake and monitoring urine output, as well as careful consideration of the type and route of fluid administered. Pharmacological treatment plays an important role, with diuretics and positive inotropes, for example.

The most common conditions of the renal and genitourinary system will now be discussed briefly.

Hydronephrosis, nephrotic syndrome and renal failure

A normal kidney consists of a cortex or the outermost part, the medulla or middle section and the pelvis. The cortex and medulla contain the nephrons that are the functional units of the kidney. The urine is produced in the nephrons and accumulates in the renal or kidney pelvis, from where it flows through the ureters to the bladder for excretion via the urethra.

Hydronephrosis refers to dilation of the renal pelvis due to an obstruction of renal flow lower down. There is accumulation of urine in the kidney and increased pressure as glomerular filtration still continues in the kidney, but there is also a decrease in measured urine output. As the pressure in the nephrons increases, the activities in the nephrons lessen. Consequently, the urine output decreases, the internal homeostasis becomes disturbed and the toxic and waste products accumulate. An obstruction can be caused by various congenital structural defects or an acquired obstruction, such as scar formation after renal surgery or chronic infection. The diagnosis will be based on the clinical features, urine analysis, blood results and a renal sonar or scan. An important warning sign would be a family history of renal problems. An antenatal diagnosis of hydro-nephrosis can be made with ultrasonography.

Nephrotic syndrome is the result of various renal problems and is characterised by proteinuria, hypoalbuminaemia, oedema and hyperlipidaemia due to damage of the glomeruli and proteins leaking into the urine during filtration. Nephrotic syndrome often precedes renal failure.

Renal failure can be acute or chronic and it is the inability of the kidneys to continue with their normal function in maintaining homeostasis. Acute renal failure is more common in newborns and chronic renal failure is associated mainly with congenital renal abnormalities and a slower deterioration. The causes of renal failure can be classified as pre-renal, intrinsic or post-renal:

▶ *Pre-renal kidney failure* is caused by problems that originate in other organs or systems that eventually cause deterioration and failure of the kidneys. Examples include congestive heart failure, hypoxia, hypotension, dehydration, sepsis and shock. Renal artery thrombosis is also classified as a pre-renal cause for the same effect of hypoperfusion, although the thrombosis is situated in the kidney.

▶ *Intrinsic kidney failure* is kidney failure due to renal cellular damage of any part of the nephron and a consequent loss of function. Causes included are prolonged pre-renal insults and congenital abnormalities such as hypoplasia, dysplasia, polycystic kidneys and nephrotic syndrome. It may also be due to chronic inflammatory causes, such

as congenital infection or pyelonephritis; vascular causes, such as renal venous thrombosis or bleeding; and necrosis of the nephrons due to asphyxia, hypoxia, acidosis, sepsis, hypotension, dehydration or nephrotoxic drugs, such as *indomethacin*, Amphotericin B®, radiologic contrast medium and the *aminoglycoside* antibiotics like *amikacin*.

▶ *Post-renal kidney failure* is caused by problems that are present lower in the genitourinary tract than the nephrons that eventually cause failure of the nephrons. The most common post-renal causes are obstructions, either congenital or acquired, that prevent flow of urine and result in hydronephrosis and subsequent renal failure.

The clinical features of renal failure include:
▶ The presence or a history of the causing factors.
▶ A decrease in urine output to less than 0.5 to 1 ml/kg per hour.
▶ The presence of general oedema.
▶ Signs and symptoms of stress, such as irritability or lethargy and reluctant feeding.
▶ Electrolyte disturbances and acidosis.
▶ Gradual deterioration of all the systems.

The blood pressure tends to remain stable with chronic renal failure, but may deviate with acute renal failure. Except when hypotension is the cause of renal failure, these deviations initially present with hypertension. As the infant's condition deteriorates the blood pressure decreases to hypotension, followed by shock (see pages 31-4 to 31-5). The diagnosis is based on the history, clinical features, discrepancies between fluid intake and urine output, urine analysis and blood analysis.

The main focus of treatment should be prevention, which implies the prevention or early treatment of the above-mentioned causes or risk factors, especially any disturbances of internal homeostasis (see page 31-3). If prevention was not possible the primary aim should be the recovery of internal homeostasis. Admission to a neonatal intensive care unit for specialised care is recommended. Interventions for renal failure include:

▶ Symptomatic support, such as respiratory ventilation.
▶ Treatment of acidosis.
▶ Strict calculations and monitoring of intake and output – including amounts of medication and insensible water loss.
▶ Ensuring adequate nutrition with careful protein calculation and sodium restriction.
▶ Avoiding the use of nephrotoxic drugs.
▶ The selective use of diuretics.
▶ Treatment of blood pressure deviations.
▶ It may be necessary to use peritoneal dialysis or haemodialysis to restore internal homeostasis.

The outcomes depend to a large extent on the cause and its reversibility. With early diagnosis and early intervention full recovery is possible if the cause is treatable. The outcome is much more severe if the cause is untreatable or the condition is prolonged. It may become long-term chronic renal failure and chronic hypertension with consequent long-term dialysis treatment. Renal failure is associated with a high mortality rate.

Infections of the renal and genitourinary system

The normal urine flow plays an important role in protecting against infection as it 'washes away' the organisms that may gain access to the urinary tract through infiltration or by entering via the urethra. This protective mechanism is enhanced by a strictly one-way urine flow from the nephrons via the ureters to the bladder and excretion through the urethra.

Infection of the renal and genitourinary system is the invasion or overgrowth of organisms in any part of the renal and genitourinary system. Common causes are congenital abnormalities of the urinary tract, dehydration, sepsis and poor hygiene of the genitals, especially in female infants.

Urinary tract infection is a bacterial, viral or fungal infection in the urinary tract, which includes the kidneys, ureters, bladder and urethra.

Cystitis is an infection of the bladder that is often caused by bacterial organisms infiltrating the bladder via the urethra, especially in females with poor genital hygiene. Infectious organisms excreted through the kidneys in the case of a systemic infection can also cause cystitis. This is especially evident when there is dehydration or other causes of hypoperfusion of the kidneys, where the urine output is reduced for prolonged periods as it encourages bacterial growth in the bladder and does not flush out the organisms. The clinical features are mainly general signs and symptoms of infection such as tachycardia, tachypnoea, restlessness and irritability.

Glomerulonephritis is an infection of the glomeruli of the nephrons. The most common cause is a systemic infection or infective organisms that spread via the blood stream to the kidneys. As the glomeruli are part of the functional units of the kidneys, such an infection will result in decreased kidney function. The consequences and the clinical features of this condition depend on the number of glomeruli affected, as well as the severity of the infection and whether it is a viral, bacterial or fungal infection (the prognosis for a bacterial infection is much better). It may even result in acute renal failure.

Pyelonephritis is an infection of the kidney and ureter, which may be unilateral or bilateral. It may be caused by a descending infection spreading from the blood and nephrons down to the bladder, or it may be an ascending infection originating from the bladder, especially as in the case of incompetent ureter valves with reflux. The clinical features may vary from general signs and symptoms of infection to symptoms of acute renal failure.

All the above-mentioned infections are easily

overlooked as infants cannot complain about pain or describe the symptoms, such as painful urination. They simply present with the general signs and symptoms of stress. Infections can, however, be more easily diagnosed if they are seen as a possible cause of stress which should be eliminated by performing a urine analysis (dipstix) in the unit. If leucocytes, proteins or blood are present in the urine, further investigations such as blood and laboratory urine analysis are necessary to identify the cause and site of the infection.

The main focus of treatment for infections should be prevention, early diagnosis and appropriate intervention, such as antibiotics for a bacterial infection, stress reduction and maintaining internal homeostasis.

The outcomes can be excellent with early and adequate treatment. If treatment is delayed, it can result in irreversible kidney damage, urinary tract obstruction with recurrent infections or sepsis and further associated complications such as disturbances of internal homeostasis.

Congenital structural defects of the renal system

The kidneys of the fetus develop during weeks 3 to 4 and the bladder is formed by week 6, followed by the nephrons at 8 weeks. Urine is passed from approximately 9 weeks of gestation, although the vascularisation of the nephrons is completed by approximately 15 weeks. The urine that is passed in utero contributes to the amount and contents of the amniotic fluid.

Congenital structural defects of the renal system refer to renal conditions that are due to abnormal development. Causes of such conditions can be inherited, such as Potter syndrome, or they can be multifactoral, as with TORCH-infections.

Congenital structural defects of the renal system may affect only one kidney (unilateral) or both kidneys (bilateral). Furthermore the abnormality may affect only the kidney/s or it can be associated with other abnormalities,

depending on the cause. Kidney abnormalities are often associated with abnormalities of other systems as the kidneys develop very early in gestation when several other organs are also in the process of development. The same cause that has an impact on the kidneys would have an impact on the other systems, as they all are in a sensitive phase of development. Structural abnormalities of the kidneys will always result in functional problems, but it is possible for one kidney to compensate for the dysfunction of the other if the problem is unilateral and only discovered later in life.

Renal agenesis is the absence of either one or both kidneys. It is possible that *unilateral renal agenesis* remains undetected, as the normal kidney can compensate for the absence of the other one unless the workload of the kidney increases, during fluid overload for example. *Bilateral renal agenesis* is usually associated with Potter's syndrome and with various other abnormalities as well. The infants are most often stillborn or die soon after birth due to pulmonary hypoplasia (see page 31-17). The diagnosis is made on the clinical features and if required, an autopsy.

Renal dysplasia is the abnormal development of the kidneys of which the most common condition is *multicystic dysplastic kidney disease*. The number of nephrons is decreased and appears as grapelike clusters or cysts filled with fluid, and the proximal ureter is stenotic or nonpatent. It is often associated with other abnormalities and results in renal failure. *Polycystic kidney disease* is also a form of renal dysplasia where the cysts are evenly distributed throughout the kidneys to give them a sponge-like appearance, with decreased amounts of nephrons resulting in renal failure. It is usually a recessive inherited condition with the cysts found in the liver, lungs and/or pancreas too.

Atresia of the ureter/s is the lack of opening of the ureter/s into the bladder by 9 weeks of gestational age. The result is complete obstruction of urine flow into the bladder and consequent accumulation of fluid in the kidney, hydronephrosis and renal failure. It can be unilateral or bilateral. *Stenosis of the ureter/s* is a partial obstruction of the ureter, either unilateral or bilateral. The outcome depends on the severity of the obstruction and can vary from being undetected to severe hydronephrosis and renal failure. A *megaloureter* is an abnormally dilated ureter in the absence of any lower obstruction of the urinary system that is often associated with recurrent pyelonephritis. *Duplication of the collecting system* is the occurrence of two ureters on one or both sides. It may be undetected, but is often associated with recurrent urinary tract infections.

Exstrophy of the bladder is a rare congenital abnormality where the bladder is visible on the outside through a defect in the lower abdominal wall.

Atresia of the urethra refers to incomplete formation of the urethra resulting in complete obstruction of urine flow out of the bladder, hydronephrosis and renal failure or even rupture of the renal tract. *Stenosis of the urethra* is a partial obstruction of the urethra of which the most common consequence is recurrent urinary tract infection.

Deformities of the urinary tract valves can either include the ureter valves entering the bladder, or the urethral valves at the bladder neck. The deformity can either result in stenosis or a partial obstruction associated with recurrent infections or urine retention, or it can be an incompetent ureter valve, resulting in urine reflux into the ureter and pyelonephritis, or an incompetent urethral valve resulting in urine leakage and incontinence.

Patent urachus is a deformity of the bladder resulting in communication between the bladder and the umbilicus with continuous leakage of urine at the umbilical base.

Congenital structural defects of the genitals

Abnormalities of the genitals include a variety of conditions of which a familiar condition is *hermaphroditis* or bisexuality where the infant possesses both female and male internal and external organs usually due to chromosomal abnormality.

Common abnormalities of male gonads are malpositioning of the urethral opening such as the *hypospadias* or opening on the lower surface of the penis, and *epispadia*, which is an opening on the upper surface of the penis. Another abnormality in males is a *congenital hydrocele*, which is the accumulation of peritoneal fluid in the scrotum due to a congenital defect.

The most common congenital abnormality of the female gonads is *fused labia* that resembles a scrotum and is found in intersex states. The diagnosis of abnormalities of the genitals is based on the clinical features and they are often associated with chromosomal or genetic disorders that may require genetic screening. Parental education, counselling and support plays an important role due to the sensitivity and stigma associated with these conditions.

Features that may be mistakenly diagnosed as congenital abnormalities of the genitals, but are associated with prematurity, are a very *prominent clitoris* of the female and *undescended testes* of the male infant.

The diagnosis of congenital structural renal and genitourinary abnormalities is based on the history of which oligohydramnios is significant, the signs and symptoms of renal failure and a kidney sonar and/or scan, or a cysto-urethrography.

The ideal would be to prevent these abnormalities but it is most often not realistic due to the early organogenesis of the renal and genitourinary system. Early diagnosis and appropriate intervention therefore should thus be the main focus of management. It usually requires admission to a neonatal intensive care unit and referral for specialist treatment. Important principles for care include careful calculation of fluid and electrolytes, maintenance of internal homeostasis, stress reduction and symptomatic support, such as with antibiotic treatment for infection, for example. Parental counselling and support are again very important.

The expected outcomes depend on the specific disorder but most have long-term implications. Some conditions like valve deformities can be surgically corrected but others may need more dramatic interventions, such as a kidney transplant for polycystic kidneys.

This section gave a brief overview of the renal and genitourinary system and the most common abnormalities, while showing the rele-vance of the system in maintaining internal homeostasis and its importance for all other systems. Read more about fluid and elec-trolyte homeostasis in order to understand the role of the kidneys in the infant's functioning, as well as the related discussions on stress reduction and blood pressure maintenance.

Haematological conditions (including infections)

The haematological system refers to the structures and functions necessary for blood production and the functions of the plasma, red blood cells, white blood cells and platelets. This section will therefore include the conditions relating to thrombi, bleeding tendencies, infections, allergies and anaphylaxis, blood group incompatibility, anaemia, polycythaemia and hyperbilirubinaemia.

The haematological system relies on the cardiovascular system for efficiency: the cardiovascular system is the transport system and the components of the haematological system are the vehicle. For that reason their relationship has to be kept in mind. It is also very important to understand the normal physiology of blood production, the clotting cascade and the inflammatory process. The assessment of the haematological system of an infant should be interpreted in conjunction with the infant's history, such as bleeding or infection, gestational age and clinical features like tachycardia, tachypnoea and skin colour. Other important considerations are the adaptation from fetal circulation to normal circulation, compensation for an increased oxygen demand and nutrition, and any other disturbance of internal homeostasis.

The special investigations used to confirm or reject a diagnosis or to monitor the progress or response to treatment include laboratory tests, such as full blood count, coagulation times, bilirubin-levels, blood grouping, Coomb's test for blood compatibility and bone marrow aspirate.

Clotting and bleeding abnormalities

In order to stop the bleeding a sequence of events or chain reactions are activated after injury to the blood pvessels. The immediate local response includes the pressure on the damaged vessels by the blood that leaked out, spasm or constriction of the damaged vessels, formation of a platelet plug and clotting of the blood. Blood clotting relies on 12 clotting factors which create the clotting cascade so each reaction activates the next clotting factor until the clot is formed to stop the bleeding. The platelets are activated by the contents of the damaged cells to form a platelet plug and then they are consumed or destroyed during their involvement in these processes. Platelets also play an important role in the shrinking of blood clots during the healing process.

Clotting and bleeding abnormalities are most often related to platelets (with or without the involvement of other clotting factors), resulting in either increased clotting of blood or bleeding tendencies. *Thrombocytosis* refers to increased levels of platelets and *thrombocytopenia* is a reduction in the number of platelets in the circulating blood.

Thrombosis

Thrombosis refers to thrombi or clots in the blood stream that cause obstruction of the blood vessel/s. The outcome of the thrombus depends on the area where the obstruction is found, for example a thrombus in the brain will result in brain damage of the area which is provided with blood by the obstructed blood vessel. Thrombus formation is often associated with iron deficiency anaemia, cerebral ischaemia, sepsis and congenital abnormalities, such as Down's syndrome and neuroblastoma. *Polycythaemia* or increased concentration of red blood cells, which is associated with high viscosity of blood, can also cause thrombosis, especially if the blood pressure is low or the baby is dehydrated. *Thrombocytosis* or increased level of platelets can contribute to the formation of thrombi, for example after a platelet transfusion.

Thrombosis can be prevented to a certain extent by maintaining the fluid and electrolyte homeostasis and blood pressure. There is, however, a controversy surrounding the treatment of thrombosis. One possibility is to administer an anticoagulant (unfractionated heparinised solution) to prevent further clotting, with the existing clot being left to dissolve through the normal physiological processes. The other option is fibrinolytic therapy (Urokinase®) to dissolve the clot, which allows quicker restoration of the blood although there is a higher risk of bleeding, especially intracranial bleeding.

Common thrombosis areas in the neonate are the renal veins, central nervous system and aorta, as well as areas of catheter-placement, such as the umbilical lines. It is characterised by decreased organ perfusion and a subsequent decrease in function of the organ. The consequences are usually severe and may eventually be associated with shock and even mortality.

Bleeding abnormalities

Bleeding abnormalities are conditions where there is a delayed or prolonged clotting response with the increased risk of blood loss and consequently further complications. It can be caused by various factors such as deficient clotting factors, thrombocytopenia, disseminated intravascular coagulation and inherited bleeding disorders.

Calcium is an important clotting factor in the clotting cascade. *Hypocalcaemia* implies a deficiency of this clotting factor, resulting in prolonged or delayed clotting. It has other critical outcomes though, such as cardiac arrest (see page 31-29). The diagnosis is based on the history and clinical features, and confirmed with plasma-calcium level results. The focus of management should be to maintain calcium homeostasis.

Haemophilia is an inherited disease which results in bleeding tendencies due to deficient clotting factors, most commonly clotting

---

Haemorrhagic disease of the newborn

Haemorrhagic disease of the newborn or vitamin K-dependent bleeding is a bleeding tendency which is due to vitamin K deficiency. Vitamin K plays an important role in the activation of four of the 12 clotting factors, namely II, VII, IX and X. The implication of a vitamin K deficiency is that the clotting cascade will be inefficient and result in a bleeding tendency. Vitamin K requires intestinal flora for synthesis in the gastrointestinal tract but the intestinal flora are absent in a newborn until enteral feeds are started. Vitamin K synthesis is delayed if enteral feeds are delayed due to illness. This bleeding tendency is characterised by the onset of localised or diffuse bleeding 24 to 72 hours after birth, if vitamin K (Konakion®) has not been administered after birth. The possibility remains that bleeding will occur two to three weeks after birth even if vitamin K was administered after birth and the infant was kept nil per mouth for a prolonged period of time. Diagnosis will be based on the history, clinical features and response to vitamin K administration. Blood results should also demonstrate decreased levels of vitamin K-dependent clotting factors. The measures to prevent bleeding tendencies in neonates include the prophylactic administration of vitamin K (Konakion®) after birth, the prevention of injuries or bruising and the maintenance of internal homeostasis.

factor VIII (*classic haemophilia*) or clotting factor IX (*Christmas disease*). In the neonatal period the main characteristic is delayed clotting of the umbilical cord or puncture sites. The diagnosis is based mainly on family history or on clinical features later in the infant's life. Treatment is based on prevention of injuries or bleeding, the replacement of the clotting factor and/or blood transfusions.

Thrombocytopenia is a significant decrease in the platelet count, which is a symptom of various conditions that result in bleeding tendency. It is characterised by petechiae; purpura; bleeding of the mucous membranes, umbilical cord, puncture sites; and any other areas at risk, namely intracranial, pulmonary or gastrointestinal areas. The diagnosis is confirmed by the history, clinical features and platelet count. Causes of thrombocytopenia may include:

▶ Impaired platelet production due to bone marrow suppression, caused by radiation or drugs such as *dexamethasone*, and bone marrow hypoplasia, such as trisomy 13 and 18.

▶ Platelet destruction due to maternal autoimmune diseases, such as idiopathic thrombocytopenic purpura, systemic lupus erythematosus, neonatal allo-immune thrombocytopenia or when maternal antibodies enter fetal circulation and destroy fetal platelets.

▶ Neonatal asphyxia is responsible for the destruction of platelet precursors.

▶ An increased consumption of platelets in the presence of infections such as TORCH-infections.

▶ Necrotising enterocolitis and sepsis.

▶ Giant haemangiomas or microvascular diseases, such as persistent pulmonary hypertension of the newborn.

The main focus of treatment should be to identify the cause and treat that, to administer thrombopoietin to stimulate platelet production, as well as to replace the platelets via platelet transfusion.

Disseminated intravascular coagulation is an acquired bleeding disorder where the platelets and clotting factors are consumed intravascularly by the release of thromboplastic material from the damaged or diseased tissue to form numerous microthrombi. The microthrombi activate the process of fibrinolysis which is an attempt to dissolve the thrombi. Active spontaneous bleeding results from the fibrinolysis leading to shock. Precipitating factors would include hypoxia, acidosis, infections, thrombocytopenia, tissue injury and shock with a high risk of mortality. The diagnosis is made based on the history and clinical features but may be confirmed with blood results for platelet count, clotting factors and coagulation times. It is of critical importance to treat the underlying cause. The follow-up treatment would involve administering fresh frozen plasma, platelet concentrations and whole blood. A blood exchange transfusion is often indicated. Additional principles of management include stress reduction (DSC) and maintenance of internal homeostasis.

Infections

Immunity is the body's protection against infection. Natural or non-specific immunity refers to characteristics of the body that contribute to protecting against infection. Intactness of the surfaces acts as a protective barrier to prevent invasion of organisms. The biochemical barriers on the surfaces protect against infection in various ways. For example, the lower pH on the skin reduces bacterial growth, vernix caseosa on the skin of a newborn has antibacterial properties and the enzymes present in mucosal secretions reduce bacteria.

The body's first line of white blood cell defence includes the macrophages and neutrophils which respond once an invasion of organisms has occurred. They are responsible for phagocytosis and the digestion of bacteria, foreign material such as foreign blood products and cellular debris. The eosinophils are white blood cells that contribute to protection against invasive agents by destroying foreign proteins through phagocytosis. The cause of the foreign proteins may be the administration of transparenteral nutrition (hyperalimentation) or blood products but they may also be living proteins such as parasites. Blood contains soluble factors such as C-reactive protein (CRP) and various enzymes that are activated by the presence of bacteria, and which in turn activate various processes to combat the infectious agents. There are also various cells in the body that have the phagocytosis ability together with their normal functions. They are found in the spleen, lymph nodes, liver, lungs and other organs. As a group they are called the reticulo-endothelial system and they contribute to protection of the specific organs.

The inflammatory response is a local response of vascularised tissue to injury or trauma irrespective of the cause, in order to protect against invasion and to enhance healing. Once the injury has occurred, the arterioles and capillaries dilate and blood flow increases to the injured area. Exudation of fluid occurs through the capillaries that are more permeable, leaving a higher concentration of blood cells in the capillaries with higher viscosity and decreased flow. The red blood cells remain central and the white blood cells outline the vessels. The white blood cells are actively transported across the vessel wall into the inflammatory focus, where phagocytosis can occur to destroy the cause (infective organisms), or to clean up the cellular debri. The result is redness, heat, swelling, pain and temporary loss of function.

The adaptive or acquired immune response refers to a specific response which is the release of antibodies or immunoglobulins against specific invasive agents, known as antigens, and the process is known as an antigen-antibody response. Immunity can also be obtained with the involvement of activated cells, T-cells and macrophages, which are responsible for the destruction of the specific antigen through direct contact or cell-antigen response. All of these responses are important for protection against infection.

Infection occurs as soon as pathogenic organisms have invaded the host, the mentioned processes fail, the person does not have the ability to destroy the organisms, and they have the opportunity to multiply. It may also occur if normal organisms of the host have the opportunity to multiply in a different location than where they are supposed to be found and the host does not have the ability to control the growth. It is also seen as infection if there is an overgrowth of normal organisms in their normal location. These organisms can be bacteria, viruses, fungi or protozoa and each of these categories has various subcategories. The impact of an infection on the infant depends on the kind of organism, as well as the specific characteristics of the particular pathogen, its location and, whether it is localised or systemic. Other significant factors are the infant's internal homeostasis status, the infant's immune status and the presence of illness or stress. Furthermore, there are characteristics of the newborn that may contribute to infection, such as his decreased antibody levels and poor response to antigens, decreased neutrophil stores and an inability to increase production of white blood cells in the presence of infection, especially if there is an increased demand for red blood cells.

A brief description of the different kinds of pathogens will now be given, but keep in mind that there is much more information available about each group.

Bacteria

Bacteria are organisms that can function independently of the infant but they use the infant's resources for metabolism and reproduction. They are often beneficial as they play an important role in the digestion of food, or the normal flora on the skin that destroy other pathogenic organisms before infiltration can occur. A bacterial infection is problematic, however, if the resources of the infant, such as oxygen and nutrients, are depleted by the bacteria, which consequently leads to cell damage. It is also a problem if the bacteria excrete harmful endotoxins or exotoxins. *Bacterial infections* may occur as a result of lowered immunity, disturbances of internal homeostasis, contamination with foreign pathogens via the placenta, touch, inhalation, invasive procedures, administration of contaminated solutions or with cantaminated breast milk.

The responses of the body to a bacterial infection include:

▶ Signs of stress.
▶ An observable inflammatory response such as swelling, redness, pain and temporary limited function.
▶ Palpable lymph nodes and a decreased function of the affected organ/s, for example, respiratory distress if it is a respiratory infection.
▶ Bacterial infections often result in abscesses with puss formation.

Bacteraemia, sepsis or *septicaemia* are conditions where the infection has been distributed throughout the body and affects all organs with a high mortality rate. The diagnosis is confirmed with blood results. The main methods of treatment are symptomatic treatment, immunological support and the administration of antibiotics.

Viruses

Viruses can be compared to pirates as they are unable to live or function on their own although they contain genetic material. *Viral infections* occur when they invade living cells and use the contents of the cells, as well as the protection of the cells, for metabolism and reproduction for their own survival at the cost of the cells. Contamination is most often through direct contact with contaminated body fluid. The infant's response to a viral infection may be asymptomatic for a period but the infant tends to deteriorate rapidly once symptoms are observable. These signs and symptoms are similar to severe stress or shock with organ failure if it is a systemic viral infection or *viraemia*. The diagnosis is confirmed with blood results. Treatment is very difficult because viruses rely on the protection of the body cells and can be targeted once the cells

burst open and before the next cells are invaded. The main focus of treatment is therefore on boosting the immune system, symptomatic treatment and the administration of antiviral drugs over a prolonged period of time.

Fungi or mycoses

Fungi or mycoses are decomposers that release enzymes to digest organic material. A *fungal infection* occurs if the fungi use the infant's nutrients or the infant's tissue as a source for digestion to the disadvantage of the host. Some fungi release toxins as a waste product of metabolism which can cause tissue damage. Fungal infections tend to be localised and if the infection is superficial it is observed as a chronic inflammatory process with tissue damage. They are most often found in dark, moist areas. A *systemic fungal infection* is extremely dangerous due to the widespread tissue damage and the consequences thereof. The most common causes of fungal infections in newborns are:

▶ Displacement of normal flora, such as *Candida albicans*, at the tip of an indwelling catheter during the invasive procedure of inserting a catheter.
▶ A lowered immune system.
▶ The overuse of antibiotics which destroys the normal bacteria that are usually responsible for controlling the fungal growth: with the consequent overgrowth of fungi.

Fungi have several characteristics that make it difficult to destroy them, such as thick cell walls and the ability to remain dormant for long periods of time. Most species reproduce with spores that have a high resistance against treatment. The main methods of treatment are symptomatic treatment, immunological support and the administration of *antimycoticum* (for example, *nystatin* for superficial infections and Amphotericin B® for systemic fungal infections). The replacement of normal intestinal flora prophylactic in association with the administration of antibiotic treatment, is a new treatment, however it is not yet common practice. The rationale is to replace the normal

Examples of common infections in neonates

	Bacterial infections
Group B streptococci	Gram-positive organism commonly found in maternal cervix, vagina, anus and urethra. Most common cause for early-onset bacterial infections in neonates. Can be fatal or responsible for permanent damage of the affected organ. Most often sensitive to *penicillin*.

Other examples of gram-positive organisms: *Staphylococcus aureus, Stapphylococcus epidemiolis, Listeria monocytogeres*

Pseudomonas aeruginosa	Gram-negative organism commonly found in moist/wet environments, e.g. air conditioners, ventilator circuits. Can be fatal in infants with low immunity. Very often resistant against antibiotics – can be sensitive to a combination of antibiotics such as amnoglycosides in combination with an anti-pseudomonas *penicillin*.

Other examples of gram-negative organisms: *Escherichia coli, Haemophilus influenzae, Neisseria gonorrhoeae*

	Fungal infections
Candidiasis caused by Candida albicans	A normal organism that can overgrow or spread systemically, especially if the infant has low immunity. Commonly responsible for oral thrush, but most often fatal if it is spread systemically. Can be sensitive to Amphotericin B® administered for 4–6 weeks.

	Viral infections
Human immunodeficiency virus (HIV)	Human retrovirus responsible for surpression of immunity and therefore accommodating opportunistic infections. Can be asymptomatic for a period of time and then become fatal. Treatment is complex and includes antiretroviral therapy, but toxic side-effects are demonstrated in neonates.

Other examples: rubella virus, cytomegalovirus (CMV), respiratory syncytial virus (RSV), herpes simplex virus (HSV), hepatitis B.

flora destroyed by antibiotics, as the normal flora contains the growing fungi.

Living parasites

Other possible infective or pathogenic agents are living parasites, such as malaria, bilharzias and worms, but those are extremely uncommon in the neonatal period. However, they become important causes of infection after discharge from hospital.

See Chapter 29 for the general principles of infection control.

Allergies and anaphylaxis

It is necessary to understand acquired or adapted immunity regarding antigen–antibody-responses in order to understand allergies and anaphylaxis. An *allergy* is a hypersensitivity to a substance or allergen with an inappropriate response on exposure to it. The substance or allergen can be anything, for example pathogenic organisms, foreign proteins such as transparenteral nutrition or formula feeding, medication, chemicals, dust particles, mites or blood products. The exact etiology of allergy is not certain, but there is an inherited tendency and it is often associated with prematurity where there was an increased risk for absorption of allergens.

The first exposure to the allergen results in the normal first line of defence to destroy it (neutrophils and macrophages). Specific, but 'wrong' immunoglobulins that have a memory and that can destroy a specific allergen are produced thereafter. The allergen is then known as an antigen. If the person is exposed to the same antigen for a second or more times, these immunoglobulins are released resulting in a dramatic response. The process is known as sensitisation and the response includes the release of histamine responsible for capillary permeability, leakage of fluid from the vessels, swelling and activation of allergic substances with redness and itchiness. Eosinophiles, a specific group of white blood cells, are produced as a contra-reaction to inactivate the allergic substances. Other signs and symptoms include skin rash, red cheeks, persistent blocked nose or sneezing, restlessness, irritability, vomiting and other signs of stress. Treatment for allergies is aimed mainly at the suppression of the response and symptomatic treatment. It can be obtained by the use of *epinephrine*, antihistamines, corticosteroids, anti-inflammatory medication and the relevant treatment for specific symptoms, such as bronchodilators for bronchospasm.

Anaphylaxis, anaphylactic shock or *anaphylactoid* reaction occurs with a serious degree of sensitisation, resulting in the generalised allergic response as described previously but with a consequent massive fluid shift out of the vessels into the interstitial space and a drop in blood pressure. The infant presents with all the signs and symptoms of shock (see pages 31-4 to 31-5), as well as oedema or swelling, sweating and sudden deterioration. Death is likely to follow if advanced resuscitation is not initiated quick enough after onset.

Newborns and allergies

It is important to bear in mind that it is uncommon to see signs and symptoms of allergies in newborns because of the sensitisation that has to take place first and the delayed ability of newborns to produce immunoglobulins. However, this is a high-risk period for initiating sensitisation with mild to severe allergic responses developing a few weeks or even months later if the infant is exposed to the allergen again. It is therefore essential to prevent infant exposure to potential allergens as far as possible.

Prevention is critical in the treatment of allergic reactions, through preventing sensitisation, preventing exposure to the allergen after sensitisation and with the prophylactic administration of corticosteroids or antihistamines. Sensitisation can be prevented if the infant is not exposed to possible allergens such as:

▶ Chemicals which can be absorbed through the skin.
▶ The inhalation of perfumes or chemicals.
▶ Unnecessary administration of medication.
▶ Unnecessary administration of foreign protein, such as cow's milk protein or any other solid foods containing protein for at least six months.
▶ Special precautions should be taken in the presence of risk factors for increased permeability, for example to use hypoallergenic formula feeds with necrotizing enterocolitis, or to replace soap products with aqueous cream on preterm skin.

Blood group incompatibility

Blood groups are distinguished by the presence or absence of specific components in the membrane of the red blood cells, of which the Rh-factor and the A/B factors are the most familiar. The presence or absence of these components is genetically inherited in various combinations: the A and B factors can be present on their own, in combination or be absent, while, at the same time, the Rh factor can be present or absent. The absence of an A or B factor is indicated as O. The presence of the Rh factor is indicated as Rh-positive (+), and the absence of the Rh factor as Rh-negative (-). The possibilities of blood groups are therefore A+, A-, B+, B-, AB+, AB-, O+ and O-.

If a person is exposed to blood containing one of the above factors that is not present in his own blood, it will be recognised as foreign material that activates the acquired or specific immune system to produce specific antibodies, and the foreign material becomes an antigen. The antigen–antibody response will result in destruction of the antigens and therefore will result in haemolysis or breakdown of the red blood cells containing the antigens (see Table 31.2 for compatibility of blood groups).

The fetus' blood group is already determined at conception and can include factors inherited from the father that may be incompatible with the maternal blood. However, the placenta functions as a barrier between the maternal and fetal circulations and prevents any exchange of red blood cells.

Blood group incompatibility is an iso-immune haemolytic anaemia caused by an antigen-antibody response against an antigen situated in the red blood cell membranes that entered the circulation of a person who does not have the antigen.

Although the placenta acts as a barrier between the fetal and maternal circulations, there are circumstances where some red blood cells can be exchanged between the maternal and fetal circulation, for example during fetal–maternal bleeding, during delivery, the rupture of an ectopic pregnancy, amniocente-

sis, external version and manual removal of the placenta. The process of antigen–antibody production or sensitisation is initiated with the first exposure if the blood groups are incompatible, without any signs or symptoms being present. Any future exposure though will result in a massive release of antibodies to destroy the red blood cells containing the antigen, known as blood group incompatibility (see Figure 31.6). The condition is referred to as *ABO-incompatibility* if the antigen is the A, B or both factors. *Rh-incompatibility* occurs when the antigen is the Rh factor. ABO- and Rh-incompatibility may be present in combination if the person does not have any of these factors and is exposed to blood containing ABO and Rh factors.

If the mother has been sensitised before, during a previous pregnancy or blood transfusion for example, and any fetal red blood cells containing the antigen enter her circulation, she will release antibodies that enter the fetal circulation and haemolyse the fetal red blood cells (see Figure 31.7). The consequences of ABO-incompatibility are most often *fetal anaemia* with reduced red blood cells and therefore reduced oxygen-carrying ability and tissue hypoxia, acidosis, shock, organ failure and death. At birth the infant presents with multi-organ failure, severe oedema, petechiae with bleeding tendencies and a pale mottled colour. Rh-incompatibility can present with the same, but often results in intra-uterine death. The condition is known as *hydrops fetalis*. Infants that are born alive are at high risk for mortality and survivors will be at risk for the complications associated with the specific organ/s that are affected. They often have neurological damage as a result of disturbances of internal homeostasis, severe hyperbilirubinaemia and kernicterus due to massive haemolysis and severe anaemia.

The diagnosis is based on the history and the clinical features and is confirmed with a positive Coomb's test result. If it could not be prevented the decision will have to be made in coordination with the parents on whether resuscitation will be implemented or not. If

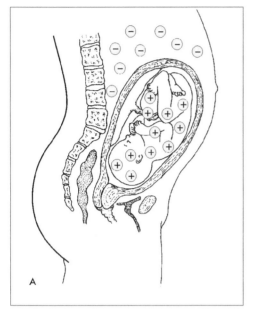

A: Mother not sensitised against baby's blood type

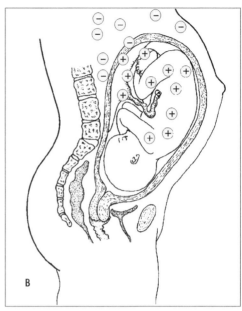

B: First exposure of mother to baby's blood after an incident

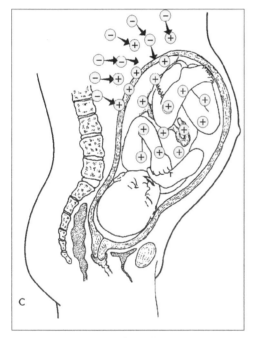

C: Maternal antibodies formed against baby's blood type

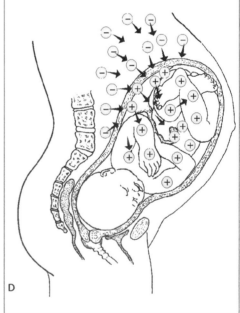

D: Maternal antibodies cross placenta and haemalyse fetal blood if any contact with fetal blood occurs (2nd exposure)

Figure 31.6 Schematic diagram of development of ABO/Rh-incompatibility during pregnancy

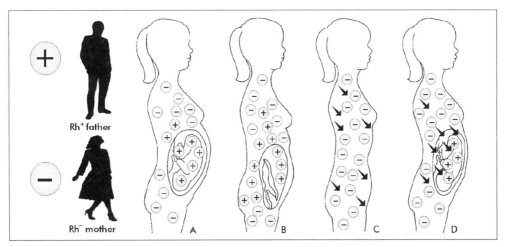

Figure 31.7 Schematic diagram of development of ABO/Rh incompatibility in follow-up pregnancy A: Mother and baby's blood is incompatible, without contact during pregnancy, B: Positive fetal blood enters maternal circulation at birth, C: Mother develops antibodies, D: First contact with incompatible fetal blood during any of the following pregnancies results in release of antibodies that cross the placenta and haemalyse fetal blood

resuscitation will be put into practice the main focus will be symptomatic and appropriate management of the organs involved, as well as an exchange transfusion as soon as possible.

Prevention is crucial, with early identification and management of the mother-at-risk, that is, the mother without the antigen/s in her red blood cells (refer to Table 31.2). Exposure of the mother to incompatible blood has to be prevented as far as possible. Appropriate prophylaxis after exposure or possible exposure to incompatible antigens is the administration of *Anti-D immunoglobulin* to the mother within 72 hours of the exposure, for example after an abortion, amniocentesis or birth. The administration of *Anti-D immunoglobulin* (antigen-antibodies) is given to destroy the antigens and therefore prevents sensitisation and the production of antibodies. Counselling the mother is very important.

These processes of bloodgroup incompatibility can also occur if an infant is exposed to

Table 31.2 Blood groups and compatibility									
Blood group of receiver	A		B		AB		O		
	Rh +	Rh -	Rh +	Rh -	Rh +	Rh -	Rh +	Rh -	
Blood group of donor									
A Rh +		X	X	X		X	X	X	
Rh -			X	X			X	X	
B Rh +	X	X		X		X	X	X	
Rh -	X	X					X	X	
AB Rh +	X	X	X	X		X	X	X	
Rh -	X	X	X	X			X	X	
O Rh +		X		X		X		X	
Rh -									

blood products that contain unfamiliar material, as with the transfusion of blood products, as previously described. The infant will be asymptomatic after the first exposure, as this will be the sensitisation process. If the infant is exposed again to blood containing the antigen, the antibodies will be released to destroy the red blood cells with the antigen. The common result is *haemolytic anaemia* and *hyperbilirubinaemia*. It can also result in an *allergic response*, followed by *anaphylaxis*.

Preventing sensitisation should be the main focus of management for this condition. It can be accomplished by the selective use of blood products, only if it is crucial for survival, and to then ensure that compatible blood groups only are administered. See Table 31.2 as a guideline.

Anaemia and polycythaemia

Red blood cells are responsible mainly for the transport of oxygen to tissue, the removal of carbon dioxide and for acting as a buffer for acid-base balance. They are produced in the bone marrow under the influence of the hormone erythropoietin. Erythropoietin is stimulated by hypoxia especially, which in turn stimulates the production of red blood cells. The requirements for the production of red blood cells include protein, iron, vitamin B_{12} and folic acid. An adult's red blood cells normally have a lifespan of 100 to 120 days, whereas those of a term infant are 60 to 90 days and those of a preterm infant are 35 to 50 days.

Anaemia

Anaemia is decreased levels of red blood cells. It is reflected in the number of haemoglobin (Hb of usually less than 13 g/dl but varies according to gestational age) or the amount of red blood cells (a red blood cell count of less than 4 mm^3).

Anaemia can be caused if more normal red blood cells are lost from the circulation than can be produced. The one way to lose red blood cells from the circulation is through bleeding. Bleeding may take place externally,

as when there is a cut, a disconnected infusion line or blood taken in large quantities for laboratory studies, or it may occur internally, as with intracranial bleeding or in any other place. Another cause of losing red blood cells can be if they are destroyed or haemolysed. Possible reasons for haemolysis are blood group incompatibility, bruising or trauma, pathogens present during septicaemia or infections, and due to some drugs.

Anaemia may also be due to a decrease in red blood cell production. This can occur if the bone marrow is suppressed, as with for example corticosteroid treatment or disturbances of internal homeostasis, with the exception of hypoxia. The red blood cell production will decrease if the amount of bone marrow available as production sites is limited as is the case with prematurity. Production of red blood cells can also be reduced if some of the requirements are lacking, if there is an iron deficiency or poor maternal diet with folic acid or vitamin B_{12} deficiency. Anaemia in preterm infants is aggravated by the short lifespan of red blood cells which increases the demand for red blood cell production, as well as the increased demand associated with growth and an increasing volume of circulating blood.

Congenital or inherited causes of anaemia include sickle cell anaemia and glucose-6-phosphate dehydrogenase deficiency, with a decreased lifespan of the red blood cells.

All the causes of anaemia will result in a *lower oxygen-carrying capacity of the blood with a decrease in oxygen delivery to the tissue*. The main compensatory mechanisms for enhancing the provision of oxygen to the tissue are tachycardia and tachypnoea. Other signs and symptoms include paleness, reduced energy or tiredness with failure-to-thrive and poor peripheral perfusion. If the condition is severe, cyanosis may also be observed with eventual cardiac failure. The diagnosis is based on the progress history and the clinical picture and may be confirmed with laboratory blood test results. The long-term outcome for anaemia depends on the severity and how the other systems are affected by the decrease in oxygen-carrying ability. The outcome may therefore be very good without any complications, with the worst case scenario being mortality.

The treatment for anaemia depends on the cause and the severity. If the infant is lethargic and unable to feed on his own within a reasonable period, he should be admitted to a neonatal intensive care unit for specialised care. General management involves reducing the oxygen demand, which is done by maintaining internal homeostasis, stress management and reducing activity. It would be helpful to include DSC principles and to rather provide nasogastric feeding until the infant's condition improves. The treatment for chronic anaemia includes replacement therapy if there is a deficiency of iron, vitamin B_{12} and folic acid. *Erythropoietin* (Eprex®) is often prescribed to stimulate red blood cell production. The treatment of acute anaemia would involve replacement treatment such as transfusion of blood products containing red blood cells (whole blood or packed cells). It is very important to consider all the ethical aspects surrounding blood transfusion before the decision is made to administer blood. These aspects include the risk of infections such as HIV and hepatitis B, as well as the possibility that blood transfusions may be deemed unacceptable for religious reasons.

Polycythaemia

Polycythaemia is an excess in circulating red blood cells (Hb usually more than 22 g/dl). It is most often caused by intra-uterine hypoxia or placental insufficiency, maternal-fetal or twin-to-twin transfusion and maternal diabetes. Polycythaemia can also occur with the hypertransfusion of blood. The problems related to this condition are mainly due to the increased viscosity of the blood with a reduced blood flow or hypoperfusion to all the organs and the risk of thrombosis, as well as hyperbilirubinaemia, and its associated complications.

The clinical presentation of the infant with polycythaemia is a reddish discolouration of the skin, in spite of hypotension and poor perfusion. Other symptoms are signs of stress and hypoperfusion of organs with deterioration of their distinguishing functions. If thrombosis is present, the symptoms will show failure of the organ affected. If kernicterus occurs as a result of hyperbilirubinaemia, the associated signs and symptoms will also be present. The long-term outcomes will be related to the complications present and can vary from full recovery without any long-term sequelae to mortality. Diagnosis will be based on the history and clinical features, as well as blood test results.

The focus of management is mainly on early diagnosis and appropriate treatment which should include supportive symptomatic treatment, stress reduction (DSC) and maintaining internal homeostasis. Exchange blood transfusion should be considered if obvious signs and symptoms are present. There is, however, controversy surrounding exchange blood transfusion, and the advantages and risks have to be considered before a decision is made.

Hyperbilirubinaemia and kernicterus

Red blood cells of preterm infants circulate approximately 35 to 50 days before they are haemolysed, while term infants' red blood cells circulate approximately 60 to 90 days before haemolysis. The haemoglobin is separated from the rest of the red blood cell

---

Hyperbilirubinaemia

Hyperbilirubinaemia is the term used to describe an increase in the levels of bilirubin in the plasma. It is not a disease but a symptom of several diseases and is commonly associated with yellow discolouration of the skin. The level of unconjugated bilirubin is interpreted on a graph according to gestational age in order to determine toxicity. *Kernicterus* is the associated complication with toxic levels of unconjugated bilirubin.

---

during haemolysis and is then further broken down into unconjugated bilirubin, iron and globin. Iron and globin will be reused for the production of new red blood cells, while the rest of the cell materials will be digested by phagocytosis. The unconjugated bilirubin, which is fatsoluble, has to be transformed into watersoluble conjugated bilirubin in order to be excreted.

Haemolysis of the red blood cells takes place in the reticulo-endothelial system, which consists of groups of cells found in the lymph nodes, spleen and liver. The unconjugated bilirubin is excreted into the blood stream where it binds to albumin in order to be transported to the liver. (Take note that the blood serum levels of bilirubin do not reflect the unconjugated bilirubin that is bound to albumin.) The unconjugated bilirubin is then removed from the albumin and taken up by the liver cells when the blood flows through the liver. The unconjugated bilirubin that is fatsoluble is converted to watersoluble conjugated bilirubin in the liver cells under the influence of a specific enzyme (glucuronyl transferase) and by using glucose and oxygen.

The watersoluble conjugated bilirubin then becomes part of the bile and it moves through the bile ducts to the small intestines, where it is excreted as part of the stools. Small amounts may also be reabsorbed into the blood stream to be excreted through the kidneys as part of the urine.

The enzyme betaglucuronidase in the small intestines has the ability to convert conjugated bilirubin back to its fatsoluble unconjugated status which can be reabsorbed from the small intestines into the blood stream. This process is called the enterohepatic circulation of bilirubin. Delayed enteral feeding or insufficient volumes of enteral feeding are contributing factors.

Increasing levels of unconjugated bilirubin may lead to it being deposited in the fatty tissue, including the subcutaneous fat. The unconjugated bilirubin can be conjugated in the superficial surfaces in the presence of ultraviolet light. Conjugated watersoluble bilirubin is reabsorbed into the blood stream and excreted by the kidneys in the urine.

Physiological jaundice

Physiological jaundice is the presence of hyperbilirubinaemia in newborns within the first week of life where it does not reach toxic levels and usually peaks on day 3 for full-term infants and day 5 to 6 for preterm infants. Newborns are born with higher levels of red blood cells as they produce more red blood cells in utero for efficient oxygenation via the placenta. The respiratory system is 'activated' at birth together with other changes for adjustment from intra-uterine to extra-uterine life, which reduces the amount of red blood cells required for efficient oxygenation. The haemolysis of the so-called extra red blood cells results in increased production of unconjugated bilirubin with other factors such as decreased liver function and increased reabsorption of bilirubin contributing to the condition. It becomes visible as an evenly spread yellow discolouration of the skin and the sclera of the eyes, while the urine appears dark yellow. The diagnosis is based on the history, such as the onset of the yellow discolouration, the clinical presentation of the infant and confirmation of increased serum levels of unconjugated bilirubin. In the case of a breastfed baby, it also has to be confirmed that the baby is receiving adequate breastmilk so as to exclude breastfeeding jaundice. It is usually treated with phototherapy (exposure of large skin surfaces to ultraviolet light or sunlight) but the serum levels should decrease even without treatment. However, it is critical to exclude the possibility of pathological jaundice.

Breastfeeding jaundice

Breastfeeding jaundice is increased levels of unconjugated bilirubin caused by the enterohepatic circulation due to *inadequate breastfeeding* with decreased fluid and caloric intake. It has an early onset, within the first two to four days of life. The bilirubin levels decrease as soon as sufficient breastmilk is provided, either by increasing the frequency of feedings or if the amount of breastmilk taken per feed increases. Supplementation with water or glucose water has to be avoided. Breastfeeding jaundice usually has an earlier onset than physiological jaundice and the serum levels of unconjugated bilirubin decrease as soon as the feeding is increased, while the amount of feeding does not influence the progress of physiological jaundice. It is very rare that the unconjugated bilirubin levels reach toxic levels.

Breastmilk jaundice

Breastmilk jaundice, on the other hand, is when there are increased levels of unconjugated bilirubin due to the *ingredients of breastmilk*. The onset is later, usually from the first four to seven days of life, but it can occur even up to two to six weeks after birth. It is associated with prolonged jaundice. The diagnosis is based on the history of the breastfed baby with late onset of jaundice, the absence of other causes such as hypo-albuminaemia or liver problems, the clinical picture of jaundice and the laboratory results. It is confirmed if breastfeeding is temporarily discontinued and replaced by formula feeding and the bilirubin levels are found to decrease rapidly. If it does not decrease rapidly within 72 hours, breastmilk is not the cause and breastfeeding can continue while further investigations are made. If it is the cause, it is still advisable to continue with breastfeeding, as there is a good possibility that although the bilirubin levels will increase again, they will be lower than previously. The final decision to continue or discontinue breastfeeding is made once the diagnosis of breastmilk jaundice is confirmed and is based on the seriousness of the condition and the mother's preference.

Pathological unconjugated hyperbilirubinaemia

Pathological unconjugated hyperbilirubinaemia refers to increased levels of unconjugated bilirubin that is due to a pathological cause, where the risk for toxic levels are high, or it lasts for more than a week in a term infant or more than two weeks in a preterm infant.

The causes of this group of conditions can be related to increased production of unconjugated bilirubin through haemolysis. Haemolysis may be the result of any of the following:
▶ Blood group incompatibility.
▶ A reaction to blood transfusion.
▶ Bruising or injury.
▶ Haemorrhage.
▶ Red blood cell disorders.
▶ Severe infection or sepsis.
▶ Medication.

Hyperbilirubinaemia may also be caused by *hypo-albuminaemia* where not enough albumin is available to bind with the unconjugated bilirubin in order to inactivate it. There are also several factors that can *prevent or reduce the binding of unconjugated bilirubin and albumin* with the same results, such as hypoxia, acidosis, asphyxia, hypothermia, infection, hypoglycaemia, starvation, stress and drugs.

Problems resulting in the *inability of the liver to convert the unconjugated bilirubin* to conjugated bilirubin, include prematurity, where there is a lack of the enzyme glucuronyl transferase. Hypotension and stress are also important reasons for decreased liver function due to the reduced perfusion of blood to the liver. Asphyxia can reduce liver function because of cell damage in the liver.

Increased enterohepatic circulation is also an important contributor to increased levels of unconjugated bilirubin. The enterohepatic circulation can be the result of increased levels of the enzyme beta-glucuronidase in the small intestine which converts conjugated bilirubin to unconjugated bilirubin, which is then reabsorbed into the blood stream. High levels of this enzyme are common in newborn infants. The enterohepatic circulation can also be increased if there is a lack of motility that prevents the excretion of the bile. Reasons for this phenomenon can be delayed feeding, too little feeding, stress, intestinal obstruction and necrotizing enterocolitis.

Inborn errors of metabolism can also lead to pathologic hyperbilirubinaemia, such as galactosemia, cystic fibrosis and maternal diabetes.

In all of the above cases, the infant will present with jaundice which is an evenly spread yellow discoloration of the skin, mucous membranes and sclera of the eyes. Other signs and symptoms are often irritability or lethargy, mild tachycardia, loss of appetite or reduced feeding. The colour of the urine changes to a dark yellow. The diagnosis is based on the history (gestational age, day of life, duration of hyperbilirubinaemia, type and amount of enteral feeding), clinical presentation and blood serum test results.

The main treatment is phototherapy (see Chapter 29) and if necessary, a referral for advanced care. Advanced care includes the treatment or elimination of the cause if possible, for example, by administering albumin for hypoalbuminaemia or surgical repair of the intestinal obstruction. It is also crucial to maintain internal homeostasis and to reduce stress for these infants. The blood serum levels of the unconjugated bilirubin are closely monitored, usually on a daily basis, and plotted on a graph to monitor progress. An exchange blood transfusion should be considered if the unconjugated bilirubin levels reach toxic levels in order to prevent kernicterus. The outcome for these infants is usually very good, without any long-term complications unless they develop kernicterus.

Kernicterus

Kernicterus is the yellow staining with neuronal injury to the basal ganglia in the brain by unconjugated bilirubin which results in encephalopathy or irreversible brain damage. It is caused by fatsoluble unconjugated bilirubin that crosses the blood–brain barrier and then deposits in the basal ganglia where it injures the brain cells. This crossing usually occurs when unconjugated bilirubin reaches toxic serum levels, which can be due to any of the previously discussed reasons for pathological hyperbilirubinaemia.

Kernicterus is initially characterised by jaundice with lethargy and hypotonia, weak suckling, a blunted Moro or startle reflex and high-pitched crying. Later signs are fever, hypertonia, upward gaze and opistotonus. There is a high mortality rate for infants with kernicterus and if they survive their outcomes may include hearing loss, cerebral palsy and mental retardation.

The diagnosis is based on the clinical picture of jaundice and neurological deterioration, and can be confirmed with high levels of unconjugated bilirubin found with biochemical laboratory tests.

The main aim of treatment is prevention by maintaining internal homeostasis, reducing stress and early phototherapy. If the unconjugated bilirubin reaches toxic levels, exchange blood transfusion may be necessary to prevent kernicterus. Once kernicterus is present the focus of care shifts to symptomatic and supportive treatment, as well as rehabilitation. The parents need to be counselled, especially regarding the long-term complications.

A broad overview has been given on the most common haematological problems found with newborns, including the conditions related to the platelets, white blood cells and red blood cells, as well as the management for these conditions. It is important to keep in mind that haematological conditions have an influence on the functioning of all the other organs or systems.

Gastrointestinal conditions

The gastrointestinal system includes all the structures necessary for the intake and transport of food, as well as its digestion and absorption in cooperation with the metabolic and endocrine systems. Together with the metabolic and endocrine systems, the gastrointestinal system is a crucial role-player in the maintenance of fluid and electrolyte homeostasis, and therefore also in maintaining internal homeostasis and growth.

The metabolic and endocrine systems are discussed on pages 31-75 to 31-80, including the important conditions relating to digestion. Nutrition, which is the functional component of the gastrointestinal system, is discussed in Chapter 30. This part of the chapter will therefore focus more on the structural abnormalities and problems relating to the intake, transport and absorption of food.

The mouth is responsible for food intake and limited digestion, as well as speech at a later stage. The oesophagus enables transport of food to the stomach and digestion takes place in the stomach and continues in the intestines. The absorption of nutrients takes place predominantly in the small intestines and water is absorbed in the large intestines. The anus controls excretion of stools. The gastrointestinal valves (oesophageal and piloric) ensure a one-directional flow of food.

See Chapter 29 for assessment of the infant and keep in mind the interrelated effects of the different systems. Take note that the term 'ileus' is often used synonymous to 'intestinal obstruction'.

Special investigations of the gastrointestinal system may be used to confirm or reject a diagnosis. A pH probe test (pH-metry) is used to study the pH of the lower oesophageal area over a 24-hour period in order to diagnose gastrointestinal reflux. Abdominal X-rays are done for observation of the bowel gas pattern, especially to determine if there is an obstruction. The structure of the gastrointestinal system, obstruction and malrotation can be observed in radiological studies with contrast medium (barium swallow and/or barium enema). Ultrasonography (sonar) is often used to diagnose anatomical abnormalities and obstructions. Biopsy of tissue may also be done.

The management of gastrointestinal problems is primarily based on:
- The prevention of congenital abnormalities with quality preconception and antenatal care, especially a well-balanced diet and withholding of toxic or damaging agents.
- Acquired abnormalities can be prevented or limited by maintaining internal homeostasis, especially oxygenation, acid-base homeostasis, fluid and electrolyte homeostasis, nutritional status and thermoregulation.
- Problems can also be prevented or limited by reducing stressors according to the Developmentally Supportive Care principles (see Chapter 29).
- Early diagnosis and intervention.
- Symptomatic or specific treatment for specific problems in association with the management of endocrine or metabolic problems, such as the correct formula feeding for the specific condition or surgical repair for intestinal obstruction.

Feeding difficulty and failure-to-thrive

Feeding difficulty and failure-to-thrive are not gastrointestinal conditions, but are symptoms of various possible problems.

Feeding difficulty is often used to describe an infant who is unable to latch, suck and/or swallow, to coordinate sucking, swallowing and breathing, or to finish the prescribed amount of feed within a reasonable time period. It may be the result of anatomical or structural problems such as cleft lip and/or palate, a large or very small tongue or an underdeveloped or small lower jaw. Another possible cause is damage of nerve supply to an area/s involved in the process of feeding. It may be caused by a lack of stimulation of the processes involved, such as with preterm or intubated infants. It may also be related to damage or suppression of the relevant part of the cerebral cortex due to medication such as sedatives, disturbances of internal homeostasis such as hypoxia, hypotension, acidosis, stress, illness or fatigue. It is of exceptional value if these infants are referred to a speech-language therapist as soon as possible.

Failure-to-thrive refers to the inability of the infant to pick up weight over a period of time and follow a normal growing curve. The underlying problems include any of the reasons for feeding difficulty, malabsorption or metabolic disorders, insufficient feeding, chronic diarrhoea, chronic vomiting, or fatigue due to illnesses such as cardiac defects or bronchopulmonary dysplasia. It is crucial to diagnose and treat the underlying cause, as well as to apply the principles of good nutrition (see Chapter 30).

Cleft lip and/or palate

The primary palate develops to form the upper lip and anterior part of the maxilla, while the secondary palate develops to form the hard and soft palates. An infant's ability to latch and suck, which is crucial for feeding, is influenced by the upper part of the mouth, which is formed together by the upper lip and hard and soft palates.

A cleft in the lip and/or the hard palate and/or the soft palate may be caused by chromosomal inheritance or multifactoral causes and it is often associated with syndromes.

A *unilateral cleft lip* is an asymmetrical upper lip, varying from a niche in the lip to a complete separation extending upward into the floor of the nose. *Bilateral cleft lip* presents with symmetrical clefts in the upper lip. It may be present on its own or be associated with a cleft hard palate and/or soft palate. A *hard or soft cleft palate* will vary in size and severity of the cleft. If it is only a cleft palate it may not be visible at all but can be felt by placing a finger in the mouth on the palate. In severe cases, a bilateral cleft lip and palate may result in nasal distortion and a deformed midface.

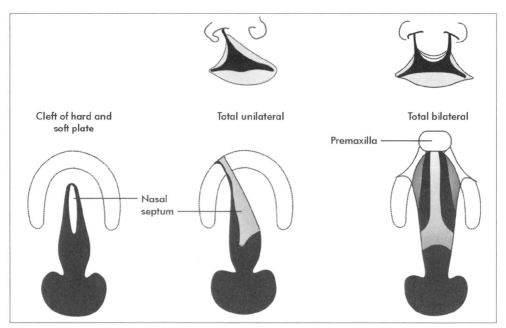

Figure 31.8 Some variations of cleft lip and/or palate

All these variations (see Figure 31.8) result in various degrees of difficulty in feeding due to an inability to create a vacuum to suck, the tendency to aspirate with feeding, an unaesthetic appearance and, in the long term, speech problems and low self-esteem. It is possible that the outcome can be without any complications at all, depending on the severity of the cleft and the success of surgical correction. However, the outcomes may be altered by associated anomalies or abnormalities.

Quality preconception and antenatal care can reduce the incidence of cleft lip and/or palate, especially by ensuring a balanced diet and avoiding teratogens. The main focus is on early appropriate management, including the prevention of aspiration, proper nutrition and referral for surgical correction. Support may include feeding with special cleft palate nipples, feeding bottles or squeeze bottles. An artificial temporary palate is often used to assist in feeding until surgical correction can be done. Parental support and education is crucial, as well as referral to a speech-language therapist.

Tracheo-oesophageal atresia and/or fistula

Variations of tracheo-oesophageal atresia and/or fistula are congenital structural defects that have a major impact on the gastrointestinal system, as well as respiratory system. It was discussed in more detail on pages 31-12 to 31-13 as part of the respiratory system.

Abdominal wall defects

The intestines, oesophagus and stomach are present and distinct by the fourth week of gestation. Muscle layers in the abdominal wall fuse from weeks 10 to 12 and cover the intestines in the abdominal cavity. When the abdominal contents protrude through an opening or weakness in the abdominal wall the condition is known as *abdominal wall defects*. The cause is probably multifactoral and it is often associated with other anomalies.

An *omphalocele, umbilical hernia* or *exomphalos* occurs if there is a abdominal wall defect with protrusion of abdominal organs into the umbilical cord. It is usually covered by a transparent peritoneal sac and with the umbilical vessels protruding into the apex of the defect. There are various sizes possible, from a small protrusion that may look like 'a fat umbilical cord', to a large protrusion of intestines and even the liver, spleen and stomach into the umbilical cord. Associated anomalies include chromosomal anomalies, cardiac defects, neurological, genitourinary and skeletal anomalies, as well as other gastrointestinal abnormalities.

Gastroschisis is the protrusion of the abdominal contents through an abdominal wall defect, usually to the right of the umbilicus. The protruding abdominal contents are usually intestines only and are not covered. Intestinal malrotation and atresia are often associated with gastroschisis but any other anomalies can also be found.

The diagnosis of abdominal wall defects will be based on the physical examination. Babies with these conditions are usually doing well after birth, unless other anomalies are present. Common long-term effects are malabsorption and intestinal obstruction. Other complications include infection, sepsis, necrosis or short bowel syndrome. Full recovery after surgical correction is possible though without further complications.

The focus of management is on early diagnosis with antenatal ultrasonography, appropriate early intervention and early referral for surgical management. If the diagnosis has already been made before birth, it is very important to arrange for the baby to be delivered through a caesarean section in a hospital where he can be admitted immediately to a neonatal intensive care unit.

After birth the protruding contents should be covered as soon as possible with warm, sterile and moist dressings (preferably normal saline) and then with a sterile plastic dressing or bag to prevent evaporation. Precautions have to be taken to prevent any pressure on the exposed intestines or kinking. The infant must be admitted to a neonatal intensive care unit for specialised care and kept nil per mouth with a nasogastric tube in situ on free drainage to prevent any bowel distension that may worsen the already compromised bowels. The maintenance of internal homeostasis is crucial, with special emphasis on thermoregulation as these infants are at risk of losing body heat easily. Fluid and electrolyte homeostasis, parental nutrition, pain management and infection control are also high priorities (see Chapter 29 on DSC). The parents will need support and reassurance as the appearance of the abdominal wall defects may be a frightening experience.

Other congenital gastrointestinal conditions

The intestines, oesophagus and stomach are present and distinct by the fourth week of gestation. Further development of these organs would include a period where the intestines turn and protrude into the umbilical cord, with the duodenum being temporarily occluded. By 10 to 12 weeks the intestines will have returned to the abdominal cavity and the rectum will have separated from the developing urinary bladder. The muscle layers of the intestines are present by 12 weeks and active absorption can then begin. From 10 to 12 weeks the fetus swallows amniotic fluid and meconium will be present from 16 weeks. The nerve supply to the intestines is completed by 24 weeks, peristalsis is present from approximately 26 weeks and the gastrointestinal tract is mature from 36 to 38 weeks. One of the main functions of the gastrointestinal tract is the transport of food through the tract.

Congenital obstructive gastrointestinal conditions may include various conditions of partial or full gastrointestinal obstruction that the infant is born with. The cause is often unknown but it may be influenced by chromosomal or genetic inheritance, multifactoral causes or teratogens, and it is often associated with syndromes.

The infant presents with associated problems once feeding is initiated. Transport of food may be interrupted due to the partial or full obstruction, the food together with the secretions will accumulate and increase in a confined space, digestion slows down and absorption decreases. The condition is aggravated by swelling due to an inflammatory process in the affected areas. It most often results in hypoglycaemia, abdominal distention and other signs and symptoms of stress. The other specific signs and symptoms are related to the area where the obstruction is situated, as well as whether it is a partial or full obstruction.

Congenital obstructive conditions of the gastrointestinal tract

A full obstruction of the upper gastrointestinal tract may be the result of an *oesophageal atresia*, which is due to the lack of or defective embryonic development of the oesophagus. It means that the feeds cannot be transported further than the oesophagus. The characteristics of this condition include continuous drooling, milk runs out of the mouth during feeding, a flat abdomen, an absence of meconium and a history of polyhydramnios. If a *tracheo-oesophageal fistula* is present in association with oesophageal atresia, the infant will also present with choking and coughing during feeding and develop chronic pneumonia (see pages 31-12 to 31-13).

A *partial obstruction of the upper gastrointestinal tract* may be the result of an *oesophageal stenosis* or *oesophageal sphincter stenosis* and can vary from severe with a clinical picture as for full obstruction of the upper gastrointestinal tract, to asymptomatic and undiagnosed.

A *full obstruction of the lower part of the gastrointestinal system* is characterised by abdominal distension, vomiting, poor feeding, signs of stress and an absence of meconium. *Atresia of the small intestines* (duodenum, jejenum or ileum) is either a blind ending of the intestine, or the lumen is obstructed by a septum of tissue. *Malrotation of the intestines* occurs as an incomplete turn of the intestines during embryonic development, which leads to it kinking and a consequent obstruction.

A *partial obstruction of the lower gastrointestinal tract* is characterised by slow onset of abdominal distension, vomiting, reduced stools or the appearance of constipation, as well as signs of stress and discomfort or even shock. It is most often as a result of a reduced diameter of the gastrointestinal lumen, as is the case with *stenosis of the large intestines*.

Hirschsprung's disease

Hirschsprung's disease or aganglionic megacolon refers to a lack of nerve cells in the distal part of the colon, due to an interruption in the nerve supply growth into the colon. Peristalsis will be absent in the affected part of the colon and there may be atrophy. The size of the colon area affected depends on at what stage of growth the interruption occurred and it is classified as low if the short lower part of the colon is affected, or high if it is a longer part. The onset and severity is worse with a high megacolon than with a low megacolon.

Anorectal malformations and meconium ileus

The *anorectal malformations* include a broad spectrum of defective anorectal development, characterised by stenosis or atresia of the anal canal, with or without a fistula between the rectum and the perineum, the vagina in females, or the urethra in males. The outcomes are commonly associated with obstruction of the lower gastrointestinal tract. Other signs and symptoms depend on the location of the malformation and the presence or absence of fistulas. An absent anus or anus imperforatum may be found with a physical examination, but it is also possible that it appears as if the anus is present, without being able to pass any stools due to an anorectal membrane. It is also possible to find meconium in the urine in the presence of a fistula.

Meconium ileus is a mechanical obstruction of the distal ileum due to the accumulation of thick tar-like meconium and it is associated especially with cystic fibrosis. It has to be differentiated from a *meconium plug* which is a temporary obstruction by meconium.

The clinical presentations of the above-mentioned conditions may be very similar. Special investigations are therefore important to confirm the diagnosis.

As gastrointestinal obstruction is usually not preventable, the main focus is on early diagnosis, appropriate intervention and referral. As soon as the first signs of gastrointestinal obstruction appear, such as abdominal distension and/or vomiting, the infant must be kept nil per mouth. In order to reduce abdominal discomfort a nasogastric tube on free drainage should also be considered. The nasogastric tube should be in situ with the outside end being left open to drain the gastric contents into a container that must be positioned lower than the stomach. The maintenance of fluid and electrolyte balance is a high priority, as well as maintaining other aspects of internal homeostasis.

The outcome depends on the specific cause of the obstruction, the location and the course of management. They may also be related to surgical results, which would include the possibility of a temporary or permanent colostomy and further surgical complications such as infection, adhesions, necrosis or short bowel syndrome. Other outcomes would include the association of these congenital gastrointestinal anomalies with other congenital anomalies and syndromes. Common long-term outcomes are malabsorption, problems with diarrhoea or constipation, bowel incontinence and delayed toilet training.

Acquired neonatal obstructive gastrointestinal conditions

All the gastrointestinal organs are formed by 12 weeks gestation and they will mature at a rapid pace until approximately 38 weeks. Maturation of the gastrointestinal tract still continues after birth for the first few years of life, but at a slow pace.

Acquired neonatal obstructive gastrointestinal conditions include the conditions responsible for partial or full gastrointestinal obstruction of which the cause is not related to embryonic development defects. These conditions usually develop after birth. The diagnosis is based on history and clinical presentation, and may be confirmed with X-rays or ultrasonography.

Meconium plug

A *meconium plug* occurs when thick meconium is responsible for a mechanical obstruction in the absence of any other abnormalities. The actual reason for it occurring is unclear but it is often associated with prematurity, hypotonic infants, sepsis and infants of diabetic mothers. The infant presents with abdominal distension, severe stress, vomiting and failure to pass meconium. The diagnosis will be confirmed if the plug is removed, usually with an enema, such as the barium enema used for investigative purposes. There should be a full recovery with no repetition of the condition.

Intussusception

Intussusception is the telescoping of a portion of the intestine into an adjacent more distal section of the intestine. It often occurs in the presence of hyperperistalsis, malrotation of the intestines or as a surgical complication. As a part of the intestines is pulled into a lower part, the blood supply is cut off, resulting in inflammation with swelling and obstruction. The swelling will worsen the pressure and contribute to hypoxia and tissue damage, resulting in necrosis of the 'trapped' intestines. The infant will present with the signs and symptoms of obstruction, as well as severe stress or shock. Immediate treatment includes pain management, nil per mouth with nasogastric tube in situ and referral for surgical treatment.

Volvulus

The twisting or 'kinking' of the intestines is known as *volvulus* and it results in a mechanical, lower gastrointestinal obstruction. It is often associated with malrotation of the intestines. The onset of the clinical picture of gastrointestinal obstruction is usually sudden, with signs of severe stress or shock.

Perforation or rupture of the intestines

Perforation or rupture of the intestines occurs as a complication of necrotizing enterocolitis, volvulus, intussusception, surgery and prolonged gastrointestinal obstruction, or with the continuation of enteral feeding in the presence of a gastrointestinal obstruction. Perforation may also occur with forced insertion of a nasogastric tube. The major problem is the risk of peritonitis due to the intestinal contents (including normal flora) leaking into the peritoneum. It presents with abdominal distension, vomiting, pain and severe stress or shock. The abdomen may also be red in appearance.

Hypertrophic pyloric stenosis

Hypertrophic pyloric stenosis is the abnormal increase in size of the pyloric valve, resulting in an occluded or partially occluded outflow of the stomach. The condition is probably inherited but it is classified as acquired because the signs and symptoms only appear from approximately three to four weeks or up to five months after birth. The typical clinical presentation is projectile vomiting within an hour of enteral feeding and the associated complications, including dehydration, electrolyte disturbances and failure-to-thrive. The diagnosis will be confirmed with palpation of the 'pyloric olive', ultrasonography and with an upper gastrointestinal contrast study (barium swallow).

These acquired conditions have to be prevented with early diagnosis and treatment of the primary causes as discussed. If it could not be prevented, the main focus should be on early diagnosis, referral to a specialised surgeon and the appropriate supportive management. Immediate supportive treatment would include nil per mouth if there were any suspicion of an obstruction and replacing fluid and electrolytes intravenously. If the baby has been given nil per mouth for more than 24 hours, nutrients have to be replaced via total parental nutrition

---

Necrotizing enterocolitis

Necrotizing enterocolitis is a common acquired condition of gastrointestinal obstruction and occurs mostly in preterm infants. It can also occur in very ill full-term infants. The condition is characterised by:
▶ Necrotic areas of the small and/or large intestines with bacterial growth.
▶ The signs and symptoms of gastrointenstinal obstruction, such as abdominal distension, vomiting and severe discomfort.
▶ Feeding intolerance.
▶ Absent or small amounts of stools passed.
▶ Stress or shock.

The cause is most probably a combination of factors, including:
▶ Prematurity.
▶ Intestinal ischaemia resulting from internal disturbances such as hypoxia, acidosis, hypothermia and hypotension.
▶ Bacterial colonisation, especially *Klebsiella, Escherichia coli, Enterobacter* and *Pseudomonas*.
▶ Oral feeding during stress/shock periods.
▶ Hyperosmotic oral feeding such as formula feeding mixed with less water than prescribed.

The occurrence in association with oral feeding is less if the infant has been fed with breast milk and higher if the infant has been fed with concentrated formula, or the feeding has been increased with more than 20 to 30 ml/kg per day.

Diagnosis for necrotizing enterocolitis may be confirmed with a physical examination, abdominal X-rays and blood test results showing acidosis, infection, electrolyte imbalances and low platelet counts. Prevention is critical and should especially focus on maintaining internal homeostasis and reducing stress (see Chapter 29 on DSC), as well stopping oral feeding if there is a risk of reduced gastrointestinal perfusion, such as hypotension or other severe disturbances of internal homeostasis. If oral feeding is stopped it has to be replaced with intravenous feeding. The infant should also be referred for urgent surgical treatment. The condition is associated with a high risk for mortality but the outcomes are usually much better if it is diagnosed and treated early.

(hyperalimentation). Other strategies will be pain management and reducing stress (see Chapter 29 on DSC). Specialist treatment is often surgical correction with pharmacological treatment such as *cisorpride*.

The outcomes of acquired gastrointestinal conditions are better with early diagnosis and appropriate interventions, and in some cases it may even be without any long-term complications. If diagnosis and treatment are delayed the outcomes will be much worse, as the condition can result in sepsis, severe electrolyte disturbances and shock, or even death. One of the complications of surgery is short bowel syndrome and consequential malnutrition, electrolyte disturbances, dehydration and failure-to-thrive.

Gastrointestinal infections

A relatively mature gastrointestinal tract is usually present at 38 weeks and it plays an important role in protecting the infant against invading toxins and pathogens because it acts as an intestinal barrier with selective permeability. Several immunological factors are also present in the intestinal tract and contribute to the protection. The risk of invasion of microbes is decreased with the normal motility of the intestines, which reduces the time allowed for bacterial growth and invasion, and bacterial growth is further reduced by an acidic pH.

The gastrointestinal tracts of all infants are more alkaline: A preterm infant's gastrointestinal tract, however, is immature, which means there is an immature intestinal barrier and fewer immunological factors of protection, resulting in an increased risk of bacterial, viral or fungal infection. Preterm infants, as well as ill neonates, have gastrointestinal tracts that are more alkaline and have reduced motility. This increases the risk of infection. Another factor that can act as a trigger for gastrointestinal infection is early enteral feeding in the presence of these risk factors, especially if there are other internal homeostasis disturbances, such as hypoglycaemia or hypotension.

Gastrointestinal infections include invasion and growth of microbes in any area of the gastrointestinal tract, or overgrowth of the normal flora. The causes are most commonly related to exposure to microbes from the external environment, such as through contaminated formula feeding or breastmilk, invasive procedures such as nasogastric tube insertion, or sucking a contaminated dummy. The use of antibiotics is a contributing factor (see page 31-55).

The signs and symptoms depend on the affected area, as well as the nature of the infecting agent (virus, bacteria or fungus) (see pages 31-55 to 31-57). *Stomatitis* or infection of the mouth is characterised by visibly infected mucosa and a reluctance to feed. *Intestinal infections* are evident with vomiting and/or diarrhoea, except for necrotizing enterocolitis that presents with vomiting, but not diarrhoea. Other signs and symptoms include the infant's general stress response, such as tachy-cardia, tachypnoea and desaturation, or even the presence of shock. *Peritonitis* is an infection of the peritoneum or mucous membrane lining the abdominal cavity and it is often a consequence of gastrointestinal perforation (see page 31-72).

The diagnosis will be based on the clinical presentation and may be confirmed with abdominal X-rays and laboratory test results, such as full blood count, CRP and microscopic culturing and sensitivity of stool specimen.

The focus of management is on implementing effective infection control principles and delaying enteral feeding in the presence of the above-mentioned risk factors. It is of critical importance to replace the fluid and nutrients by alternative means if enteral feeding is withheld. Maintaining internal homeostasis and reducing stress is also crucial. It is recommended to administer antibiotics if it is a bacterial infection, and antimycotic treatment is recommended for a fungal infection, such as *nystatin* for fungal stomatitis. The use of prophylactic antibiotic treatment, however, is a controversial (see page 31-55).

Full recovery without any complications is possible if the gastrointestinal infection has been diagnosed and treated early. The risk for systemic infection increases if treatment is delayed or if other disturbances of internal homeostasis are evident. The outcomes for fungal and viral infections are usually worse than bacterial infections. Possible complications of gastrointestinal infections include perforation of the intestines with peritonitis, disturbances of internal homeostasis (especially fluid and electrolyte disturbances), sepsis and even mortality.

The gastrointestinal conditions discussed in this section mainly involve structural and acquired conditions. It is important to interpret these conditions in conjunction with the endocrine and metabolic conditions, as well as general nutrition (see Chapter 30).

Endocrine and metabolic systems

The endocrine system encompasses the hormonal glands and hormones, with all their various functions, while the metabolic system refers to the metabolic processes and the enzymes responsible for them. Both systems play a crucial role in the development and maturation of all the organs of the fetus, as well as the growth, development, maintenance and repair of damaged tissues that continue after birth.

The neurological, endocrine and metabolic systems are interdependent and closely related, which means any disturbance in the one, will lead to disturbances of the others. Together they are to a great extent responsible for maintenance of internal homeostasis of the individual.

The main anatomical components of the endocrine system include the hypothalamus, pituitary gland, pineal gland, thyroid gland, parathyroid gland, thymus, adrenal glands, pancreas and ovaries (female) or testes (male). (Refer to a relevant textbook for revision.)

The functions of the endocrine system are related to the specific hormones and their target cells and they include:
▶ Homeostasis of blood glucose
▶ Growth and development
▶ Acid-base status
▶ Fluid and electrolyte status
▶ Blood pressure maintenance
▶ Thermoregulation
▶ Stress response, emotions and alertness
▶ Efficiency of musculo-skeletal function
▶ Skin function
▶ Feeding and nutrition

The hypothalamus can be seen as the control mechanism of the endocrine system, as well as the link between the neurological system and the endocrine system, where integration takes place of all information regarding sensory input, higher brain functions, emotions and internal homeostasis. The effects of hormones are usually systemic and widespread and seldom located to a specific area.

The metabolic system relies heavily on the endocrine system for proper functioning, which includes:
▶ The different glands responsible for the production, secretion and activities of enzymes.
▶ The digestion and metabolism of the carbohydrates, lipids, proteins, vitamins and a lot of the minerals, and therefore regulating blood glucose balance, thermoregulation, acid-base balance, cellular functioning, as well as growth and development.

The metabolic system's effects are also widespread and involve all systems. Requirements for metabolism include living cells, oxygen, water, enzymes, various nutrients for the various metabolic pathways, as well as various electrolytes and minerals. More energy and heat is released if metabolism increases, but the consumption of nutrients and oxygen will increase too, with an increased demand on the respiratory and cardiovascular systems. The amount of waste products also rises if the metabolic rate increases, which amplifies the workload on the lungs, liver and kidneys to get rid of the waste products.

Although nearly all the glands are completely developed by week 12 gestation, the fetus depends mainly on maternal hormones and metabolism, as well as placental function for clearing waste products. Endocrine or metabolic disoreders of the mother, for example maternal diabetes mellitus or hyperthyroidism, will therefore have an important impact on fetal development, growth and maturation.

Abnormalities of the endocrine system in an infant are usually related to either of the following conditions:
▶ Hyposecretion of a hormone with a decrease in or lack of its related function/s.
▶ Hypersecretion of the hormone/s with an enhanced effect of the particular functions.

Abnormalities of the metabolic system are often related to the absence of an enzyme with a subsequent interruption of the related metabolic process or pathway. The clinical presentation of the affected baby is usually vague, widespread and involves several organs. A diagnosis is usually made through a process of elimination, and investigations are done to confirm or eliminate the most obvious conditions responsible for the particular clinical picture of the baby until the last possible causes left are endocrine or metabolic conditions. Once an endocrine and/or metabolic condition is suspected, special investigations can be done to eliminate or confirm the diagnosis based on the serum-levels of the specific hormones, such as thyroid hormones, cortisol, growth hormones, insulin or the suspected enzymes. Urine or blood analysis tests can also be performed for the levels of specific waste products of metabolism, which is often referred to as metabolic screening. Other investigations include chromosomal and genetic screening.

Screening for endocrine or metabolic abnormalities

If an infant presents with widespread abnormalities that affect various organs with slow or sudden deterioration in condition, screening should be considered for endocrine or metabolic abnormalities. Screening focuses first on the common conditions, but if the results are negative further investigations are necessary to eliminate the more uncommon conditions too. If it cannot be done at a specific hospital or clinic, the infant should be referred for specialised care.

These investigations are very specific, highly specialised and expensive, therefore they are usually not done routinely. A cheaper and simple metabolic screening system for the common metabolic disorders will probably be available in South Africa in the near future.

There is a wide variety of conditions relating to the endocrine or metabolic system of newborns but only the most common conditions will be reviewed.

Blood glucose disturbances

Blood glucose homeostasis is crucial for normal cell function and for its role in aerobic metabolism, and therefore for its role in energy release, especially in the brain. Homeostasis is maintained with a delicate balance between the increase of blood glucose levels on the one hand, versus the decrease of blood glucose levels on the other. Normal blood glucose levels are 3,0 mmol/l (40 mg/dl) to 12 mmol/l (150 mg/dl).

Blood glucose increases with the intake of glucose, for example with oral feeding or intravenous nutrition, or with the metabolic production of glucose under the influence of various hormones. These hormones include:
- Glucagon from the pancreas.
- Growth hormones from the pituitary gland.
- The stress-related hormones, namely cortisol and the catecholamines from the adrenal gland.

Blood glucose decreases if the glucose stores are depleted, as seen in preterm infants, or through insulin secretion. Insulin, which is secreted by the pancreas, decreases blood glucose by increasing metabolism, as well as through growth and therefore the utilisation of glucose. Growth hormones can also reduce blood glucose levels through the increased use of glucose for growth.

Hyperglycaemia

Hyperglycaemia or increased levels of blood glucose can be the result of either an increased intake of glucose, such as with hyperalimentation, a lack of efficient insulin secretion (referred to as *hypoinsulinism*), or due to stress and the increased production of glucose by the stress hormones. It may also be caused by prematurity with a lack of sensitivity of the hypothalamus for high blood glucose levels and therefore there is less response to release hormones that decrease the blood glucose levels.

The main problem with hyperglycaemia is the hyperosmotic effect it has, especially in the brain. Hyperosmotic effect is the ability to draw water out of the cells towards the glucose into the blood stream, which dehydrates the cells. Glucose will be excreted in the kidneys if the levels are high, again followed by water and thus leading to dehydration of the baby. A contributing problem of hyperglycaemia is that it is initially asymptomatic until there are complications, such as hypovolaemic shock. It also seems that the fluid shift in the brain contributes to intraventricular bleeding. The diagnosis is based on glucose in the urine and by measuring high blood glucose levels.

The appropriate management of hyperglycaemia includes reducing the glucose intake by replacing the intravenous fluid with a dextrose-free solution, such as Normal saline 0.9% or Ringer's lactate. If the blood glucose levels remain high, the attending physician may consider the administration of insulin.

Hypoglycaemia

Hypoglycaemia or decreased levels of blood glucose may be the result of decreased glucose intake when there is delayed or insufficient feeding. It can also be decreased when the glucose stores are depleted, for example, because of the lack of brown fat and subcutaneous fat in preterm infants, or the stress associated with an increase in consumption of glucose. Other causes may be the inability of the baby to produce glucose from other nutrients and this is associated with disturbances of internal homeostasis or increased levels of insulin, such as with an overdosage of insulin. *Temporary hyperinsulinism* can also be the result of a diabetic mother where the infant has excreted insulin in utero as a response to increased maternal hyperglycaemia and continues to excrete insulin after birth in the absence of hyperglycaemia.

The main problem with hypoglycaemia is the lack of 'fuel' for metabolism and therefore the lack of energy release. All the systems are affected with a subsequent decrease in function. The neurological system presents with lethargy, tremors, jitteriness and high-pitched crying and if the condition worsens there will be floppiness, unresponsiveness or seizures.

Other signs and symptoms include respiratory distress, poor feeding and absorption, decreased kidney function and weakness. A diagnosis can be confirmed by measuring the blood glucose levels. Hypoglycaemia should be corrected by administering glucose in the form of oral feeding if the baby does not present with symptons of stress, or intravenously with *dextrose,* as prescribed. If the blood glucose remains low, the attending physician may consider *glucagon* administration, although *glucagon* is contraindicated in preterm infants.

Prevention of blood glucose disturbances includes proper routine screening for early detection, at least once when the physical examination is done. Oral feeding has to be initiated as soon as possible – already at birth if the infant's condition allows it. If early feeding is not possible, replacement of nutrition with intravenous supplements should be initiated. It is important to adhere to the following guidelines:

▶ Calculate the amount of feeding or intravenous fluid accurately (see Chapter 30).
▶ To ensure accuracy, administer *all* intravenous fluids through an infusion pump.
▶ Reduce the oxygen and glucose demands through stress reduction (DSC) and pain management, as well as by maintaining internal homeostasis.

The outcome will depend on the duration and degree of the condition. It often contributes to further disturbances of internal homeostasis but it can be reversed. If the blood glucose disturbances are not properly managed or they are prolonged, it may result in permanent damage, especially of the brain, and even shock or death.

Other endocrine conditions

The endocrine system is a very complex system, involving several glands that have various functions. A deficiency or overproduction of any of the hormones can be inherited, or due to defective development of the gland, or due to damage by other factors such as an ischaemic incident. Endocrine conditions can also be caused by overstimulation or a fall in stimulation due to the maternal hormones. The outcomes are most often widespread and of a serious nature, and will depend, as with the clinical presentation, on the functions of the hormones involved.

Hypothyroidism and hyperthyroidism

The thyroid hormones are responsible for stimulating the metabolism which results in heat production and increases in nerve conduction, muscle tone and heart contractility. They also contribute to the maturation of the lungs, gastrointestinal system and liver, as well as the growth of bones, skin and brain. All these effects will increase the demand for oxygen and feeding, resulting in a decrease in weight gain.

Hypothyroidism refers to a temporary or permanent condition, which is characterised by a decrease in the levels of thyroid hormones. There are several causes but those of particular importance after birth are:

- A lack of iodine intake via feeding.
- Iodine excess through skin absorption from antibacterial ointment.
- Suppression of the thyroid gland by, for example, exposure to radiographic contrast agents.
- Maternal hyperthyroidism.
- Inherited congenital hypothyroidism.

Hypothyroidism is characterised by hypothermia, poor muscle tone or floppiness, poor feeding, hypotension, poor maturation of the lungs with a tendency to develop hyalin membrane disease and poor bone growth. However, there is an increase in weight gain because of the lowering of the metabolism. The diagnosis will be confirmed with low blood serum levels of the thyroid-related hormones. The management would include the pharmacological replacement of the hormones (thyroxine) or the iodine, as well as symptomatic treatment through maintaining thermoregulation, supporting cardiac contractility with *inotropes* and lowering the oxygen and

nutrient demand by reducing stress. Infants who suffer from this condition can be assisted with feeding by using a teat with an easier flow.

Hyperthyroidism is the condition where there are increased levels of thyroid hormones. Though it is uncommon in newborns, it can be inherited or acquired through an overdose of thyroid hormones during hormone replacement therapy for hypothyroidism. The characteristics of congenital hyperthyroidism are mainly the result of increased metabolism and therefore include small-for-date, hyperthermic and 'hungry' infants with relatively mature lungs. Other signs and symptoms include gastrointestinal overstimulation with vomiting and diarrhoea, cardiac stimulation with tachycardia, arrhythmias and congestive heart failure, hyperactivity, irritability and increased muscle tone, tremors or convulsions. The diagnosis may be confirmed with high serum levels of thyroid-related hormones.

Management for this condition involves suppression of the thyroid gland with pharmacological agents, or partial surgical removal of the thyroid gland in rare cases because there is the risk of developing hypothyroidism. Symptomatic treatment plays an important role, such as maintaining thermoregulation, nutrition, respiratory support, treatment for cardiac overstimulation through digitalis or beta-adrenergic blockers, and sedation for tremors or convulsions.

Hypercalcaemia and hypocalcaemia

Calcium homeostasis is a very important function of the endocrine system as calcium plays a role in several functions, including impulse conduction in the nervous system, muscle contraction, growth, blood clotting, and bone and teeth formation. The thyroid and the parathyroid glands, which maintain plasma calcium levels within normal limits, control the balance.

Calcium levels are *increased* by parathormone from the parathyroid gland, which stimulates calcium absorption from the gastro-intestinal tract, reabsorbs calcium in the kidneys and decalcifies bone. Calcium absorption is also increased by a low gastro-intestinal pH and the presence of proteins in the gastrointestinal tract, as well as activated vitamin D (which is activated by parathormone).

Calcium levels are *decreased* by a thyroid hormone called calcitonin, which reduces the reabsorption of calcium in the kidneys with an increase in excretion of calcium in the urine. Calcitonin also stimulates the calcification of bone and withdraws calcium from the plasma in the process.

Hypercalcaemia or increased levels of plasma calcium may be caused by overtreatment or excessive intake of calcium or Vitamin D. Inherent or temporary congenital *hyperparathyroidism* is possible if the mother had hypoparathyroidism. In maternal hypothyroidism the infant had to compensate in utero with the increase in production of parathormone because of the lack of maternal parathormone, which continues for days to weeks after birth. Inherited congenital hyperparathyroidism is a life-long condition. The common signs and symptoms of hypercalcaemia include hypotonia, weakness, irritability, poor feeding, constipation, vomiting, bradycardia, increased urine output and dehydration. It also causes calcifications with the signs and symptoms showing deterioration of the affected organ. The long-term effect is thick bone density, but it can be lethal before thick bone density is observed and calcifications in the brain can result in permanent brain damage.

The management of hypercalcaemia focuses on restricting the intake of calcium and vitamin D, with a calculated increase in phosphate, as well as the use of diuretics and hydration in order to excrete calcium. Supportive treatment should focus on neurological, cardiac and respiratory management with added emphasis on stress reduction.

Hypocalcaemia or decreased levels of plasma calcium can be caused by poor calcium intake as with delayed feeding, an alkaline gastrointestinal pH, vitamin D deficiency and prematurity. Preterm infants have limited calcium stores or bone, and their parathyroid gland often lacks sensitivity for hypocalcaemia. Temporary *congenital hypoparathyroidism* can occur if the mother had hyperparathyroidism with increased levels of parathormone, which suppressed the baby's parathyroid gland in utero and for a period after birth. Inherited congenital hypoparathyroidism ia a permanent condition. The common signs and symptoms of hypocalcaemia include jitteriness, excitability, stridor, convulsions and cardiac arrhythmias. If it persists, poor bone density and fractures may occur and the outcomes can be life threatening.

The main focus of management is on replacement of calcium, gluconate and vitamin D by feeding or intravenous replacement, and to support the systems that need assistance, including stress reduction and maintaining internal homeostasis.

The endocrine conditions discussed previously are the most common endocrine disorders, but there are many more that can have devastating effects.

Inborn errors of metabolism

Metabolism refers to various activities that take place in the cells to break down substances or to build new substances, as well as to release energy and heat for all the bodily functions to continue. It is critical for growth, repair, adaptation, homeostasis and for maintaining life. Enzymes under the influence of hormones control metabolism and it takes place in specific sequences, known as metabolic pathways. The fetus depends on the maternal and placental function in utero but has to rely on his own metabolism after birth.

Inborn errors of metabolism refer to congenital metabolic disorders where an enzyme is absent, resulting in the disruption of a metabolic pathway. There are more than 300 metabolic disorders, examples of which include *G6PD-deficiency, galactosaemia, phenylketonuria* and *maple syrup disease*.

The outcomes would depend on the

particular disrupted pathway. It can result in an accumulation of toxic waste products, incomplete or vulnerable cells forming, the metabolism slowing down with a lack of energy production, or a lack of metabolism and therefore accumulation of damaging substances such as drugs. The common problem is the presence of some factor that causes damage to cells, organs or the whole body.

The common signs and symptoms are tachypnoea, tachycardia, poor feeding, failure-to-thrive, arrhythmias, cardiac failure, hypertonicity or hypotonicity, seizures, jaundice and unusual odours or colour. After birth the condition usually starts as vague, non-specific problems that do not respond to treatment, followed by progressive deterioration.

The treatment and the long-term outcomes depend on how early the diagnosis is made and the treatment possibilities for the particular condition. Some cases may have a favourable prognosis with permanent replacement therapy and the baby can lead a relatively normal life, while other conditions may be lethal without any possible treatment.

A brief overview has been provided on endocrine and metabolic disorders. It should be remembered, however, that they affect all other systems and are an integral part of all bodily functions, but can easily be overlooked. It is therefore important for midwives to be aware of the possibility of endocrine or metabolic disorders if the clinical picture of the infant is vague and widespread with various organs being affected. If the common and obvious causes are eliminated, such as hypoglycaemia or hyperglycaemia, it may be necessary for further investigations or referral for specialised management.

Conditions of the special senses: The ears and vestibular system

The ears are part of the neurological system but they are discussed separately because of the highly specialised function of this sense.

The anatomy of the ears can be divided into three categories: the external or outer ear, middle ear and inner ear. The main function of the external and middle ear is the conduction of sound. In the inner ear, the cochlea is responsible for the reception of the sound impulses and their conduction to the cerebral cortex, while the vestibular system influences balance.

Special investigations that are used for diagnostic purposes include the various methods to determine responsiveness to sound, such as auditory brainstem response (ABR) or evoked otoacoustic emissions (EOAEs). The most common vestibular investigation is the 'doll's eye' test, where the infant's head is slowly moved from the one side to the other side. A normal vestibular response would be that the eyes move to the opposite direction of rotation.

Congenital malformations of the ears

The external ear is already formed by 8 weeks, it develops in the upper part of the neck and ascends as the mandible is developing to be at eye level at approximately 12 weeks. The external ear is initially soft and pliable and becomes firmer when cartilage develops from 34 to 38 weeks gestation.

Congenital malformations of the ear are structural defects due to developmental problems. *Low-set ears*, when the upper part of the ears are lower than the level of the outside corners of the eyes, has been associated with various inherited or multifactoral congenital disorders, such as Down's syndrome, congenital rubella syndrome and fetal alcohol syndrome. If low-set ears are observed, it is important to assess the infant for the presence of other deformities associated with congenital disorders or syndromes. Prevention is often possible with quality preconception and antenatal care, such as preventing TORCH infections and radiation, as well as withholding of alcohol, nicotine and drugs. If exposure to harmful substances could not be ruled out, the low-set ears are seen as an important indicator of congenital abnormalities, but it does not need any treatment as such. The management of the baby in general will be determined by the other signs and symptoms present.

Microtia or small ears, and *auricular appendages*, are often inherited, but not associated with congenital syndromes. The appendages can be removed surgically for aesthetic reasons.

Conductive hearing loss

Sound is normally transmitted from the external ear canal through the tympanic membrane to the three bones of the middle ear and to the inner ear. The bones in the middle ear are surrounded with air of which the pressure is maintained equal to the outside air pressure via the Eustachian tube, in order to allow conduction of the sound waves from the tympanic membrane to the inner ear.

Conductive hearing loss refers to partial or complete loss of the ability to hear due to the lack of conduction of sound or interference in sound transmission up to the inner ear. The interference may occur if there is an obstruction in the outer ear canal or an injury to the tympanic membrane, but it is uncommon in newborns. *Inherited otosclerosis* (congenital rigid middle ear bones) and chronic infection of the middle ear or *otitis media* causes the joints of the bones of the middle ear to be rigid, which can also result in interference with sound conduction. If the bones are surrounded by fluid, as with a middle ear infection for example, or if the air pressure in the outer ear and middle ear differs, as with a blocked Eustachian tube, temporary conductive hearing loss is present. It results in muffled or faint sounds heard with bone conduction through the skull and temporal bones. It is difficult to identify conductive hearing loss in infants but it may be picked up as a lack of

response to sound. It is also possible that the lack of response is due to other reasons, such as prematurity or illness, leading to misdiagnosis. However, any sign of hearing loss should not be ignored, as early referral and treatment or surgery may prevent permanent hearing loss and developmental delays.

Prevention is thus very important with early recognition of risk factors such as otitis media or family history, and appropriate treatment (such as with antibiotics for otitis media). Early diagnosis of hearing loss is strongly recommended as part of a routine screening programme, followed by early referral for specialised treatment such as audio- and speech-language therapy and an ENT surgeon. The routine screening programme is currently available in most private institutions in South Africa but not yet in governmental institutions. Monitoring developmental milestones and communication is very important, as well as parental education and support.

Sensorineural hearing loss and central auditory dysfunction

The sound that is conducted from the middle ear is transmitted to the cochlea in the inner ear which is filled with fluid and contains the Corti-organs. This is where the sound waves are converted to neurological impulses for conduction to the cerebral cortex for interpretation. The inner ear is formed from about 4 weeks gestation, the fetus responds to sound at approximately 17 weeks and by 24 weeks the auditory apparatus is complete and fully functional, but maturation continues to term.

Sensorineural hearing loss

Sensorineural hearing loss is partial or complete loss of hearing as a result of injury or defective functioning of the hearing components of the inner ear. It is often the result of cochlear damage due to disturbances of internal homeostasis such as acidosis, hypoxia and hyperbilirubinaemia, as well as loud sounds and the use of ototoxic drugs, such as *aminoglycocide* antibiotics and diuretics. Preterm infants' risks are also higher for damage of the cochlear hair cells as a result of these risk factors, as well as because of the sensitivity of the cochlear hair cells during the developmental phase. Injury is irreversible and permanent with various degrees of deafness.

Central auditory dysfunction

Central auditory dysfunction refers to the inability of the cerebral cortex to interpret the sounds correctly and therefore demonstrates decreased or complete loss of interpretation of sound, observed as deafness. It is most often the result of a cerebral injury.

Sensorineural hearing loss and central auditory dysfunction may be genetic or associated with congenital syndromes, such as fetal alcohol syndrome, congenital infections (especially TORCH-infections), and congenital abnormalities of the head and neck, such as encephalocele. Both result in a poor or inappropriate response to sound, bone conduction is not helpful and a hearing aid does not improve the quality of sound heard. The degree of hearing loss may vary greatly. The diagnosis is confirmed with auditory brainstem response (ABR) or evoked otoacoustic emissions (EOAEs).

Prevention of the risk factors is crucial and often possible, by preventing TORCH infections, reducing noise levels in all areas were babies are present (see Chapter 29 on DSC) and by monitoring drug levels of ototoxic drugs. The next important step is early diagnosis and referral (ENT surgeon and audio- and speech-language therapy) for specialised treatment. Parental education and support is critical if there is any risk of the infant having hearing loss, as they have to manage the condition in the long term.

Vestibular dysfunction

The vestibular system develops from four weeks after conception and it is functional at approximately 21 weeks. It consists of the three semicircular ducts that are responsible for balance and contain hair cells that are filled with fluid. The movement of the fluid with any positional changes is observed by the hair cells as impulses and converted to the cerebral cortex for interpretation, together with visual and other impulses in order to create a motor response for maintaining balance.

Vestibular dysfunction refers to a defect or damage to the vestibular part of the inner ear, resulting in balance disturbances. It is often caused by:

◗ Congenital infections, such as TORCH-infections.
◗ Disturbance of internal homeostasis, such as acidosis and hypoxia.
◗ Sudden movement or sudden positional changes ('premie-flip').

The hair cells of the vestibular system are sensitive for the same factors as the cochlear hair cells, except they have a sensitivity for sudden movement instead of sound. Overstimulation results in stress for the infant or even damage to the vestibular hair cells. Vestibular dysfunction is difficult to observe in the neonatal phase but it results in motor developmental delays where balance plays a part. In the neonatal phase vestibular dysfunction will result in a stress response with any positional changes, most often with slow recovery thereafter.

Although it is not really possible to diagnose vestibular dysfunction in the neonatal period, it is crucial to be aware of it and prevent it as it can result in irreversible damage of the vestibular system. It can be prevented by maintaining internal homeostasis, reducing stress and especially by avoiding sudden movement (such as 'premie-flip'). Early diagnosis, referral for specialist treatment (occupational or physiotherapy) and parental education are very important if the above-mentioned risk factors are present. For this reason the parents need to be sensitive to the issues of balance abnormalities or developmental delays, such as gross motor development.

Infections of the ear

Because they are not exposed to the external environment the middle ear and inner ear are usually well protected against infection. The Eustachian tube, which connects the middle ear and the nasopharynx, is relatively short in an infant and more horizontal than in an adult. It has less connective tissue which makes the middle ear more susceptible to microbes entering from the nasopharynx via the Eustachian tube. The inner ear is completely protected from the external environment but it is rich in blood supply, which provides an access point for microbes via the systemic circulation.

Infections of the ear refer to infiltration and growth of microbes, most often caused by the systemic spreading of microbes and decreased immunity. The following categories of infection may be evident:

▶ *Otitis externa* or infection of the outer ear is usually the result of contact with microbes in the external environment, such as chorio-amnionitis or soiled linen.
▶ *Otitis media* or infection of the middle ear can be due to feeding reflux through the Eustachian tube if the infant is fed in a supine position.
▶ *Otitis interna* or infection of the inner ear is usually caused by systemic spreading from another infection site, especially if the immune system is compromised.

Ear infections cause tremendous pain and discomfort, which manifest in a very irritable infant. Infants with otitis media are often more comfortable in an upright position. If the infection is not resolved, it can lead to permanent cell damage in those areas and with subsequent hearing loss. The outcome of prolonged otitis media is often permanent conductive hearing loss, while otitis interna leads to sensorineural hearing loss.

Prevention of infection by maintaining internal homeostasis and therefore boosting the immune system should be the primary focus. Otitis media can be prevented by feeding an infant in a half upright position and not putting the baby on his back too soon after feeding. Spreading of infection can also be limited with the early diagnosis and treatment of infections anywhere else, such as with antibiotics for bacterial infections.

The main conditions relating to the ears were briefly discussed in this section but it must be emphasised that more detailed information can be found in advanced neonatal textbooks. Also remember that problems of the ears and vestibular system should always be interpreted together with any information regarding the neurological system.

Conditions of the special senses: Eyes

The eyes are part of the neurological system but will be discussed separately because they are highly specialised. The anatomy of the eyes refers mainly to the eyeballs with all their related structures, namely, the eyelids, conjunctiva, retina, lacrimal system, extra-ocular muscles and the bony socket. The main function of the eyes is vision but several factors have an impact on the eyes and their functioning, including internal homeostasis and gestational age. Abnormalities of the eyes most often result in malfunctioning of various degrees, such as abnormal eye movement, excessive tearing and lubrication of eyes, closure of eyelids, vision loss and other abnormalities.

Congenital malformations of the eyes

The eyeballs and lenses develop from the fourth week after conception and except for the retina, they are completely formed by 13 weeks. From week 6 the eyelids develop, fusing at about 10 weeks and separating at about 26 weeks gestation.

Congenital malformations or defective development of the eyes may be chromosomal, such as Trisomy 13, or associated with teratogenic or multifactoral factors, like congenital rubella syndrome, cytomegalovirus, toxoplasmosis and fetal alcohol syndrome.

Anophthalmos is the absence of the eyeballs and lenses and means complete blindness. The eyelids are present and appear sunken. *Microphthalmos* refers to excessively small eyes and subsequent vision disturbances. Both conditions can be diagnosed with the physical assessment of the eyes. These disorders are irreversible but not life threatening. The degree of vision loss in the case of microphthalmos can vary from slight to total blindness but the appearance of the infant may be of great concern for the parents and necessitate counselling and/or plastic surgery, such as an eye prosthesis.

The most important aspect of the management of congenital eye conditions is the prevention by quality preconception and antenatal care, especially the prevention of TORCH infections, withholding alcohol during pregnancy and a balanced diet, including vitamin E. If it could not be prevented, early diagnosis and referral become very important, especially in association with other congenital abnormalities or syndromes.

Retinal conditions: Retinoblastoma and retinopathy of prematurity

The retina develops from the fourth week of gestation and is completed by approximately 22 weeks, except for the blood supply which is completed by 40 to 44 weeks.

Retinoblastoma is a relatively common malignant tumour on the retina and the condition may be inherited, usually in both eyes, or non-heredity where only one eye is usually affected. It is important to refer the infant to an ophthalmologist as soon as possible if the eyes appear to be abnormal on assessment, which is if the eyes are uneven, dull or if there is any other reason for concern. The outcome of retinoblastoma depends on the degree of infiltration and the stage at which specialist treatment was administered. It is often associated with blindness and a high mortality rate due to metastasis.

Retinopathy of prematurity refers to abnormal growth of blood vessels into the retina and it is associated with prematurity. When an infant is born preterm, the retinal layers will be formed but the blood supply development would not yet have completed. These growing blood vessels are very vulnerable. The acute phase of retinopathy of prematurity would be the interruption of vascularisation or growth of the blood vessels, caused by hyperoxia, hypoxia, hypercapnoea, acidosis, hypoperfusion, blood pressure fluctuations and several other internal disturbances, as well as exposure to bright lights. It is followed by the chronic phase with scarring of the area where the growth stopped and then continuation of the growth of the blood vessels but into the gel in the eyeball. This can be followed with detachments of the retina and different degrees of permanent vision loss. The diagnosis will be confirmed with an eye examination done preferably by a paediatric ophthalmologist. If the above-mentioned risk factors are present, the infant should at least be referred to a paediatric ophthalmologist after discharge.

The most crucial part of management is the prevention of any of the risk factors, especially preterm birth and the prevention of internal homeostasis disturbances, in particular the prevention of high levels of oxygen in the blood. If oxygen is administered to the infant, his saturation levels must not exceed 95%. Protection against bright lights can be done by manipulating the environment as discussed in Chapter 29 on Developmentally Supportive Care principles. If prevention was impossible, early diagnosis and referral for specialist treatment is crucial.

Cataracts

The lens of the eye is biconvex and transparent and it refracts light to enable focusing on an object for sharp imaging.

Cataract refers to an opaque lens of the eye. The amount of light entering through the pupil to produce an image on the retina is therefore limited, resulting in various degrees of vision loss and consequential developmental delays. During the physical examination of the eye, the pupil will appear to be white in colour. It is associated with autosomal inheritance and congenital syndromes, such as Down's syndrome, Pierre Robin syndrome and Crouzon's syndrome, congenital infections (especially the TORCH-infections) and metabolic disorders such as galactosaemia.

If possible at all, it is crucial to prevent the etiological factors, such as TORCH infections. If not, early diagnosis and referral to a paediatric ophthalmologist for specialist treatment is essential. The treatment usually entails surgical removal of the lens. Outcomes with specialist treatment may vary depending on the extent of the cataract, the age at which removal is done, as well as other associated abnormalities.

Abnormal eye movement: Strabismus and nystagmus

The eyeballs are moved in the orbit by six groups of muscles into the different directions. Maturation of the eyes will include the ability to coordinate the movement of the eyes as smooth equal movements at about three to five months after birth.

In the first month of infancy it is common to find a lack of coordination between the two eyes during movement, which can mistakenly be misdiagnosed as strabismus. *Strabismus* is an abnormal eye alignment or squint. It is the result of developmental abnormalities or cerebral trauma, or it may be associated with other congenital abnormalities. If there is a sudden onset of strabismus, it is crucial to eliminate the possibility of increased intracranial pressure or cerebral trauma that can be diagnosed with sonar, CT-scan or MRI. If strabismus is present from birth and persists after three months, it may need referral and surgical correction.

Nystagmus is a rhythmic oscillation of one or both eyes and it can be associated with developmental defects of the eyes, ischaemic, toxic or compressive neurological disorders and chromosomal abnormalities. These conditions are associated with neurological and/or eye disorders because they influence the smooth motor coordination of the muscle groups responsible for eye movement. The nystagmus itself is not harmful, but it is important to refer the baby for investigations of possible underlying problems, if present, as it can be an indicator of further disorders.

Nasolacrimal duct obstruction

The tear glands produce tears, while the eyelids use the tears to lubricate the cornea and conjunctiva and the nasolacrimal duct drains the fluid to the nasopharynx.

Nasolacrimal duct obstruction refers to an inability of the lacrimal duct to drain the tears into the nasopharynx, either because of a congenital atresia or obstruction, or because of infection or inflammation. Continuous tearing is the result and there is a tendency to develop eye infections. Eye hygiene is therefore very important and if indicated, massaging from the eye towards the nose on a regular basis (three to six hourly) would be beneficial. It seldom needs surgical correction as there is usually spontaneous recovery.

Eye infections

The eyes are well protected under normal circumstances with the tears being antimicrobial and washing away dirt, thereby contributing to natural infection control. Infection is also controlled through the conjunctival reflex that closes the eyelids and increases tearing when they are touched. The eyes are further protected by the barriers between the inside of the eye and the external environment.

Eye infections are microbes invading and

growing in or on the eye structures, which may occur before, during or after birth. It could also be through direct contact or via systemic infection of microbes from another infected site. Decreased immunity and disturbances of internal homeostasis may contribute to the severity of the infection.

Conjunctivitis or infection of the conjunctiva and *chorioretinitis* or infection of the retina, are the most common eye infections. The infection leads to a local inflammatory response with redness, swelling and pain, as well as a general stress response. Conjunctivitis usually has a yellowish secretion and the outcomes depend on the severity of the infection, the duration and the efficiency of the treatment. It can vary from an absence of any complications to loss of vision or even an eye. The severe outcomes are usually associated with viral and fungal infections and/or poor immunity, and chorioretinitis. Diagnosis will be made on the appearance and confirmed with a specimen obtained for culture from the conjunctiva, as well as blood cultures for chorioretinitis.

Eye infections can often be prevented, for example with early treatment of chorioamnionitis, birth by caesarean section if the mother has a severe vaginal infection, prophylactic administration of antibiotic ointment (such as *chloromycetin*) if indicated and appropriate infection control after birth, as well as maintaining an optimal internal homeostasis to maximise immunity. If it is not possible to prevent it, bacterial conjunctivitis should be treated with local antibiotic eye ointment and chorioretinitis should be treated with systemic antibiotics. Refer to pages 31-55 to 31-56 on treating viral and fungal infections.

The conditions of the eyes that were briefly discussed are the most common in the newborn period but there are many more. It is very important to read this section in conjunction with the neurological system and to remember that it is a specialised discipline so there is emphasis on referring any problems observed. Further reading may be done on the topic in advanced neonatal care textbooks.

References

Als, H., Duffy, F. H. & McNulty, G. B. 1996. Effectiveness of individualized neurodevelopmental care in the newborn intensive care unit (NICU). *Acta Paediatric Supplement,* 416:21–30.

American Heart Association. 1997–1999. *Paediatric Advanced Life Support.* Part of professional educational program of the American Heart Association.

Askin, D. F. 1997. Interpretation of neonatal blood gases, Part 1: Physiology and acid-base homeostasis. *Neonatal Network,* 16 (5):17–28.

Balaguru, D., Artman, M. & Auslender, M. 2000. Management of heart failure in children. *Current Problems in Pediatrics,* 30:5–30.

Bergman, N. 1998. Introducing kangaroo-mother care. *Pedmed,* September/October 9–10.

Blackburn, S. 1995. Hyperbilirubinemia and neonatal jaundice. *Neonatal Network,* 14 (7):15–24.

Blackburn, S. T. 1996. Research utilization: Modifying the NICU light environment. *Neonatal Network,* 15(4):63–66.

Blass, E. M. & Smith, B. A. 1992. Differential effects of sucrose, fructose, glucose and lactose on crying in 1–3-day-old human infants: Qualitative and quantitative considerations. *Developmental Psychology,* 28(5):804–810.

Broadhead, J. M., Parra, D. S. & Skelton, P. A. 2001. Emerging multiresistant organisms in the ICU: Epidemiology, risk factors, surveillance and prevention. *Critical Care Nursing,* 24(2):20–29.

Brouillette, R. T. & Waxman, D. H. 1997. Evaluation of the newborn's blood gas status. *Clinical Chemistry,* 43(1):215–221.

Christianson, A. L. 1994. Folic acid and prevention of spinal bifida and other neural tube defects. *Micronutrients,* March 56–59.

Christianson, A. L. 2000. Medical genetics in primary health care. *Indian Journal of Pediatrics,* 67(11):831–835.

Deacon, J. & O'Neill, P. 1999. *Core curriculum*

for neonatal intensive care nursing. Second edition. Philadelphia: Saunders.

Delport, S. D. 2002. Acquired pulmonary disorders causing respiratory distress in the term newborn infant. *Geneeskunde/The Medicine Journal*, April 41–44.

Dietch, J. S. 1993. Periventricular–intraventricular hemorrhage in the very low birth weight infant. *Neonatal Network*, 12(1):7–15.

Flores, M. 2003. Ibuprofen: Alternative treatment for patent ductus arteriosus. *Neonatal Network*, 22(2):27–31.

Gale, G., Franck, L. & Lund, C. 1993. Skin-to-skin (kangaroo) holding of the intubated premature infant. *Neonatal Network*, 12(6):49–57.

Hadley, G. P. 1998. Neonatal transport. *Trauma and Emergency Medicine*, August/September 40–44.

Harper, J., Oranje, A. & Prose, N. 2000. *Textbook of paediatric dermatology*. London: Blackwell Science.

Harrison, V. C., Keet, M. P. & Shore, S. C. L. 1996. *The newborn baby*. Third edition. Cape Town: Juta & Co. Ltd.

Inder, T. E. & Volpe, J. J. 2000. Mechanisms of perinatal brain injury. *Seminars in Neonatology*, 5:3–16. http://www.idealibrary.com.

Isaacs, D. & Moxon, E. R. 1991. *Neonatal infections*. Oxford: Butterworth/Heinemann.

Jee, L. D. 2001. Urinary tract infections in children. *Geneeskunde/The Medicine Journal*, September 16–20.

Jones, M. W. & Bass W. T. 2003. Perinatal brain injury in the premature infant. *Neonatal Network*, 22 (1):61–69.

Jorgensen, K. M. 1999. Pain assessment and management in the newborn infant. *Journal of PeriAnasthesia Nursing*, 14(6):349–356.

Jorgensen, K. M. 2000. *Developmental care of the preterm infant, a concise overview*. Second edition.http://www.childmed.com.

Kirsten, D. 1996. Patent ductus arteriosus in the preterm infant. *Neonatal Network*, 15(2):19–25.

Loo, K. K., Espinosa, M., Tyler, R. & Howard, J. 2003. Using knowledge to cope with stress in the NICU: How parents integrate learning to read the physiologic and behavioural cues of the infant. *Neonatal Network*, 22(1):31–37.

Lorenz, J. M. 1997. Assessing fluid and electrolyte status in the newborn. *Clinical Chemistry*, 43(1):205–210.

Lund, C. H., Osborne, J. W., Kuller, J., Lane, A. T., Wright Lott, J. & Raines, D. A. 2001. Neonatal skin care: Clinical outcomes of the AWHONN/NANN evidence-based clinical practice guideline. *Journal of Obstetric, Gynecologic and Neonatal Nursing*, 30(1):41–51.

Marieb, E. N. 1998. *Human anatomy and physiology*. Fourth edition. California: Benjamin/Cumings Publishing Co.

McGrath, J. M. 2000. Developmental physiology of the neurological system. *Central Lines (NANN)*, 16(4):1–16.

McLachlan, J. 1995. *Medical embryology*. Wockingham: Addison-Wesley.

Merenstein, G. B. & Gardner, S. L. 1998. *Handbook of neonatal intensive care nursing*. Fourth edition. Missouri: Mosby.

Millar, A. J. W. & Rode, H. 2001. Neonatal intestinal obstruction. *Geneeskunde/The Medicine Journal*, July 39–44.

MRC Unit for maternal and infant health care strategies, PPIP users & National Departement of Health. 2001. *Saving babies 2001, Second perinatal care survey of South Africa*. http://www.ppip.co.za

Penschaszadeh, V. B., Christianson, A. L., Giugliani, R., Boulyjenkov, V. & Katz, M. 1999. Report: Community genetics. *Community genetics*, 2:196–201.

Premji, S. S. & Bosco, P. 2000. Gastointestinal function and growth in premature infants: Is non-nutritive sucking vital? *Journal of Perinatology*, 1:46–53.

Seaman, S. L. 1995. Renal physiology, Part II: Fluid and electrolyte regulation. *Neonatal Network*, 14(5):5–8.

Taylor, D. 1994. *Pediatric opthalmology.* Boston: Blackwell Scientific Publications.

Thomas, K. 1994. Thermoregulation in neonates. *Neonatal Network,* 13(2):15–22.

Van Den Ende, J. 1999. An introduction to clinical microbiology. Unpublished seminar.

Vargo, L. 1998. The basics of neonatal ECG interpretation. *Neonatal Network,* 17(8):7–16.

Warren, I. M., Quinn, C. & Ghaus, K. 2000. Step by step guide: Non-invasive care, assisting the philosophy. *Eme-med in association with Journal of Neonatal Nursing,* http://www.eme-med.co.uk.

Index

Please note: Page numbers in *italics* refer to tables and figures.